汉英中医学精要

主编 梁晓春 孙 华

主译 朴元林 吴群励 张 文

编者（按姓氏笔画排序）

尹德海 包 飞 田国庆 朴元林

孙 华 吴群励 张 文 张孟仁

郝伟欣 徐慧媛 梁晓春 董振华

中国协和医科大学出版社

图书在版编目（CIP）数据

汉英中医学精要／梁晓春，孙华主编. —北京：中国协和医科大学出版社，2014.7
ISBN 978-7-5679-0061-5

Ⅰ．①汉…　Ⅱ．①梁…②孙…　Ⅲ．①中医学-汉、英　Ⅳ．①R2

中国版本图书馆 CIP 数据核字（2014）第 060326 号

汉英中医学精要

主　　编：梁晓春　孙　华
责任编辑：吴桂梅　顾良军

出版发行：中国协和医科大学出版社
　　　　　（北京东单三条九号　邮编 100730　电话 65260378）
网　　址：www. pumcp. com
经　　销：新华书店总店北京发行所
印　　刷：北京佳艺恒彩印刷有限公司

开　　本：889×1194　　1/16 开
印　　张：35.5
字　　数：1300 千字
版　　次：2015 年 1 月第 1 版　　2015 年 1 月第 1 次印刷
印　　数：1—3000
定　　价：112.00 元

ISBN 978-7-5679-0061-5

Essentials of Traditional Chinese Medicine
Chinese-English Bilingual Version

Editor-in-Chief   Liang Xiaochun   Sun Hua

Translators-in-Chief Piao Yuanlin Wu Qunli Zhang Wen

Contributors and translators (Listed in the order of strokes of their Chinese surnames)

Yin Dehai	Bao Fei	Tian Guoqing
Piao Yuanlin	Sun Hua	Wu Qunli
Zhang Wen	Zhang Mengren	Hao Weixin
Xu Huiyuan	Liang Xiaochun	Dong Zhenhua

Peking Union Medical College Press

内 容 提 要

　　《汉英中医学精要》中英文对照教材是北京协和医学院中医教研室组织编写的。本书以中国协和医科大学出版社出版的《中医学》为蓝本进行精选，尽可能地将中西医结合的理念和内容贯穿其中，旨在使留学生学习并掌握与西医完全不同的中医系统思维方法，掌握中医学的基本知识、基础理论、中药、方剂等。在教材内容上，增加了中西医理论体系的特点、形成和发展的差异等；在教材结构上，把脏腑的生理功能和病理辨证合二为一；在治则和治法方面把"调整阴阳"作为治疗疾病的总纲，把"治病求本"作为治疗疾病的指导思想。针灸部分突出理论联系实际，重点介绍了经络、腧穴、刺灸法、针灸的治疗原则和配穴处方。本教材语言表达简明扼要，通俗易懂，执简驭繁，译文准确流畅。本教材主要适用于国外医学生、交换学者学习中医，对于国内医学生、自学考试者及西学中人员也有参考价值。

Introduction

The Chinese-English bilingual textbook *Essentials of Traditional Chinese Medicine* is compiled by the Teaching and Research Section of Traditional Chinese Medicine (TCM) of Peking Union Medical College. The textbook is refined and based on the book *Traditional Chinese Medicine* published by Peking Union Medical College Press. We tried our best to embody the concept and content of the integration of TCM and Western medicine, aiming to impart the international students not only the basic knowledge, basic theories, medicinals and formulas of TCM but also the systematic ways of thinking of TCM, which are totally different from Western medicine. In the aspect of the content, the textbook added the difference in the characteristics of theoretical structure, formation, and development of both of TCM and Western medicine theories. In the aspect of the structure of the textbook, we combined both the physiological functions and pathological differentiations as a whole; in the parts of therapeutic rules and treatments, we set "adjusting yin and yang" as the general rule and made "treating the root" as the guiding thought of treatments; in the part of acupuncture, we focused on the combination of the theory and practice, mainly introduced the meridians and collaterals, acupuncture points, needling and moxibustion manipulations, and therapeutic principles and prescriptions of acupuncture. The expression of the textbook is concise and easy to understand, which is good to solve the difficulty with simple methods, and the translation is accurate and fluent. The textbook is mainly suitable for international medical students and exchanging scholars to study TCM. Also it is of reference value to domestic medical students, persons preparing for self-teaching examinations, and Western medicine staff learning TCM.

前　言

北京协和医学院每年都接受国外大学（如哈佛、UCSF）的学生来交流学习，其中不乏对中医充满好奇和兴趣的学生，而中医教研室没有专门供留学生使用的教材，临床教学存在一定的难度。为此，中医教研室编写了这本《汉英中医学精要》以满足临床教学需要。

《汉英中医学精要》编写的宗旨是：在总体构思上，力争保持中医学的系统性和完整性，突出其针对性和实用性。在教材内容上，注重理论联系实际，精选了中医基础理论、中医诊断、辨证、中药、方剂及针灸治疗，增加了中医传统医德教育，分析了中西医理论体系之异同，并附有临床辨证分析典型病例。在教材结构上，把脏腑的生理功能和病理辨证合二为一，这样可以起到事半功倍的效果；在治则和治法部分把"调整阴阳"作为治疗疾病的总纲，把"治病求本"作为治疗疾病的指导思想，这样对"正治反治"、"病治异同"、"标本缓急"等起到提纲挈领的作用；针灸部分图文并茂，重点介绍了经络，腧穴，刺灸法，针灸的治疗原则和配穴处方。在语言表达上，力求简明扼要，通俗易懂，译文准确流畅。

为了确保教材编写及译文的质量，我们参考了近几年的中文版及中英文对照的《中医学》教材及讲义，汲取了各版教材的精华，对教材的编写理念、结构、体例等方面进行了探索性改革；对教材内容、结构和体例进行了数次修改，反复推敲，力争实现教材内容的整体优化，达到系统性、科学性、完整性、创新性及译文准确性的完美结合。

本教材的英文部分主要由朴元林、吴群励两位博士，以及《中国结合医学杂志》张文女士完成。由于编者水平有限，时间仓促，教材中难免存在偏颇甚至谬误的地方，敬祈读者指正。

本教材的完成得到了北京协和医学院的教学改革立项课题资助，得到了中国协和医科大学出版社的鼎力相助。谨致谢忱！

《汉英中医学精要》编委会

2014 年 1 月

Essentials of Traditional Chinese Medicine
Chinese-English Bilingual Version

PREFACE

Peking Union Medical College receives international students from overseas universities such as Harvard University and UCSF every year. Many international students have great interest on Traditional Chinese Medicine (TCM). Since the Teaching and Research Section of TCM in our college does not have a suitable textbook for international students, there is difficulty in clinical teaching. Thus, we compiled this Chinese-English bilingual textbook—*Essentials of Traditional Chinese Medicine* to meet the need of clinical teaching.

The compiling aim of the Chinese-English bilingual textbook— *Essentials of Traditional Chinese Medicine* is as follows: in the aspect of general structure, we tried to keep the systematicness and integrity of TCM and emphasize on its well-directing and practicality; in the aspect of the content of the textbook, we emphasized on the connection of theory and practice, selected basic theories of TCM, diagnosis of TCM, differentiation of syndromes, traditional Chinese pharmacy, formula study and acupuncture treatment, added the traditional ethics education of TCM, analyzed the difference in theoretical systems between TCM and Western Medicine, and attached classic cases of clinical differentiation of syndromes; in the aspect of the structure of the textbook, we combined both physical functions and pathological differentiations as a whole, which can achieve half work and whole success. In the parts of therapeutic rules and treatments, we set "adjusting yin and yang" as the general rule and made "treating the root" as the guiding thought of treatments, which enlisted and summarized the contents of "routine treatment and paradoxical treatment," "same treatment for different diseases and different treatments for the same disease" and "treatment based on tip and root, acute and chronic." In the part of acupuncture, we enriched both the content and the figures, and focused on meridian and collateral, acupuncture points, needling and moxibustion manipulations, and therapeutic principles and prescriptions of acupuncture. As to the expression, we tried our best to make it concise and easy to understand, and the translation accurate and fluent.

In order to ensure the quality of the compilation and the translation of the textbook, we referred recent textbooks and teaching materials in both Chinese and Chinese-English bilingual versions, and absorbed the essence of each textbook. Moreover, we tried to reform the concepts, structures and styles of the compilation of the textbook. We carefully deliberated and revised the content, structures and styles of the textbooks for many times, and tried our best to make the whole content of the textbook optimized, and strived to achieve a perfect combination of systematicness, scientificity, integrity, innovation and accuracy of the translation.

The English version of the textbook is mainly completed by Dr. Piao Yuanlin, Dr. Wu Qunli and Ms. Zhang Wen from *Chinese Journal of Integrative Medicine*. Due to the limitation of our capabilities and time constraints, inevitably there are biases even errors in the textbook. We sincerely wish the readers point them out and correct them.

The completion of the textbook has been funded by Peking Union Medical College's Teaching Reform Project Grant, together with the kind help of Peking Union Medical College Press. Hereby, we would like to express our gratitude to them.

Editorial Board of the *Essentials of Traditional Chinese Medicine*

January, 2014

目录 Contents

第一章　中医学绪论

灿烂辉煌的中华文明孕育了博大精深的中医药文化，从伏羲制九针、神农尝百草开始，逐渐形成了包括经络文化、诊疗文化、本草文化、养生文化等在内的完整的中医药理论体系。在历史的长河中，古巴比伦医学、印度医学和中医学被称为人类最早形成体系的三大传统医学，前两者虽比中医药学发展要早，但现在仅存一些零散的理论和疗法，唯有中医学以其独特完整的理论体系和卓越的临床疗效，屹立于世界医学之林。中医学是中华民族在长期医疗生活实践中积累总结而成的，曾对中华民族的繁衍昌盛做出过巨大的贡献。时至今日，中医学仍然为人类医疗和保健发挥着重要的作用。

第一节　中医学的发展历程

人类漫长的进化过程就是人类生活与生产的知识和技能不断积累和发展的过程。早在远古时代，我们的祖先为了生存和繁衍，在觅食充饥及与疾病斗争的过程中，积累了一些原始医疗保健的知识。从"伏羲制九针"、"神农尝百草"、"伊尹治汤液"这些经典的传说中就足以证明这一点。

春秋战国时期，中国社会急剧变化，政治、经济、文化都有显著发展。"诸子蜂起，百家争鸣"，学术思想空前活跃，元气论、自然观和阴阳五行学说等在战国末年已具雏形。秦汉之际，《黄帝内经》、《难经》、《神农本草经》、《伤寒杂病论》等医学经典著作相继问世，标志着中医理论体系的初步形成。

晋至隋唐，我国现存最早的针灸学专著《针灸甲乙经》由晋·皇甫谧编撰而成；隋·巢元方编撰了我国第一部病因病机证候学专著《诸病源候论》。唐朝政治稳定，文化繁荣，医药学也进入了快速发展的轨道，中医学海纳百川，融合来自印度、波斯等国外医学知识，成为当时世界医学中心。《新修本草》成为世界上最早由国家制

CHAPTER ONE   INTRODUCTION
TO TRADITIONAL CHINESE MEDICINE

The splendid civilization of China has bred the great and profound culture of traditional Chinese medicine(TCM), which can be dated back to the period of Fuxi who invented needle therapy and Shennong who tasted and discovered hundreds of herbs. From them on, the complete TCM theory system has been gradually developed, including meridian and collateral culture, diagnosis and treatment culture, materia medica culture, and life nurturing culture. TCM, ancient Babylonian medicine, and ancient Indian medicine are regarded as the earliest three great systematic traditional medicines which enjoy the longest history. However, only TCM has still been standing out in the medicines of the world with its unique and integrated theoretical system and prominent clinical curative effects; on the contrary, the other two medicines, though developed earlier, only leaves us some fragmented theories and therapies. TCM gradually comes into being after summarization and accumulation of generations of Chinese people in the long period of living and medical treatment practices. Even now, it still plays a significant role in medical treatment and health care.

Section 1   Development of TCM

The lengthy evolution of humanity is in company with the continuous accumulation and development of living and production knowledge and skills. As early as ancient times, for survival and reproduction, our ancestors built up some primitive health care knowledge during the course of hunting for food and struggling with diseases, which can be manifested by these classic legends of Fuxi Making Needle Therapy, Shennong Tasting Hundreds of Herbs, and Yiyin Making Herb Decoction.

During the Spring and Autumn Period and Warring State Period, dramatic changes took place in China, with remarkable advances in politics, economy and culture. Academic thoughts were unparalleledly active in the atmosphere of "Contention of a Hundred Schools of Thoughts by their Exponents." Under such circumstance, Theory of Source Qi, View of Nature and Yin-Yang Theory, and Five Phase came into being with prototypes in the late Warring State Period. Between Qin Dynasty and Han Dynasty, a series of classic TCM masterpieces came out in succession like *Huangdi's Internal Classic*, *Classic of Difficult Issues*, *Shennong's Classic of Materia Medica*, and *Treatise on Cold Damage and Miscellaneous Diseases*, marking the preliminary formation of theoretic system of TCM.

During Jin Dynasty, Sui Dynasty, and Tang Dynasty, a lot of great TCM monographs were compiled like *A-B Classic of Acupuncture and Moxibustion* by Huangfu Mi of Jin Dynasty, the earliest existing treatise on acupuncture and moxibustion; and *Treatise on the Pathogenesis and Manifestations of All Diseases* by Chao Yuanfang of Sui Dynasty, the first book on the causes, pathogenesis and syndrom of diseases in the history of China. TCM attained rapid development in Tang Dynasty due to its political stability and prosperous culture. During this period, TCM absorbed and integrated the foreign medicines such as India and Persia, turning China then into the world medicine center. *Tang Meteria Medica* was the earliest and first officially issued medical classic in the world. Meanwhile, all the clinical subjects experienced booming

定颁布的官方药典。同时临床各科蓬勃发展，外科手术发展亦至鼎盛。孙思邈编撰《备急千金要方》和《千金翼方》，可称我国第一部医学百科全书；王焘的《外台秘要》集唐以前医学之大成。

宋至金元，是医学发展的重要时期。宋元时期，预防天花的人痘术开创了免疫学的先河；宋慈的《洗冤录》达到了古代法医学的顶峰；官办药局的《太平惠民和剂局方》对配方进行了严格规范；针灸铜人的铸造、《铜人腧穴针灸图经》的编撰使针灸教学有所遵循。金元时期出现"古方今病不相能"的思潮，涌现出一些不同的学派，活跃了医坛学术气氛，并在某些方面取得了突破。具有代表性的有"金元四大家"：刘完素提出"百病多因于火"，治疗主张以寒凉为主，被称为"寒凉派"；张从正认为凡病皆因"邪"而生，"邪去则正安"，成为独树一帜的"攻下派"；李杲强调"内伤脾胃，百病由生"，治疗以补益脾胃为主，被誉为"补土派"；朱震亨倡导"阳常有余，阴常不足"，推崇养阴药，后世医家尊为"养阴派"。诸家见解，虽各有偏颇，但在不同程度上丰富了中医学理论，推动了中医学术的发展。

明清时期，中医药学发展出现了革故鼎新的趋势。吴有性创立了"戾气学说"；李时珍的《本草纲目》走向世界；张景岳的命门学说《景岳全书》独树一帜；王肯堂的诊疗规范《证治准绳》启封问世，这些著作对宋、金、元、明以来医学各领域众多进展在总结归纳的基础上进行了创新。清代的主要医学成就是温病学说的形成：叶天士创立温病学说及卫气营血辨证；薛生白深入论述了湿热病的病因、病机及治法；吴鞠通独创三焦分治纲领；王孟英集前贤温病学说之大成，对暑、湿、火三气辨证从理论到治疗推向了一个新的阶段。被西方医学界称为中国近代解剖学家的清代医家王清任勇于革新，他的《医林改错》改正了古籍中人体解剖方面的错误，肯定了"灵机记性不在心在脑"，并发展了瘀血理论，创制了许多治疗瘀血病证的有效方剂，丰富了中医学的宝库。另外，清代西方医药开始传入中国，出现了中西汇通思想，代表人物如清初著名学者方以智，他所著的《医学汇通》、《通雅》等，引进了西方传教士带来的有关人体解剖、生理的一些新知识，为后来中西医汇通派的形成打下了一定的基础。

鸦片战争后，"欧风东进"，西方医学在中国迅速传播，中西汇通思想不断滋长，队伍不断扩大，被称为中西汇通派。代表人物有唐宗海、朱沛文、恽铁樵、张锡纯等，主张"采西人之所长，以补吾人之所短"，确立了衷中参西的汇通原则。到了民国，国民党政府试图以立法方式，废止中医。在《规定旧医登记案原则》中采取了釜底抽薪的办法，提出不准中医办学，使其后继无人，以达到中医消亡之目的。正是由于中医学自身不容忽视的医疗价值和一大批仁人志士的奋力抗争，才得以顽强生存下来。

development, among which surgery reached its peak.*Essential Prescriptions Worth a Thousand Gold for E-mergencies* and *Supplement to the Essential Prescriptions Worth a Thousand Gold* both written by Sun Simi-ao were the first medical encyclopaedias of China.*Medical Secrets of an Official* by Wang Tao embodied all the achievements before Tang Dynasty.

Song, Jin and Yuan Dynasties are another important period in the history of TCM development. During this period, poxinoculation preventing against variola was created, a token of the start of immunology. Records for *Washing Away of Wrong Cases* written by Song Ci were the peak masterpiece on forensic medicine in the ancient time.*Prescriptions from the Great Peace Imperial Grace Pharmacy* compiled by government-run bureau of compounding made strict specifications on recipes. The foundry of bronze acupuncture figure and compilation of *Illustrated Manual of Acupuncture Points of the Bronze Figure* provided a good basis for teaching the acupuncture and moxibustion. Even in Jin and Yuan Dynasties, there emerged the ideological trend of "the ancient recipes cannot totally cure the diseases nowadays," under which there sprung up some different schools of thoughts, activating the atmosphere of medical field and achieving great breakthroughs in some aspects. The four eminent physicians in Jin and Yuan Dynasties were the representatives of the thoughts. Liu Wansu believed that "fire and heat" were the main causes of a variety of diseases and that diseases should be treated with drugs cold and cool in nature, so his theory was known as the "school of cold and cool" by the later generations; Zhang Congzheng believed that all diseases were caused by exogenous pathogenic factors and advocated that pathogenic factors should be driven out by means of diaphoresis, emesis and purgation, so his theory was known as the "school of purgation;" Li Gao held that "internal impairment of the spleen and stomach would bring about various diseases" and therefore emphasized that the most important thing in clinical treatment should be to warm and invigorate the spleen and stomach, so he was regarded as the founder of the "school of reinforcing the earth;" and Zhu Zhenheng believed that "yang is usually redundant while yin is frequently deficient" and the body "is often abundant in yang but insufficient in yin," so his theory was known as the "school for nourishing yin." Though these opinions were biased or partial, they enriched TCM theory to some extent and promoted the development of TCM.

In Ming and Qing Dynasties, there had a revolutionary tendency in TCM development. Wu Youxing created the "epidemic pathogen theory." Li Shizhen compiled *Compendium of Materia Medica*, which enjoys a high reputation in the world. Zhang Jingyue set up the unique "life gate theory" in his own *Complete Works of Jingyue*. And Wang Kentang produced *Standards of Syndrome Identification and Treatment*, specifying the standards of diagnosis and treatment. All the works were innovated on the basis of summarization of the medical developments created since Song Dynasty in all aspects. The creation of theory of Warm Disease Study presented the principal medical achievement in Qing Dynasty. Ye Tianshi originated the theory of warm disease study and Defense, Qi, Nutrient and Blood syndrome differentiation. Xue Shengbai deepened expatiation of the causes, pathogenesis and therapy of dampness-heat diseases. Wu Jutong created Principle of Triple Energizer Partition Treatment. And Wang Mengying pushed the theory and treatment of syndrome differentiation of summer, dampness and fire pathogens to a new height on the basis of the former physicians. Wang Qingren, a physician in Qing Dynasty, revered as the anatomist in the modern times of China by Western medicine, worked out *Correction of Errors in Medical Classics*, in which he braved to correct the errors in human anatomy recorded in ancient books and pointed out "memory came out from the brain rather than from the heart." Besides, he developed the theory of blood stasis and invented many effective formulas to cure blood stasis, enriching the TCM treasure-house. In Qing Dynasty, the Western medicine began to be introduced into China and combined with TCM, as a result of which there came out Fang Yizhi, the famous scholar in early Qing Dynasty. As the representative of the integration of traditional and Western medicine, he wrote *Combination of Western and Chinese Medicine* and *Standards of Integration of*

中华人民共和国成立以后，中医学才枯木逢春。在党的中医政策的指引下，全国中医高等院校先后成立，培养了大量的中医及中西医结合人才；医疗机构和研究院所茁壮成长，学术研究取得了令人瞩目的成果。如：中国中医研究院屠呦呦教授等"青蒿素的发明"，征服了恶性疟疾，为世界热带医学作出了杰出的贡献，被称为"20世纪下半叶最伟大的医学创举"及"中国的第五大发明"；韩济生院士等"针刺镇痛原理的研究"阐明了针刺镇痛的机制，证明了针刺穴位能够刺激中枢神经中镇痛化学物质释放，从而起到镇痛作用，为针灸走出国门提供了科学的依据；陈可冀院士等"血瘀证及活血化瘀研究"明确了"血瘀证"的科学内涵，提高了治疗心脑血管疾病的临床水平；吴咸中院士等"急腹症与通里攻下法研究"，揭示了"六腑以通为用"的真谛，降低了急腹症的手术率；张亭栋教授、陈竺院士等"砷制剂治疗白血病"，完善了白血病的治疗，打开了中医药走向世界的大门。还有中国特色的恶性肿瘤的治疗模式，"带瘤生存"的治疗理念；小夹板固定治疗骨折，"动静结合、内外兼治、筋骨并重"的治疗方法，有助于功能恢复，并能节省费用的治疗优势，等等，不胜枚举。这些研究及成果不仅印证了古老中医药治疗的科学性，而且还得到了国际社会的认可。

第二节　中医学的特点

一、整体观念

整体观念就是强调在观察分析和研究处理问题时，要注重事物本身所存在的统一性、完整性和联系性。中医学的整体观念是关于人体自身的整体性及人与自然和社会环境的统一性的认识。

（一）人体自身的统一性

中医学认为人体是一个有机整体，是以五脏为核心，与六腑互为表里，通过经络与体表、形体、官窍相联系的有机统一的整体。具体体现在以下四个方面：

1. 人体结构　人体是由若干脏腑器官所组成的，这些脏腑器官是不可分割、相互联系的，任何局部都是整体的一个组成部分。如"舌为心之苗"、"口为脾之窍"等。

2. 基本物质　组成各脏腑器官并维持其功能活动的物质是同一的，即精、气、血、津、液，这些物质分布并运行于全身，以保证全身脏腑器官的功能活动。如"气为血之帅、血为气之母"、"精血互生"、"气随津脱"等。

3. 功能活动　人体组织结构和基本物质的统一性，决定了各种不同功能活动之

Traditional and Western Medicine, in which he introduced the new knowledge about human anatomy and physiology brought in by Western preachers, therefore laying the foundation for formation of the Huitong School (school combining the TCM and Western medicine).

After the Opium War, European thoughts flowed into and affected China. The Western medicine was soon spread in China to nourish the Huitong School and expand their team, represented by Tang Zonghai, Zhu Peiwen, Yun Tieqiao, and Zhang Xichun, who advocated "supplementing the weakness of TCM with the advantages of Western medicine" and established the principle of integration of TCM and Western medicine. During the Republic of China period, the Kuomintang government once tried to abolish TCM through legislation. They put dramatic measures in an attempt to eliminate TCM like forbidding running the TCM schools in *Provisions on Principle of Registration of Old Medicine*. However, it was due to the eminent medical values of TCM and the arduous struggle of upright scholars that TCM survived tenaciously.

After the foundation of the People's Republic of China, the TCM blossomed again. Under the guidance of the TCM policies made by the Communist Party, a group of TCM colleges, universities, and institutes were successively founded, cultivating plenty of both TCM and integrated traditional and Western medicine talents. Under such circumstance, the medical agencies and institutes throve and achieved remarkable academic research. For instance, artemisinin invented by Professor Tu Youyou and her team of China Academy of TCM has an effective treatment of malignant malaria, greatly contributing to the tropical medicine in the world and therefore, reputed as "the Greatest Medical Innovation in Latter Half of 20th Century" and "the Fifth Invention of China." Research on Acupuncture Analgesia Principle by Academician Han Jisheng clarified the mechanism of acupuncture analgesia, demonstrating that acupuncture of points can stimulate the release of analgesia chemical substances in central nerves so as to reduce pain, therefore, providing scientific bases for spreading acupuncture in the world. Research on Blood Stasis Syndrome and its Therapeutic Method of Activating Blood and Resolving Stasis by Academician Chen Keji and his team explicated blood stasis syndrome scientifically, raising the medical technology level of treating cardiovascular diseases. Research on Acute Abdomen and its Therapeutic Method of Expelling Pathogen in the Interior through Purgation by Academician Wu Xianzhong indicated the concept that the six bowels must keep its dredging function and lessened the operation rate of acute abdomen. Treatment of Leukemia with Arsenic Preparation created by Professor Zhang Tingdong and Professor Chen Zhu consummated the treatment of leukemia and opened the door for the TCM to the world. In addition, the mode of treating malignant tumor, therapeutic concept of survival with tumor; fracture treatment through splintage and therapy of "combination of dynamic and static, the internal and the external, and muscle and bones," all of which had Chinese characteristics, enjoyed the advantages of helping recuperation of functions of the body and saving treatment costs. All of these researches and achievements further confirmed the scientificity of these old treatment methods of TCM and push TCM to the world.

Section 2   Characteristics of TCM

Concept of Holism

Concept of holism means that people should stress the unitarity, integrity and interaction of objects when observing, analyzing, studying and dealing with problems. Concept of holism of TCM refers to cognition of the wholeness of the human body and of the unity of man, nature and the social environment.

Unitarity of Human Body

TCM regards the human body as an organic whole, with the five viscera (a collection term for the heart, liver, spleen, lung and kidney) as the core inside, corresponding with the six bowels (a collective

间密切的联系性。它们互根互用，协调制约，相互影响。如血液的生理功能的实现，要靠心、肝、脾、肺、肾共同协调完成，包括心主血脉、肺朝百脉、肝调血量、脾生血液及精血互生。

4. 诊断治疗　中医认为人体在生理功能上相互协调，在病理上也相互影响。在诊断上，察外知内，根据外在病变表现推测内在脏腑的病理变化，综合分析辨证；在治疗上，强调从整体进行调节，注重因时、因地、因人制宜。

（二）人与自然界的统一性

"天食人以五气，地食人以五味"。自然界的一切变化都可以直接或间接影响着人体的机能活动，在正常变化的范围内，人体可以作出相应的生理性适应，但若变化过大超出人体所能适应的限度，或者人体适应能力下降时，就可能成为疾病。这就是中医所谓"天人相应观"。它具体体现在自然环境对功能活动的影响等不同方面。

1. 季节气候对人体生理的影响　四季春温、夏热、长夏湿、秋凉、冬寒是正常的气候变化，人体的生理功能也随之而变化，称之为适应性调节。正如《灵枢·五癃津液别》说："天暑衣厚则腠理开，故汗出……天寒则腠理闭，气湿不行，水下留于膀胱，则为溺与气。"

2. 昼夜晨昏变化对人体生理的影响　中医学认为，在一日之内，随着昼夜晨昏阴阳消长的变化，人体的阴阳气血也进行相应的调节，与之相适应。如《素问·生气通天论》说："故阳气者，一日而主外，平旦人气生，日中而阳气隆，日西而阳气已虚，气门乃闭。"这种人体阳气白天趋于体表、夜间潜于内里的运动趋向，反映了人体随昼夜阴阳二气的盛衰变化而出现适应性调节。

3. 地域气候对人体生理的影响　地理环境和生活习惯的不同，在一定程度上也影响着人体的生理活动和脏腑功能，进而影响体质的形成。如江南多湿热，人体腠理多稀疏；北方多燥寒，人体腠理多致密。生活在这样的环境中，一旦易地而处，环境突然改变，初期多感不太适应。但人体也能进行相应的调节和适应，经过一段时间的锻炼，大都能够适应。

人对生存的自然环境的适应不是消极的、被动的，而是积极的、主动的。随着科学技术的发展，人们对客观世界的认识逐渐深入，人类自身不仅能主动地适应自然，而且能在一定程度上改造自然、美化环境，使大自然为人类服务。

term for the gallbladder, stomach, large intestine, small intestine, urinary bladder and triple energizers) outside and linked with the body surface, constituent and orifices of sense organs through meridian and collateral. It can be embodied in the following four aspects:

1. In terms of the human body structure, it is composed of different viscera and bowels. All these organs are inseparable and interconnected one another and are the integral parts of the whole body. For example, heart opens at the tongue and spleen opens at the mouth, etc.

2. In terms of the fundamental substance, the materials to build up the physical structure and maintain body functions are identical, namely essence, qi, blood, and fluid and humor. These substances spread and move throughout the whole body to ensure the normal functional activities of the organs. For example, "qi is the commander of blood and blood is the origin of qi, " "essence and blood are generated and transformed from each other, "and "qi will collapse if the body fluids deplete. "

3. In terms of functional activity, the unitarity of body structure and fundamental substance decides the close correlation of the different functions of organs, which mutually interdepend with and promote, coordinate with and restrict one another. For instance, to realize physiological function of blood, it needs the cooperation of the heart, liver, spleen, lung and kidney. As the heart controls blood circulation, all the vessels converge in the lung, the liver regulates blood volume, the spleen generates blood, and the essence and blood can alternate each other.

4. In terms of diagnosis and treatment, TCM regards the organs and their functions cannot only inter-coordinate physiologically but also inter-influence pathologically. So when diagnosing, inspection of the exterior manifestations will enable one to understand the interior conditions and then to analyze and differentiate the syndrome in an all-around way. While making treatment, emphasis on holism should be laid as well as suiting treatments to different conditions in terms of time, place, and patients.

Unitarity of Human Beings and Nature

"The sky provides men with five kinds of qi(wind, heat, dampness, dryness and cold) and the earth provides men with five kinds of flavors(acid, bitter, sweet, pungent and salty) from the earth." All the changes in the nature can directly or indirectly affect the functional activities of the human body. If these changes are within the normal range, human body can adjust itself to adapt them. But if they are beyond the extent human body can adapt to, or when the acclimatization of human body declines, then they will cause various diseases. It is "the philosophy of correspondence between nature and human" that TCM holds, which embodies in the aspects of how the natural environment affects the functional activities of human body.

1. The seasons and climates have impacts on the physiological functions of the human body. As for normal climate, spring is marked by warmth, summer by heat, late summer by dampness, autumn by dryness and winter by cold. The human body is no exception and it also makes corresponding changes according to it, which is called as accommodation. *Miraculous Pivot* described this as "The muscular interstices are open when one puts on more clothes in summer, that is why there is sweating…the muscular interstices are closed when it becomes cold, that is why dampness cannot be excreted and water is retained in the bladder to form urine or to cause retention of urine. "

2. The changes of day and night also affect the human body. TCM regards that yin, yang, qi, and blood regulate themselves to adapt the changes of yang rising in the morning and daytime and yin rising in afternoon and in the nighttime, as set forth in *Plain Questions* "Yang flows around the surface of the skin in the daytime. It is generated and rises in the morning, thrives at midday, weakens and hides inside with the sweat pores closing in the afternoon." This movement tendency of yang reflects the accommodation human body makes according to the changes of yin in the nighttime and yang in the daytime.

3. Besides, the differences in geographic environments and life styles also influence the physiological

（三）人与社会环境的统一性

人体的生命活动，不仅受到自然环境变化的影响，而且受到社会环境的制约。政治、经济、文化、宗教、法律、婚姻、人际关系等社会因素，会通过与人的信息交换影响着人体各种生理、心理活动和病理变化，而也在认识世界和改造世界的交流中，维持着生命活动的稳定、有序、平衡、协调。一般来说，良好的社会环境、融洽的人际关系，可使人精神振奋、积极上进、心情愉快，气血调和，阴阳平衡；若社会环境不佳，人际关系恶劣，家庭纠纷、亲人离别等不良事件就会使人压抑、紧张、焦虑，气血不和，阴阳失衡。另外，如果社会环境、经济状况及社会地位的骤变也会导致人的精神情志的紊乱，从而影响人体脏腑的功能而致某些身心疾病的发生。

二、辨证论治

辨证论治是中医学的特点和精华。辨证论治包括辨证和论治两大方面：辨证是确定治则治法的前提和依据；论治则是在辨证的基础上，确定治疗原则、选择治疗的具体手段和方法，并加以实施，治疗的效果又是检验辨证正确与否的依据。

辨证——即采用望、闻、问、切等诊法所收集的资料，包括症状和体征，在中医理论指导下，通过分析综合，去粗取精，去伪存真，辨清疾病的原因、性质、部位、发展阶段及邪正之间的关系等，最后概括、判断为某种性质的证。因此，辨证的过程就是对病人做出正确、全面判断的过程，或者说通过分析综合找出主要矛盾的过程。

论治——即是根据辨证的结果，选择和确定相应治疗原则和治疗方法的过程，也就是研究和实施治疗的过程。

中医认识和治疗疾病，是从症状入手，通过四诊手段，分析综合，审证求因。找出疾病的本质，确定治疗方案。例如头痛，由于病因不同，除头痛以外可表现出一些不同的特征，如外感头痛，可伴有恶寒、发热、脉浮等症；若血瘀头痛，可出现舌质紫暗、脉涩等症。如此方能避免治疗用药的盲目性，减少失误，提高疗效。

and functional activities of the human body to some extent and therefore lead to different constitutions. For example, the muscular interstices of residents living in the regions south of the Yangtze River are mostly rare and loose due to its damp and heat climate, while the muscular interstices of residents living in the northern part of China are often dense and compact due to its dry and cold climate. One will feel acclimatized at the beginning in case of the sudden change of the living environment or place, but will soon adapt to it with the adjustment of the human body.

Man often makes an adjustment actively and positively rather than negatively and passively to adapt to the natural environment in which he lives. With further development of science and technology, and the deep understanding of the objective world, human can initiatively adapt himself to the nature and transform the nature to a certain degree so as to beautify the environment and make it serve him better.

Unitarity of the Human Body and the Social Environment

The vital movements of the human body are affected by the changes of natural environment and restricted by the social environment. The social factors like politics, economy, culture, religions, law, marriage and interpersonal relations will bring about the psychological, physiological and pathological changes through conducting information exchange with human body. Meanwhile, they keep the life of human body evolving in a stable, well-organized, balanced, and harmonious way through the interchange activities of understanding and remoulding the world. Generally speaking, favorable social environment and harmonious interpersonal relations can make one happy, positive, and energetic and gain the qi-blood harmony as well as the yin-yang equilibrium. On the contrary, unfavorable social environment, worse interpersonal relations and other unhappy affairs such as family quarrels and parting of the family are apt to result in depression, nervousness, anxiety, qi-blood disharmony and yin-yang imbalance. In addition, the sudden and dramatic changes in social environment, economic status and social status can give rise to the disturbance of spirit and emotions, therefore, cause some spiritual or physical diseases by impacting the functions of the internal organs.

Treatment Based on Syndrome Differentiation

Treatment based on syndrome differentiation is the feature and essence of TCM, which is composed of syndromes differentiation and treatment. Syndrome differentiation is the precondition and basis of identifying therapeutic rules and methods. While treatment means to determine the principles of treatment, choose and carry out concrete therapies based on syndrome differentiation. And treatment effect is the proof to test the validity of syndrome differentiation.

Syndrome differentiation is a process under the guidance of TCM theory that doctors collect the information of a disease through the four examinations(inspection, listening and smelling, inquiry, and palpation)including all symptoms and signs, then analyze and generalize the location, cause and nature of the disease, the relation between the pathogenic factors and the healthy qi as well as the nature of the pathological changes of the disease at a certain stage, and finally make judgment of the properties of the syndromes based on this information. So the process of syndrome differentiation is also the course of making accurate and all-around judgment of a disease, or finding out the principal contradiction through a comprehensive analysis.

Treatment refers to the process of selecting and determining the corresponding therapeutic principles and methods according to the result of syndrome differentiation. In another word, it is the course of studying and implementing therapy.

The TCM doctors understand and treat diseases through comprehensively analyzing the syndromes gathered from the four examinations, probing into the nature of the disease from all etiologic factors collected based on differentiation, and determining the corresponding treatment option. For example, headache

第三节　中医和西医理论体系之异同

中西医理论体系的形成与发展离不开特定的东西方文化背景。东方文化的认知方法是经验和直觉,从整体上来认识和处理包括疾病和生命等复杂事物和问题;而西方文化的认知方法则是实证加推理。也就是说中医学是经验的归纳,而西医学是实验的总结;中医看到的是模糊的整体,而西医看到的是清晰的局部。从理论构建来看,中医学采用宏观形象,而西医学采用微观观察;从思维方法来看,中医学应用辩证思维,而西医学应用逻辑思维;在认识方法上,中医学是取类比象,而西医学是实体解剖;在知识应用上,中医学以辨证论治为核心,而西医学以辨病论治为基础;中医是治疗有病的人,重视人的整体变化;而西医是治疗人的病,关注病的病理特征。可以说中医是关于人的生命过程及其运动方式的相互关联的学说,它以促进人的自我实现、自我发展、自我和谐为宗旨,强调生命动态的"形神合一";追求自然环境的"天人合一"。尽管东西方医学是两种完全不同的理论体系,但事实上,中医和西医有很多相似之处。中医思维模式主要是从宏观辩证的角度来认识人体的生理病理过程,而西医主要从微观分析的角度来研究人体的生命和疾病。虽然两者的方法不同,但都应用了比较、分类、类比、归纳演绎、分析综合的方法。如中医的"揆度奇恒"、"司外揣内"、"援物比类"等都是逻辑思维方法的具体应用,而西医的"鉴别诊断"、"疾病分类"、"动物造模"和"诊断性治疗"等也采用了逻辑思维方法。正如前卫生部部长陈竺院士所言:中医强调"阴阳平衡",与现代系统生物学有异曲同工之妙;中医强调"天人合一",与现代西方科学讲的健康环境因素十分相似;中医强调"辨证施治",类似于西方医学通过药物遗传学为每一个病人找到最适合的药;中医的复方理论,实际上就是现在的西方治疗学越来越强调的各种疗法的综合使用。因此了解中西医理论之异同,打破中西医之间的壁垒,东西方两种认知力量汇聚是现代医学向更高境界提升和发展的一种必然趋势。

can manifest different symptoms according to different pathogenesis. If the headache is caused by external contraction, it often presents an aversion to cold, fever and floating pulse. And if it is caused by blood stasis, it often accompanies the signs of dark tongue and rough pulse. Only in this way, can the errors in making treatment and prescriptions be reduced and the curative effects improved.

Section 3   Similarities and Differences between the Theoretical Systems of the Western Medicine and TCM

The theoretical systems of the Western medicine and TCM derive from the Western culture and oriental culture, respectively. In the oriental culture, people perceive the objects through experience and intuition. They recognize and deal with the complicated objects and problems like diseases and life in a holistic sense. In the Western culture, people perceive objects through demonstration and ratiocination. In another word, the TCM derives from the generalization of experiences, while the Western medicine derives from summarization of experiments. TCM sees the vague wholeness whereas the Western medicine observes the clear and specific parts. From the angle of theoretic structure, TCM uses macro image, while the Western medicine utilizes micro observation. From the prospective of thinking method, TCM applies dialectical thinking, whereas the Western medicine applies logical thinking. From the view of cognition method, TCM is based on analogy, whereas the Western medicine is based on anatomy. From the point of knowledge application, TCM takes the treatment based on syndrome differentiation as the core, while the Western medicine takes the treatment based on disease identification as the base. In the aspect of treatment, TCM treats the patient and focuses on the holistic changes of the patient, while the Western medicine treats the diseases of the patient and concerns the pathological characteristics of the disease. TCM is the theory on the correlation of the life course and its mode of motion. It follows the tenet of promotion of self-realization, self-development, and self-harmony, emphasizes harmonization between soma and spirit of the dynamic life, and pursues for the harmonization of man and the nature. Though they are the two totally different theoretical systems, the Western medicine and TCM actually share a lot of similarities. TCM primarily recognizes the physiology of the human body and the pathology of diseases in the macro and dialectical view, while the Western medicine studies the life and diseases in the view of micro analysis. In spite of differences in adopting the methods, they both apply comparison, classification, analogy, deduction and conclusion, analysis, and summarization. For example, "assessment of the normal and abnormal(determining the extent to which an individual is exhibiting abnormal characteristics which may be indicative of a disease or pathological condition), ""judging the inside from the observation of the outside, "and"deduction of a disease by comparing and analogizing it with the similar one"stressed in TCM are the concrete application of logic thinking methods, while"differential diagnosis, " "assortment of diseases, " "animal model establishing, " and"diagnostic treatment" adopted in the Western medicine are also the application of logic thinking methods. As Academician Chen Zhu, former Minister of Ministry of Health of P.R.China once said, TCM stresses the equilibrium between yin and yang, which has the similarity with the modern systematic biology. TCM emphasizes the harmonization between man and the nature, which is similar with the health environmental factors set forth by the modern Western science. And TCM focuses on treatment based on syndrome differentiation, which is like pharmacogenetics that the Western medicine considered as the most proper medicines for each patient. The complex prescription of TCM is actually the combination of all therapies the Western medicine stresses nowadays. To understand the differences and similarities of the Western medicine and TCM, to break barriers between them and to converge the cognitive methods of both the Western medicine and TCM is the inevitable tendency of the modern medicine, through which it can further promote and develop.

第四节　传统医德的现代价值

中医传统医德反映了广大劳动人民的利益和愿望，是中国传统文化中最为宝贵的精神财富之一。传统医德闪耀着人性与理性的光芒，崇尚"生命至重，惟人最尊"的信念；倡导"医乃仁术、济人为本"的思想；坚持"医贵乎精，仁术济世"的精神；恪守"贵义贱利，自正己德"的准则。数千年来这些传统医德成为医生规范自我、独善其身、鞭策奋进的精神动力。其内容丰富涉猎广泛，其主要内容包括"诚于品德，精于专业，勇于探索，融于同道"等方面。

一、诚于品德、精于专业

在祖国医学史上，"苍生大医"层出不穷。如战国时期的扁鹊、汉代的张仲景、唐代的孙思邈、明代的李时珍、清代的王清任等，他们以崇高医德和杰出成就成为医界楷模。孙思邈在《千金要方·大医精诚》中明确提出了医生必须恪守的道德准则："凡大医治病，必当安神定志，无欲无求，先发大慈恻隐之心，誓愿普救含灵之苦。若有疾厄来求救者，不得问其贵贱贫富，长幼妍媸，怨亲善友，华夷智愚，普同一等，皆如至亲之想；亦不得瞻前顾后，自虑吉凶，护惜身命。见彼苦恼，若己有之，深心凄怆，勿避艰险、昼夜、寒暑、饥渴、疲劳，一心赴救，无作功夫形迹之心。"意思是说，医生诊治疾病时应当精神安宁、神志专一，不可以有任何私心杂念，要怀有一颗仁爱之心，要有为病人除病解难之志，对病人应当一视同仁、不分贵贱，急病人之所急、想病人之所想，一心赴救；不可计较个人得失，不可顾虑个人安危。又如：明代名医陈实功提出为医者要做到"一戒重富嫌贫，二戒行为不俭，三戒图财贪利，四戒玩忽职守，五戒轻浮虚伪"。还有徐大椿的《医学源流论》告诫为医者不要做"立奇方以取异；或用僻药以惑众；或用参茸补热之药以媚富贵之人；或假托仙佛之方，以欺愚鲁之辈；或立高谈怪论，惊世盗名；或造假经伪说，瞒人骇俗；或明知此病易晓，伪说彼病以示奇"的庸医。

作为医生只有仁爱救人之心，没有济世救人之术，"济世活人"也就会成为空话。《医学集成》要求："医之为道，非精不能明其理，非博不能至其约。"为了施行仁术，医生不但要刻苦学习，而且要不耻下问，提高医术。王世雄在《回春录序》中也说："医者，生人之术也，医而无术，则不足生人。"叶天士更是入木三分地指出："术不精则无异于杀人。"他在临终时告诫后人："医可为而不可为，必天资能悟，语书万卷，而后可借术济世。不然，鲜有不杀人者，是以药饵为刀刃也。"汉代张仲景"感往昔之沦丧，伤横夭之莫救"，为了济世救人，乃"勤求古训，博采众

Section 4   Modern Value of Traditional Medical Ethics

As one of the most precious intellectual treasures of the traditional cultures of China, the traditional TCM ethics reflects the interests and desire of the working people. Shining beautiful light of humanity and rationality, it holds the concept of "life is the most important and human should be the most honorable," advocates the thought of "medicine is a humane art" and "the obligation of a doctor is to helping the patient," adheres to the spirit of "mastering excellent medical skills and holding noble ethics to benefit the mankind," and follows the criterion of "cherishing righteousness and justice rather than benefits and profits, and raising the morality by strict self-discipline." For thousands of years, these excellent traditional medical ethics has been the spiritual impetus of the doctors in enhancing their medical skills and their personal morality. The traditional medical ethics covers an extensive scope, primarily in the aspects of "faithful quality, professional medical skills, braveness in exploration, and harmony with peer reviews."

Faithful Quality and Professional Medical Skills

There springs out innumerable outstanding doctors with high morality revered as "Empyreal Doctor", such as Bian Que of the Warring States Period, Zhang Zhongjing of Han Dynasty, Sun Simiao of Tang Dynasty, Li Shizhen of Ming Dynasty, and Wang Qingren of Qing Dynasty. All of them had set good examples for the doctors with the lofty medical ethics and great achievements. Sun Simiao once definitely set forth the code of ethics for doctors in the chapter of Medical Morality of his book *Great Doctors of Essential Prescriptions Worth a Thousand Gold for Emergencies*. That is "Generally speaking, when the well-qualified doctors treat patients, they are usually calm and concentrated without any desire and avarice. They first have great sympathy for the patients and then are determined to save people from the suffering. If patients come to ask for help, they should not treat them differently by seeing whether they are rich or poor, old or young, beautiful or ugly, enemy or friend, Chinese or foreigners, and foolish or wise. They should treat all the patients like their close relatives. In treating patients, they should not think over and over for themselves and pay too much attention to the protection of their own life. Being doctors, they should regard the patients' suffering as their own and have deep sympathy for them. Confronted with danger, they should not try to avoid it. No matter in the daytime or night, in the winter or summer, and no matter when they are hungry or thirsty, and tired or exhausted, they should work for the patients heart and soul, without any delay or regardless of personal thought for gain or loss." Chen Shigong, a famous doctor of Ming Dynasty, put forward that the doctors should keep away from such notions and behaviors as care for the rich and discrimination of the poor, misconduct, avarice, malpractice and truancy, frivolity and hypocrisy. In addition, Xu Dachun, a famous physician of Qing Dynasty, also warned in his work of *Theory of Medical Origins* that "the doctors should get away from the conducts of making themselves different from other doctors by prescribing the uncommon herbs, confusing peoples with unfamiliar herbs, pleasing the rich and the nobles with ginseng, cartialgenous and other rare medicinals, deceiving illiterates with witchcraft, building up reputation by writing weird information, cheating others by fabricating the classic works and showing off the skills by naming the common diseases as uncommon ones."

A doctor should be equipped with both merciful heart and excellent medical skills; otherwise, to save lives and benefit mankind will be a totally empty talk. It stated in *Compendium of Medicines* that "the doctors should intensify their study to master the medical principles and cover a wide range of works to make the correct prescriptions." To put their kindness into practice, the doctors should work hard and grasp every chance to learn from others so as to raise their medical skills. Wang Shixiong wrote in his *Preface of Rejuvenation Record* that "doctors were the people to save lives, without excellent medical skills, they could

方"，撰写了《伤寒杂病论》，创立了六经辨证，为中医辨证施治奠定了基础。孙思邈认为医学是"至精至微之事"，"学者必须博极医源，精勤不倦，不得道听途说"，提出了"省病诊疾，至意深心；详察形候，纤毫勿失，处判针药，无得参差"。他直到白发暮年还手不释卷，"一事长于己者，不远千里，伏膺取决"，终成苍生大医。

二、勇于探索、融于同道

一名"苍生大医"还应该是科学的实践者、真理的追求者。神农尝百草"一日而遇七十毒"，为的就是"令民有所避就"；华佗创造麻沸散，刮骨疗伤，开颅剖腹，为的是探索未知解除病痛；李时珍远涉深山旷野，访问名医宿儒，博采民间验方，集中国药学之大成，为的是造福生民，民族昌盛；王清任革故鼎新，亲自观察尸体结构，绘制脏腑图谱，开宗正义地推出《医林改错》，为的是后人有所遵循，不至于南辕北辙。西方医学传入中国后，唐宗海、张锡纯等中西汇通的实践等，都是勇于探索、追求科学的典范。北京中医药大学任应秋老师经常对学生讲："学问多半都是一望无涯的汪洋大海，不具备一点牺牲精神，甘冒风险，战胜惊涛骇浪，坚定地把握着后舵，航船是不可能安全达到彼岸的。"先人已为后人树立了勇于探索，不畏艰苦，为医学献身的光辉典范。每个学生都应该努力学习，积极探索，在医学的道路上孜孜以求。

"苍生大医"还必须具备尊重同行的品德。孙思邈《备急千金要方》中指出："为医之法，不得多语调笑，谈谑喧哗，道说是非，议论人物，炫耀声名，訾毁诸医，自矜己德。"并说，有的人"偶然治瘥一病，则昂头戴面而有自许之貌，谓天下无双。此医人之膏肓也。"即作为一名医生应当谦虚谨慎，不可以随便谈说别人的短处，以炫耀自己的名声，甚至诽谤攻击其他医生，借以夸耀自己的功德；偶然治好了一个病人，就骄傲自满、目中无人，医生是绝不准许有这种行为。一名优秀的医生，应当"捐众贤之砂砾，掇群才之翠羽"，时时处处谦虚谨慎，尊重同行，精求医理，博采众长。明代著名外科学家陈实功在《外科正宗》中说："凡乡井同道之士，不可轻侮傲慢。与人切要谦和谨慎，年尊者恭敬之；有学者师事之；骄傲者逊让之；不及者荐拔之。如此自无谤怨，信和为贵也。"明仪龚廷贤《万病回春·云林暇笔》中也对医生不尊重同行的行为给予严厉的批评。他说总有一些"无行之徒，专一夸己之长，形人之短。每至病家，不问疾疴，唯毁前医之过，以骇患者"，这是非常不道德的行为。

（梁晓春）

not rescue lives in spite of cherishing merciful desire."Ye Tianshi elaborated on the principle that"without excellent medical skills,a doctor may turn into a killer even though he is kindhearted."To remind the later generations,he cautioned before he died that"the doctors must be those talented with high comprehension. Before practicing their medical skills,they must read through a great number of books and works,or they will be killers with medicines as knives."It was with the same emotion and awareness that Zhang Zhongjing of Han Dynasty read a lot of ancient medical classics and finally compiled *Treatise on Febrile and Miscellaneous Diseases* by absorbing their essences and created Six-Meridian Syndrome Differentiation,which laid a solid foundation for treatment based on syndrome differentiation.Sun Simiao regarded iatrology as the most precise and delicate skills,which required its practitioners to refer to a plenty of the medical books and therefore understand the principles of medical sciences rather than listening to others. On this basis,he proposed"the doctor should concentrate when making examination and diagnosis,and then made the prescription or performed needles strictly in accordance with the symptoms."Following this code,he studied hard even at his old age and finally became a great doctor immortally.

Braveness in Exploration and Harmony with Peer Reviews

An"Empyreal Doctor"is also a practicer of science and pursuer of truth.Shennong neglected the danger of being killed by poison and tasted hundreds of herbs with the aim of distinguishing them for people.Hua Tuo invented Mafei San(Chinese ancient narcotic drug),scrapped bones and conducted craniotomy and laparotomy in order to explore the unknown and to relieve the patients from pain and diseases.Li Shizhen walked to visit prestigious doctors and distinguished scholars living in mountain and remote areas and collected the folk recipes for the purpose of benefiting people and prolonging their lives.Wang Qingren observed the structure of corpses, drew the atlas of the viscera bowels,and wrote *Correction of the Errors of Medical Works* with the purpose of correcting the wrong concepts of the ancestors and providing the offspring with the correct one.After the Western medicine was introduced into China,Tang Zonghai,Zhang Xichun and other doctors,in pursuit and exploration of science,combined the Western medicines with TCM,therefore setting examples for the later generations.Ren Yingqiu,a teacher of Beijing University of Chinese Medicine often educated his students"knowledge is the endless sea and one wouldn't get to its coast unless she/he is brave enough to take adventure and conquer the waves and firmly hold the helm."There are a lot of splendid examples in the medical history that bravely greeted challenges,explored sciences and therefore dedicated themselves to medicines.So each of the students should work hard and explore actively along the medical road.

"Empyreal Doctors"should also respect the other doctors.Sun Simiao pointed out in *Valuable Prescriptions for Emergency* that"the doctors should be equipped with the quality of being humble and cautious,avoiding taking about failings of others to show off his knowledge and slandering other doctors to brag about his own merits."Meanwhile,he added that"a doctor should abstain from such conducts as conceit and complacency."A brilliant doctor should be modest and prudent,respect other doctors,refine medical theory and learn from others openheartedly.Chen Shigong,the famous surgical doctor stated in *Orthodox Manual of External Medicine* that"a doctor should not despise other doctors in villages and countryside.On the contrary,he should be humble and prudent and respect the elders and seniors,learn from the experienced ones,even show respect for the arrogant ones,and help those juniors to improve their skills and recommend them if there was an opportunity.If a doctor can abide by this principle and good faith, then he will get respects from others."Gong Tingxian of Ming Dynasty also made rigorous criticism on the misconduct of disregarding other doctors in his *Rejuvenation of illness*,in which he said that"there were always some wicked doctors who often exaggerated the merits of their own and defamed others in front of the patients so as to frighten the patients and raise their own reputation."

(Wu Qunli   Zhang Wen)

第二章　阴阳五行学说

阴阳学说萌生于商周，成熟于战国与秦汉之际，是古人探求宇宙本原和解释宇宙变化的一种世界观和方法论，属于中国古代唯物论和辩证法的范畴。春秋战国时期以后，医学家开始将阴阳学说引入中医学领域，成为中医理论体系的重要组成部分，用以说明生命的起源、人体组织结构、生理功能和病理变化，并指导临床诊断和治疗。

第一节　阴阳学说

一、阴阳的基本概念

阴阳，是对自然界相互关联的某些事物或现象对立双方属性的概括。阴阳学说认为"阴阳者，万物之能始也"。"天地合而万物生，阴阳接而变化起"。

阴阳学说认为宇宙间凡属相互关联且又相互对立的事物或现象，或同一事物内部相互对立的两个方面，都可以用阴阳来概括分析其各自的属性。如天与地、日与月、水与火、寒与热、升与降、明与暗等。一般来说，凡是运动的、外向的、上升的、温热的、无形的、明亮的、兴奋的都属于阳；相对静止的、内守的、下降的、寒冷的、有形的、晦暗的、抑制的都属于阴。如以天地而言，则"天为阳，地为阴"，由于天气清轻向上故属阳，地气重浊凝滞故属阴。以水火而言，则"水为阴，火为阳"，由于水性寒而润下故属阴，火性热而炎上故属阳。以物质的运动变化而言，"阳化气，阴成形"，物质从有形化为无形的过程属于阳，由无形凝聚成有形的过程属于阴。阴和阳的相对属性引入医学领域，将人体中具有中空、外向、弥散、推动、温煦、兴奋、升举等特性的事物及现象统属于阳，而将具有实体、内守、凝聚、宁静、凉润、抑制、沉降等特性的事物和现象统属于阴。如脏为阴而腑为阳，精为阴而气为阳，营气为阴而卫气为阳等等。

但是事物的阴阳属性在某种意义上又是相对的，一方面，阴阳无限可分，即阴阳之中可

CHAPTER TWO   YIN-YANG THEORY AND FIVE-PHASE THEORY

Yin-yang theory sprouted in Shang and Zhou Dynasties and matured between the Warring States Period, Qin Dynasty, and Han Dynasty. It is a world view and methodology that the ancient chinese people explored the origin of the universe and explained the changes of the universe, so it belongs to the category of ancient Chinese materialism and dialectics. After the Spring and Autumn Period and the Warring States Period, this theory was introduced into TCM and became the important integral part of TCM theory, which interpreted the origin of life, body structure, physiological functions and pathological changes of human body and was used to guide the clinical diagnosis and treatment.

Section 1   Yin-Yang Theory

Basic Concepts of Yin and Yang

Yin and yang are the general descriptive terms for the two opposite, complementary, and inter-related cosmic forces found in all matter in nature. Yin-yang theory regards "yin and yang are the origins of all things in the universe" and "all the things are generated from the interaction of yin and yang, which comes into being after the separation of the heaven and the earth."

Yin-yang theory states that all the two opposite and interrelated things or phenomena in the universe or the two opposite aspects of a thing can be summarized and categorized as yin and yang, for example, heaven and earth, sun and moon, water and heat, cold and heat, ascending and descending, brightness and dimness, etc. Generally speaking, those with the basic nature of motion, outward and upward directions, heat, intangibility, brightness and excitement, pertain to yang; while those with the basic nature of stillness, inward and downward directions, cold, tangibility, dimness and inhibition, pertain to yin. For instance, the heaven is yang while the earth is yin because the heavenly qi is clear, light, and rising whereas the earth qi is heavy, turbid, and sluggish. Water belongs to yin while fire belongs to yang because water has the property of cold and moisture whereas fire has the property of heat and ascending. From the angle of motion and change of substances, yang produces the invisible qi while yin constitutes the visible parts. So the course of turning substances from tangible to intangible belongs to yang; and on the contrary, the process of agglomerating the intangible to be the tangible substances belongs to yin. When this theory was introduced into TCM, the parts or phenomena of human body characterized by hollowness, outward, dispersion, promotion, warming, and excitement are all sorted as yang; while the parts or phenomena of human body featuring tangibility, inwardness, cohesion, tranquility, coldness and moist, depression and descending are all categorized as yin. For example, the five viscera belong to yin while the six bowels belong to yang, essence belongs to yin while qi belongs to yang, and nutrient qi belongs to yin while defense qi belongs to yang.

再分阴阳，即所谓阴中有阳，阳中有阴。例如：昼为阳，夜为阴。而白天的上午与下午相对而言，则上午为阳中之阳，下午为阳中之阴；夜晚的前半夜与后半夜相对而言，则前半夜为阴中之阴，后半夜为阴中之阳。由此可见，自然界中相互关联又相互对立的事物可以概括为阴阳两类，事物内部又可分为阴和阳两个方面，而每一事物内部的阴或阳的任何一方，还可以再分阴阳。故《素问·阴阳离合论》说："阴阳者，数之可十，推之可百，数之可千，推之可万，万之大，不可胜数，然其要一也。"另一方面，阴阳的属性在一定条件下可以相互转化。如属阴的寒证在一定条件下可以转化为属阳的热证；属阳的热证在一定条件下也可以转化为属阴的寒证。病变寒热性质的改变，其证候的阴阳属性也随之改变。再如人体气化过程中，精属阴，气属阳；精代谢为能量（气），为阴转化为阳；消耗能量而获得营养物质（精）的产生，为阳转化为阴。

二、阴阳的变化规律

阴阳学说的核心是阐述阴阳之间的相互关系及其通过这些关系来认识自然界万物生长、发展和变化的内在机制和规律。阴阳的变化规律主要有以下几个方面（图2-1）：

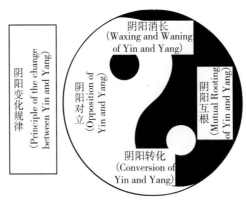

图 2-1 太极图

（Figure 2-1 Diagram of the Universe）

（一）阴阳对立

是指阴阳双方存在对立和制约的关系。自然界一切事物或现象都存在着相互对立的阴阳两个方面，如上与下、左与右、天与地、动与静、出与入、升与降、昼与夜、明与暗、寒与热、水与火等等。阴阳双方既是对立的，又是统一的，统一是对立的结果。如自然界阴阳的对立制约：春夏之所以温热，是因为春夏阳气上升抑制了寒凉之气；秋冬之所以寒冷，是因为秋冬阴气上升抑制了温热之气的缘故。同此，在人体中的阳气能推动和促进机体的生命活动，加快新陈代谢，而人体中的阴气能调控和抑制机体的代谢和各种生命活动，阴阳双方相互制约而达到协调平衡，则人体

However, the nature of yin and yang of things is relative in a sense. On one hand, yin and yang can be divided *ad infinitum* as yin exists in yang and yang exists in yin. For example, the daytime is yang, while the nighttime is yin. As for the daytime, the morning belongs to yang within yang, while the afternoon belongs to yin within yang. As to the nighttime, the time from nightfall to midnight belongs to yin within yin, while the time after midnight belongs to yang within yin. It shows that those interrelating with and opposite to one another in the universe can be summarized and categorized as yin and yang, the two opposite aspects of one thing or phenomenon can also be classified into yin and yang, and even the yin aspect or yang aspect can be further divided into yin and yang, as defined in *Plain Questions*, "yin and yang can be divided *ad infinitum*, but their essence is yin and yang, which is generated from Taiji, the harmony of two aspects of a thing." On the other hand, yin and yang can be mutually converted into each other under certain condition. The cold syndrome characterized by yin property can be turned into heat syndrome featuring yang property in certain circumstances, and vice versa. The yin or yang property of the syndrome of a disease varies with the change of the property of cold or heat of the pathology. As for human body, essence is yin while qi is yang, but during the course of transformation, essence is metabolized into energy (qi), which is the conversion from yin to yang; and the transformed energy or qi flow to help generate nutrient substances (essence), which is the conversion from yang to yin.

Principle of the Change between Yin and Yang

The core of yin-yang theory is to elaborate the relations between yin and yang and then adopt it to explain the intrinsic mechanism and principle of growth, development and change of all things in the universe. The principle of the change between yin and yang is as follows:

Opposition of Yin and Yang

It means that yin and yang are mutually opposing, repelling, and contending. All things or phenomena in the natural world have the opposing and restrictive aspects, such as top and bottom, left and right, heaven and earth, motion and quiescence, entering and existing, ascending and descending, day and night, brightness and dimness, cold and heat, and water and fire, etc. Yin and yang are opposite and unitive, with unity being the result of oppositeness. In terms of oppositeness and restriction of yin and yang in the natural world, the climatic change of the four seasons can be taken as the example. It is warm in spring and hot in summer because yang qi rises in spring and summer and restricts the cool and cold qi of autumn and winter. It is cool in autumn and cold in winter because yin qi rises in autumn and winter and restricts the yang qi of spring and summer. In the same way, yang qi of the human body can promote and motivate the vital activities of human body and accelerate the metabolism; while the yin qi of human body can adjust and restrict such activities and metabolism. Such mutual restriction between yin and yang can balance the vital activities of human body and make people healthy and orderly, as described in *Plain Questions*, "harmony of yin and yang contributes to the body and mental health."

Mutual Rooting of Yin and Yang

It means that yin and yang are the precondition of existence of each other. In another word, there will be no yin without yang or there will be no yang without yin, as stated in the annotation of *Plain Questions* by Wang Bing, "yang roots in yin and yin derives from yang, and yang cannot be generated without yin and yin cannot be formed without yang." In the natural world, heat belongs to yang while cold belongs to yin, cold will not exist if there is no heat, and vice versa. The heaven belongs to yang and the earth belongs to yin. There will be no earth if there is no heaven. So yang exists in yin and yin exists in yang. As for human body, it is stated in *Plain Questions* "yin remains inside to act as a guard for yang, while yang stays outside

生命活动健康有序。即《素问·生气通天论》所谓"阴平阳秘，精神乃治"。

（二）阴阳互根

是指阴阳双方互为存在的前提和条件，也就是说，阴阳双方都以对方的存在而存在。正如王冰注《素问·生气通天论》说："阳气根于阴，阴气根于阳，无阴则阳无以生，无阳则阴无以化。"在自然界中，热为阳，寒为阴，没有热也就无所谓寒，没有寒也就无所谓热；天为阳，地为阴，没有天也就无所谓地，所以说阳依存于阴，阴依存于阳。在人体，《素问·阴阳应象大论》说："阴在内，阳之守也；阳在外，阴之使也。"指出阳以阴为基，阴以阳为偶；阴为阳守持于内，阳为阴役使于外，阴阳相互为用，不可分离。

《素问·阴阳应象大论》曰："阴生阳长，阳杀阴藏。"就是说，阳依赖于阴而存在，阴依赖于阳而存在。倘若由于某些原因，阴和阳之间的互根关系遭到破坏，就会导致"孤阴不生，独阳不长"，甚则"阴阳离决，精气乃绝"而死亡。如果人体阴阳之间的互滋互用关系失常，就会出现"阳损及阴"或"阴损及阳"的病理变化。

（三）阴阳消长

是指阴阳双方始终处于动态的平衡之中，如阴消阳长，阳消阴长，阴阳消长是阴阳运动变化的一种形式，而导致阴阳出现消长变化的根本原因在于阴阳之间存在着的对立制约与互根互用的关系。以四时气候变化而言，从冬至春及夏，气候从寒冷逐渐转暖变热，这是"阳长阴消"的过程；由夏至秋及冬，气候由炎热逐渐转凉变寒，这是"阴长阳消"的过程。以人体的生理活动而言，白天阳气盛，故机体的生理功能以兴奋为主；夜晚阴气盛，故机体的生理功能以抑制为主。子夜一阳生，日中阳气隆，机体的生理功能由抑制逐渐转向兴奋，这是"阳长阴消"的过程；日中至黄昏，阴气渐生，阳气渐衰，机体的生理功能也由兴奋逐渐转向抑制，这是"阴长阳消"的过程。由此可以看出，阴与阳之间的互为消长是不断进行着的，是绝对的；而阴与阳之间的平衡则是相对的，是动态的平衡。

（四）阴阳转化

是指阴阳双方在一定条件下可向各自相反的方向转化，阳可以转化为阴，阴可以转化为阳。如果说阴阳消长是量变的过程，那么，阴阳转化就是质变的过程。

任何事物都处在不断地运动变化之中。《素问·天元纪大论》所说的"物生谓之化"，是指事物由小到大的发展阶段；"物极谓之变"，是指事物发展到极点，由盛到衰，向它反面转化的阶段。正如《素问·阴阳应象大论》曰，"重阴必阳，重阳必阴"、"寒极生热，热极生寒"以及"寒甚则热，热甚则寒"，就是指阴阳消长变化发展到"极"的程度，就要向它的反面转化。以疾病来说，阴阳的转化常常表现为在一定条件下表证与里证、寒证与热证、虚证与实证的相互转化。如急性热病（如

to serve as an actor of yin."It indicates that yin is the base of yang while yang is the source of yin;yin provides substances for yang in the interior while yang defends against pathogens of yin in the exterior;and yin and yang are interdependent and inseparable.

Yang's existence depends on yin while yin's subsistence relies on yang,as stated in *Plain Questions* "yang grows with the increase of yin,and yin declines with decreasing of yang."If the interdependence between yin and yang is destroyed for some reasons,then such situation will occur that"neither yang nor yin will grow without each other";even worse,it will lead to death as the result of"dissociation of yin and yang and extinction of the vital essence."If yin and yang of human body can not support each other,then the pathological change of"detriment to yang affects yin"or"detriment to yin affects yang"will occur.

Waxing and Waning of Yin and Yang

Yin and yang coexist in a dynamic equilibrium in which one waxes while the other wanes.Growth and decline are the way that yin and yang move.The root cause of such motion lies in their relations of opposition,restriction and interdependence.Take the seasonal and climatic variations for example,it gets warmer from winter to spring,and hotter from spring to summer,which is the process of"yang waxing and yin waning."Conversely,it gets cooler from summer to autumn and colder from autumn to winter,which is the process of"yin waxing and yang waning."As for physiological functions of the human body,it becomes excited and dynamic during the daytime,when yang qi is exuberant;and gradually quiet during the nighttime,when yin qi is abundant.Yang begins to grow from the midnight and becomes exuberant at midday, so the human body turns from quiet and depressed to dynamic and excited,which is the course that yang grows and yin declines.Yin starts to grow at midday and become abundant in the dusk,so the human body turns from dynamic to static,which is the course that yin grows and yang declines.It can be concluded that the motion of yin and yang is permanent and absolute,while the balance between yin and yang is relative and dynamic.

Conversion of Yin and Yang

It means under given conditions,either yin or yang may transform into its opposite side.That is to say yin may be transformed into yang and yang into yin.If the waning and waxing relation between yin and yang can be regarded as a process of quantitative change,then the inter-transformation between yin and yang is a qualitative change.

All things are in constant motion and change,as described in *Plain Questions* "the growth of things means transformation,"which refers to the development of things growing from a small beginning into a mighty force;and"change takes place when things develop to extremity,"which means things will develop in the opposite direction when they become extreme.As *Plain Questions* stated,"extreme yin turns into yang,while extreme yang turns into yin"and"extreme cold brings on heat,while extreme heat brings on cold."It means yin and yang will go reversely when they develop to their extremity respectively.With regard to diseases,the mutual of transformation of exterior syndrome and interior syndrome,cold syndrome and heat syndrome,excess syndrome and deficiency syndrome,is the embodiment of yin-yang conversion. For example,the acute pyreticosis(like severe pneumonia)presents the excess heat syndrome with high fever,red complexion,cough and pant,heavy breath,polydipsia,rapid and full pulse;but if the extremely overabundant heat impairs the healthy qi so that the healthy qi cannot subdue the pathogenic factors,then the deficiency cold syndrome with pale complexion,cold limbs,listlessness,extremely weak pulse(such as shock)will suddenly turn up.It is a good example to show the yang syndrome of extreme heat(high fever) converts into the yin syndrome of cold.In addition,people with constitutional exuberant yang will manifest the yin cold syndrome of aversion to cold when attacked by cold,but it will turn into the yang heat because

重症肺炎等），表现为高热、面红、咳喘、气粗、烦渴、脉数有力等，属于阳实热证。邪热极盛，耗伤正气，可致正不胜邪，而突然出现面色苍白、四肢厥冷、精神萎靡、脉微欲绝（如休克等）一派虚寒表现的阴证，就是由于热极（高热）的阳证转化为阴寒证的实例。又如阳盛体质的人感受风寒，出现恶寒等阴寒证，但由于寒邪束表，阳气闭而化热，则有外寒转化为内热的阳热证。上述两个病例中，前者的热毒极重，后者的寒邪外束，即是促成阴阳相互转化的内在必备条件。

　　阴阳之间的这些关系及其运动规律彼此互相联系，互相影响。阴阳的对立互根是阴阳最普遍的规律，事物之间的阴阳两个方面通过对立制约而取得了平衡协调，通过互根互用而互相促进，不可分离。阴阳消长是在阴阳对立制约、互根互用基础上表现出的量变过程，阴阳转化则是在量变基础上的质变，是阴阳消长的结果。阴阳的动态平衡由阴阳之间的对立制约、互根互用及其消长转化来维系，而阴阳自和表达了其自动维持和自动恢复这一动态协调平衡的能力与趋势。如果阴阳的这种动态平衡遭到了破坏，又失去了自和的能力，在自然界就会出现反常现象，在人体则会由生理状态进入病理状态，甚至导致死亡。

三、阴阳学说在中医学中的应用

　　阴阳学说渗透于中医学的各个方面，构筑了中医学理论体系的基本框架。以阴阳学说来解释和说明人体的组织结构、生理功能、病理变化，并指导临床诊断和治疗。

（一）说明人体的组织结构

　　人体是一个有机整体。组成人体的所有脏腑经络形体官窍，既是有机联系的，又都可以根据其所在部位、功能特点划分为相互对立的阴阳两部分。从人体部位来说，体表属阳，体内属阴。就其四肢内外侧来说，四肢外侧为阳，四肢内侧为阴。以脏腑来分，五脏属里，藏精气而不泻，故为阴；六腑属表，传化物而不藏，故为阳。由于阴阳之中复有阴阳，所以分属于阴阳的脏腑形体官窍还可以再分阴阳。如五脏分阴阳：心肺居于上属阳，而心属火，主温通，为阳中之阳；肺属金，主肃降，为阳中之阴。肝、脾、肾居下属阴，而肝属木，主升发，为阴中之阳；肾属水，主闭藏，为阴中之阴；脾属土，居中焦，为阴中之至阴。

（二）说明人体的生理功能

　　中医学认为人体正常的生命活动是阴阳两个方面对立制约、互根互用和消长转化，维系着协调平衡的结果。例如物质和功能之间的关系，物质属阴，功能属阳；气为阳，血为阴。生、长、壮、老、已的整个生命过程，是由精血所化之气来推动和调控的。脏腑经络的功能，是由贮藏和运行于其中的精、气、血做为基础的。精、血藏于脏腑之中，主内守而属阴，气由精血所化，运行于全身而属阳。精、血与气

wind-cold fettering the exterior lead to the blocked yang qi of transforming into the interior heat. The aforementioned two cases are both the examples of yin-yang conversion. The extremely severe heat toxin in the former case, and cold fettering the exterior in the latter case are the intrinsic and essential conditions for promoting the conversion between yin and yang.

All of the relations and motion patterns of yin and yang also influence one another. Relation of opposition and interdependence between yin and yang is their most common principles. The aspects of yin and yang of an object can reach balance and harmony through their relations of opposition and restriction, and promote each other and become inseparable through their relation of interdependence. Waxing and waning of yin and yang is the course of quantitative change on the basis of their relation of opposition, restriction and interdependence; while conversion of yin and yang is the qualitative change based on the quantitative change. The dynamic balance of yin and yang is maintained by their relations of opposition, restriction, interdependence, waxing and waning, and conversion; while the automatic harmony between yin and yang exhibits their ability to automatically maintain and recover the dynamic balance and coordination. If such dynamic balance between yin and yang and their ability to automatically harmonize with each other is destroyed, people will get ill and even die.

The Application of Yin-Yang Theory in TCM

The yin-yang theory permeates all aspects of the theoretical system of TCM. It serves to explain the organic structure, physiological functions, and pathological changes of the human body; in addition, it guides the clinical diagnosis and treatment.

Explicating Body Structure

Anatomically, TCM holds that the human body is an integrated whole, in which all the viscera and bowels, meridians and collaterals, and body constituents and orifices of sense organs are interrelated with one another and can be classified into yin and yang from the aspects of their locations and functions. From the aspect of body position, the exterior is yang while the interior is yin. With regard to the four limbs, the outside of the limbs is yang while the inside of them is yin. In terms of the viscera and bowels, the five viscera belong to the interior and yin, in charge of storing the vital essence; while the six bowels belong to the exterior and yang, responsible for transporting and transforming the living substances. As there is yang within yin and yin within yang, all these internal organs and orifices of sense organs belong to yin category or yang category can be further divided into yin and yang. Among the five viscera, the heart and lung locate in the upper part of the body, so they both belong to yang. In addition, the heart is pertaining to fire and takes charge of warming and freeing, so it belongs to yang within yang; the lung is pertaining to gold and governs purification and down-sending, so it belongs to yin within yang. The liver, spleen and kidney all locate in the lower part of the body, so they all belong to yin. But the liver is pertaining to wood and governs up-bearing and effusion, so it belongs to yang within yin; the kidney is pertaining to water and governs closing and storing, so it belongs to yin within yin; and the spleen is pertaining to the earth and locates in the middle energizer, so it belongs to extreme yin within yin.

Explicating Physiological Functions of the Human Body

TCM regards the normal life activities of the human body as the result of mutual opposition and restriction, interdependence, waxing and waning, and conversion, which work together to maintain the harmony and balance of the human body. Take the relationship between the function and substance for example. The function pertains to yang while substance to yin. Qi belongs to yang while blood belongs to yin. The whole life process of birth, growth, strongness, old age, and death is under the control and regulation of qi

的相互资生、相互促进，维持了脏腑经络形体官窍的功能活动稳定有序。若人体内的阴阳二气不能相互为用而分离，人的生命也就终止了。

（三）说明人体的病理变化

"阴平阳秘"是健康的保证，而阴阳失衡就是疾病的根源。常见的阴阳失衡有以下四个方面。

1．阴阳偏盛　指阴或阳的一方偏于亢奋的病理状态。如《素问·阴阳应象大论》指出："阳胜则热，阴胜则寒。"阳胜，是指机体阳气亢盛所致的一类病证。由于阳气的特性为热，故说"阳胜则热"。如温热之邪侵犯人体，可出现高热、烦躁、面赤、脉数等"阳胜则热"的热证。阴胜，是指机体阴气偏盛所致的一类病证。由于阴气的特性是寒，故说"阴胜则寒"。如寒邪直中太阴，可出现面白形寒、脘腹冷痛、泻下清稀、舌质淡苔白、脉沉迟或沉紧等"阴胜则寒"的寒证。

2．阴阳偏衰　指阴或阳的一方偏于虚弱的病理状态。如《素问·调经论》指出："阳虚则寒，阴虚则热。"阳虚，指机体阳气不足所致的一类病证，是由于阳气不足、温煦失司，不能制约阴寒而出现虚寒征象。阴虚，指机体阴津不足所致的一类病证，是由于阴津亏损，濡润不足，不能制约阳热而出现虚热征象。

3．阴阳互损　是指在阴或阳偏衰到一定程度时，会出现阴损及阳、阳损及阴的阴阳互损的病理状态。当阳虚至一定程度时，因阳虚不能生阴，继而出现阴虚的现象，称为"阳损及阴"。同样，当阴虚至一定程度时，因阴虚不能生阳，继而出现阳虚的现象，称为"阴损及阳"。阳损及阴或阴损及阳，最终都导致"阴阳两虚"。这种阴阳两虚并不是阴阳双方处于低水平的平衡状态，同样存在着偏于阳虚或偏于阴虚的不同。如由精虚无以化气而导致气虚的阴损及阳，属以阴虚为主的阴阳两虚；由气虚无力生血而致血虚的阳损及阴，属以阳虚为主的阴阳两虚。

4．阴阳转化　在临床上，不同的病理状态，在一定条件下可以相互转化。如《素问·阴阳应象大论》曰"重阴必阳，重阳必阴"、"寒极生热，热极生寒"，即指这类的病理变化。"重"和"极"就是阴阳转化的必要条件。如外感热毒之邪，出现高热，治疗不及时就会出现四肢厥冷等阴寒之证。

generated from the essence and blood. The functions of viscera and bowels, meridians and collaterals depend on the substances of vital essence, qi and blood storing and transporting in them. The essence and blood store in the viscera and bowels dominating defending internally, so they belong to yin; while qi generates from the essence and blood circulating along the whole body, so it belongs to yang. The essence, blood, and qi, through mutual interdependence and promotion, maintain all the viscera and bowels, meridians and collaterals, body constituents and orifices of sense organs of the human body to work steadily and in order; the life will come to the end if yin and yang in the body become independent and separated from each other.

Explicating Pathogenic Changes of the Body

"Equilibrium of yin and yang" is the guarantee of health, while imbalance between them is the source of diseases. The disharmony of yin and yang primarily covers four aspects as follows:

1. Abnormal exuberance of yin or yang

It refers to any pathological change marked by yin or yang higher than the normal level due to yin pathogens or yang pathogens, as specified in *Plain Questions*, "predominance of yin leads to the disease of yang and predominance of yang results in the disease of yang." Exuberance of yang refers to the syndrome caused by overabundant yang qi. As yang is characterized by heat, so predominance of yang gives rise to heat syndrome. Invasion of warm heat in the human body often leads to heat syndrome with the symptoms of high fever, dysphoria, red complexion, and rapid pulse. Exuberance of yin refers to the syndrome caused by excess of yin qi. As yin qi has cold features, predominance of yin brings on cold syndrome. If cold strikes the spleen directly, it often manifests as the cold syndrome with pale complexion, fear of cold, abdominal cold pain, diarrhea, light tongue with white coating, and slow and sunken pulse or sunken and tight pulse.

2. Abnormal debilitation of yin or yang

It refers to any pathological change marked by yin or yang lower than the normal level due to deficiency of yin or yang of the human body, as described in *Plain Questions*, "yang asthenia (or deficiency) leads to exterior cold and yin asthenia (or deficiency) brings on interior heat." Yang deficiency refers to the syndrome caused by insufficient yang qi in the body. Deficient yang qi cannot exert its warming function and constrain yin cold, so there emerges the sign of deficiency cold. Yin deficiency refers to the syndrome caused by insufficient yin fluid in the body. Impairment of yin fluid cannot well moisten and nourish the body and restrict yang heat, so there emerges the manifestation of deficiency heat.

3. Mutual detriment of yin and yang

It refers to yin deficiency affecting yang or yang deficiency affecting yin when deficiency of yin or yang develops to a certain extent. Detriment of yang affects yin means when yang deficiency develops to a certain degree, and yin deficiency occurs as the result of insufficient yang failing to generate yin. Detriment to yin affects yang means when yin deficiency develops to a certain degree, yang deficiency turns up as the result of insufficient yin failing to generate yang. Both of them will eventually result in a deficiency of both yin and yang, which do not mean that yin and yang are both in the low-level but in a balanced status. In the case of deficiency of both yin and yang, there still exists relative exuberance of deficiency of yin or yang. If detriment to yin affects yang is due to qi deficiency arising from deficient essence failing to be transformed into qi, then it is categorized into the deficiency of both yin and yang with the relative predominance of yin deficiency. If detriment to yang affects yin derives from blood deficiency ascribed to deficient qi failing to generate blood, then it is classified into the deficiency of both yin and yang with the relative predominance of yang deficiency.

4. Mutual transformation between yin and yang

（四）指导疾病诊断

阴阳学说用于疾病的诊断，如《素问·阴阳应象大论》指出："善诊者，察色按脉，先别阴阳"。

通过望、闻、问、切四诊所收集的各种资料，包括即时的症状和体征，以阴阳理论辨析其阴阳属性，表、热、实属于阳；里、虚、寒属于阴。从色泽的明暗辨别阴阳，一般来说，色泽鲜明为病属于阳；色泽晦暗为病属于阴。从气息分辨阴阳，通常来看语声高亢洪亮、多言而躁动者，多属实、属热，为阳；语声低微无力、少言而沉静者，多属虚、属寒，为阴。从动静喜恶判断阴阳，临床出现躁动不安属阳，蜷卧静默属阴；身热恶热属阳，身寒喜暖属阴等。从脉象观察阴阳，以部位分，寸为阳，尺为阴；以动态分，则至者为阳，去者为阴；以至数分，则数者为阳，迟者为阴；以形状分，则浮大洪滑为阳，沉涩细小为阴等等。

（五）指导疾病治疗

疾病的根本是阴阳失衡，治疗的关键就是调节阴阳，补其不足，泻其有余，使之恢复相对平衡。主要内容包括有以下三个方面。

1. 指导养生　养生最根本的原则就是要"法于阴阳"，即遵循自然界阴阳的变化规律来调理人体之阴阳，使人体中的阴阳与四时阴阳的变化相适应，以保持人与自然界的协调统一。

2. 确定治则治法　阴阳失调是疾病的基本病机，而偏盛偏衰和互损又是其基本表现形式，因而恢复阴阳平衡是治疗疾病的基本原则之一。

3. 归纳药物的性能　药物性能由药物的气（性）、味和升降浮沉来决定。按照阴阳来分，温、热性的药物属阳，寒、凉性的药物属阴；药味辛、甘、淡的属阳，酸、苦、咸的属阴；药物在体内趋于升浮作用的属阳，趋于沉降作用的属阴。

Clinically, the different pathological conditions can be transformed into each other under certain conditions, as set forth in *Plain Questions*, "extreme cold leading to heat and extreme heat resulting in cold" and "extreme yin turning into yang and extreme yang changing into yin." Extreme is the prerequisite of mutual conversion between yin and yang. For example, high fever caused by external contraction of heat will present the cold syndrome like reversal cold of the extremities if it is not treated in time.

Guiding Diagnosis of Diseases

Yin-yang theory is applied to diagnose diseases, as defined in *Plain Questions*, "a skilled diagnostician should first differentiate between yin and yang when inspecting the complexion and feeling the pulse."

The doctor collects all the data, including the temporal symptoms and signs of the time, through the four examinations (inspection, listening and smelling, inquiry and palpation), then differentiates and analyzes the nature of the disease, yin or yang in accordance with yin-yang theory. The exterior syndrome, heat syndrome and excess syndrome belong to yang; while the interior syndrome, cold syndrome and deficiency syndrome belong to yin. During the differentiation and analysis of yin or yang from the brightness or darkness of complexion, bright complexion indicates the disease belongs to yang syndrome, while dark complexion reveals the disease belongs to yin syndrome. With respect to breath and voice, usually, the patients in loud voice, talkative and fidgeted have the excess, heat and yang syndrome; while the patients in lower and weak voice, often silent or quiet manifest deficiency, cold and yin syndrome. Judging in light of behaviors, dysphoria belongs to yang while cowering and quietness belongs to yin; fever and aversion to heat belongs to yang, while cold and preference of warm belongs to yin. As for pulse, Cun Pulse belongs to yang and Chi Pulse belongs to yin from pulse position, coming pulse belongs to yang and going pulse belongs to yin from movement tendency of pulse, rapid pulse belongs to yang and slow pulse belongs to yin from speed of pulse. In addition, floating, large, surging, and slippery pulses belong to yang, and sunken, uneven, thin, and small pulses belong to yin from pulse shape.

Guiding Treatment of Diseases

Diseases originate from an imbalance between yin and yang, the treatment should concentrate on regulating yin and yang by supplementing the deficiency and discharging the excess until they meet balance. It includes three aspects as follows:

1. Guiding life nurturing

Following the example of yin and yang is the essential principle for life nurturing. In another word, people must regulate the body's yin and yang following the natural change of yin and yang, so as to make the yin and yang of the body in compliance with that of the seasons and to guarantee the harmony and unity of human and the nature.

2. Determining diagnostic and therapeutic principles

Imbalance between yin and yang is the basic pathogenesis of any disease, which manifests as deficiency or excess of yin or yang, or mutual impairment of yin and yang. So recuperating the balance between yin and yang is one of the basic principles in treating diseases.

3. Generalizing properties and functions of drugs

The properties and functions of medicinals are determined by their qi(nature), flavors, and their ascending, descending, floating and sinking tendencies. Medicinals with the nature of warmth and hot belong to yang, while medicinals with the nature of coolness and cold belong to yin. Medicinals with the flavors of pungency, sweetness, or lightness belong to yang, while medicinals with the flavors of sourness, bitterness, or saltiness belong to yin. Medicinals tending to produce ascending and floating actions in the body belong

第二节 五 行 学 说

五行学说认为，宇宙间的一切事物都是由木、火、土、金、水五种基本物质所构成的。自然界各种事物的发展变化，都是这五种物质不断运动和相互作用的结果。宇宙间的一切事物都可用五行的特性进行演绎、推论和归类。五行之间的生克乘侮关系是各种事物普遍联系的基本法则。五行学说运用到中医学领域后，作为一种思维方法贯穿于中医学理论体系的各个方面，用以说明人体的生理功能及病理变化，并指导疾病的诊断和治疗，成为中医学理论体系的重要组成部分。

一、五行的特性

古人在长期的生活实践中，通过长期观察，对木、火、土、金、水五种物质的特性进行了归纳，并作出演绎分析，以这五种物质的抽象特性来推演各种事物的五行属性。现结合《尚书·洪范》的记载，将五行特性分述如下：

木的特性："木曰曲直"。所谓"曲直"，是以树干曲曲直直地向上、向外伸长舒展的生发姿态来形容其具有生长、升发、条达、舒畅等特性的事物及现象。凡具有这类特性的事物或现象，都可归属于"木"。

火的特性："火曰炎上"。所谓"炎上"，是指火具有温热、升腾、向上的特征。因此，凡具有温热、升腾等特性的事物或现象，均可归属于"火"。

土的特性："土爱稼穑"。"稼"指播种，"穑"指收获。所谓"稼穑"，指土地可供人们播种和收获食物。延伸而言，凡具有生化、承载、受纳特性的事物或现象，均可归属于"土"。由于农耕生产方式影响，古人对"土"特别重视，故有"土载四行"、"万物土中生，万物土中灭"以及"土为万物之母"等说法。

金的特性："金曰从革"。"从革"本意颇为费解，今人认为有"变革"之意。引申为肃杀、潜降、收敛等。凡具有这类特性的事物或现象，皆可归属于"金"。

水的特性："水曰润下"。所谓"润下"，是指水具有滋润和向下的特性。凡具有寒凉、滋润、向下、静藏等特性和作用的事物或现象，均可归属于"水"。

二、事物属性的五行归类

五行学说对事物属性的归类推演，是以天人相应为指导思想，以五行为中心，以空间结构的五方、时间结构的五季、人体结构的五脏为基本框架，将自然界的各种事物和现象以及人体的生理病理现象，采用"取象比类"和"推演络绎"的方法，按其属性进行归纳。凡具有生发、条达、调畅等性质和作用者，统属于木；具有温

to yang, while those tending to produce descending and sinking actions belong to yin.

Section 2   Five Phase Theory

Five phase theory regards that all things in the universe are made up of five basic phases, namely wood, fire, earth, metal, and water, and that the development and change of all things are the result of the constant movement and interaction of these five phases. All things in the universe can be deduced and summarized with the characteristics of the five phases. Engendering, restraining, overwhelming, and rebellion of the five phases are the basic rule through which all things relate to one another. After introduced to TCM, the five phase theory has been carried into and as a way of thinking through all aspects of the theoretical system of TCM, to specify the physiological function and the pathological changes of human body, guide the diagnosis and treatment of diseases, therefore, being the integral part of the theoretical system of TCM.

Characteristics of the Five Phases

Chinese ancestors made a long-term observation on the five substances—wood, fire, earth, metal, and water in the long course of their living and working, and then analyzed and deduced their characteristics. According to it, everything in nature is attributed to one of the five phases on the bases of its abstract features. Here are the detailed properties of the five phases in accordance with the record in *Shangshu*.

Characteristic of wood: "Wood is characterized by growing freely and peripherally." This refers to the outward and upward extension and stretching of the trunks, which is used to describe the objects or phenomena characterized by growing, ascending, developing and soothing freely. So anything or phenomenon with such characteristics is attributed to the category of wood.

Characteristics of fire: "Fire is characterized by flaming up." Flaming up means that fire has the characteristics of warming, rising and ascending. Thereby, anything or phenomenon with the functions of warming and rising is attributed to the category of fire.

Characteristics of earth: "Earth is characterized by cultivation and reaping." So anything or phenomenon with the functions of generating, transforming, supporting and receiving is attributed to the category of earth. In addition, influenced by the farming production mode, Chinese ancestors attached special importance to earth. Thereby, there emerged prevailing sayings of "earth carrying the other four phases," "all things in the world originate from and finally return to the earth," and "earth is the mother of all things."

Characteristics of metal: "Metal is characterized by change." Nowadays, it is regarded that metal has the revolutionary functions of descending, purifying and astringent. Hence everything or phenomenon has those features is attributed to the category of metal.

Characteristics of water: "Water is characterized by moistening and downward flowing." Therefore anything or phenomenon of the functions of cooling, moistening, and moving downward is attributed to the category of water.

Categorization According to the Five Phases

Under the guiding ideology of correspondence between the nature and human, taking the five phases as the core, and the five directions (the east, south, west, north, and the central) in space structure, the five seasons (spring, summer, autumn, winter, and late summer) in time structure, and the five viscera (the heart, liver, spleen, lung and kidney) in human body as the basic framework, the five phase theory general-

热、炎上等性质和作用者，统属于火；具有承载、生化等性质和作用者，统属于土；具有收敛、肃降等性质和作用者，统属于金；具有寒凉、滋润、向下等性质和作用者，统属于水。五行学说将人体的生命活动与自然界的事物和现象联系起来，形成了人体内外互相关联的五行结构系统，用以说明人体的生理病理现象及人与自然环境的统一性。如日出东方，东方属木，人体的肝喜条达与木的升发、条达特性相似，故将东方、肝归属于木，这就是取类比象法。根据已知的某些事物的五行归属，推演归纳其他相关的事物的方法是推演络绎法。如已知肝属木，由于肝合胆，主筋膜，其华在爪，开窍于目，因此可推演络绎出胆、筋、爪、目归属于木。如表 2-1 所示。

表 2-1 自然界与人体的五行分类简表

自然界						五行	人体				
五味	五色	五化	五气	五方	五季		五脏	五腑	五官	五体	五志
酸	青	生	风	东	春	木	肝	胆	目	筋	怒
苦	赤	长	暑	南	夏	火	心	小肠	舌	脉	喜
甘	黄	化	湿	中	长夏	土	脾	胃	口	肉	思
辛	白	收	燥	西	秋	金	肺	大肠	鼻	皮	悲
咸	黑	藏	寒	北	冬	水	肾	膀胱	耳	骨	恐

三、五行学说的生克乘侮

五行学说认为五行之间不是孤立的、静止的，而是密切联系和运动变化着的。以五行间的相生、相克等关系来探索和阐释事物间的相互联系和相互协调，同时还以五行相乘和相侮来探索和阐释事物间的协调平衡被破坏后的相互影响。

（一）相生相克

五行"相生"，是指五行中某一行事物对于另一行事物具有促进、助长和资生作用。五行相生的规律和次序是：木生火、火生土、土生金、金生水、水生木。所谓"相克"，是指五行中某一行事物对于另一行事物具有抑制、约束、削弱等作用。五行相克的规律和次序是：木克土、土克水、水克火、火克金、金克木。这种联系体现为"生中有克"和"克中有生"。只有这样，自然界才能维持协调有序，人才能维护其生理状态。正如张介宾说："造化之机，不可无生，亦不可无制。无生则发育无出，无制则亢而为害。"

根据生克次序，对五行中的任何一行来说，都存在着"生我"、"我生"和"克我"、"我克"四个方面的联系。就木而言：木之"生我"者为水，"我生"者为火，"克我"者为金，"我克"者为土。而"生我"和"我生"在《难经》中被喻为

izes all things and phenomena in the world and the physiological and pathological conditions of human body in accordance with their properties using the methods of analogism and deduction. All those have the characteristics or functions of growing, ascending, developing, and soothing are classified into wood. All those have the characteristics or functions of warming and ascending are sorted as fire. All those have the characteristics or functions of bearing, generating, and transforming are categorized as earth. All those have the characteristics or functions of astringency, purification, and down-sending are classified into metal. And all those have the characteristics or functions of cooling, moistening, and downwards are classified into water. In this way, it connects the life activities with the objects and phenomena in the nature, and forms an interrelated body system based on the five phases, so as to explicate the physiological and pathological phenomena of human body as well as the unitarity between human beings and the natural environment. For instance, the sun rises in the east and the east belongs to wood, which is characterized by growing, rising, and soothing. In human body, the liver likes smoothing, so the east and the liver are both classified into wood. This is the analogism. Deduction refers to deduce and generalizing the five-phase properties of other objects on the basis of the known object. For example, as known, the liver belongs to wood, so it can be deduced and concluded that the gallbladder, tendons, fingers and eyes which are all attributed to wood as the liver is connected with the gallbladder, controls the sinews, opens at the eyes and nourishes the nails (Table 2-1).

Table 2-1   Classifications of the Nature and Human Body on the Basis of Characteristics of Five Phases

Natural world						Five phases	Human body				
Five flavors	Five colors	Five transfo-rmations	Five climates	Five directions	Five seasons		Five viscera	Five bowels	Five sense organs	Five body constituents	Five emotions
Sourness	Green	Generation	Wind	The east	Spring	Wood	Liver	Gallbladder	Eyes	Sinew	Anger
Bitterness	Red	Growth	Sum-merheat	The south	Summer	Fire	Heart	Small intestine	Tongue	Vein	Joy
Sweetness	Yellow	Transfor-mation	Damp	The central	Late summer	Earth	Spleen	Stomach	Mouth	Muscle/flesh	Thought
Pungency	White	Harvest	Dryness	The west	Autumn	Metal	Lung	Large intestine	Nose	Skin	Sorrow
Saltiness	Black	Storage	Cold	The north	Winter	Water	Kidney	Bladder	Ears	Bone	Fear

Engendering, Restraining, Overwhelming, and Rebellion of the Five Phase Theory

The five phase theory regards that the five phases are neither isolated nor static, but closely correlated and dynamic. It explores and illuminates the inter-association and inter-coordination of all things through inter-engendering and inter-restraining of the five phases, as well as the interplay due to the damage of such harmony and balance through overwhelming and rebellion of the five phases.

Engendering and Restraining

Engendering of the five phases refers to the promotion, facilitation, and generation of one phase to its sequential phase. Its discipline and sequence are as follows: wood engenders fire, fire engenders earth, earth engenders metal, metal engenders water, and water engenders wood. Restraining of the five phases refers to the restriction, control, and impairment of one phase to another phase. It follows a circular order: wood restrains earth, earth restrains water, water restrains fire, fire restrains metal, and metal restrains

"母"和"子"。"生我"者为"母"，"我生"者为"子"。"克我"和"我克"又称作"所不胜"和"所胜"。"克我"者即"所不胜"，"我克"者即"所胜"。可见五行中任何一行都受着其他四行的不同影响，任何一行又可以不同方式影响其他四行。

（二）相乘相侮

五行相乘，实为五行之间过度的"相克"。相乘的次序与相克相同，即木乘土、土乘水、水乘火、火乘金、金乘木。导致五行相克异常而出现相乘的原因一般有三：①所不胜行过于亢盛，因而对其所胜行的制约太过，使其虚弱。如木过亢，则过度克制其所胜土，导致土虚弱不足，称为"木亢乘土"。临床上所见的剧烈的情志变化引起的脾胃功能失调，一般属此种情况。②所胜行过于虚弱，其所不胜行则相对偏亢，故所胜行也受到其所不胜行的制约而出现相乘。如木虽然没有过亢，但土已经过于虚弱不足，木对土来说属相对偏亢，故土也受到木的较强的克制而出现相乘，称为"土虚木乘"。临床上所见的慢性胃病因情绪变化的发作，多属此种情况。③既有所不胜行的过于亢盛，又有其所胜行的虚弱不足，则出现较重的相乘。如既有木的过亢，又有土的虚弱不足，则两者之间则出现更为严重的相乘，一般称为"木乘土"。临床上所见的肝气郁结或上逆，而脾胃功能早已虚弱不足，则易发生较重的"肝气乘脾"病理变化，病人的病情也较重。

五行相侮，是指其中的一行对其"所不胜行"的反向制约，又称"反克"。故相侮的次序与相克、相乘相反。依次顺序为木侮金，金侮火，火侮水，水侮土，土侮木。引起五行相克异常而产生相侮的原因，一般也有三：①所胜行过于亢盛，不仅不受其所不胜行的制约，反而反向克制其所不胜行，因而出现相侮。如木过于亢盛，不但不受其所不胜金的制约，反而反过来欺侮金，一般称为"木火刑金"。就是临床上常见的肝火犯肺证，即属此种情况。②所不胜行虚弱不足，而其所胜行则相对偏亢，故所不胜行必然受到其所胜行的反向克制而出现相侮。如金虚弱不足，而木相对偏亢，金不但不能制约木，反而被木反向克制，一般称为"金虚木侮"。临床所见的慢性肺病（如肺痨）常因情绪剧烈变化而加重或发作，即属此种情况。③既有所胜行的过于亢盛，又有其所不胜行的虚弱不足，易出现较为严重的相侮。如既有金的虚弱不足，又有木的过于亢盛，相侮则较为严重，一般称为"木侮金"。临床所见的既有慢性肺病长期不愈，肺气已虚，又有较为强烈的情绪刺激，肝气正亢，因而发作为较为深重的病证，一般属于此种情况。

相乘与相侮，都属于不正常的相克现象，既有联系，又有区别。两者的区别在于，相乘是按五行相克次序的克制太过，相侮则是与相克次序相反方向的克制异常。两者的联系在于，发生相乘时，有时也可同时出现相侮；发生相侮时，有时也可同

wood. Engendering and restraining of the five phases embody each phase is promoted while restricted at the same time. Only in this way can the universe maintains the harmonious and orderly development, and can man preserve its physiological status, as stated by Zhang Jiebin: "Nothing can live without the function of promotion or restriction. As without generation, there would be no growth and development; without inter-restriction, there will inevitably be hyperactivity that consequently bringing about harm."

According to the order of engendering and restraining, each of the five phases is marked by such relations as "being engendered" and "engendering" as well as "being restrained" and "restraining." Take wood as an example, it is engendered by water and engenders fire, is restrained by metal and restrains earth. In *Classic of Difficult Issues*, it terms the phase of "engendering" and "engendered" as "mother" and "child" respectively. Each phase is the "child" of the phase that engenders it and the "mother" of the one it engenders. Meanwhile, it defines the phase of "restraining" and "restrained" as "winner" and "loser" respectively. It reveals that any phase of the five is influenced by the other four and meanwhile affects the other four in different ways.

Overwhelming and Rebellion

Overwhelming among the five phases is actually the excessive restraining among the five phases. It has the same sequence as restraining, namely wood overwhelms earth, earth overwhelms water, water overwhelms fire, fire overwhelms metal, and metal overwhelms wood. Generally, there are three situations leading to overwhelming as the result of abnormal restraining among the five phases:

1. The restraining phase is too excessive and exerts too much restriction on the restrained one to weaken the latter. For example, if wood overacts, it will overwhelm earth, the restrained one, and lead to weakness and deficiency of earth, which is called as "wood overwhelming earth due to its excess." The dysfunction of the spleen and stomach due to the acute emotional changes generally can be attributed to this reason.

2. The restrained phase is too weak that the restraining phase relatively too active, then the restrained one will be restricted by the restraining one, therefore leading to overwhelming. For instance, even when wood is normal, it can still overwhelm the earth if the latter is too weak and deficient, which is termed as "earth being overwhelmed by wood due to its weakness and deficiency." Clinically, relapse of chronic gastropathy as the result of emotional changes can mostly be owed to this reason.

3. The serious over-restraining will occur when the restraining phase is too excessive and the restrained phase is too weak. For example, if wood is excessive and earth is too weak, the severe over-restraining between them will turn up, which is defined as "wood over-restraining earth." Clinically, the stagnation or reverse flow of the liver qi, together with the weak and deficient spleen and stomach is apt to give rise to serious pathological change of "the liver qi over-restraining the spleen."

Rebellion among the five phases refers to the restraining opposite to that of the normal restraining sequence of the five phases, also known as "reverse restraining," namely wood rebels mental, metal rebels fire, fire rebels water, water rebels earth, and earth rebels wood. Generally, there are also three situations brining about rebellion caused by the abnormal restraining among the five phases:

1. The restrained phase is excessive and reverses to restrict the restraining one rather than being restricted, therefore, resulting in rebellion. For example, if wood is excessive, it will reserve to restrain metal rather than being restrained by the latter, which is generally termed as "wood-fire impairing metal." Clinically, the liver-fire attacking the lung is among the situation.

2. When the restraining phase is too weak and deficient and the restrained phase is relatively over-abundant, the restraining phase will inevitably reverse to be restricted by the restrained one, therefore

时伴有相乘。两者皆用于阐释疾病的病理变化（图 2-2）。

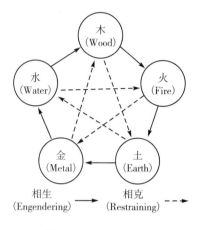

图 2-2　五行生克图

（Figure 2-2　Engendering and Restraining of the Five Phases）

四、五行学说在中医学中的应用

五行学说在中医学的应用，主要是以五行的特性来分析归纳人体脏腑、经络、形体、官窍等组织器官和精神情志等各种功能活动，构建以五脏为中心的生理病理系统，进而与自然环境相联系，建立天人一体的五脏系统，并以五行的生克制化规律来分析五脏之间的生理联系，以五行的生克乘侮等关系来阐释五脏病变的相互影响，指导疾病的诊断和防治。

（一）阐述人与自然的关系

五行学说渗透到中医学中，以五脏为中心，推演络绎整个人体的各种组织结构与功能，将人体的形体、官窍、精神、情志等分归于五脏，并将自然界的五方、五气、五色、五味等与人体的五脏联系起来，建立了以五脏为中心的天人一体的五脏系统，将人体内外环境联结成一个密切联系的整体。五脏的功能不是孤立的，而是互相联系的。中医学借助五行以探索五脏生理功能之间的内在联系，即相互资生和制约关系。如以肝为例，《素问·阴阳应象大论》云："东方生风，风生木，木生酸，酸生肝，肝生筋……肝主目"。《素问·金匮真言论》指出，"东方青色，入通于肝，开窍于目，藏精于肝，其病惊骇，其味酸，其类草木……是以知病之在筋也"，这样把自然界的东方、春季、青色、风气、酸味等，通过五行的木与人体的肝、筋、目联系起来，构筑了联系人体内外的肝木系统，体现了天人相应的整体观念。

（二）说明五脏的生理功能

五行学说将脏腑分别归属于五行，并以五行来说明各脏的生理特性。如木有生

leading to rebellion. For instance, if metal is too weak and deficient and wood is relatively excessive, metal will fail to restrain wood and reverse to be restricted by wood, which is generally known as "metal being rebelled by wood due to its deficiency." Clinically, relapse or aggravation of chronic lung disease(like tuberculosis) due to acute emotional changes can be ascribed to such reason.

3. Serious rebellion will occur when the restrained phase is hyperactive and the restraining element is too weak and deficient. For instance, weakness and deficiency of metal together with an overabundance of wood will produce serious rebellion, which is termed as "wood rebelling metal." Clinically, the severe diseases caused by lung qi deficiency arising from the chronic lung disease and excessive liver qi resulting from intense emotional irritations can be put down to this cause.

Overwhelming and rebellion are both abnormal restraining situations, which are connected with and different from each other. The difference between them is that overwhelming refers to excessive restraining in line with the abnormal restraining sequence, while rebellion refers to the reverse sequence. The connection between them is that overwhelming will lead to counter restraining, while the latter is often accompanied by the former. Both overwhelming and rebellion can be applied to illustrate the pathological changes of diseases.

Application of the Five Phase Theory in TCM

The five phase theory is primarily applied in TCM to analyze and conclude the functional activities of viscera and bowels, meridians and collaterals, body constituents and orifices of sense organ, as well as the mental activities and emotions, according to the features of the five phases. It helps to build the physiological and pathological mechanism focusing on the five viscera and, on this basis, further associates the human beings with the natural environment to build the five viscera system integrating human beings with the nature. In this way, it analyzes the physiological connections among the five viscera in the principles of inter-engendering, inter-restraining and inter-conversion of the five phases, and expounds the interrelation of the pathological changes of the five viscera according to their relations of inter-engendering, inter-restraining, overwhelming, and rebellion.

Elaborate the Relation between Man and the Nature

Totally involved in the whole system of the TCM, the five phase theory radiates from its center, the five viscera to deduce the constituents and functions of human body, and classifies body constituents, orifices of sense organ, mental activities and emotions into each of them, connects them with the five directions, five climates, five colors, and five flavors, respectively, therefore building the great five viscera system integrating man with the nature and the inner part of the body with the external environment. The functions of the five viscera are not isolated, but closely related. By virtue of the five phases, the TCM has been exploring the intrinsic relations of the physiological functions of the five viscera, namely the relation of inter-promotion and inter-restriction. Take the liver as an example. As described in *Plain Questions*, "the east direction corresponds to the wind, the wind promotes the growth of the wood, the wood matches the sour flavor, the sour flavor nourishes the liver, and the liver promotes the health of sinews······the liver governs the eyes;" "the east in the direction corresponds to the green in the color, the liver in the five viscera, the eyes in the orifices, the sour in the flavour, and grass and wood, with its essence stored in the liver; When there is something wrong with the liver qi, it will cause fright······it can judge there is something wrong with the sinews." The liver is associated with the east in the direction, spring in the season, green in the color, wind in the climate, sour in the flavor, and sinews and eyes in human body constituents, so as to form a liver wood system linking the interior of human body with the exterior environment according to its

长、升发、舒畅、条达的特性，肝属木，故肝喜条达而恶抑郁，有疏通气血、调畅情志的功能；火有温热、向上的特性，心主血脉，"禀阳气"为五脏之主，故心属火。土性敦厚，有生化万物的特性，脾主运化水谷、化生精微以营养脏腑形体，为气血生化之源，故脾属土。金性清肃、收敛，肺具有清肃之性，以清肃下降为顺，故肺属金。水具有滋润、下行、闭藏的特性，肾有藏精、主水功能，故肾属水。

（三）阐释五脏的相互关系

五行学说运用五行生克制化理论来说明脏腑生理功能的内在联系，即五脏之间存在着既相互资生又相互制约的关系。

1. 以五行相生说明五脏之间的资生关系　肝生心即木生火，如肝藏血以济心，肝之疏泄以助心行血；心生脾即火生土，如心阳温煦脾土，助脾运化；脾生肺即土生金，如脾气运化，化气以充肺；肺生肾即金生水，如肺之精津下行以滋肾精，肺气肃降以助肾纳气；肾生肝即水生木，如肾藏精以滋养肝血，肾阴资助肝阴以防肝阳上亢。

2. 以五行相克说明五脏之间的制约关系　肾制约心即水克火，如肾水上济于心，可以防止心火之亢烈；心制约肺即火克金，如心火之阳热，可以抑制肺气清肃太过；肺制约肝即金克木，如肺气清肃，可以抑制肝阳的上亢；肝制约脾即木克土，如肝气条达，可疏泄脾气之壅滞；脾制约肾即土克水，如脾气之运化水液，可防肾水泛滥。

3. 以五行制化说明五脏之间的协调平衡　依据五行学说，五脏中的每一脏都具有生我、我生和克我、我克的生理联系。五脏之间的生克制化，说明每一脏在功能上因有他脏的资助而不至于虚损，又因有他脏的制约和克制，而不至于过亢；本脏之气太盛，则有他脏之气制约；本脏之气虚损，则又可由他脏之气补之。如脾（土）之气，其虚则有心（火）生之，其亢则有肝（木）克之；肺（金）气不足，脾（土）可生之；肾（水）气过亢，脾（土）可克之。这种制化关系把五脏紧紧联系成一个整体，从而保证了人体内环境的统一。

（四）解释五脏的病理传变

五行学说可用于解释某些病理状况，特别是用以说明病理情况下脏腑间的某些相互影响。这种相互影响，被称之为"传变"。可分为相生关系的传变和相克关系的传变两类（图2-3）。

1. 相生关系的传变　是指病变顺着或逆着五行相生次序的传变。它可归纳成"母病及子"和"子病及母"两种类型：

（1）母病及子：是指病变由母脏累及到子脏。例如：肾属水，肝属木，水能生木，故肾为母脏、肝为子脏；肾病及肝，就是母病及子。临床常见的肝肾阴虚、肝

relation with the wood in the five phases. It is the reflection of the holistic concept of correspondence between the nature and human.

Explicate the Physiological Functions of the Five Viscera

The five phase theory categorizes the five viscera into five phases respectively and explicates the physiological features of each viscus, based on the characteristics of the five phases. For example, the wood is characterized by growing, ascending, developing, and soothing; and the liver likes dispersing and hates being depressed, so the liver corresponds to the wood, which can regulate qi and blood circulation and soothe the mental states. The fire is characterized by warming and upward rising; and the heart governs blood circulation and receives yang qi, so the heart, the lord of the viscera, corresponds to the fire. The earth can grow all the plants and feeds all the animals; and the spleen takes charge of transporting and transforming water and food, and turns them into the essence to nourish the viscera and bowels, so the spleen corresponds to the earth. The metal has the feature of descending, purifying, and astringent; and the lung is responsible for purification and down-sending, so the lung corresponds to the metal. Water is characterized by moistening, downbearing, and storing; and the kidney governs storing essence and water metabolism, so the kidney corresponds to the water.

Expound the Interrelation of the Five Viscera

The five phase theory expounds the intrinsic relation of the physiological functions of the viscera by its rule of inter-engendering, inter-restriction and inter-conversion.

1. Explain the inter-promoting relations of the five viscera by the five phase theory of inter-engendering. The liver engenders the heart or the wood engenders the fire: the liver stores blood and provides it to the heart, and meanwhile the liver's function of free coursing can help the heart to circulate blood. The heart engenders the spleen, or the fire engenders the earth: the heart yang warms the spleen to facilitate its function of transportation and transformation. The spleen engenders the lung or the earth engenders the metal: the spleen transports and transforms the water and food and turns them into essence to nourish the lung. The lung engenders the kidney or the metal engenders the water: the lung's essence and fluid descends to enrich the kidney essence, and the depurative downbearing of lung qi helps the kidney to absorb qi. The kidney generates the liver, or the water generates the wood: the kidney stores the essence to nourish the liver blood, and the kidney yin supplements the liver yin to prevent ascendant hyperactivity of liver yang.

2. Explain the restriction relations of the five viscera by the five phase theory of inter-restraining. The kidney restrains the heart, or the water restrains the fire: the kidney water circulates upward to moisten the heart and prevent the hyperactivity of the heart fire. The heart restrains the lung, or the fire restrains the metal: the warm heart fire can restrict the lung from being over-descending. The lung restrains the liver, or the metal restrains the water: the lung qi down-sends to restrain ascendant hyperactivity of liver yang. The liver restrains the spleen, or the wood restrains the earth: the liver qi stretches to sooth the stagnation of the spleen qi. The spleen restrains the kidney, or the earth restrains the water: the spleen qi transports and transforms the water to restrain the kidney water from flooding.

3. Explain the coordination and harmony of the five viscera by the five viscera theory of inhibition and generation. According to the theory, each viscus can engender and restrain the other viscera and can be engendered and restrained by other viscera. The generation, restriction, inhibition, and transformation among the five viscera make sure that each viscus can function soundly by being nourished by its engendering viscus from being deficient and being restricted by its restraining viscus from being excessive. Each viscus' qi will be restricted by that of its restraining viscus when it is excessive and supplement by that of

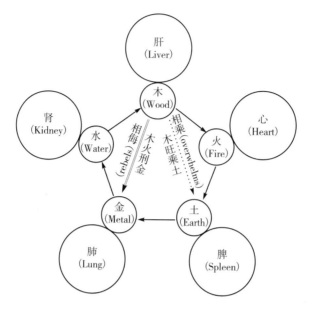

图 2-3 脏腑五行图

（Figure 2-3 Chart of Five Phases Applied in Viscera and Bowels）

阳上亢证，就是由于肾阴不足，不能滋养肝木而导致的"水不涵木"，就是母病及子的结果。

（2）子病及母：又称"子盗母气"，即病变由于脏影响到母脏。例如：肝属木，心属火，木能生火，故肝为母脏、心为子脏；心病及肝，就是子病累母。临床常见的心肝血虚证，就是因心血不足累及肝血亏虚的"子病及母"之虚证；因心火亢盛引动肝火而形成心肝火旺证属"子病及母"之实证。另外还有子脏盛导致母脏虚的虚实夹杂病变，如肝火亢盛，下劫肾阴，以致肾阴亏虚的病变即是。

2. 相克关系的传变 是指病变顺着或逆着五行相克次序的传变，包括"相乘"与"相侮"两种类型。

（1）相乘：指相克太过为病。其原因不外乎一行过强，一行过弱。五行太过相乘，如以木克土为例：正常情况下，木能克土，土为木之所胜。若木气过于亢盛，对土克制太过，可致土的不足。这种由于木的亢盛而引起的相乘，称为"木旺乘土"。五行不及相乘，仍以木克土为例，正常情况下，木能制约土；若土气不足，木虽然处于正常水平，土仍难以承受木的克制，因而造成木乘虚侵袭，使土更加虚弱。这种由于土的不足而引起的相乘，称为"土虚木乘"。

（2）相侮：指反克为病。指逆着原先相克次序的病理传变，其原因亦不外乎一行太盛，一行太虚。以肺肝关系为例，正常情况下，肺可制约肝，但在某些病理情况下，如肺虚或肝旺，反倒出现了肝来侮肺，表现为"木亢侮金"就是肝火犯肺的

its engendering viscus when it is deficient.For example,when the spleen(earth)qi is deficient,it will be supplemented by the heart(fire)qi through its engendering function(the heart fire engenders the spleen earth),when the spleen qi is excessive,it will be restrained by the liver(wood)qi through its restraining function(the liver wood restrains the spleen earth);when the lung(metal)qi is deficient,the spleen (earth)qi will tonify it;when the kidney(water)qi is excessive,the spleen(earth)qi will restrict it.Under the engendering and restraining relation,the five viscera are closely connected to be a whole and guarantee the integrity of the interior of our body.

Clarify the Pathological Transmutation of the Five Viscera

The five phase theory can be applied to explain the pathological status,especially the interaction the disease causes on the viscera and bowels.This interaction is called as transmission and transmutation, which includes the transmutation resulting from inter-engendering,and the one arising from inter-restraining(Figure 2-3).

1. Transmutation resulting from inter-engerdering refers to the disease being transmitted from the ill viscera or bowels to the other viscera or bowels in or against the sequence of engendering of the five phases,which can be classified into"the disease of the mother-organ involving the child-organ"and"disease of the child-organ affecting the mother-organ."

(1)"The disease of the mother-organ involving the child-organ"refers to the pathology of the engendering viscus involving its being engendered viscus.The kidney disease affecting the liver is one of the examples.Kidney pertains to water,liver pertain to wood,and water can engender wood,so the kidney(the mother viscus)will affect the liver(its son viscus)when it is ill.Liver-kidney yin deficiency syndrome and syndrome of ascendant hyperactivity of liver yang are such the cases,caused by deficient kidney yin failing to nourish the liver wood.

(2)"The disease of the child-organ affecting the mother-organ"is also known as"the child viscus stealing its mother viscus' qi."It refers to the pathology of the child viscus affecting its mother viscus.The heart disease affecting the liver is one of the examples.Liver pertains to wood,heart pertains to fire,and wood can engender fire,so the heart(the child viscus)will affect the liver(its mother viscus)when it is ill. Syndrome of heart-liver blood deficiency is such the case,a deficiency syndrome caused by deficient heart blood resulting in the liver blood deficiency.Syndrome of excessive heart-liver fire is another case,but an excess syndrome is caused by hyperactive heart fire arousing the liver fire.In addition,some of the deficiency-excess complexes,which are caused by the child viscus excess leading to the mother viscus deficiency,belong to this kind of case,such as hyperactive liver fire robbing the kidney yin and leading to kidney yin deficiency.

2. Transmutation of diseases resulting from inter-restraining refers to the disease being transmitted from the ill organ to the other one or against the sequence of restraining of the five phases,which are composed of"overwhelming"and"rebellion."

(1)Overwhelming refers to the pathological status caused by excessive restraining.Such situation occurs when one phase is too excessive or the other is too deficient.Take wood restraining earth as an example,normally the wood restrains the earth properly.However,when the wood is superabundant,it will overwhelm the earth and lead to the earth deficiency.In this case,it is called as"wood overwhelms earth due to its excess."Still take wood restrains earth as an example to analyze overwhelming due to deficiency.When the earth is deficient,it still cannot bear the restriction from wood even though the wood just works normally.In this case,it will lead to wood invading the deficient earth and making it more deficient,which is known as"wood overwhelms earth due to earth deficiency."

病理传变。又如正常情况下，金克木，木克土，但当木过度虚弱时，则不仅金来乘木，而且土也会因木的衰弱而"反克"之。这种现象，称为"木虚土侮"。

（五）指导临床治疗

五行学说用于指导治疗，具体可体现在以下几方面：

1. 指导控制疾病的传变　一脏之病常可波及他脏而使疾病发生传变。因此，治疗时，除需对已病之脏进行治疗外，还应在五行生克理论指导下，调整各脏之间的相互关系，防止疾病进一步传变。如肝脏有病，肝气太过，木旺每易乘土，此时常应先健脾防其传变；脾胃不弱则不易传变，肝病也就容易痊愈。"见肝之病，则知肝当传之于脾，故先实其脾气"，就是指提早治疗未病之脏防止传变。

2. 指导确定治则与治法　根据相生规律确定治疗原则，包括"虚则补其母"和"实则泻其子"。补母，是指一脏之虚证，不仅须补益本脏以使之恢复，同时还要依据五行相生的次序，补益其"母脏"，通过"相生"作用而促其恢复。如肝血不足，除须用补肝血的药物（如白芍等）外，还可以用补肾益精（如何首乌等）的方法，通过"水生木"的作用促使肝血的恢复。泻子，是指一脏之实证，不仅须泻除本脏亢盛之气，同时还可依据五行相生的次序，泻其"子脏"，通过"气舍于其所生"的机制，以泻除其"母脏"的亢盛之气。如肝火炽盛，除须用清泻肝火的药物（如龙胆草、黄芩等）外，还可用清泻心火（如黄连、莲子心等）的方法，通过"心受气于肝"、"肝气舍于心"的机制，以消除亢盛的肝火（图2-4）。

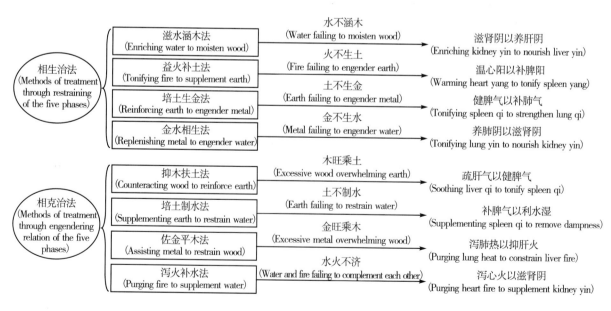

图 2-4　五行在治疗中的应用

（Figure 2-4　Schematic Diagram of Five Phases Applied in Treatment）

（梁晓春）

(2)Rebellion refers to the diseases caused by reversed restraining, or the transmutation against the normal sequence of the restraining.Such situation occurs when one phase is too excessive or the other is too deficient.Take the relation between the liver and the lung as an example, normally the lung restrains the liver; however, when such pathological changes occur like lung deficiency or liver excess, the liver will rebel to restrain the lung, therefore, leading to liver fire invading lung, also known as "wood rebels metal due to wood excess. "Still, normally metal restrains wood and wood restrains earth. But when the wood is too deficient, not only metal will overwhelm wood but also earth will rebel it, which is named as "earth rebels wood due to wood deficiency".

Guiding Clinical Treatment

The application of five phase theory to guide clinical treatment is embodied from the following aspects:

1. Control transmission and transmutation of the diseases

The disease of one viscus may be transmuted by affecting the other viscera, so it is necessary to regulate all the viscera under the guidance of five phase theory on engendering and restraining while focusing on treating the affected viscus.Only in this way can the disease prevent from being transmitted.According to the principle of excessive wood overwhelming earth, when the liver disease is detected, spleen should be reinforced to prevent it from being affected by the liver disease due to excessive liver qi.The sound and strong functions of the spleen and stomach can ward off such transmutation and help to recover the function of the liver. "When detecting the liver disease, a qualified physician ought to strengthen the spleen qi as the liver disease will affect the spleen, "which is an example of reinforcing the still sound organ in advance to fend off the transmutation.

2. Identify the therapeutic principles and therapeutic methods

The therapeutic principles made according to the rule of engendering are known as "to reinforce the mother-organ in case of deficiency" and "to purge(or reduce)the child-organ in case of excess. "Reinforcing the mother-oragan refers to treating and recovering the deficient organ by tonifying its mother-organ in the engendering sequence of the five phases while treating the affected organ.For example, liver blood deficiency can be cured either by replenishing the liver blood with the liver-blood-generating drugs like *radix paeoniae alba* or by tonfiying the kidney essence with the drug like *polygonum multiflorum*, based on the principle of "promoting the wood by reinforcing the water. "Purging the child-organ refers to treating and recovering the affected organ by purging the excessive qi of its child-organ in the engendering sequence of the five phases while purging the excessive qi of the affected organ, which is based on the mechanism of "the organ qi is able to be relieved by purging the qi of its child-organ. "For instance, the intense liver fire can be cleared either by purging the liver fire with liver-fire-purging drugs like *radix gentianae* and *radix scutellariae* or by purging the heart fire with the drugs like *rhizoma coptidis* and lotus plumule, based on the mechanism of "liver qi engendering heart qi. "(Figure 2-4)

(Wu Qunli   Zhang Wen)

第三章 病因病机

　　能够破坏机体相对平衡状态而引发疾病的各种因素，称之为病因。中医的病因包括了外感性致病因素、内伤性致病因素、继发性致病因素和其他致病因素四大类。病机是指疾病的发生、发展及变化的机制。病邪作用于人体，产生全身或局部的各种各样的病理变化。多数疾病的病机不外乎正邪相争、气机失常及阴阳失调等。

第一节　病　因

一、外感致病因素

　　外感致病因素来源于自然界，多从人体肌表、口鼻侵及机体而发病。包括六淫、疠气等。

（一）六淫

　　风、寒、暑、湿、燥、火是六种自然界正常的气候变化，有利于万物的生长、繁衍，一般不易使人发病。如果气候变化异常，六气发生太过或不及，或非其时而有其气（如春天当温而反寒，冬季当凉而反热），以及气候变化过于急骤（如暴寒、暴暖），超出了机体的适应能力，就会导致疾病的发生。六气成为致病的因素而称为"六淫"。不属正气，所以又有"六邪"之称。

　　1. 风　风是春天的主气，但四季皆有风，故风邪致病又不局限于春季。风邪的性质及致病特点：

　　（1）风为阳邪，其性开泄，易袭阳位：风邪具有轻扬、升发、向上、向外的特性，故属于阳邪；其性开泄，是指风邪易使腠理疏泄而开张。正因其能轻扬、升发，并善于向上、向外，所以风邪致病，常伤及人体的上部（头面）、阳经和肌表，使皮毛腠理开泄，出现头痛、汗出、恶风等症状。《素问·太阴阳明论篇》说："伤于风

CHAPTER THREE   ETIOLOGY AND PATHOGENESIS

The cause of disease, or etiology, refers to the factors that damage the relative dynamic equilibrium and result in disease. In TCM, the cause of disease covers exogenic pathogenic factor, internal pathogenic factor, secondary pathogenic factor, and other pathogenic factors. Mechanism of disease refers to the mechanism by which disease arises and develops, the same as pathogenesis. The invasion of pathogenic factors can lead to the occurrences of various pathological changes throughout human body. The pathogenesis of most diseases is struggling between the healthy qi and the pathogenic qi, or disorder of qi movement and disharmony of yin and yang.

Section 1   Cause of Disease

Exogenic Pathogenic Factors

External pathogenic factors come from the nature, which invade the human body via the body surface, mouths, and noses. Such factors include six excesses and pestilent qi, etc.

Six Excesses

Wind, cold, summerheat, dampness, dryness, and fire are the normal climatic changes of nature, benefiting the growth and reproduction of all things. Under normal conditions, they will not cause diseases. However, when they are excessive or deficient, or when they take place in wrong time (like cold in spring when it ought to turn warmer, or hot in winter when it ought to be cold), or change too sharply (such as sudden cold or sudden warm), or when the body resistance is too weak to adapt to the climatic changes, these six climatic changes will turn into pathogenic factors and attack the human body. Then the six climatic phenomena will be regarded as six excesses, also known as six exopathogens because they are not normal qi any more.

1. Wind

Though the wind is the primary climatic characteristic of spring, it also exists in other seasons, so diseases resulted from wind is not limited to occur in spring. Wind has the nature and pathogenic characteristics as follows:

(1) Wind belongs to yang pathogen, characterized by upward and outward dispersion, and it tends to attack the yang parts of the body.

Wind belongs to yang pathogen because it has the feature of lightness, rise, upwards, and outwardness. Its nature of upward and outward dispersion means it tends to open and discharge striae. Due to its light, rising, upward, and outward characteristics, it often hurts the upper part of human body (head and face), yang meridians and body surface, and opens and discharges skin, hair and striae, therefore, manifesting the symptoms of headache, sweating, and aversion to wind just as described in *Plain Questions* "the patients suffering from wind have the symptoms in the upper part of body."

者，上先受之。"

（2）风性善行而数变："善行"是指风性善动不居，具有行无定处、病位游移的特点。如风邪导致之"痹证"，临床症状就可出现疼痛走窜不定，亦称之为"行痹"或"风痹"；"数变"是指风邪致病具有变幻无常和发病迅速的特性而言，如风疹块（荨麻疹）起病急速、发无定处、此起彼伏、时隐时现的特点。

（3）风为百病之长：风为百病之长，是指风邪为六淫之邪的首要致病因素，其余外邪常依附于风而侵犯人体，如外感风寒、风热、风湿、风燥等证。古人甚至将风邪作为外感致病因素的总称。故《素问·骨空论篇》说："风者，百病之始也"。

（4）风性主动：动即动摇不定。风性主动指风邪致病具有动摇不定的特征。凡眩晕、震颤、抽搐、颈项强直、角弓反张、两目上视等动的症状，都属风证。

2. 寒　寒为冬季主气，故寒邪致病多见于冬季。由于淋雨涉水，或汗出当风，或贪凉露宿，以及屋内空调过凉，亦是寒邪的致病途径，故其他季节也可由寒致病。寒邪的性质及致病特点：

（1）寒为阴邪，易伤阳气：寒为阴气盛的表现，故其性属阴，阴邪伤及阳气，导致阳气失去正常的温煦、气化作用，可出现阳虚阴盛的寒证。如外寒侵袭肌表，卫阳被遏，就会出现恶寒发热、无汗、鼻塞、流清涕等症；寒邪直中脾胃，脾阳受损，便可见脘腹冷痛、呕吐、腹泻等症。

（2）寒性凝滞，主痛：凝滞，即凝结阻滞不通。寒性凝滞，即指寒邪侵入，易使气血津液凝结、经脉阻滞，不通则痛，故寒邪伤人多见疼痛症状。正如《素问·痹论篇》说："痛者，寒气多也，有寒故痛也"。

（3）寒性收引："收引"，有收缩牵引之意。寒性收引，即指寒邪侵袭人体，使气机收敛，腠理、经络、筋脉收缩而挛急。如寒邪侵及肌表，毛窍腠理闭塞，卫阳被郁不得宣泄，可见恶寒、发热、无汗等；寒客经络关节，则经脉收缩拘急，甚则挛急作痛，屈伸不利，或冷厥不仁等。寒入厥阴经，可见少腹拘急不仁。

3. 暑　暑为夏季的主气，为火热之气所化，主要发生于夏至以后、立秋之前，有明显的季节性。暑邪与温、热及火属同一类的病邪，它们的区别在于程度与季节的不同。暑邪致病，有伤暑和中暑之别。起病缓、病情轻者为"伤暑"；发病急、病情重者为"中暑"。暑邪的性质及致病特点：

（1）暑为阳邪，其性炎热：暑为盛夏火热之气所化，火热属阳，故暑邪为阳邪。夏季气候炎热，暑邪随其炎热之势，较其他季节的火热之邪更为炽盛，即暑邪伤人多表现为一系列阳热症状，如高热、心烦、面赤、脉洪大等。

（2）暑性升散，伤津耗气：升，即升发、向上。暑为阳邪，其性升发，故易上扰心神或侵犯头目，见头昏、目眩、面赤等症。"散"，指暑邪侵犯人体，可致腠理

（2）Wind is apt to move in frequent change.

"Aptness to move"refers to its characteristic of keeping moving and therefore changing the locations of disease,such as moving impediment caused by wind,which manifests as continuous changes of pain locations,so also termed as"moving impediment"."Frequent change"means it remains changing and develops quickly,like wheal(urticaria),which has the characteristics of breaking out quickly and spreading from one place to another while the former recovers.

（3）Wind is the leading pathogenic factor in causing various diseases.

It is the primary pathogenic factors of the six excesses and often cooperates with and leads other exogenous evils to invade the human body to cause disease like external contraction of wind cold,wind heat, wind dampness,and wind dryness.In the ancient time,exogenous pathogenic factors were even all termed as wind as depicted in *Plain Questions* "wind is the origin of all diseases."

（4）Wind tends to migrate.

Migration refers to destabilizing."Wind tends to migrate"means that the diseases caused by wind has the characteristic of destabilizing,with the symptoms of sway such as dizziness,tremor,hyperspasmia,stiff neck,opisthotonus,and upward-staring eyes.

2. Cold

Cold is the leading climatic characteristic of winter,so diseases caused by cold often occur in winter. However,it also breaks out in other season due to the misconducts like being wetted by rain or water,exposure to wind while sweating,sleeping outside or in the cold environment,or low temperature of air conditioning,all of which are also the ways that cold invades the human body.Here is the nature and pathogenic characteristics of cold evil.

（1）Cold belongs to yin evil and easily injuries yang qi.

As yin qi,cold is the manifestation of yin qi exuberance.Cold easily injuries yang qi,therefore,damaging the functions of warming and transforming of yang qi,and leading to the cold syndrome of yang deficiency and yin excess.When exogenous cold attacks the human body surface and obstructs defense yang, such symptoms as fever with aversion to cold,adiaphoresis,stuffy nose,and clear nasal discharge come out.If cold directly strikes the spleen and stomach,it will damage the spleen yang along with the symptoms of cold pain in the abdomen and stomach,vomiting and diarrhea and etc.

（2）Cold tends to stagnate by nature,resulting in pain.

Stagnation refers to coagulation and blockage.Stagnation of cold means invasion of cold evil often leads to stagnation of qi,blood,fluid and humor,and blockage of meridians.As the obstruction often causes pain,the diseases originating from cold evil accompany the symptom of pain,as stated in *Plain Questions* "pain is the feature of cold excess,so pain is often caused by cold evil."

（3）Cold tends to contract by nature.

Contraction refers to convergence and shrinking.Contraction of cold demonstrates that an invasion of cold evil will result in contraction of qi as well as the contraction and spasm of striae,meridians and collaterals.For example,when cold attacks the surface of human body,blocks skin and striae,and constrains defense yang from diffusion and discharge,such symptoms as fever,aversion to cold,and adiaphoresis come out.When cold stays in meridians,collaterals and joints,the meridians and collaterals contract and it even leads to spasm and pain,manifested as hardness to stretch,cold or numbness.In addition,when cold attacks liver meridian,there comes out with the symptom of lower abdominal contracture.

3. Summerheat

Summerheat is the leading climatic characteristic of summer,generated from fire.It primarily emerges between the summer solstice and the beginning of autumn,so it has distinct seasonal characteristic.Summerheat,warm,heat and fire belong to the same kind of pathogenic factors,but occur in different degrees

开泄而多汗；汗出过多，气随津泄，不仅伤津，而且耗气，故见口渴喜饮、尿赤短少、气短、乏力；若气津耗伤太过，清窍失养，可见突然昏倒、不省人事。

（3）暑多挟湿：暑季除气候炎热外，且常多雨而潮湿，热蒸湿动，故暑邪为病，常兼挟湿邪而侵犯人体。其临床特征除发热、烦渴等暑热症外，常兼见四肢困倦、胸闷呕恶、大便溏泻而不爽等湿阻症状。

4．湿　湿为长夏主气。长夏即农历六月，时值夏秋之交，为一年中湿气最盛的季节。湿邪为病，有外湿、内湿之分。外湿多由气候潮湿或涉水淋雨、居所潮湿等所致；内湿则是由于脾失健运、水湿停聚而成。湿邪的性质和致病特点：

（1）湿为阴邪，易损伤阳气，阻遏气机：湿为重浊有质之邪，侵入最易留滞于脏腑经络，阻遏气机，使脏腑气机升降失常，经络阻滞不畅，可见胸膈满闷、小便淋涩不畅、大便不爽。湿为阴邪，易伤脾阳，脾阳不振，纳运失司，水湿停滞，常见脘痞腹胀、食欲减退、腹泻、尿少、腹水等症。

（2）湿性重浊："重"，即沉重、重着，指湿邪致病，出现以沉重感为特征的临床表现。如头身困重、四肢酸楚沉重等。若湿邪外袭肌表，困遏清阳，清阳不升，则头重如束布帛；湿邪阻滞经络关节，阳气不得布达，则可见肌肤不仁、关节疼痛重着等，称之为"湿痹"或"着痹"。"浊"，即秽浊不清，指湿邪为患，易呈现分泌物和排泄物秽浊不清的现象。如湿滞大肠，则大便溏泄、下痢脓血；湿浊下注，则小便浑浊、妇女白带过多；湿邪浸淫肌肤，则可见湿疹等。

（3）湿性黏滞：湿邪致病，以黏腻停滞为特点。主要表现在两个方面：一是症状的黏滞性，如排泄物和分泌物多滞涩不畅。湿滞大肠，则大便排泄不爽或里急后重；湿阻膀胱，则小便滞涩不畅或尿频涩痛；湿浊内蕴，则见口黏口甘、舌苔厚滑黏腻等。二是病程的缠绵性。因湿性黏滞，易阻气机，气不行则湿不化，故起病隐缓，病程较长，反复发作或缠绵难愈，如湿温、湿疹、湿痹（着痹）等。

（4）湿性趋下，易袭阴位：湿邪为重浊有质之邪，属阴，而有趋下之特点。人体下部亦属阴，故湿邪为病，多易伤及人体下部，如水肿、湿疹等病以下肢较为多见。此外，湿邪下注致病，如淋病、尿浊、带下、腹泻、痢疾等，都为湿性趋下、易袭阴位特点的体现。

5．燥　燥为秋季的主气，又称"秋燥"，具有干燥、收敛等特性。秋季一派秋凉而劲急干燥的气候，故秋季多燥病。燥邪伤人，多自口鼻而入，首犯肺卫，发为外燥病证。燥邪为病可由相兼的寒热邪气的不同又有温燥、凉燥之分。初秋尚有夏末之余热，燥热相合，发为温燥证；深秋又有近冬之寒气，燥寒相合，则发为凉燥证。燥邪的性质和致病特点：

（1）燥性干涩，易伤津液：燥邪属阳，易伤阴液。燥邪为病，可见各种阴津亏

and seasons and causes the diseases to different extent. Diseases caused by summerheat are divided into "heat injury" characterized by late onset and mildness, and "heat stroke" featuring quick breakout and severity. Here is the nature and pathogenic characteristics of summerheat.

(1) Summerheat belongs to yang evil which has the characteristic of torridness.

Summerheat is generated from heat fire of midsummer, which belongs to yang, so summerheat is yang evil. Summerheat is much more serious in the hot summer than in other seasons, so a patient is injured by it primarily manifests a series of yang heat symptoms of high fever, dysphoria, red face and surging, and big pulse.

(2) Summerheat has the property of upward dispersion, so it injuries fluid and consumes qi.

Upward dispersion refers to upward rising. As yang evil, summerheat has a feature of ascending, so it is apt to disturbing inner mind or affecting head and eyes with the symptoms of dizziness, vertigo, and red face. Dispersion means invasion of summerheat opens striae and leads to excessive sweating, during which qi collapses due to fluid depletion, followed by a series of symptoms of thirst and desire to drink, short and red urine, short breath and fatigue. If excessive fluid and qi is consumed, there is not enough fluid to nourish the clear orifices (including the ears, nose and throat) and the symptoms of sudden faint and unconsciousness will turn up.

(3) Summerheat is likely to be mixed with dampness. As the summer season features heat, much rain and moist, summerheat often mixes with dampness to harm the human body, presenting the clinical summerheat symptoms of fever and polydipsia, and concurrently dampness blockage symptoms of heavy and weak limbs, chest distress, vomiting nausea, and grimy sloppy stool.

4. Dampness

Dampness is the climatic characteristic of the wettest late summer in the lunar June, the alternative period of summer and autumn. Dampness evil can be classified into exogenous dampness caused by humid climate, exposure to rain or water or wet living condition, and endogenous dampness resulting from dysfunction of the spleen in transportation and retention of water-dampness. Dampness has the property and characteristics as follows:

(1) Dampness belongs to yin evil, which impairs yang qi and obstructs qi movement. As heavy and turbid evil, dampness tends to stay and stagnate in internal organs and meridians and collaterals, therefore, blocking qi movement, disturbing the ascending and descending movement of the internal organs, and retarding circulation of meridians and collaterals, in company with the symptoms of full and stuffy chest diaphragm, urine retention and sloppy stool. In addition, dampness is apt to injury the spleen yang, leads to devitalized spleen-yang failing to transport and transformation, and the formation of water-dampness stagnation, accompanied by the symptoms of distension and depression in the stomach and abdomen, decreasing appetite, diarrhea, oliguria and ascites, etc.

(2) Dampness has the feature of heaviness and turbidness.

Heaviness is the leading manifestation of the diseases caused by dampness, such as heavy head, body, and limbs. If dampness invades the surface of the human body and obstructs the clear yang from rising, the symptom of heavy head which is like being bundled with cloth will come out. When it stays in meridians, collaterals and joints and blocks yang qi from spreading, it will lead to numbness and arthralgia, termed as "dampness impediment" or "fixed impediment." Turbidness refers to unclearness. It means the patient attacked by dampness often has the symptoms of having turbid and dirty secreta and excreta. Retention of dampness in large intestine can result in sloppy and loose stool and dysentery with pus and blood. Descending turbid dampness is able to give rise to turbid urine and leukorrhagia of women. Invasion of dampness evil into skin may bring about eczema.

(3) Dampness has the feature of stickiness and stagnation.

虚、滞涩的证候，如口鼻干燥、咽干口渴、皮肤干涩甚则皲裂、毛发不荣、小便短少、大便干结等。

（2）燥易伤肺：肺为娇脏，喜清润而恶燥。肺主气司呼吸，直接与自然界大气相通，且外合皮毛，开窍于鼻。故燥邪伤人，多从口鼻而入，最易伤肺，出现干咳少痰，或痰黏难咯，或痰中带血，甚则喘息胸痛等肺津受伤的症状。此外，肺与大肠相表里，肺津耗伤，大肠失润，传导失司，可现大便干涩不畅等症。

6. 火（热）及火证　火为热之极，常将二者并称。火旺于夏季，其他季节气温骤高亦可化为火热之邪，伤人致病。火热邪气致病有内外之分：属外感者，多是直接受温热邪气侵袭，如风热、燥热、湿热等；属内生者，则常由脏腑阴阳气血失调，阳气亢盛而成，如心火、肝火、胃火等。火热之邪的性质和致病特点：

（1）火（热）为阳邪，其性趋上：火热之性燔灼、升腾，故为阳邪。"阳胜则热"，故火邪致病多见高热、烦渴、汗出、脉洪数等症。火性趋上，故火热之邪易侵害人体上部，尤以头面部更著，出现目赤肿痛、咽喉肿痛、口舌生疮糜烂、牙龈肿痛、耳内肿痛或流脓等症。

（2）火热易扰心神：心属火，火热致病，易犯心经，扰动心神。轻者心神不宁而心烦、失眠；重者可神不守舍，出现狂躁不安，或神昏、谵语等症。故《素问·至真要大论篇》说："诸躁狂越，皆属于火。"

（3）火热易伤津耗气：火热之邪，最易迫津化汗外泄，或直接灼煎津液，使人体阴津耗伤。临床表现除热象显著外，往往伴有口渴喜冷饮、咽干舌燥、小便短赤、大便秘结等津伤阴亏的征象。同时，阳热太盛，伤津耗气，气随汗泄，临床可兼见体倦乏力、少气懒言等气虚症状，重则可致全身津气脱失的气脱证。

（4）火热易生风动血："生风"，是指火热之邪侵犯人体，燔灼肝经，耗劫津液，筋脉失养失润，易引起肝风内动的病证。又称"热极生风"。临床表现为高热神昏、四肢抽搐、两目上视、角弓反张等。"动血"，指火热之邪入于血脉，易灼伤脉络，迫血妄行，导致各种出血证，如吐血、衄血、便血、尿血、皮肤发斑、妇女月经过多、崩漏等。

（5）火邪易致疮痈：火邪入于血分，可聚于局部，腐蚀血肉，发为痈肿疮疡。《灵枢·痈疽》说："大热不止，热胜则肉腐，肉腐则为脓……故命曰痈。"由火毒壅聚所致之痈疡，其临床表现以疮疡局部红肿热痛为特征。

The diseases caused by dampness show the characteristics of stickiness and stagnation, which primarily manifest in two aspects. The first is the sticky and stagnant symptoms such as sloppy excrement and secretion, hardness to excrete stool and tenesmus in case of retention of dampness in the large intestine; short and frequent urine in case of retention of dampness in the bladder; and sticky sensation and sweet taste in the mouth, slippery, thick and greasy tongue coating in case of internal retention of turbid dampness. The second is lingering course of disease. The diseases caused by dampness like dampness-warmth syndrome, eczema, and dampness impediment (fixed impediment) usually have latent and slow onset and long and lingering course; they are hard to be healed and easy to recur. It is due to the characteristics of stickiness and stagnation of dampness, which blocks qi movement from circulating and results in dampness retention.

(4) Dampness is apt to descend and attack yin parts of the human body.

Dampness belongs to yin evil characterized by heaviness and turbidness and downwardness. As the yin part of human body, the lower parts are often apt to be hurt by dampness. For example, dropsy and eczema which often emerge in the legs and feet. The diseases like gonorrhea, turbid urine, morbid leucorrhoea, diarrhea and dysentery, resulting from dampness, demonstrate the above-mentioned feature of dampness.

5. Dryness

Dryness is the leading climatic characteristic of autumn, also known as autumn dryness, which features dryness and convergence, so dryness often occurs in autumn. It often hurts the human body by entering into the body from mouth and nose to invade the lung and defense qi. As a result, there has the symptom of external dryness. Dryness can be divided into warn dryness and cool dryness based on which kind of evil they complex with, cold or heat. Warn dryness often takes place in early autumn when dryness is easy to complex with afterheat of the summer; while cool dryness often occurs in the late autumn when dryness tends to complex with cold of winter. Here are the nature and characteristics of dryness.

(1) Dryness, characterized by dryness and astringency, is apt to deplete fluid.

Dryness belongs to yang evil and easy to injury yin fluid. Diseases caused by dryness often accompany the symptoms of yin and fluid deficiency and astringency like dry mouth, nose and throat, thirst, dry and even chapped skin, lusterless hair, short and less urine and dry stool, etc.

(2) Dryness tends to injure the lung.

Lung is the tender organ which prefers moisture rather than dryness. Lung in charge of respiration, governing skin and hair and opening at nose directly connects with outside air, so dryness often hurts people by coming in from mouth and nose and injuring the lung, followed with a series of lung-fluid deficient symptoms of dry cough with little phlegm, sticky sputum hard to be coughed up, bloodstained sputum or gasping and chest pain. In addition, as the lung stands in interior-exterior relationship with the large intestine, the depletion of lung fluid will lead to dryness and malfunction of the large intestine, therefore resulting in dry and astringent stool and etc.

6. Fire(heat) and fire syndrome

Fire is the extreme heat, so it is often mentioned together with heat. Fire activates in summer, but if the temperature suddenly rises sharply in other seasons, then it will come up with fire. Diseases caused by fire can be divided into the one arising from exogenic pathogen and the other one from endogenic pathogen. The former results from direct invasion of warm and heat like wind heat, dry heat and damp heat; and the latter comes into being because of yin-yang imbalance and qi and blood disorder of the internal organs as well as yang qi excess like heart fire, liver fire and stomach fire. Fire has the property and features as follows:

(1) Fire(heat) belongs to yang evil featuring ascending.

Fire(heat) is apt to burn and rise, so it is termed as yang evil. "Predominance of yang generates heat," so the diseases caused by fire often present the symptoms of high fever, fidget and thirst, sweating,

（二）疠气

疠气，指一类具有强烈致病性和传染性的外感病邪。在中医文献中，疠气又称为"疫毒"、"疫气"、"异气"、"戾气"、"毒气"、"乖戾之气"等，是有别于六淫而具有强烈传染性的外感病邪。

疠气可以通过空气传染，经口鼻侵入致病；也可随饮食、蚊虫叮咬、虫兽咬伤、皮肤接触等途径传染而发病。如痄腮（腮腺炎）、烂喉丹痧（猩红热）、疫毒痢、白喉、天花、肠伤寒、霍乱、鼠疫以及疫黄（急性传染性肝炎）、流行性出血热等，都属感染疠气引起的疫病。

1. 疠气的致病特点

（1）发病急骤，病情危笃：一般而言，由于疠气多属热毒之邪，其性疾速，而且常挟毒雾、瘴气等秽浊之邪侵犯人体，故其致病比六淫更显发病急骤，来势凶猛，变化多端，病情险恶。因而发病过程中常出现发热、扰神、动血、生风、剧烈吐泻等危重症状。《温疫论》述及某些疫病，"缓者朝发夕死，重者顷刻而亡"，足见疠气致病来势凶猛，病情危笃。

（2）传染性强，易于流行：疠气具有强烈的传染性和流行性，可通过空气、食物等多种途径在人群中传播。当处在疠气流行的地域时，无论男女老少、体质强弱，凡触之者，多可发病。疠气发病，既可大面积流行，也可散在发生。

2. 疠气的发生与流行因素

（1）气候因素：自然气候的反常变化，如久旱、酷热、洪涝、湿雾瘴气、地震等，均可孳生疠气而导致疾病的发生。霍乱等病的大流行与此类因素有关。

（2）环境因素：环境卫生不良，如空气、水源、食物等受到污染，均可引起疫病发生。如麻疹、疫毒痢、疫黄等病。

（3）预防因素：由于疠气具有强烈的传染性，人触之者皆可发病。若预防隔离工作不力，也往往会使疫病发生或流行。

（4）社会因素：社会动荡不安，或战乱不停，或工作环境恶劣，生活极度贫困，则疫病容易不断发生和流行。若国家安定，且注意卫生防疫工作，采取一系列积极有效的防疫和治疗措施，疫病即能得到有效的控制。

surging and rapid pulse, etc. Fire tends to rise upward, so fire is prone to invade and hurt the upper parts of the human body especially the head, with the symptoms of red, swelling and achy eyes, swelling and sore throat, mouth and tongue ulcer, swelling and aching gum, swelling, achy and even suppurated ears, etc.

(2) Fire(heat) is inclined to disturb the mind.

Heart is pertaining to fire, so fire evil is inclined to attack the heart channel and disturb the mind in company with the symptoms of light unease like dysphoria and insomnia, and of heavy vesania such as coma, and delirious speech as described in *Plain Questions* "all the vesania syndromes result from the invasion of fire."

(3) Fire(heat) tends to injury fluid and qi.

Fire(heat) evil is apt to turn fluid into sweat and discharge it or directly burn fluid to consume yin, with the clinical manifestation of fluid-deficient syndrome like thirst and preference of cold drinks, dry mouth and tongue, red and short urine and constipation besides high fever. In addition, the excessive fire depletes fluid and consume qi by discharging sweat, so it will concurrently presents the qi deficiency syndrome of weakness, tiredness, lack of qi and no desire to speak, or even the heavy syndrome of qi collapse arising from total depletion and loss of both of fluid and qi.

(4) Fire(heat) is apt to engender wind and cause bleeding.

Fire(heat) is apt to engender wind means invasion of fire is apt to cause the syndrome of liver wind by burning liver meridian, consuming fluid and humor, de-nourishing and de-moistening meridians, also known as extreme heat giving rise to wind, with the clinical manifestations of high fever with coma, hyperspasmia of limbs, eyes staring upward and opisthotonus and etc. Bleeding means invasion of fire evil in blood vessels is inclined to injure vessels and accelerate the circulation of blood, thus resulting in various hemorrhage syndromes like hematemesis, hemorrhinia, hemafecia, hematuria, skin blotches, and menorrhagia, metrorrhagia and metrostaxis of women.

(5) Fire is apt to bring about sore and abscess.

Fire getting into the blood aspect often gathers in a fixed part and erodes the adjacent flesh and blood to generate abscess, swelling, sore and ulcer, as depicted in *Miraculous Pivot* "long-lasting extreme heat leads to heat excess and then corruption of flesh, which finally turns into abscess···, so termed as carbuncle." The sore and ulcer resulting from convergence and retention of fire toxin has the clinical feature of red, swelling, hot, and ache of the skin around ulcer.

Epidemic Pathogens

Epidemic pathogens refer to those exogenic pathogens easily leading to epidemic diseases. In TCM documents, epidemic pathogens are often termed as epidemic pathogenic toxin, poison qi, etc. It is a kind of exogenic pathogen with strong contagiosity and different from six excesses.

Epidemic pathogens can spread through the air and infect people through mouth and nose, or it can cause diseases through diet, mosquito sting, animal bite, skin contact, etc. Such diseases cover mumps(parotitis), scarlet fever(scarlatina), fulminant dysentery, diphtheria, smallpox, ileotyphus, cholera, pestis, epidemic yellow(acute infectious hapatitis), and epidemic hemorrhagic fever.

1. Features of diseases caused by epidemic pathogens

(1) Sudden onset and serious disease

The epidemic pathogens, mostly as heat toxin, have a characteristic of sudden onset and often invade us together with other dirty and turbid evils like toxic smog and miasma, so they cause diseases much more quickly, acutely, severely and changefully than the six excesses. Due to these characteristics, the diseases caused by them often manifest the severe symptoms of fever, spirit disturbance, acceleration of blood circulation, vomiting and diarrhea, and so on, as described in *Treatise on Pestilence*: "the patients suffering from

二、内伤性致病因素

（一）七情

七情，是指喜、怒、忧、思、悲、恐、惊七种正常的情志活动，一般情况下这些情志变化不会致病。只有强烈持久的情志刺激，超越了人体的生理和心理适应能力，七情才会成为致病因素，故也称之为"七情内伤"。七情致病特点：

1. 直接伤及内脏　七情是机体对内外环境变化所产生的复杂心理反应，以内脏精气为物质基础。因此，七情过激致病，可直接伤及内脏。如心在志为喜，过度高兴则伤心；肝在志为怒，过度恼怒则伤肝；脾在志为思，过度思虑则伤脾；肺在志为悲，过度悲伤则伤肺；肾在志为恐，过度惊恐则伤肾。

2. 影响脏腑气机　七情致病主要影响脏腑气机失常，气血运行紊乱，出现相应的临床表现。如《素问·举痛论篇》说："……百病生于气也，怒则气上，喜则气缓，悲则气消，恐则气下……惊则气乱……思则气结。"

（1）怒则气上：怒为肝之志，过怒可导致肝气疏泄太过，气机上逆，甚则血随气逆，并走于上。临床主要表现为头胀头痛、面红目赤、呕血甚则昏厥猝倒。

（2）喜则气缓：喜为心之志，过度喜乐可导致心气涣散不收，重者心气暴脱或神不守舍。临床可见精神不能集中，甚则神志失常、狂乱，或见心气暴脱的大汗淋漓、气息微弱、脉微欲绝等症。

（3）悲则气消：悲为肺之志，过度悲伤可导致肺失宣降及肺气耗伤。临床常见意志消沉、精神不振、气短胸闷、乏力懒言等症。

（4）思则气结：思为脾之志，过度思虑伤心脾，导致心脾气机郁滞、运化失职的病机变化。临床可见精神萎靡、反应迟钝、不思饮食、腹胀纳呆、便溏等症状。

（5）恐则气下：恐为肾之志。恐，是一种胆怯、惧怕的心理反应。长期恐惧或突然意外惊恐，皆能导致肾气受损，肾气不固，气陷于下，可见二便失禁、精遗、骨痿等症。恐惧伤肾，精气不能上荣，则心肺失其濡养，水火升降不交，可见胸满腹胀、怵惕不安、夜不能寐等症。

（6）惊则气乱：指猝然受惊伤心肾，导致心神不定，气机逆乱，肾气不固的病机变化。临床可见惊悸不安，慌乱失措，甚则神志错乱，或二便失禁。《素问·举痛论篇》说："惊则心无所倚，神无所归，虑无所定，故气乱矣。"

情志内伤引起的病理变化是相当复杂的，既可单一情志伤人，也可两种以上情志交织伤人而出现一脏或多个脏腑损伤的症状。临床中还要全面综合分析，以进行正确判断。

such epidemic diseases die in the same day, and even worse, some of them die at the moment when they are infected," which pointed out the acuteness and severeness of such diseases.

(2) Strong infectiousness and epidemicity

Epidemic pathogens have strong infectiousness and epidemicity. They can spread through air, food, and other pathways. Most people in epidemic regions, men or women, strong or weak, can be infected when attacked. The epidemic pathogens can cause diseases in a large area or in some places.

2. Occurrence and epidemic factors of epidemic pathogens

(1) Climatic factor: Abnormal climate like long-lasting drought, extreme heat, flood, miasma caused by wet smog and earthquake can breed epidemic pathogens and cause epidemic diseases such as pandemic cholera.

(2) Environment factor: Poor environmental sanitation like polluted air, polluted water, and polluted food can give rise to epidemic diseases such as measles, fulminant dysentery, and epidemic yellow (acute infectious hepatitis).

(3) Preventative factor: As epidemic pathogens have strong infectiousness, the failure of preventative quarantine measures will help it to spread.

(4) Social factors: Such factors as turbulent society, continuous war chaos and poor working environment and extremely impoverished living conditions also contribute to the occurrence and epidemic of epidemic diseases. On the contrary, such epidemic diseases can be effectively controlled in the stable countries where the governments pay attention to epidemic prevention and take a series of active and effective prevention and treatment measures.

Endogenic Pathogenic Factors

Seven Emotions

Seven emotions refer to the seven normal emotional activities including joy, anger, anxiety, thought, sorrow, fear, and fright. These emotional changes generally do not result in diseases. However, they may become pathogenic factors when there is strong and everlasting emotional stimulus beyond physiological and psychological adaptability, so it is also termed as internal injuries due to emotional disorder. Seven emotional pathogens have the characteristics as follows:

1. Directly injure the internal organs

Seven emotions are the complicated psychological reactions to the changes between interior environment and exterior environment, with essence of the viscera (the heart, liver, spleen, lung and kidney) as the materials base, so overreaction of seven emotions can directly injure the viscera. For example, the heart corresponds to joy in the emotion, but extreme joy will hurt the heart; the liver corresponds to anger in the emotion, but rage will impair the liver; the spleen corresponds to thought in the emotion, but too much thought will damage the spleen; the lung corresponds to sorrow in the emotion, but extreme sorrow will injure the lung; and the kidney corresponds to fright in the emotion, but excessive fright will impair the kidney.

2. Affect the vital qi of the internal organs

The extremity of the seven emotions leads to disorder of qi movement of the internal organs and then the disorder of qi and blood circulation, therefore presenting a series of related clinical symptoms, as set forth in *Plain Questions* "… All diseases are caused by the disorder of qi, which ascends in case of rage, becomes slack in case of extreme joy, consumes in case of excessive sorrow, sinks in case of fear, goes turbulent (disorder) in case of fright and knots in case of pensiveness."

(1) Rage leading to qi ascending: Anger corresponds to the liver, but rage will result in excessive discharge of liver qi and reversely lead qi or even blood to ascend, with the clinical symptoms of fullness of

（三）饮食

1. 饮食不节 过饥，摄食不足，气血生化乏源，久则气血不足，脏腑失养，功能活动衰退，抗病力弱等；过饱或暴饮暴食，导致脾胃难于消化转输而致病。此外，若饮食无度，也易导致脾胃损伤。

2. 饮食不洁 进食不洁净的食物如进食陈腐变质，或被疫毒、寄生虫等污染的食物，可引起多种肠胃病，如痢疾、霍乱等；还可发生食物中毒或某些传染性疾病，轻则脘腹疼痛，呕吐腹泻；重则毒气攻心，神昏谵语，甚至导致死亡。

3. 饮食偏嗜 饮食偏寒偏热，或饮食五味有所偏嗜，或嗜酒成癖等，均可导致人体阴阳失调，或导致某些营养物质缺乏而引起疾病。

（四）劳逸

1. 过劳 包括劳力过度、劳神过度和房劳过度三个方面。劳力太过而伤气，损伤内脏的精气，导致脏气亏虚，功能减退。常见如少气懒言、体倦神疲、喘息汗出等；过度劳力而致形体损伤，主要是筋骨、关节、肌肉的运动，如果长时间用力太过，则易致形体组织损伤，久而积劳成疾。劳神过度，是指思虑太过，劳伤心脾而言。用神过度，长思久虑，则易耗伤心血，损伤脾气，以致心神失养，神志不宁而心悸、健忘、失眠、多梦和脾失健运而纳少、腹胀、便溏、消瘦等。房劳过度，又称"肾劳"，是指性生活不节，房事太过，或妇女早孕多育等。症见腰膝酸软、眩晕耳鸣、精神萎靡、性功能障碍；妇女可见月经失调，带下过多、不孕不育等。此外，房劳过度也是导致早衰的重要原因。

2. 过逸 过度安逸，可致气血运行不畅，脾胃等脏腑功能衰减，可见食少、乏力神疲，肢体不强，抗邪无力，动则心悸、气短、汗出等；脾失健运，水湿不化，痰浊内生。此外长期用脑过少，不善思考，可致神气衰弱，常见精神萎靡、健忘、反应迟钝等。

head, headache, red face and eyes, haematemesis, and even faint.

(2) Joy leading to qi slack: Joy corresponds to the heart, but extreme joy will loosen heart qi with the clinical manifestations of distraction, deliriums and derangement, or even desert it suddenly, with the symptoms of dripping sweat, weak breath and extremely weak pulse.

(3) Sorrow leading to qi consumption: Sorrow corresponds to the lung, but excessive sorrow will lead to failure of the lung in diffusion, prurificaton and down-bearing, and finally consumption of lung qi, with the clinical symptoms of despondence, dispiritedness, short breath, chest distress, debility, and no desire to speak, etc.

(4) Thought leading to qi stagnation: Thought corresponds to the spleen, but too much thought will give rise to stagnation of the activities of the heart qi and spleen qi and dysfunction of the spleen in transportation and transformation, clinically presenting the symptoms of listlessness, slow response, poor appetite, abdominal distension, and loose stool.

(5) Fear leading to qi sinking: Fear, a psychological reaction to timidity and dread, corresponds to the kidney, but long-lasting fear or sudden or unexpected fear will harm the kidney qi and un-consolidate kidney qi so as to make it sink, with the symptoms of urinary and fecal incontinence, spermatorrhea, and atrophic debility of bones. In case of fear impairing the kidney, the vital essence fails to ascend to nourish and moisten the heart and lung, so such symptoms as full chest and abdominal distention, anxiety, unease and sleeplessness at night will come out, as the result of the disorder of ascending and descending of water (kidney) and fire (heart) and the failure of their communication.

(6) Fright leading to qi turbulence: The sudden and unexpected fright will injure the heart and the kidney, therefore bring about absentmindedness, reversion and disorder of qi activity and unconsolidation of the kidney qi, clinically manifesting the symptoms of palpitation, fluster, disturbance, and even mind disorder or urinary and fecal incontinence, as represented in *Plain Questions* "fright will lead to the unconsolidation of the heart qi, unrest and anxiety of mind, so qi disorders."

Extremity of the seven emotions gives rise to quite complicated diseases, which can be caused by one or the combination of several emotions, therefore impairing one or the several related internal organs. To make correct judgment (diagnosis) and treatment, the comprehensive and all-around clinical analysis should be made.

Diet

1. Irregular diet

The excessive hungriness or intake of less food, from which the qi and blood is transformed, will lead to the deficiency of qi and blood, de-nourishment and hypofunction of the viscera and bowels, and weakening of disease-resistance. But overfeeding or gluttony will increase the burden of the spleen and stomach in digesting and transforming the food and therefore result in diseases. Eating too much is apt to injure the spleen and stomach.

2. Unclean diet

Eating the unclean food like rotten or bad food, or food polluted by epidemic pathogens or parasites can cause various gastrointestinal diseases like dysentery and cholera, lead to food poisoning or even infect some communicable diseases, with the symptoms of abdominal pain, vomiting and diarrhea, or even coma, delirious speech or even death, arising from the invasion of poisonous air (evil qi) into the heart.

3. Diet predilection

Habitual preference of hot or cold foods, or one flavour to others, or alcoholomania will cause the diseases due to imbalance of yin and yang or lack of some nutrients.

Labor and Rest

1. Overstrain

三、继发性致病因素

继发于其他疾病过程而产生的致病因素，故称"继发性病因"。

（一）痰饮

1. 痰饮的形成　痰饮是人体水液代谢障碍所形成的病理产物。稠浊者称为痰，清稀者称为饮。两者同出一源，故并称为痰饮。痰可分为有形之痰和无形之痰。有形之痰，是指视之可见，闻之有声的痰液。无形之痰，是指只见其征象，不见其形质的痰病，包括瘰疬、痰核及停滞在脏腑经络等组织中的痰。痰饮多由六淫、饮食失宜、劳逸过度、七情内伤等，使与水液代谢有关的脏腑如肺、脾、肾、三焦等气化功能失调，导致水液代谢障碍、水津停滞所致。

2. 痰饮的致病特点　痰饮一旦产生，致病广泛，全身各处，无处不到，如《杂病源流犀烛·痰饮源流》说："其为物，则流动不测，故其为害，上至巅顶，下至涌泉，随气升降，周身内外皆到，五脏六腑俱有……故痰为诸辨之源，怪病皆由痰成也。"由于痰饮引起病症繁多，故有"百病多由痰作祟"之说。

痰饮病症分为痰证和饮证。根据痰停留的部位不同，其临床特点亦不同。如痰滞在肺，可见喘咳咯痰；痰阻于心，心血不畅，而见胸闷心悸；痰迷心窍，则可见神昏、痴呆；痰火扰心，则发为癫狂；痰停于胃，胃失和降，可见恶心、呕吐、胃脘痞满；痰在经络筋骨，则可致瘰疬痰核，肢体麻木，或半身不遂，或成阴疽流注等；痰浊上犯于头，可见眩晕、昏冒；痰气凝结咽喉，则可出现咽中梗阻，吞之不下、吐之不出之病症。根据饮停留的部位不同，其临床特点亦不同：饮在肠间，则肠鸣沥沥有声；饮在胸胁，则胸胁胀满、咳嗽气促引痛，称"悬饮"；饮在膈上，则咳喘气逆，不能平卧，其形如肿，称为"支饮"；饮溢肌肤，则见肌肤水肿、无汗、身体疼重，称"溢饮"。痰饮由水湿停滞聚集而成，故具有湿邪致病的特点，如大多有沉重、秽浊、黏滞不爽的症状。同时所致疾病均有病势黏滞缠绵，病情容易反复，病程相对较长。

Overstrain includes three aspects of excessive labor, consumption of too much energy and sexual overstrain(sex excessive).Excessive labor impairs the essential qi of the internal organs, thus leading to deficiency of the qi of the internal organs and hypofunction of these organs, with the manifestations of lack of qi and no desire to speak, tiredness, heavy breath and sweating.It is apt to injure the human body, especially muscles, bones and joints.Excessive labor for a long time tends to impair tissues of the body or even lead to physical disability.Consumption of too much energy means long-lasting and excessive contemplation hurts the heart and spleen.Permanent excessive contemplation is inclined to deplete the heart blood and impair the spleen qi, with the symptoms of palpitation, amnesia, insomnia and dreaminess as the result of heart de-nourishment, and eating less, abdominal distention, loose stool and emaciation as the consequence of failure of the spleen in transformation and transportation.Sexual overstrain, also termed as kidney overstrain, refers to too frequent sexual intercourse, or early pregnancy or many births of women, presenting the symptoms of weakness at waist and knees, dizziness and tinnitus, listlessness, and sexual dysfunction, and also menstrual disorder, morbid leucorrhoea and infertility.In addition, sexual overstrain also plays a significant role in senilism.

2. Over-relaxation

Over-relaxation(sitting or sleep) is prone to retard circulation of the blood and dysfunction of the spleen and stomach in company with the symptoms of eating less, tiredness, feeble limbs, weak resistance, palpitation, short breath and sweating.It also leads to dysfunction of the spleen in transportation so as to fail to evaporate and transport dampness and form phlegm.Meanwhile, long-lasting relaxation of the brain is apt to result in inactivity of the brain, listlessness, amnesia and slow response, etc.

Secondary Pathogenic Factors

The pathogenic factors which are secondary in diseases are termed as secondary pathogenic factors.

Phlegm and Retained Fluid

1. Formation of phlegm and retained fluid

Coming from the same source, phlegm and retained fluid are the pathological products caused due to dysbolism of body fluid.Phlegm refers to thick and turbid pathological product while retain fluid refers to the clear and thin one.Phlegm is divided into visible one and invisible one, with the former referring to material sputum that can be seen or heard, and the latter referring to those only with the syndromes of phlegm diseases like struma, subcutaneous nodule and sputum stagnating in the internal organs and channels.Phlegm and retained fluid often arise from six excesses, improper diet, overstrain and over-relaxation and internal injuries caused by seven emotions, which contribute to the internal organs(such as the lung, spleen, kidney and the triple energizer)fail to transform and metabolize water and fluid, therefore resulting in dysbolism and retention of water and fluid.

2. Characteristics of phlegm and retained fluid as pathogenic factors

Once phlegm and retained fluid comes into being, they will flow to anywhere of the body and give rise to a wide range of diseases, as described in *Analysis of the Source and Cause of Miscellaneous Diseases* "Once coming into being, phlegm and retained fluid will flow with circulation of qi to anywhere from the top of the head to the feet, from skin and muscles to the internal organs···so phlegm is the primary pathogenic factor of many diseases and all strange diseases can be originated from phlegm."As phlegm and retained fluid causes a large range of diseases, there is a saying that"all diseases can be owed to phlegm and retained fluid."

Phlegm and retained fluid refer to two different syndromes: phlegm syndrome and retained fluid syndrome.There are different clinical manifestations in accordance with where phlegm stays.For example, phlegm stagnating in the lung causes asthma, cough and coughing up phlegm; phlegm stagnating in the

（二）瘀血

1. 瘀血的形成 瘀血为血液运行障碍、停滞所形成的病理产物。包括离经之血，滞留于经脉、四肢及脏腑之中而未能消散之血液。瘀血是疾病过程中形成的病理产物，又是某些疾病的致病因素。形成原因有气虚、气滞、血寒等致使血行不畅；另有气虚统摄血液不利，或火热迫血妄行，或外伤，致使血溢脉外而为瘀。

2. 瘀血的致病特点 瘀血致病特点极为复杂，可随着瘀血阻滞的部位不同而不同。如瘀阻于心，则胸闷、心前区绞痛、唇青舌紫，瘀血化热则可神昏发狂等；瘀阻于肺，可见胸痛、气促、咯血；瘀阻于肝，可见胁痛、胁下痞块；瘀阻于肠胃，可见吐血或黑便；瘀阻于胞宫，经行不畅，可见痛经、月事不调、经色紫暗有块，或见崩漏；瘀阻于肢体肌肤，可见局部肿痛青紫；瘀阻于脑，脑络不通，可致突然昏倒、不省人事，或留有严重的后遗症，如痴呆、语言謇涩等。瘀血致病证候虽多，但有共同的特点表现：疼痛，或为刺痛，或为刀割，痛处拒按、固定不移，多于夜间加剧；肿块，瘀血不散，久之形成肿块。外伤瘀血，伤处则见青紫色血肿；瘀血积于体内、四肢，患处可及肿块，位置固定，称为癥积；出血，血色多呈紫暗色，或夹有血块；另外可见面色黧黑，口唇及指端紫暗，皮肤甲错，舌色紫暗或有瘀斑，舌下青紫。

（三）结石

1. 结石的形成 结石是指体内某些部位形成并停滞为病的砂石样病理产物或结块。常见的结石有泥砂样结石、圆形或不规则形状的结石、结块样结石（如胃结石）等。结石的成因较为复杂，有些机制目前尚不清楚。比较常见的因素有：饮食不当，饮食偏嗜。喜食肥甘厚味，影响脾胃运化，蕴生湿热，内结于胆，久则可形成胆结石；湿热下注，蕴结于下焦，日久可形成泌尿道结石。若空腹食柿，影响胃的受纳和通降，可形成胃结石。另为外情志不遂，肝气郁结，疏泄失职，胆汁郁结，排泄受阻，日久亦可形成结石。此外，某些地域的水质中含有过量的矿物及杂质等，也可能是促使结石形成的原因之一。

2. 结石的致病特点

（1）多发于肝、肾、胆、胃、膀胱等脏腑：肝气疏泄，关系着胆汁的生成和排泄；肾气的蒸化，影响尿液的生成和排泄，故肝、肾功能失调易生成结石。肝、肾有管道与胆及膀胱相通，而胃、胆、膀胱等管腔性器官，结石易于停留。故结石为病，多为肝、胆、肾、膀胱结石和胃结石。

（2）病程较长，病情轻重不一：结石多为湿热内蕴，日渐煎熬而成，故大多数结石的形成过程缓慢而漫长。由于结石的大小不等，停留部位不一，故临床症状表

heart slows down the circulation of the heart blood, with the manifestations of chest distress and palpitation; phlegm blocking the heart leads to coma and aphronesia(dementia) ; phlegm-fire disturbing the heart causes daftness; phlegm staying in stomach results in stomach qi rising in company with the symptoms of nausea, vomiting and epigastric fullness; phlegm retaining in channels, muscles and bones brings about scrofula, subcutaneous nodule, numb limbs, or hemiplegia, suppurative osteomyelitis and deep multiple abscess; turbid phlegm perturbing the head gives rise to dizziness and mental confusion; and phlegm and qi coagulating in throat causes pharynx obstruction from swallowing in and spitting out. There also betray different manifestations in line with where retained fluid stays. For instance, retained fluid staying in the intestines causes borborygmus; retained fluid staying in chest and hypochondrium leads to abdominal distention and breath shortness and pain when coughing, which is also termed as "pleural fluid retention;" retained fluid staying above the diaphragm results in cough, gasp, reversed flow of qi and inability to lie on the back, swelling body, which is also defined as "thoracic fluid retention;" and retained fluid spreading around the skin manifests hydropic skin, no sweat, achy and heavy body, which is named as "subcutaneous fluid retention." Phlegm and retained fluid both arise from stagnation and aggregation of water and dampness, so the diseases caused by them are often characterized by heaviness, turbidness, stickiness, lingering and aptness to relapse.

Blood Stasis

1. Formation of blood stasis

Blood stasis is the pathological product caused by dysfunction of blood circulation and stagnation of blood, including the blood flowing out of their original vessels and stagnating in channels, limbs, and the internal organs. Blood stasis is the pathological product coming into being in the course of the diseases. It is also the pathogenic factor causing some kinds of diseases. Blood stasis is the result of qi deficiency, qi stagnation and blood cold, all of which slow down circulation of the blood. It is also the result of inability of weak qi in governing blood, or extreme heat abnormally accelerating circulation of blood, or trauma, all of which drive the blood to come out of the vessels.

2. Characteristics of blood stasis

Blood stasis has very complicated characteristics in causing diseases and varies with where the blood stasis stagnates. Blood stasis stagnating in the heart leads to chest distress, colic in precordium, blue lip and purple tongue, and coma and delirium as the result of blood stasis turning into heat. Blood stasis stagnating in the lung results in chest pain, shortness of breath and hemoptysis. Blood stasis stagnating in the liver gives rise to hypochondriac pain and lumps in hypochondria. Blood stasis stagnating in the stomach and intestines manifests the symptoms of hematemesis and black stool. Blood stasis blocking the uterus generates dysmenorrhea, disorder of menstruation and dark menses with lumps, or metrorrhagia and metrostaxis. Blood stasis stagnating in the skin and limbs brings about swelling, sore, and cyanosis. And blood stasis obstructing the brain causes sudden faint and coma, or the severe sequelas like aphronesia and difficulty in speaking as the result of damage of brain collaterals. In spite of a variety of symptoms of the diseases caused by blood stasis, there are the same manifestations like pain, prickling or lancination(stabbing pain), fixed in the same spot and aggravated by pressure and in the nighttime, as well as lumps deriving from the long-time indispersible blood stasis. Blood stasis is caused by trauma presents the manifestation of dark hematoma in the wounded part. When blood stasis stays in the body and limbs, the lump will emerge and fix in the affected part, which is termed as aggregation-accumulation. Dark blood or blood lumps often occur in haemorrhagia. In addition, dark face, lips and finger tips, squamous and dry skin, dark tongue sometimes with ecchymosis, and purple sublingual are also the manifestation of blood stasis.

Calculus

1. Formation of calculus

现差异很大。一般来说，结石小，病情较轻，有的甚至无任何症状；结石过大，则病情较重，症状明显，发作频繁。

（3）阻滞气机，损伤脉络：结石为有形实邪，停留体内，势必阻滞气机，影响气血津液运行，如局部胀痛、水液停聚等。重者，结石嵌顿于狭窄部位，如胆道或输尿管中，气血严重郁阻，常出现腹部绞痛；若损伤脉络，可致出血（如尿血等）。

四、其他致病因素

（一）外伤

枪弹、刀斧、持重努扭等均可造成外伤。轻者引起局部皮肤肌肉瘀血肿痛、出血，或骨折、脱臼等；重则可伤及内脏或出血过多，危及生命。此外，枪弹、金刀伤及皮肤肌肉，治疗不当或再感邪毒，以致溃烂化脓为"金疮"。

（二）烧烫伤

沸水、沸油、烈火、高温物体或气体等均可造成烧烫伤，属火毒致病。轻者引起局部肌肤出现红肿热痛或起水疱；重则可因面积过大，或伤及肌肉组织过深，导致津液大伤，脱水休克，或火毒内攻脏腑，出现烦躁不安、发热、少尿等症，甚至导致死亡。

Calculus is the sandstone-shaped pathological product or agglomeration formed and stagnated in some parts of the body.Sand-shaped,round and irregularly shaped calculus and agglomerated calculus(such as stomach calculus)are the common ones.The cause of formation of calculus is so complicated that some of the mechanism still remain unknown,but improper diet and diet predilection are the common causes.Predilection of greasy,sweat,and strong-flavored food is apt to affect functions of the spleen and stomach in transportation and transformation,and engenders damp-heat,which agglomerates in the gallbladder to form biliary calculus.Downward flow of damp-heat to gather in the lower energizer is prone to produce urinary calculus.Eating persimmon when hungry tends to affect the functions of the stomach for absorbing food and drink and propelling them downward and therefore results in stomach calculus.Besides,depression leading to stagnation of the liver qi will affect the free coursing function of the liver qi,and then bile stagnates and can not excrete smoothly and finally result in calculus.In addition,excessive minerals and impurities in the water in some areas can also lead to calculus.

2. Characteristics of calculus

(1)Calculus is apt to occur in the liver,kidney,gallbladder,stomach,and the urinary bladder

The normal flow of the liver qi helps generate and activate bile,and evaporation of the kidney qi contributes to generation and discharging of urine,so dysfunctions of the liver and kidney are apt to produce calculus.The liver and kidney have the ducts to link them with gallbladder and bladder respectively and the calculus is apt to stay in the lumen organs like stomach,gallbladder and bladder,so most of calculus diseases are those of hepatic calculus,gall-stone,kidney stone,bladder calculi,and stomach stone.

(2)Long disease course

Most of calculus come into being in a long period as they are mostly caused by damp-heat inside, which finally becomes stones after being steamed for a long time.The diseases caused by calculus betray a series of clinical symptoms varying with the size and position of the calculus.In a general way,small calculus presents light symptoms or even no syndrome at all,while large calculus leads to serious diseases with obvious manifestations,which are apt to frequent relapse.

(3)Block qi and impair channels and collaterals

As the tangible pathogen,calculus,once staying in the body,is bound to obstruct qi and affect the circulation of qi,blood,fluid and humor,with the symptoms of distention,pain and retention of water.If the calculus retains in the narrow parts like biliary tract or ureter,it will seriously obstruct the blood and qi, manifesting the symptoms of abdominal colic;or impair the collaterals and lead to haemorrhage like hematuria,etc.

Other Pathogenic Factors

Trauma

Trauma can arise from bullet,knives,axes,carrying heavy things and twisting,etc.In a light case,it will cause blood stasis,distention,pain and hemorrhage of the skin and the muscle around the trauma,or bone fracture and dislocation.In a severe case,it will injure the internal organs or lead to serious hemorrhage to threat the life.In addition,the malpractice or infection of wounds caused by bullet,knife or axe will fester and suppurate and turn into"metal sore".

Burns and scalds

Boiling water,boiling oil,blazing fire and high-temperature objects or gas all can lead to burns and scalds,so they belong to fire poison.In a light case,it will cause red,swelling,hot and pain or blister around the wounded skin.In a serious case,it will injure the muscle in a large scale or in depth to bring about serious impairment of body-fluid,deprivation of body fluid and shock;or retrocession of fire toxin into the internal organs in company with the symptoms of dysphoria,fever,oliguria and even death.

（三）冻伤

过度寒冷，低温的环境下，可使机体发生冻伤，属寒毒致病。局部性冻伤，多发生在手足、耳郭、鼻尖及面颊等易暴露的部位。寒性收引，主凝滞，故而受伤部位初始苍白、冷麻，继之肿胀、青紫、痒痛；血瘀不畅，肌肤失养，故而冻处易溃破腐烂。全身性冻伤，多为阴寒过盛，阻遏阳气，失其温煦与推动作用，可见体温下降、面色苍白、唇舌肢末青紫、反应迟钝、呼吸微弱、脉微欲绝等阳衰之证，此时如不及时救治则可导致死亡。

（四）虫兽伤

虫兽伤包括毒虫、毒蛇、疯狗及野兽等对人体的伤害。这种伤害轻则局部损伤，出现瘙痒、肿痛、破溃、出血等；重则损及内脏，或出血过多而死亡。毒蛇咬伤，可见全身中毒症状，不及时治疗，可致死亡。疯狗咬伤，可发生"狂犬病"，此为危重之症，多不治而亡。

第二节　病　　机

中医病机学是根据以五脏为中心的藏象学说，把局部病变同机体全身状况联系起来，从机体内部脏腑经络之间的相互联系和制约关系，来探讨疾病的发生、发展和转归，从而形成了注重整体联系的病机观。概括起来，主要包括邪正相争、阴阳失调、气机紊乱等基本规律。

一、正邪相争

邪正相争，是指在疾病的发生过程中，机体的抗病能力与致病邪气之间相互斗争。在疾病的发生复杂过程中，始终贯穿着正气与邪气之间的盛衰转化。疾病过程就是正邪相争及其盛衰变化的过程。

（一）正邪相争与发病

正气不足是发病的内在因素。在正常情况下，人体脏腑功能协调，气血充盈，卫外固密，足以抗御邪气的侵袭，病邪便难以侵入，此为"正气存内，邪不可干"。邪气对疾病的发生亦有重要作用。没有邪气的侵袭，机体一般不会发病，并且在一定的条件下，邪气甚至起主导作用，如高温、高压电流、化学毒剂、枪弹杀伤、毒蛇咬伤等，此时即使正气强盛，也难免不被伤害。疫疠在特殊情况下，常常成为疾病发生的决定性因素，因而导致了疾病的大流行。

正邪相搏的胜负，决定疾病的发生与否。正胜则邪退，机体不受邪气的损害，无临床症状和病理体征，即不发病；邪胜则正衰，机体受损，出现临床症状和病理体

Cold Injuries

Excessive cold in cryogenic environment is easy to cause cold injuries, so it is regarded as cold toxin. The partial cold injuries often occur in hands, feet, pinnas of ears, tip of nose and cheek and other part exposed outside. Cold is characterized by contraction and stagnation, so the part injured by cold is pale, cold and numb before turning swelling, dark, itchy and achy. The wounds injured by cold are apt to rupture and decay as a result of stagnation of the blood and dystrophy of skin. Systemic frostbite is a result of excessive cold which blocks yang from warming and pushing forward, with the yang-deficient syndrome of dropping of body temperature, pale face, dark mouth, tongue and the end of limbs, slow response, weak breath and weak pulse. It will lead to death without timely treatment.

Bites of Insects or Animals

Such injuries refer to the bites of poisonous insects, venomous snakes, rabid dogs and wild animals. In a light case, it will cause partial injury in company with the symptoms of itch, sore pain, fester and haemorrhage, etc. In a serious case, it will result in death by seriously damaging the internal organs or bleeding excessively. Bites of venomous snakes will present the symptoms of systemic poisoning and lead to death without prompt treatment. Bites of rabid dogs will give rise to hydrophobia, most of which are extremely serious and cannot be cured and die finally.

Section 2   Pathogenesis

Pathogenesis of TCM is visceral manifestation theory based on the five viscera (the heart, liver, spleen, lung and kidney). It is a pathogenetic concept focusing on the relations of the whole body, which links the pathological changes of the special parts with the situation of the whole body and then discuss the occurrence, development, and prognosis of a disease from the interrelation and mutual restriction among the internal organs and meridians and collaterals. In summary, it includes the key basic principles like the struggle between the healthy qi and pathogenic qi, yin-yang disharmony and disorder of qi, etc.

Struggle between the Healthy Qi and Pathogenic Qi

Struggle between the healthy qi and pathogenic qi refers to the mutual struggle between disease-resistance of the body and pathogenic factors in the course of a disease. Healthy qi and pathogenic qi run through the complicated course of a disease and vary with the changes of exuberance and debilitation. So the course of a disease is also the process of healthy qi struggling with pathogenic qi and their transformation from rising to falling.

Struggle between the Healthy Qi and the Pathogenic Qi and Pathogenesis

Deficiency of the healthy qi is the intrinsic factor leading to a disease. Under normal circumstances, the viscera and bowels harmonize with one another to generate sufficient healthy qi and blood and spread them around the body and form the defensive qi to resist the invasion of evil qi, known as "with sufficiency of healthy qi inside, pathogenic factors have no way to invade the body." Pathogenic qi is also the important factor causes the disease. Without the invasion of pathogenic qi, people are unlikely to be infected with a disease. Under some circumstances, the pathogenic qi even play a leading role in a disease, such as high temperature, high-voltage current, chemical poison, wound caused by bullet and bite of venomous snakes, which will impair the body even though people have sufficient healthy qi. In special situations, the epidemic disease often plays a decisive role in the onset of a disease which becomes pandemic soon.

Whether a disease occurs relies on the result of the struggle between the healthy qi and pathogenic qi. If the healthy qi expels the evil, then the body will be protected from being injured by the evil qi, so there are no clinical symptoms and physiological signs. If the evil qi defeats the healthy qi, then the disease

征，即疾病发生。中医学就从这两个方面的辩证关系出发，建立了发病学的基本观点，既强调了人体正气在发病上的决定作用，又不排除邪气的致病条件，这是中医发病学的基本特点。

（二）正邪盛衰与病邪出入

疾病过程中，正、邪两种力量并非固定不变，而是在其相争的过程中，双方力量对比上发生着消长盛衰的变化。

1. 表邪入里　是指外邪侵入机体，停留于肌表而引发表证，而后内传入里，转化为里证的病理传变过程。说明疾病发展，病情加重。病邪由表入里，大多是由于正气不足，或邪气过盛，致使正不胜邪，邪气入里；或由于失治、误治，表邪不衰，传变入里。如：外感风温初起时，仅出现发热恶寒、头痛鼻塞、运化、咽喉疼痛、脉浮数等表热证，继而出现但热不寒、口渴汗出、咳嗽咯黄痰、脉滑数等邪热壅肺之里证，此为表热证转化为里热证，即表邪入里。

2. 里邪出表　是指病邪由里透达于表的传变过程。此为正气逐渐恢复，邪气逐渐衰败，正气驱邪出表。里邪出表预示疾病趋愈，病情好转。如热邪致病，内热炽盛，出现口渴烦热、舌红苔黄、脉洪大等里热症状，然汗出而热解，说明邪气由里出表，机体即可恢复健康。

（三）正邪盛衰与虚实变化

疾病过程中正邪相争的运动变化贯穿于疾病发展变化的全过程。体内邪正双方力量对比的盛衰，决定着患病机体的虚与实两种不同的病理变化。实证是指邪气的致病力强盛而正气的抗病能力未衰，临床上出现一系列病理性反映比较剧烈的、有余的证候。实证常见于外感六淫和疠气致病的初期和中期，或由于湿、痰、水饮、食积、瘀血等病理产物滞留体内而导致的病证；虚证是指正气虚损，临床上表现一系列虚弱、衰退和不足的证候。虚证常见于疾病的后期和慢性疾病过程中。

在复杂的疾病发生过程中，邪正双方力量的对比经常发生变化，因而疾病在一定条件下也可发生由实转虚和因虚致实的病理变化。例如，病本在表，由于治疗不当，护理失宜，导致病情迁延不愈，正气日损，可逐渐出现肌肉消瘦、纳呆食少、面色不华、气短乏力等肺脾功能衰减之虚象，此为由实转虚；又如由于脏腑生理功能低下，产生了气滞、瘀血、痰饮、水湿等实邪停留体内为害，此为由虚转实。

will occur and the body will be impaired with some clinical symptoms and physiological signs. It is from the dialectical relations between these two aspects that TCM establishes the basic concept of pathogenesis—the basic concept both stressing the decisive role of the healthy qi of the body in defending diseases and considering the requirement of pathogenic factors. It is the basic feature of pathogenesis of TCM.

Vicissitude of Healthy Qi and Pathogenic Qi and Inwardness and Outwardness of Pathogenic Qi

During the course of a disease, the healthy qi and pathogenic qi remain changed to cause their exuberance and debilitation during the struggle.

1. Exterior pathogen entering the interior

It refers to the physiological course of a disease turning from the exterior syndrome caused by the invasion of the exogenous pathogen in the surface into the interior syndrome resulted from the inward invasion of the disease. It indicates the development and aggravation of the disease. The inward invasion of the exterior pathogen mostly owes to either the deficiency of the healthy qi or excess of the pathogenic qi, as a result of which the healthy qi fails to expel the evil and leads to the inward invasion of the evil; or lack of timely treatment and mis-treatment, as a result of which the still excessive exterior pathogen transmits to the interior. For example, a patient who suffers from exogenous febrile disease often has the exterior heat syndrome of fever and aversion to cold, headache, stuffy nose, a sore throat, superficial and rapid pulse at the beginning, followed by the pathogenic heat retenting in the lung syndrome of only fever without chill, thirst, sweating and coughing up yellow sputum, and rapid and slippery pulse, which manifest that the exterior pathogen has transferred into the interior.

2. Interior pathogen moving out to the exterior

It refers to the process of pathogenic factor turning from the interior into the exterior. It indicates the gradual recovery of the healthy qi and wane of the pathogenic qi; as a result, the healthy qi expels the pathogenic qi to the exterior. Therefore, interior pathogen moving out to the exterior presages the improvement of a disease. The diseases caused by heat evil often have the manifestation of excessive endogenous heat, with the symptoms of thirst, red tongue, yellow tongue coating, and surging pulse. However, the heat discharging with sweat demonstrates that the pathogenic qi turns from the interior to the exterior and the patient will recuperate soon.

Vicissitude of Healthy Qi and Pathogenic Qi and Transformation of Deficiency and Excess

The motion changes during the struggle between the healthy qi and pathogenic qi run through the whole course of a disease. Vicissitude of the healthy qi and pathogenic qi determines the two physiological changes of deficiency and excess in the body of patients. Excess syndrome refers to a series of drastic and excessive physiological manifestations resulting from the struggle between the strong pathogenicity of pathogenic qi and the proportional disease-resistance of healthy qi. It often appears at the beginning or in the middle of the course of diseases which caused by the six excesses or epidemic pathogens. It also refers to the syndromes arising from stagnation of such pathological products as damp, phlegm, retained fluid, dyspepsia, and blood stasis. Deficiency syndrome refers to a series of the clinical syndromes of weakness, regression and shortage as the result of deficiency or loss of the healthy qi. It often emerges in the late stage of the course of a disease or in the chronic diseases.

During the course of the complicated diseases, the power and the strength of the healthy qi and pathogenic qi often changes, so the diseases can be transferred from the excess syndrome to the deficiency syndrome or reversely. For instance, a excessive exterior disease can be turned into a deficient disease in case that it does not get proper and timely treatment and nursing, which leads to delay of curing the disease, gradual impairment of the healthy qi and weakening of the spleen and stomach with the symptoms of amyotrophy, indigestion, dark complexion, short breath and tiredness, etc. On the contrary, the weak functions

（四）正邪盛衰与疾病转归

在疾病的发生、发展过程中，由于邪正双方的斗争，其力量对比不断发生消长盛衰的变化，这种变化对疾病转归起着决定性的作用。在疾病过程中，正气奋起抗邪，正气渐趋强盛，而邪气渐趋衰减，疾病向好转和痊愈方向发展的病机变化，此为正胜邪退；若疾病过程中，邪气亢盛，正气虚弱，机体抗邪无力，疾病向恶化、危重，甚至向死亡方面转化，此为邪胜正衰。此外，疾病过程中，邪正双方势均力敌，此时，出现正邪对峙，或正虚邪恋，或邪气去而正气未复。某些急性疾病慢性化，或留下后遗症，或慢性病久治不愈均与此有关。

二、阴阳失调

阴阳失调是阴阳之间失去平衡协调的总称，是疾病发生、发展变化的内在根据，是疾病的基本病机之一。

（一）阴阳盛衰

1. 阳盛则热　阳盛是指机体在疾病过程中所出现的阳气病理性偏亢、脏腑经络机能亢进、机体反应性增强、邪热过剩的病理变化。

阳盛则热的病机特点是阳盛而阴未虚或亏虚不明显，临床表现为实热证。阳以热、动、燥为其特点，故阳气偏盛则表现为壮热、烦躁、舌红苔黄、脉数等热证，故曰"阳盛则热"。由于阳的一方偏盛会导致阴的一方相对偏衰，所以除上述临床表现外，同时还会出现口渴、小便短少、大便干燥等阴液不足的症状。

2. 阴盛则寒　阴盛是指机体在疾病过程中所出现的阴气病理性偏盛、脏腑经络机能障碍或减退、机体反应性下降、热量耗伤过多、阴寒过盛以及代谢产物积聚的病理变化。

阴盛则寒的病机特点是阴盛而阳未虚或虚损不甚，临床表现为寒证。阴以寒、静、湿为其特点，故阴偏盛则表现为形寒、肢冷、喜暖、口淡不渴、苔白、脉迟等寒证，故曰"阴盛则寒"。由于阴的一方偏盛会导致阳的一方相对偏衰，所以除上述临床表现外，同时还会出现恶寒、溲清、便溏等阳气不足的症状。

3. 阳虚则寒　阳虚是指机体在疾病过程中所出现的阳气虚损、失于温煦、机能减退或衰弱的病理变化。形成阳偏衰的主要原因，多由于先天禀赋不足，或后天饮食失养，或劳倦内伤，或久病损伤阳气所致。阳虚则寒，虽也可见到面色㿠白、畏寒肢冷、舌淡、脉迟等寒象，但还有喜静蜷卧、小便清长、下利清谷等虚象。

阳虚则寒与阴盛则寒，不仅在病机上有所区别，而且在临床表现方面也有不同：前者是虚而有寒，后者是以寒为主，虚象不明显。

4. 阴虚则热　阴虚是指机体在疾病过程中所出现阴气不足、阴不制阳、阳气相

of the internal organs are apt to give rise to stagnation of sthenic pathogenic products like stagnant qi, blood stasis, phlegm, retained fluid and water damp in the body, therefore turning from an asthenic disease to a sthenic one.

Vicissitude of Healthy Qi and Pathogenic Qi and Prognosis of the Disease

The struggle between the healthy qi and pathogenic qi at the onset and during the development of a disease is prone to bring about vicissitudes of the power and strength of the two sides, which makes a decisive role in the further prognosis of the disease. During the course, if the healthy qi rises to resist the pathogenic qi and gradually increases to impair the latter, it will lead to improvement of or recovery from the illness, which reveals the healthy qi defeating the pathogenic qi. But if the pathogenic qi becomes excessive to weaken the healthy qi and its disease-resistance, then it will result in aggravation of the illness or even the death of the patient, which manifests the pathogenic qi triumphs over the healthy qi. In addition, if the healthy qi and pathogenic qi are even in power and strength, it will cause the confrontation of these two kinels of qi, or asthenic healthy qi with pathogen lingering, or the pathogenic qi vanished with the healthy qi unrecovered. Moreover, it is also one of the causes that some acute diseases turn into the acute ones or generate the sequels or that some of the chronic diseases are uneasy to be cured after long treatment.

Yin-yang Disharmony

Yin-yang disharmony refers to a general term for all kinds of pathological changes due to imbalance and incoordination of yin and yang. It is the intrinsic basis of occurrence, development and transformation of a disease and one of the basic pathogenesis of a disease.

Exuberance and Debilitation of Yin and Yang

1. Predominance of yang gives rise to heat syndrome

Yang excess refers to the pathological changes occurring in the course of a disease, including hyperactivity of yang, hyperfunction of the viscera and bowels and meridians and collaterals, increase in reactiveness of the body and excessive pathogenic heat.

Yang excess generating heat syndrome is characterized by the overabundance of yang without deficiency of yin or with light deficiency of yin, clinically manifesting excessive heat syndrome. Yang is characterized by heat, dynamic and dryness, so yang excess presents the heat syndrome of high fever, dysphoria, red tongue with yellow tongue coating, and swift pulse, so termed as "predominance of yang gives rise to heat syndrome." In addition, as the yang excess also leads to the deficiency of yin, it also accompanies the yin-deficient syndrome of thirst, short and little urine and dry stool.

2. Predominance of yin brings on cold syndrome

Yin excess refers to the pathological changes occurring in the course of a disease, including hyperactivity of yin, hypofunction or dysfunction of the viscera and bowels and meridians and collaterals, and excessive pathogenic yin, decline of reactiveness of the body, and accumulation of metabolism as the result of consumption of too much heat and excessive yin.

Excessive yin generating cold syndrome is characterized by the overabundance of yin without deficiency of yang or with light deficiency of yang, clinically manifesting excessive cold syndrome. Yin is characterized by cold, static and wet, so yin excess presents the cold syndrome of cold limbs, preference of warm, tastelessness and aposia, white tongue coating and slow pulse, so termed as "predominance of yin brings on cold syndrome." In addition, as the yin excess also leads to yang deficiency, it also accompanies the yang-deficient symptoms of aversion to cold, clear urine and loose stool, etc.

3. Yang deficiency leads to cold

Yang deficiency refers to the pathological changes of hypofunction of the internal organs as the result of the deficiency and loss of warming yang during the course of a disease. The formation of yang deficiency

对偏盛的病理变化，临床表现为虚热证，故曰"阴虚则热"。由于阴液不足以及滋养、宁静功能减退，以致阳气相对偏盛。如五心烦热、骨蒸潮热、面红目赤、消瘦、盗汗、咽干口燥、舌红少苔、脉细数无力等，即是阴虚则热的表现。

阴虚则热与阳盛则热的病机不同，其临床表现也有所区别：前者是虚而有热，后者是以热为主，虚象并不明显。

（二）阴阳互损

阴阳互损，是指在阴或阳任何一方虚损的前提下，病变发展影响到相对的一方，形成阴阳两虚的病理变化。

1. 阴损及阳　由于阴液亏损，阳气生化而不足，或无所依附而耗散，导致阳气不足，从而在阴虚的基础上又出现阳虚，形成了以阴虚为主的阴阳两虚的病理变化。例如，临床常见的遗精、盗汗、失血等慢性消耗性病证，严重地耗伤了人体阴精，因而化生阳气的物质基础不足，发展到一定阶段就会出现自汗、畏冷、下利清谷等阳虚之候。

2. 阳损及阴　由于阳气虚损，无阳则阴不能生，导致阴液的生化不足，从而在阳虚的基础上又出现阴虚，形成了以阳虚为主的阴阳两虚的病理变化。例如，临床上常见的水肿一病，其病机主要为阳气不足，温煦推动不利，水液停滞，溢于肌肤所致。但其病变发展，则又可因阳气不足，化生功能减退，出现形体消瘦、烦躁，甚则筋无所养而抽搐等阴虚症状，转化为阳损及阴的阴阳两虚证。

（三）阴阳格拒

阴阳格拒是由于某些原因引起阴或阳的一方偏盛至极，而壅遏于内，将另一方排斥于外，迫使阴阳之间不相维系所致。阴阳格拒是阴阳失调中比较特殊的一类病机，包括阴盛格阳和阳盛格阴两方面。表现为真寒假热或真热假寒等复杂的病理现象。

1. 阴盛格阳（真寒假热）　是指阴寒过盛，阳气被格拒于外，出现内真寒外假热的一种病理变化。如寒性疾病发展到严重阶段，临床上除有阴寒过盛之面色苍白、精神萎靡、畏寒蜷卧、小便清长、下利清谷、脉微细欲绝等症状外，又见身反不恶寒（但欲盖衣被）、面颊泛红、口渴（但喜热饮）等假热之象。

2. 阳盛格阴（真热假寒）　是指邪热过盛，深伏于里，阳气被遏，闭郁于内，不能透达于外，出现真热假寒的一种病理变化。如热性病发展到极期，临床上除有阳热极盛之面红、气粗、心胸烦热、胸腹扪之灼热、口干舌燥、舌红等症状外，又见四肢厥冷（但不喜加衣被）、表情淡漠、困倦懒言等假寒之象。

is primarily due to insufficiency of natural endowment, or improper diets, or injuries of the internal organs arising from tiredness, or impairment of yang as a result of suffering a disease for a long time. Though it also has the cold syndrome of bright pale complexion, fear of cold, cold limbs, pale tongue and slow pulse, it also manifests the deficient syndrome of preference of quietness and curling up, clear abundant urine and clear-food diarrhea, etc.

Cold syndrome caused by deficiency of yang is different from that caused by excessive yin in terms of pathogenesis and clinical manifestations. In the former case, the cold arises from asthenia, while in the latter case, the cold is the main syndrome, without too obvious asthenic syndrome.

4. Yin deficiency leads to heat

Yin deficiency refers to the pathological changes of relative hyperactivity of yang due to the failure of yin in restricting yang as the result of insufficient yin qi during the course of a disease, clinically manifesting deficiency-heat syndrome, so known as "yin deficiency leads to heat." Insufficient yin fluid and weakening of its nourishing and static function will lead to the relative overabundance of yang qi, with the symptoms of vexing heat in the chest, palms and soles, bone-steaming tidal fever, red face and eyes, emaciation, night sweating, dry throat and mouth, red tongue with little tongue fur and weakly thin and swift pulse, etc.

Heat syndrome caused by yin deficiency is different from that caused by excessive yang in terms of pathogenesis and clinical manifestations. In the former case, the heat arises from asthenia, while in the latter case, the heat is the main syndrome and without obvious asthenic syndrome.

Mutual Detriment of Yin and Yang

Mutual detriment of yin and yang refers to the pathological changes of deficiency of both yin and yang as the result of aggravation of the deficiency of one party.

1. Detriment to yin affects yang

It refers to the pathological change of dual deficiency of yin and yang with priority to yin deficiency as the result of consumption of yin fluid failing to generating and carrying yang qi and then leading to secondary yang deficiency based on primary yin deficiency. For example, spermatorrhea, night sweating, hemorrhage and other chronic consumptive symptoms will seriously deplete yin fluid. Therefore, the material base for engendering and transforming of yang qi is insufficient. And when it develops to a certain stage, a series of yang deficiency symptoms like spontaneous perspiration, fear of cold and clear-food diarrhea will come into being.

2. Detriment to yang affects yin

It refers to the pathological change of dual deficiency of yin and yang with priority to yang deficiency as the result of consumption of yang qi failing to generating and transforming yin fluid and then leading to secondary yin deficiency based on primary yang deficiency. For example, the primary pathogenesis of edema is due to insufficient yang qi failing to warm and carry the fluid, which leads to it stagnating in the body and then overflowing to the skin. But with its aggravation, yin deficiency symptoms like emaciation, dysphoria and hyperspasmia will occur as the result of weakening functions of generating, transforming and nourishing of yang qi due to its deficiency. Even worse, it may turn into the syndrome of dual deficiency of both yin and yang arising from detriment to yang affecting yin.

Repulsion of Yin and Yang

Yin-yang repulsion refers to a serious pathological state in which extremely excessive yin or yang in the interior forces the other side to spread outward and lose their interaction. It is a special pathogenesis caused by yin-yang disharmony, including exuberant yin repelling yang and exuberant yang rebelling yin, which manifests a complicated pathological phenomena including true cold with false heat and true heat with false cold.

1. Exuberant yin repelling yang(true cold with false heat)

（四）阴阳转化

在疾病发展过程中，阴阳失调还可表现为阴阳的相互转化。

1. 由阳转阴　疾病的本质为阳气偏盛，但阳气亢盛到一定程度，就会向阴的方向转化。如某些急性外感性疾病，初期可以见到高热、口渴、胸痛、咳嗽、舌红、苔黄等一些热邪亢盛的表现，属于阳证。由于治疗不当或邪毒太盛等原因，可突然出现体温下降、四肢厥逆、冷汗淋漓、脉微欲绝等阴寒危象。

2. 由阴转阳　疾病的本质为阴气偏盛，但阴气亢盛到一定程度，就会向阳的方向转化。如感冒初期，可以出现恶寒重发热轻、头身疼痛、骨节疼痛、鼻塞流涕、无汗、咳嗽、苔薄白、脉浮紧等风寒束表之象，属于阴证。如治疗失误，或因体质等因素，可以发展为高热、汗出、心烦、口渴、舌红、苔黄、脉数等阳热亢盛之候。

（五）阴阳亡失

1. 亡阳　是指机体的阳气发生突然脱失，而致全身机能突然严重衰竭的一种病理变化。一般地说，亡阳多由于邪盛、正不敌邪、阳气突然脱失所致；也可由于素体阳虚、正气不足、疲劳过度等多种原因，或过用汗法、汗出过多、阳随阴泄、阳气外脱所致。慢性消耗性疾病的亡阳，多由于阳气的严重耗散、虚阳外越所致，其临床表现多见大汗淋漓、手足逆冷、精神疲惫、神情淡漠，甚则昏迷、脉微欲绝等一派阳气欲脱之象。

2. 亡阴　是指由于机体阴液发生突然性的大量消耗或丢失，而致全身功能严重衰竭的一种病理变化。一般地说，亡阴多由于热邪炽盛，或邪热久留，大量煎灼阴液所致。其临床表现多见汗出不止而黏、四肢温和、渴喜冷饮、身体干瘪、皮肤皱折、眼眶深陷、精神烦躁或昏迷谵妄、脉细数疾无力，或脉洪大按之无力。

亡阴和亡阳，在病机和临床征象等方面，虽然有所不同，但由于机体的阴和阳存在着互根互用的关系。阴亡，则阳无所依附而浮越；阳亡，则阴无以化生而耗竭。故亡阴可以迅速导致亡阳，亡阳也可继而出现亡阴，最终导致"阴阳离决、精气乃绝"，生命活动终止而死亡。

It refers to the pathological changes of true cold with false heat as the result of the excessive cold yin repelling yang to the exterior.Such situation will occur when the cold disease deteriorates to a serious extent,clinically not only with the true cold symptoms of pale complexion,listlessness,fear of cold and curling up,clear abundant urine,clear-food diarrhea,thin and weak pulse,but also with the false heat symptoms of not aversion to cold(but want to put more clothes or cover quilt),red cheek and thirst(only like hot water).

2. Exuberant yang repelling yin(true heat with false cold)

It refers to a pathological change of true heat in the interior with pseudo-cold manifestations.The cause is the heat is so excessive and lurks so deeply inside the body that it leads to yang qi being contained and obstructed in the interior and then failing to permeate to the exterior smoothly and thoroughly. Such situation will occur when the heat disease deteriorates to the extreme,clinically not only with the true heat symptoms of red complexion,rough breath,dysphoria,scorching thorax-abdomen,dry tongue and mouth,and red tongue,but also with the pseudo-cold manifestations of cold limbs(but not want to put clothes or cover quilt),indifferent expression,tiredness,sleepiness and un-desire to speak.

Mutual Conversion of Yin and Yang

Mutual conversion of yin and yang is another manifestation of yin-yang disharmony in the development of a disease.

1. Conversion from yang to yin

Although excessive yang is the cause of a disease,it will be converted into yin when getting to the peak.For example,some of the acute diseases caused by the exogenetic pathogens manifest some excessive heat symptoms of high fever,thirst,check pain,coughing,red tongue with yellow fur at the beginning, which belongs to yang syndrome.But it finally will present the dangerous cold-yin syndrome of sudden drop in body temperature,cold limbs,cold sweat and extremely weak pulse in case of improper treatment or serious invasion of the pathogens.

2. Conversion from yin to yang

Although excessive yin is the cause of a disease,it will be converted into yang when getting to the peak.For example,in the beginning of the cold,it often accompanies the wind-cold fettering the exterior syndrome of heavy aversion to cold but light fever,headache and body pain,joint pain,stuffy and running nose,anhidrosis,coughing,thin and pale fur and floating and tight pulse,which belongs to yin syndrome. But it will present the excessive heat symptoms of high fever,sweat,dysphoria,thirst,red tongue with yellow fur and rapid pulse in case of improper treatment or other factors like of constitution.

Collapse of Yin and Yang

1. Collapse of yang

It refers to a pathological change where yang qi is suddenly exhausted,resulting in abrupt failure of bodily functions.Generally,collapse of yang is often due to failure of the healthy qi to defeating the excessive pathogens and sudden depletion of yang.It also can be owed to constitutional yang weakness,insufficient of the healthy qi,overfatigue,or excessive diaphoresis therapy resulting in too much sweating and then yang qi exhaustion outside along with yin depletion.In the chronic wasting diseases,collapse of yang primarily arises from severe yang consumption and its floating outside,mostly with the clinical manifestations of profuse perspiration,cold limbs,fatigue,indifferent expression,and even with coma and extremely weak pulse and etc.

2. Collapse of yin

It refers to a pathological change caused by sudden massive depletion or loss of fluid leading to a serious collapse of bodily functions.Generally,collapse of yin is often due to excessive heat,or pathogenic heat stagnating to consume a great quantity of yin-fluid,with the clinical manifestations of dripping and

三、气机失调

气机失调是指疾病过程中，由于致病因素的作用导致脏腑气机即升降出入运动失调的病理状态。临床中气机失调病变不外乎升降不及、升降太过、升降反常三类。

1. 升降不及　是指由气机升降作用减弱所产生的病理状态。多由脏腑虚弱，运行无力，或气机阻滞，运行不畅所致。如脾气主升，肺主肃降，脾虚则清阳不升，而头晕、便溏；肺虚则失宣肃，而呼吸少气，咳嗽气促；大肠传送糟粕，以通为顺，如腑气不足，传导不利，可出现糟粕停滞而便秘。以上均为升降不及所致。

2. 升降太过　是指气机升降作用过强，超出了正常范围所产生的病理状态。如胃、小肠、大肠均以通为顺，但通降太过，就会出现大便溏泻，甚则滑脱不禁；又如肝气主升，若升发太过，则可出现肝气上逆、肝阳上亢、肝火上炎等证。

3. 升降反常　是指气机升降运行与其正常趋势相反所产生的病理状态，即当升反降、当降反逆。如脾气不升，中气下陷，则见泄泻、脱肛、胃或子宫下垂；胃气不降，则见呃逆、嗳气甚则呕吐等症；肝气不疏，则见肝气郁结。

（郝伟欣　徐慧媛）

sticky sweat, warm limbs, thirst and preference of cold drinks, withered body, wrinkling skin, deep-sunk eyes, dysthesia, or coma and delirium, and weak, thin, rapid pulse, or surging pulse but no signal when pressed.

Yin and yang inter-dependent with and mutual promotes each other. Collapse of yin deprives yang of material base and leads to floating of yang, while collapse of yang deprives yin of material source and results in exhaustion of yin. So the collapse of yin or yang can quickly bring about collapse of the other side and finally gives rise to death because of dissociation of yin and yang and exhaustion of the vital essence.

Disorder of Qi Movement

Disorder of qi movement refers to a pathological state of the disorder of movements (upward, downward, inward and outward) of the viscera and bowels due to the pathogenic factors. It clinically manifests as insufficiency of ascending and descending, or excess of ascending and descending, or abnormality of ascending and descending.

1. Insufficiency of ascending and descending

It refers to a pathological state of the dysfunction of qi in ascending and descending, which primarily arises from too weakness of the viscera and bowels to move or stagnation of qi unable to flow smoothly. For example, since the spleen governs ascending and the lung governs descending, spleen deficiency will leads to the failure of rising yang, with the symptoms of dizziness and loose stool, while the lung deficiency will result in the failure in descending qi in company with asthenic breathing, cough and shortness of breath. As the large intestine controls transportation and discharging of dross and should be kept unobstructed, qi deficiency of it will give rise to retard of transportation and constipation as the result of stagnation of dross. All the above cases are the results of insufficiency of ascending and descending.

2. Excess of ascending and descending

It refers to a pathological state of hyperfunction of the viscera and bowels in ascending and descending. For instance, as the large intestine and the small intestine both govern emptying the dross, hyperfunctions of them will lead to diarrhea and even slippage of stool. And the liver governs ascending, its ascending excessively can bring about the syndromes of liver qi flow upward, ascendant hyperactivity of liver yang and liver fire flaming upward.

3. Abnormality of ascending and descending

It refers to a pathological state of reverse motion of qi movement. For example, descending when it should have ascended and ascending when it should have descended. The failure of upwardness of spleen qi and sinking of the middle qi causes diarrhoea, rectocele, gastroptosis and hysteroptosis. Failure of downwardness of stomach qi leads to hiccup, belching, and even vomiting. Failure of dispersion of liver qi generates stagnation of liver qi.

(Wu Qunli   Zhang Wen)

第四章　四诊八纲及辨证

第一节　四　　诊

四诊，是指望、闻、问、切四种诊病的方法。四诊是中医学独具特色的诊断疾病方法，各有其独特作用，临床中必须综合运用，才能为正确认识疾病所用，称之为"四诊合参"。

一、望诊

望诊是医生用眼睛观察病人的神、色、形、态、舌象及分泌物和排泄物等变化，获得诊断疾病之依据，并判断、估计疾病的轻重、性质以及预后的一种诊病手段。望诊须在充足的自然光线下进行，结合病情，有步骤、有重点地仔细观察。一般分全身望诊和局部望诊。

（一）全身望诊

全身望诊主要是通过观察病人的精神、面色、形态等整体表现，从而对病性的表里、寒热、虚实与病情的轻重缓急产生总体认识。

1. 望神　神，广义是指人体生命活动的外在表现，狭义是指神志、意识、思维活动。望神，即是通过观察人体生命活动的整体表现来判断病情。通过观察神的变化，推测病人精气的盛衰、病情的轻重、疾病的发展、预后及转归。神的表现一般分为四种：

（1）有神：表现为神志清楚，表情自然，面色荣润，目光明亮，语言清晰，反应灵敏，精力充沛，呼吸匀畅，体态自如，肌肉丰满等。表示正气充足，脏腑功能未衰，或病情轻浅，预后良好。

（2）少神：精神不足，动作迟缓，气短懒言，反应迟钝，面色不华。提示正气

CHAPTER FOUR   FOUR EXAMINATIONS, EIGHT PRINCIPLES, AND SYNDROME DIFFERENTIATION

Section 1   Four Examinations

The"four examinations"is a collective term for inspection,listening and smelling,inquiry,and palpation.It is the unique diagnostic method of TCM,each having its own specific functions.Comprehensive application of the four examinations is highly valued because it is the premise of making accurate acquaintance and diagnose of a disease,which also known as"correlation of all four examinations."

Inspection

Inspection is one of the four diagnostic examinations,including observing the patient's mental state, facial expression,complexion,physical condition,condition of the tongue and secretions,from which the basic information of a disease can be obtained and then the seriousness,nature,and prognosis of the disease can be judged and estimated.Inspection should be conducted in sufficient natural light.When conducting an inspection,doctors should combine the patient's condition with careful observations and focuses in a good procedure.It is composed of inspection of the whole body and inspection of special parts of the body.

Inspection of the Whole Body

Inspection of the whole body means to get a general understanding of the disease,including its nature of exterior or interior,cold or heat,and deficiency or excess as well as its conditions,through observing the whole manifestations of the patient such as the mental state,facial expression,complexion,and physical conditions.

1. Inspection of vitality

In a broad sense,the vitality refers to the outward manifestations of human life activities.In the narrow sense,it refers to the mental spirit,consciousness and thinking activities.Inspection of the vitality means to estimate the condition of a disease through observing the overall manifestations of life activities. Through observing the changes of the vitality,doctors can conclude not only the condition of the essential qi(exuberance or debilitation)but also the status(mild or severe),development and prognosis of the disease.The vitality consists of the four parts as follows:

(1)Presence of vitality has the manifestations of normal mental state,natural facial expression,ruddy complexion,luminous eyes,articulation,prompt and flexible action,vigorousness,smooth breathing,and plump muscles,all of which present the sufficiency of the healthy qi and normal functions of the viscera and bowels,or the mild disease with a good prognosis.

(2)Lack of vitality presents low spirit,slow action,short breath and no desire to speak,blunted response and lusterless complexion.It is often seen in the deficiency syndromes indicating insufficiency of the healthy qi and dysfunction of the viscera and bowels.

不足，脏腑功能失调，见于虚证。

（3）失神：表现为神识不清，或神昏谵语，或面色晦暗，目光呆滞，呼吸异常，循衣摸床，撮空理线，手撒尿遗，是精损气亏的表现。

（4）假神：是指患者出现精神暂时好转的假象。常见于大病、久病、重病的病人，已到病危阶段，突然出现精神好转，语言洪亮。此为精气衰竭已极，阴不敛阳，阳气无所依附而外越之象。古人将其比喻为"残灯复明"、"回光返照"。

2. 望色   望色是指通过观察病人皮肤的颜色光泽变化来了解病情的诊病方法。

皮肤色泽是脏腑气血的外荣。颜色的变化可反映不同脏腑的病证和疾病的不同性质；光泽的变化即肤色的荣润或枯槁，可反映脏腑精气的盛衰。由于面部气血充盛，且皮肤薄嫩，色泽变化易于显露，故望色主要指望面部的色泽。正常人面色微黄，红润而有光泽。由于体质禀赋的不同，气候条件与生活环境等因素，亦可出现偏红、偏白的差异，只要是荣润光泽即为正常。病色是指人体在疾病状态时的面部色泽主要有青、黄、赤、白、黑五种。

（1）白色，主虚、主寒、主血虚证：白色为气血虚弱不能荣养面部的表现。如面色㿠白而浮肿，多为阳气不足；面色淡白而消瘦，多属营血亏损；面色青白，多为寒证；面色苍白，多属阳气虚脱，或失血过多；若突然面色苍白，冷汗淋漓，多为阳气暴脱之危证。

（2）赤色，主热证：赤色为热盛之证。血得热而行，热盛则血脉充盈，血色上荣，故面色赤红。热证有实热、虚热之别。实热证可见满面通红，多伴发热、口渴、便秘等；虚热证仅见两颧嫩红，多伴午后发热、盗汗、五心烦热等。此外，若在病情危重之时，面红如妆者，多为戴阳证，是精气衰竭、阴不敛阳、虚阳上越所致，属真寒假热之证。

（3）黄色，主虚证、湿证：黄色是多为脾失健运、水湿不化，或水谷精微不得化生气血，致使肌肤失于充养所致。如面色淡黄多属脾胃气虚；面色发黄而且虚浮，多属脾虚失运，湿邪内停所致。黄而鲜明如橘皮色者，属阳黄，为湿热熏蒸所致；黄而晦暗如烟熏者，属阴黄，为寒湿郁阻所致。

（4）青色，主寒证、主痛证、主瘀血证、主惊风证：青色为经脉阻滞，气血不通之象。寒主收引主凝滞，寒盛而留于血脉，则气滞血瘀，故面色发青；经脉气血不通，不通则痛，故青色也可见于痛证。如面色青黑或苍白淡青，多属阴寒内盛；面色青灰，口唇青紫，多属心血瘀阻，血行不畅；小儿面色青紫，以鼻柱、两眉间及口唇四周明显，是惊风先兆。

（5）黑色，主肾虚证、水饮证、血瘀证：黑为阴寒水盛之色。肾阳虚衰，水饮

(3) Loss of vitality manifests unconsciousness, coma and delirium, dark complexion, dull looking, abnormal breath, carphology, uracratia, all of which show the essence impairment and qi deficiency.

(4) False vitality refers to pseudo appearance of the transient improvement in spirit of the patient. It often emerges in the critical stage of patients with serious or long-term diseases, with manifestations of sudden loud speaking and good spirit. Such phenomena indicate the extreme exhaustion of the essential qi and yin failing to restrain yang, which floats upward. It was called as "the last flicker of life in a dying man," or "the last radiance of the setting sun" in the ancient time.

2. Inspection of complexion

Inspection of the complexion is the diagnostic method used to know the condition of a disease through observing the patient's changes of brightness and color of the skin.

Color and luster of skin is the outward manifestation of the blood and qi in the viscera and bowels. The change of skin color can reflect the different syndromes of the internal organs and the nature of diseases. While the change of skin luster refers to the bright or withered condition of the complexion, which can show the status, exuberance or debilitation, of the essential qi of the internal organs. As the changes of color and luster can be easily exposed in the face where there is the thinnest and tenderest skin and filled with qi and blood, inspection of the complexion primarily refers to observe the color and luster of the face. The healthy people have ruddy but little yellowish and lustrous facial complexion. The bright and lustrous facial complexion is the manifestation of health even though it is a little bit white or red due to the physical conditions, constitutional factors, climatic conditions and living environments. Morbid complexion refers to the five primary morbid facial complexions in the course of disease, namely blue, yellow, red, pale, and dark color.

(1) Pale complexion

It is the manifestation of deficiency syndrome, cold syndrome, and blood deficiency syndrome.

Pale complexion manifests the blood and qi cannot nourish and moisten the face due to their deficiency. Bright pale complexion with dropsy presents the deficiency of yang qi. Pale white complexion with emaciation mostly reveals the depletion of nutrient blood. Bluish white complexion manifests cold syndrome. Pale complexion often shows the collapse of yang qi or loss of excessive bleeding. The occurrence of sudden pale complexion and cold profuse perspiration are the critical manifestations of violent collapse of yang qi.

(2) Red complexion

It is the manifestation of heat syndrome, particularly the excessive one, as heat accelerates the circulation of blood and facilitates it to flow upward to nourish and moisten the face. Heat syndrome is composed of excess heat and deficiency heat. Excess heat syndrome often shows flush red all over, often concurrently with fever, thirst, and constipation. While deficiency heat syndrome presents pink cheeks, often concurrently with afternoon fever, night sweating and vexing heat in the chest, palms, and soles. In addition, the face as red as blushed with powders manifests the upcast yang syndrome in the critical stage of a serious disease. It indicates the exhaustion of the essential qi and yin failing to restrain yang so that the deficient yang becomes outcast. It belongs to the syndrome of true cold with false heat.

(3) Yellow complexion

It is the manifestations of the deficiency syndrome and dampness syndrome.

Yellow facial complexion arises from the failure of the spleen in transporting and transforming water and dampness, or its failure in transforming the water and food essence into qi and blood so that the skin cannot get nourished. Yellowish facial complexion often manifests the deficiency of the spleen and stomach qi. Yellow facial complexion with edema presents internal retention of dampness as the result of the spleen failing in transportation. The yellow complexion as bright as orange peel can be seen in yang jaundice re-

不化，气血不畅，经脉肌肤失于濡养故见黑色。面色黧黑，兼见唇甲紫暗，多为肾阳衰微，阴寒凝滞或心血瘀阻；目眶周围色黑，眼睑浮肿，多为肾虚水泛；面黑而肌肤甲错，多为瘀血；面色青黑，且剧痛者，多为寒凝瘀阻。

3．望形态

（1）望形体：是指通过观望人体外形和体质，以测知内在脏腑状况的方法。

1）胖瘦：形体肥胖，气短无力，多为脾失健运，痰湿内蕴之证；形体瘦弱，皮肤枯燥，若瘦而食少为脾胃虚弱。

2）浮肿：面部、肢体浮肿而腹胀为水肿证；腹胀大如裹水、脐突是臌胀之证。

3）瘦瘪：大肉已脱，肌肤干瘪，为重病之恶病质。小儿面黄肌瘦，胸廓畸形，或囟门迟闭等，多为疳积之证。

（2）望动态：是通过观察病人的动静姿态及形体动作，进行诊断疾病的一种方法。

1）动静：喜动者多为阳证、热证、实证。其表现为卧时面常向外，或仰卧伸足，揭衣弃被，不欲近火，坐卧不宁，烦躁不安等；喜静者多为阴证、寒证、虚证。其表现为卧时面常向内，或蜷缩成团，不欲转身，喜加衣被，向火取暖。

2）咳嗽：坐而仰首，难于平卧，呼吸气粗，喘促痰多，多属肺有痰热，肺气上逆之实证；喘促气短，动则喘甚，平卧喘憋，多属肺虚或肾不纳气证；身肿心悸，气短咳喘，喉中痰鸣，多属肾虚水泛，水气凌心证。

3）抽搐：为动风之象。四肢拘挛，项背强直，角弓反张，伴高热烦渴者，多为热盛动风；面色萎黄，精神萎靡者多为血虚风动；手指震颤蠕动，头颈动摇不定者，多为肝肾阴虚，虚风内动。

4）偏瘫：一侧手足举动不遂即半身不遂，口眼㖞斜，语言不利，属中风偏枯证。常见于脑血管意外等。

5）痿躄：足膝软弱无力，行动不灵，多为痿证；手足屈伸困难或肿胀，属风寒湿痹。

sulting from a combination of damp and heat. While dark yellow complexion as smoked can be seen yin jaundice resulting from stagnation of cold and dampness.

(4) Blue complexion

It is the manifestation of cold syndrome, pain syndrome, blood stasis syndrome or infantile convulsion.

Blue complexion is the manifestation of blockage of meridians and collaterals and obstruction of qi and blood. As cold leads to contraction and stagnation, when the excessive cold stays in the vessels, it will retard the circulation of blood and qi, and lead to qi stagnation and blood stasis, and then the blue facial complexion appears. The blockage of qi and blood in the meridians and collaterals gives rise to pain, so blue complexion also presents pain syndrome. Dark blue facial complexion or pale and light blue facial complexion mostly manifest the extreme interior yin cold. The teel grey facial complexion with cyan and purple lip mostly indicates the syndrome of heart blood stasis and obstruction of blood circulation. The dark blue facial complexion is the sign of infantile convulsion if it occurs in a child, especially obvious on the sides of the nasal septum, between eyebrows and around lips.

(5) Dark complexion

It is the manifestation of kidney deficiency syndrome, fluid-retention syndrome, and blood stasis syndrome.

Dark complexion manifests the extreme yin cold and excessive water retention. Dark facial complexion occurs as the result of deficient kidney yang failing to warm and transform the water and fluid or stagnation of qi and blood failing to nourish the meridians, muscle and skin. Dark facial complexion concurrently with dark lips and nails presents the debilitation of kidney-yang, stagnation of yin cold, or heart blood stasis. Dark complexion in the periocular area with puffiness of the eyes manifests the syndrome of kidney deficiency and water flood. Dark facial complexion together with encrusted skin is mostly the sign of blood stasis. And dark facial complexion with violent pain is often the embodiment of cold stagnation and blood stasis.

3. Inspection of physical condition

(1) Inspection of body constituent

It is a method to infer and acquire the conditions of the internal organs through observing the shape and constitution.

Fatness and thinness: fatness with short breath and weakness manifests the syndrome of phlegm and dampness retention inside due to the spleen failing to transportation. Thinness with dry skin and intake of little food presents the syndrome of spleen-stomach weakness.

Edema: puffy face and limbs together with abdominal distension is the embodiment of edema. It is the tympanites if the abdomen is as big as it is fully filled with water with outward swelling of the umbilicus.

Shriveling: muscle atrophy with dry and shriveled skin is embodiment of the cachexia of the severe disease. Emaciation with sallow complexion, thoracocyllosis, or late closing of fontanelle is the manifestation of mild (infantile) malnutrition with accumulation.

(2) Inspection of actions

It refers to the observation of the gestures and actions of the patient.

Movement and quietness: Preference of movement often arises from the yang syndrome, heat syndrome and excess syndrome, characterized by facing outward or stretching feet when sleeping, willing to undress and unwilling to cover with quilt, keeping away from fire or hot places, restlessness, dysphoria, etc. While preference of quietness is often ascribed to the yin syndrome, cold syndrome and deficiency syndrome, characterized by facing inward, cowering up or willing to cover more quilt when sleeping, or preference to fire or hot places.

Cough: Symptoms like sitting with head up, hardness to lie on the back, heavy breath, panting with

（二）局部望诊

局部望诊是在整体望诊的基础上，根据病情或诊断需要，对病人身体某些具体部位进行重点、细致地观察，进而了解疾病本质。

1. 望头面部

小儿头部囟门凹陷或迟闭，多为先天不足；囟门高突，多为热邪亢盛，见于脑髓有病；头摇不能自主者，为肝风内动之兆；面肿见于水湿泛滥，或风邪热毒；腮肿为风温毒邪；口眼㖞斜，多为中风。

2. 望五官

（1）望目：眼部内应五脏，如目眦血络属心、白睛属肺、黑眼属肝，瞳子属肾，眼泡属脾。故望眼可了解五脏的情况。

1）目色：如目眦赤，为心火；白睛赤，为肺火；白睛现红络，为阴虚火旺；全目赤肿，为肝火或肝经风热；眼睑红肿糜烂，为脾胃湿热或肝经湿热；白睛色黄，为黄疸，属湿热或寒湿；白睛青蓝，为肝风或虫积；目眦淡白，为血虚；目眶周围见黑色，为肾虚水泛之水饮病，或寒湿下注的带下病。

2）目态：目窠浮肿，眼皮发亮，为水湿之泛；目窝凹陷，是阴液耗损之征，或因精气衰竭所致；眼球突起而喘，为肺胀；眼突而颈肿，则为瘿病；目睛上视，不能转动，或双眼上斜、直视，多见于惊风、痉厥或精脱神衰之重证。

（2）望鼻：主要反映肺与脾胃的情况。鼻头色赤，或伴有丘疹者（酒糟鼻），多因肺脾热盛、湿热蕴结所致；色白为气虚血亏之证；色黄为里有湿热；色青多为痛证；色黑为水气内停。鼻翼煽动频繁，呼吸喘促者，称为鼻煽。如久病鼻煽，为肺肾精气虚衰之危证；新病鼻煽，多为肺热；鼻梁溃陷见于梅毒；鼻柱崩坏、眉毛脱落见于麻风病。

（3）望耳：主要反映肾与肝胆的情况。色红明润，耳部饱满而润泽，耳内皮肤干湿适中，为肾精充足。色白多属寒证；色青而黑多主痛证；耳轮焦黑干枯，多为肾精亏极；耳轮萎缩为肾气竭绝之危候；耳旁红肿疼痛多为肝胆火热；耳内疼痛或流脓多为胆经有热或肝胆湿热；久病血瘀可见耳轮甲错。

much phlegm often result from the excess syndrome of heat phlegm in the lung and lung qi ascending counterflow.Panting and short of breath which aggravates on exertion,suffocation when lying on the back are pertain to the syndrome of lung deficiency or syndrome of kidney failing to absorb qi.Edema,palpitation,short breath,panting,and phlegm rale in the throat are often the result of the syndrome of kidney deficiency with water flood and water qi intimidating the heart.

Convulsions:It is the sign of wind engendering.Symptoms like spasm of limbs,stiffness of neck and back,opisthotonos,fever,and thirst often arise from the syndrome of extreme heat engendering wind.Sallow complexion and listlessness are the manifestation of blood deficiency engendering wind.Trembling and wriggling fingers and wavering head and neck are often the results of syndrome of liver-kidney yin deficiency engendering wind.

Hemiplegia:Symptoms like paralysis of one side of the body,facial paralysis and barylalia result from wind-stroke hemiplegia syndrome,which often occur in patients with cerebrovascular accident.

Leg flaccidity:Weak and feeble feet and knees and inflexibility in action often belong to wilting disease,while hardness to stretch hands or feet,or puffy hands and feet are the manifestation of impediment disease caused by a combination of wind,cold,and dampness.

Inspection of Special Parts of the Body

Inspection of special parts of the body is to make a focused and careful observation on the specific parts of the patient's body on the basis of the inspection of the whole body so as to make clear the nature of the disease,according to the need of state of illness or diagnosis.

1. Inspection of face and head

Fontanel sinking or closing late is the manifestation of congenital deficiency.Outward swelling of the fontanel presents the excessive pathogenic heat and there is something wrong with encephala.Unconscious head tremor is the sign of liver wind.Puffy face occurs in the syndrome of water-dampness flood or wind with heat toxin.Mumps is the result of the syndrome of wind warm toxin.Facial paralysis is the manifestation of wind-stroke syndrome.

2. Inspection of five sense organs

(1)Inspection of the eyes:The eyes correspond with the five viscera and can reflect the conditions of them.the canthus corresponds with the heart,white of the eye with the lung,dark of the eye with the liver,pupil with the kidney,and eyelids with the spleen.So doctors can know the conditions of the five viscera by inspection of the eyes.

Color of the eyes:it is the sign of heart fire if the canthus becomes red,the sign of lung fire if the white of eye turns red,and the sign of yin deficiency with effulgent fire if there is some red streak on the white of the eyes.It is the manifestation of liver fire or liver wind heat if the whole eye is red and swelling; the manifestation of dampness-heat in the spleen and stomach or dampness-heat in the liver meridian if the eye lids are red,swelling and anabrotic;the manifestation of jaundice,caused by the dampness-heat or cold-dampness syndrome if the white of eye becomes yellow;the manifestation of liver wind or worm accumulation in case of blue sclera;the manifestation of blood deficiency in case of light white of the canthus; and the manifestation of retained fluid syndrome caused by kidney deficiency with water flood,or vaginal discharge disease arising from cold-dampness pouring downward if the periphery of the eye socket is black.

Status of the eyes:it is the manifestation of flood of water and dampness if the eyelids are swollen and bright;the manifestation of yin and fluid consumption or essential qi debilitation if there is sunken eye;the manifestation of lung distention if the eye balls protrude with panting;the manifestation of goiter if the eye balls protrude and the neck is swollen;the manifestation of infantile convulsion,convulsive syncope,or collapse of essence and spirit if the eyes stare upward straightly,or eyes incline upward and stare straight-

（4）望唇与口：唇口主要反映脾胃的情况。正常唇色为红而鲜润。若唇色深红，属实、属热；唇色深红而干焦者，为热极伤津；唇色嫩红为阴虚火旺；樱桃样红为煤气中毒；唇色淡白，多属气血两虚；唇色青紫者常为阳气虚衰、血行郁滞的表现；口唇干枯皲裂，为津液已伤唇失滋润；唇口糜烂，多由脾胃积热、热邪灼伤；唇内溃烂，其色淡红，为虚火上炎；唇边生疮，红肿疼痛，为心脾积热；口角㖞斜，见于中风；口腔溃疡，为脾胃郁热或阴虚内热；睡时流涎，多属脾虚或脾胃有热。

（5）望齿龈：主要反映肾与胃的情况。牙齿干燥不泽，为津液已伤；齿燥如枯骨，为肾精枯竭；牙齿黄垢，为胃浊熏蒸；牙齿松动稀疏，齿根外露，多属肾虚或虚火上炎；牙齿有洞腐臭，为龋齿，为脾胃湿热；龈色淡白，为血虚不荣；红肿或兼出血多属胃火上炎；齿龈腐烂，流腐臭血水者，是牙疳病，多为脾胃湿热。

（6）望咽喉：咽喉主要反映肺、胃与肾的情况。咽喉红肿而痛，多属肺胃积热；红肿而溃烂，有黄白腐点，是热毒深极；鲜红娇嫩，肿痛不甚者，属阴虚火旺；咽部两侧红肿突起如乳突，称乳蛾，为肺胃热盛、外感风邪凝结而成；咽间有灰白色假膜，擦之不去，重擦出血，随即复生者，为白喉，为外感疫病之毒与气血相搏而成。

3. 望颈项躯体　颈前瘿瘤，为气结痰凝；颈侧颌下，累累如串珠，谓之瘰疬，多由虚火灼津而成痰核，亦可因感受风火时毒，导致气血壅滞、结于颈项；若伴角弓反张，多为肝风内动，或热极生风；见鸡胸者，多因先天不足、后天失养，骨骼失于充养；胸似桶状，咳喘、羸瘦者，是风邪痰热、壅滞肺气所致；肋间饱胀，咳则引痛，常见于饮停胸胁之悬饮证；乳房局部红肿，甚至溃破流脓的，为乳痈，多因肝失疏泄、乳汁不畅、乳络壅滞而成；腹皮绷急、胀大如鼓者，称为臌胀，多为气滞或水停之证；腹部凹陷如舟者，称腹凹，多见于久病脾胃之气大亏。

ly.

(2) Inspection of the nose: the status of the nose can reflect the conditions of the lung, spleen, and stomach. It is the manifestation of heat in the lung and spleen, or dampness-heat coagulation if the tip of the nose is red with papules (acne rosacea); the manifestation of qi and blood deficiency if it is white; the manifestation of interior dampness-heat if it is yellow; the manifestation of pain syndrome if it is blue; and the manifestation of interior water qi retention if it is dark. Nose incitement with panting is termed as nasal flap. Long-term nasal flap is often caused by the serious syndrome of essential qi debilitation of the lung and kidney; while new onset of nasal flap is often caused by lung heat; sunken and festered bridge of the nose presents syphilis; and collapse of nasal septum with madema presents leprosy.

(3) Inspection of the ears: the status of the ears can reflect the conditions of the kidney, liver, and gallbladder. It is the indication of sufficiency of the kidney essence if the ears are bright red, full and lustrous with moderate moisture in the endothelium skin. It is the manifestation of cold syndrome if the ears are white; the manifestation of pain syndrome if they are dark; the manifestation of extreme debilitation of kidney essence if the helixes are dry and dark; the critical manifestation of kidney qi collapse if the helixes shrinks; the manifestation of syndrome of heat-fire of liver-gallbladder if peripheries of the ears are red, swollen and achy; the manifestation of syndrome of heat in gallbladder meridian and dampness-heat of liver-gallbladder if there is pain or suppuration in the inner ears; and the manifestation of blood stasis if the helixes is encrusted.

(4) Inspection of the lips and mouth: the status of the lips and mouth can reflect the conditions of the spleen and stomach. The lips should be bright, red, and lustrous normally. It is the manifestation of excess syndrome and heat syndrome if the lips are dark red; the manifestation of extreme heat injuring fluid if they are dark red and dried; the manifestation of yin deficiency with effulgent fire if they are pink; the manifestation of carbon monoxide poisoning if they are cherry red; the manifestation of qi and blood deficiency if they are pale; and the manifestation of yang deficiency and blood stasis if they are dark blue. It is the manifestation of injury of fluid if they are dry and cracked; the manifestation of accumulated heat of the spleen and stomach if they are eroded; the manifestation of deficiency fire flaming upward if they are pinks with fester inside the mouth; the manifestation of accumulated heat of heart-spleen if there is red, swollen, and achy ulcer around the lips; the manifestation of wind-stroke syndrome if there is deviated mouth; the manifestation of spleen-stomach heat stasis or yin deficiency with internal heat if there is dental ulcer; and the manifestation of spleen deficiency or spleen-stomach heat if the patient drools when sleep.

(5) Inspection of the gingival: the status of the gingival primarily reflects the conditions of the kidney and stomach. It is the manifestation of fluid and humor impairment if the teeth are dry and lusterless; the manifestation of kidney essence exhaustion if the teeth are extremely dry; the manifestation of stomach turbidity steaming if there is yellow tartar; the manifestation of kidney deficiency or deficiency fire flaming upward if the teeth become loose and sparse; the manifestation of dental decay and spleen-stomach dampness-heat if there is tooth hole with rancidity; the manifestation of blood deficiency if the gingiva is light white; the manifestation of stomach fire flaming upward if the gingiva is red and swollen with bleeding; and the manifestation of cancrum oris and the syndrome of spleen-stomach dampness-heat if the gingiva is cankered and flows rancid blood.

(6) Inspection of the throat: the status of the throat primarily reflects the conditions of the lung, stomach and spleen. It is the manifestation of lung-stomach accumulated heat if it is red, swollen, and achy; the manifestation of extreme heat toxin if it is red and swollen with yellow and white rotten dots; and the manifestation of yin deficiency with effulgent fire if it is bright red with little swell and achiness. The tonsillitis, the inflammation of the palatine tonsils sometimes covered with a yellowish white secretion like milk, is the manifestation of extreme heat of lung and stomach together with invasion of exogenic pathogenic wind. It is

4. 望皮肤

（1）色形：皮肤面目俱黄，多为黄疸；皮肤青紫，多见于中毒；皮肤虚浮肿胀，按之可凹陷，多属水湿泛滥；皮肤粗糙如鳞，抚之涩手，称"皮肤甲错"，常见于血瘀或阴虚血燥；皮肤干瘪枯槁，多为津液耗伤；皮肤呈大片红肿，色赤如丹者，名"丹毒"，多由风热、肝火或湿热所致。

（2）斑疹：点大成片，色红或紫，平摊于皮肤，摸之不碍手，消失后不脱皮，为之斑。点小如粟，高出肤面，扪之碍手，消失后有脱皮，为之疹。斑疹多为温热之邪郁于肺胃，内迫营血所致。斑疹分布均匀，疏密适中，颜色红活润泽，松浮于皮肤表面为顺证；如若斑疹分布稠密不均，紧束有根，其色紫暗，压之不易褪色，色如鸡冠为逆证，预后不良。

（3）痘疮：皮肤起疱，形似豆粒，故名曰"痘疮"。常伴有外感证候，包括天花、水痘等；若见水疱，如带状簇生，称之为"缠腰龙"、"串腰龙"，见于带状疱疹，为湿热蕴积或肝郁化火所致。

（4）痈毒疔疖：若皮肤赤色如丹砂，边缘清楚，热痛相伴，或形如云片，上有粟粒小疹，发热作痒，并向周围浸润，或伴渗出流水，皮肤破溃，此为丹毒；皮肤瘙痒小疹，夹有脓疱，黄水淋漓，此为湿毒；若局部红肿，高出皮肤，根部紧束，此为痈；漫肿无头，坚硬不红，此为附骨疽；初起呈粟米状，根部坚硬，麻木或发痒，顶部起白头，疼痛较剧，此为疔；形如豆粒梅核，红热胀痛，起于浅表，继而顶部有脓头，此为疖。痈毒疔疖多为湿毒所致。

5. 望毛发　头发多而浓密色黑且润泽，是肾气充盛的表现。发稀疏不长，是肾气亏虚所致；发黄干枯，久病落发，多为精血不足所致；若发脱油腻，多为湿热所致；若突然出现片状脱发，称为"斑秃"、"鬼剃头"，为血虚受风或紧张惊吓所致；青少年脱发，多因肾虚或血热。

the manifestation of diphtheria if there is false grey thin coating,which cannot be removed,or will bleed if rubbed heavily and then appears again.The diphtheria is often caused by the struggle between external epidemic pathogen and the healthy qi and blood.

3. Inspection of the neck and body

It is the manifestation of qi stagnation and phlegm coagulation if there is goiter and tumor in the front of the neck;the manifestation of scrofula if there is a string of galls under the jaw at the side of the neck, which is caused by deficiency fire burning the body fluids into phlegm or infection of wind-fire epidemic pathogen leading to obstruction of qi and blood;the manifestation of liver wind or extreme heat engendering wind if it occurs opisthotonos;the manifestation of congenital deficiency and lack of nutrients which leads to de-nourishment of bones if pigeon breast appears;the manifestation of wind evil and heat phlegm obstructing lung qi if there are symptoms of barrel shaped check,cough,panting and emaciation;the manifestation of pleural fluid retention due to excess fluid retained in the side of the thorax if the symptoms of intercostals distention and stretching pain during cough;the manifestation of liver's failing in free coursing and milk obstruction in the breast collaterals if acute mastitis occurs,with the symptoms of the red and swollen breast even with festers;the manifestation of qi stagnation or water retention if there is tympanites, characterized by the severely distended abdomen like a drum accompanied by a somber yellow discoloration of the skin and prominent veins on the abdominal wall.It is the manifestation of spleen-stomach qi exhaustion resulting from long-term diseases if there is scaphoid belly.

4. Inspection of the skin

(1)Color and shape:it is the manifestation of jaundice if the skin,face,and eyes are all yellow;the manifestation of intoxication if the skin is dark blue;the manifestation of edema resulting from water-dampness flood if the skin is swollen and has pits when pressed;the manifestation of blood stasis or yin deficiency and blood dryness if there is encrusted skin,which feels like scale when touched;the manifestation of fluid and humor depletion if the skin is dry and shriveled;and the manifestation of wind heat,liver fire or dampness-heat if erysipelas occurs,the large scale of bright red and swollen skin.

(2)Macula:petechiae refer to the red or purple even spots dotted in a large scale of the skin and leave no encrustation when disappearing.While eruption refers to prominent millet-shaped spots and leave encrustation when disappearing.Macula often arises from warm-heat evil obstructing in the lung and stomach and expelling the nutrient blood overflowing the vessels.It is the manifestation of favorable syndrome indicating a positive prognosis if the macula is red and lustrous and evenly scattered in the surface of the skin;while it presents the unfavorable syndrome indicating a negative prognosis if the macula is as red as cockscomb or dark purple and unevenly or densely crowded in the skin,with color unchanged when pressed.

(3)Smallpox:it refers to bean-shaped blebs in the skin such as smallpox and chicken pox,which is often accompanied with the syndrome of external contraction.Herpes zoster,and acute eruptive disease characterized by severe pain along the girdled distribution of clustered vesicles,is arising from accumulation of dampness-heat or depressed liver qi transforming into fire.

(4)Abscess,deep-rooted boil and furuncle:it is the erysipelas if the affected skin is as red as cinnabar,with clear-cut margin,hot and painful concurrently,some scales of skin are like clouds with millet-shaped hot,itchy papule on them,or there are the festers on the skin infiltrating into the surrounding.It is the dampness toxin if the affected skin is itchy with some papules and pustules on it,excreting yellow liquid from them.It is the abscess if the affected skin is red and swollen and prominent from the surface,with the root clustering together.It is the suppurative osteomyelitis if the affected skin is swollen and hard but not red.It is the deep-rooted boil if there are millet-shaped,itchy papules on the skin at the beginning, with their roots stiff and white spot on the tops,and having severe pain.And it is the furuncle if there are

（三）望排出物

排出物指排泄物和分泌物。包括痰、涎、涕、唾、呕吐物、二便及经、带、汗液等。望排出物就是审察其色、质、形、量等变化，以了解有关脏腑的病变及邪气性质。

1. 望痰　痰液色白清稀，为寒痰；痰黄而黏稠，或质坚有块者，为热痰；痰清稀而多泡沫者，为风痰；痰白滑而量多、易于咳出者，为湿痰；痰少而黏，难于咳出，为燥痰。若干咳无痰，或咳嗽阵作，有少量泡沫痰，亦属肺燥；痰中带血，色鲜红，为热伤肺络；咳吐脓血痰液，味腥臭，或吐脓痰如米粥者，为肺痈。

2. 望涕　涕是由鼻黏膜分泌的黏液，有润泽鼻窍的功能。鼻流清涕者，为外感风寒、肺气失宣所致；鼻流浊涕者，为风热袭表犯肺、肺失清肃所致；若久流浊涕不止，为鼻渊，为风火热毒郁蒸鼻窍所致。

3. 望呕吐物　呕吐物清稀，无酸臭味者，为胃寒证；呕吐物秽浊，有酸臭味者，为胃实热证；呕吐不消化食物，其味酸腐者，多属食积；呕吐频作，物无酸腐，伴见胁满、叹气者，多因肝气不舒、横逆犯胃；呕吐黄绿色苦水，多为肝胆湿热或肝经郁火；呕吐鲜血或紫暗有块，夹有食物残渣，多属胃有积热或肝火犯胃；呕吐脓血者，属胃痈。

（四）望小儿指纹

望小儿指纹，是通过观察小儿示指掌侧前缘浅表浮露络脉的色泽与形态变化来诊查病情的方法。三岁以下小儿诊脉困难，常以诊指纹代之，指纹与诊寸口脉具有相似的诊断意义。示指第一节属风关，第二节属气关，第三节属命关（图4-1）。正常指纹，黄红相兼，隐现于风关之内。

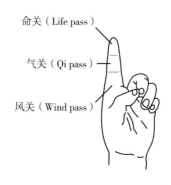

命关（Life pass）
气关（Qi pass）
风关（Wind pass）

图4-1　小儿风、气、命三关

（Figure 4-1　Wind pass，Qi pass，and Life pass in infantile finger）

bean-shaped,red and swollen papules with hot distending pain on the surface of the skin at the beginning, and then there appear pus on the tops.In most cases,they are all caused by dampness toxin.

5. Inspection of the Hair

Thick,lustrous and black hair is the manifestation of sufficiency of kidney qi.Sparse and short hair is the manifestation of kidney-qi deficiency.Dry yellow hair and hair loss in chronic diseases are the signs of insufficient essence and blood.Alopecia with greasy hair is mostly the result of dampness-heat syndrome. Alopecia areata,a sudden hair loss in a specific area,is often caused by blood deficiency with wind,or by tension or being frightened.It is the manifestation of kidney deficiency or blood heat if alopecia occurs in youths.

Inspection of Discharge

Discharge refers to excrement and secretion,including sputum,drool,snivel,spittle,vomitus,stool and urine,menses,leucorrhea,and sweat.Inspection of discharge is to obtain the conditions of the visceral and bowels and the nature of pathogens through observing the color,character,shape and volume of the discharge.

1. Inspection of sputum

The thin and white sputum belongs to cold sputum;the thick and yellow sputum belongs to heat sputum.The clear and dilute sputum with froth belongs to wind sputum.A lot of white and slippery sputum which is easy to be coughed up belongs to dampness phlegm.Little but sticky sputum which is hard to be coughed up belongs to dry phlegm.Coughing up no sputum or intermittent cough with little frothy sputum is the manifestation of lung dryness.Sputum with bright red blood is the embodiment of heat injuring lung vessels.And coughing with stinking purulent bloody sputum or spitting purulent sputum is the manifestation of lung abscess.

2. Inspection of nasal discharge

Snivel is the mucus excreted by nasal mucosa,which can moisten the nasal orifice.The clear snivel is the manifestation of external contraction of wind cold and obstruction of lung qi.The turbid snivel is the manifestation of wind heat attacking the exterior and the lung so that the lung fails to depurate and descend.The long-term turbid snivel,the manifestation of sinusitis,is caused by wind-fire-heat-toxin obstructing the nasal orifice.

3. Inspection of Vomitus

The clear and thin vomitus without sour and foul odors is the manifestation of stomach cold syndrome. The turbid vomitus with sour and foul odors is the manifestation of excessive stomach heat.Vomiting undigested food with sour and foul odors is the manifestation of food accumulation.Frequent vomiting accompanies with the fullness of hypochondrium and sigh are the manifestations of depressed liver-qi insulting the stomach.Vomiting yellow and green bitter bile is the manifestation of liver-gallbladder dampness-heat or depressed-fire in liver meridian.Vomiting fresh blood or dark blood with blood clots and residue of food is the manifestation of accumulated heat of stomach or liver fire insulting the stomach.And vomiting purulent blood is the manifestation of stomach abscess.

Inspection of Infantile Finger Venules

It is a method of diagnosing infantile diseases through observing the color,luster and shape of superficial venules floating on the surface of the front palmaris of the index finger.It is very difficult to feel the pulse of the infants under three years old,so inspection of the finger venules is conducted on these children.For the infants,the inspection of finger venules has the similar diagnostic meaning with feeling Cunkou pulse,with the first segment of the index finger belongs to wind pass,the second to qi pass and the third to life pass(Figure 4-1).The normal finger venules combine red and yellow and loom in wind bar.

指纹浮现明显者，多为病邪在表；指纹沉而不显者，多为病邪在里；色鲜红者，多外感风寒；色紫红者，多为热证；色青者主风、主惊、主痛；色紫黑者，多为血络瘀闭，病情危重。指纹细而浅淡者，多属虚证；粗而浓滞者，多属实证。指纹显于风关，表示病邪清浅；过风关至气关者，为邪已深入，病情较重；过气关达命关者，为邪陷病深；若指纹透过风、气、命三关，一直延伸指端者，即所谓"透关射甲"，提示病情危重。

（五）望舌

望舌即舌诊，是中医学中最具特色的诊断方法之一。舌诊对了解疾病本质，指导辨证论治有很大价值，在中医诊法中占有重要位置。

1. 舌与脏腑的关系　舌通过经络直接或间接与五脏相连，有"舌为心之苗，又为脾之外候"之说。另外，足太阴脾经、足少阴肾经、足厥阴肝经、手少阴心经均连于舌。正常的舌苔是由胃气上蒸所生，胃气的盛衰，可从舌苔的变化上反映出来。由此可见，舌与脏腑经络有着密切的关系。在长期的临床实践中，前人发现舌面的特定部位与相应的脏腑有一定的联系：舌尖主心肺、舌中主脾胃、舌根主肾和舌边主肝胆（图4-2）。若某一脏腑发生病变，舌面相应的部位就会反映出来。这种分部诊察舌象的方法对判断脏腑病变具有一定的参考价值。

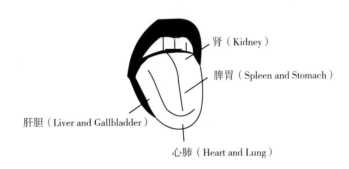

图 4-2　舌诊部位分属图

（Figure 4-2　Relationship between the Tongue and the Viscera and Bowels）

2. 舌诊的方法与注意事项

（1）望舌要点：光线充足，以室内自然柔和的光线为佳；自然伸舌，舌体放松，充分暴露舌体，不可过力伸舌，避免舌体紧张、卷缩，伸舌时间不应过长；先看舌苔，二看舌质；依舌尖、舌中、舌根及舌两边的顺序进行观察，并注意有无染苔。

（2）正常舌象：淡红舌、薄白苔，即舌质淡红明润，舌体胖瘦适中，柔软灵活；舌苔薄白均匀，干湿适中，不黏不腻，揩之不去。

It is the manifestation of pathogens locating in the exterior if the finger venules appear obviously and the manifestation of pathogens locating in the interior if they sink. Bright red finger venules present the syndrome of external contraction of wind cold; purple finger venules indicate heat syndrome; blue finger venules manifest syndrome of wind, fright and pain; and dark purple finger venules manifest obstruction of blood stasis, one kind of critical disease. The shallow and light finger venules present deficiency syndrome; while thick and broad ones present excess syndrome. It exhibits as exterior pathogen and mild disease if the finger venules only appear in wind pass; the internal invasion of pathogen and the serious disease if they penetrate to the qi pass from the wind pass; and retention of pathogen in the interior and the more serious disease if they cross the wind pass to the life pass. When the finger venules pass through wind pass, qi pass and life pass and extend to the finger nail, namely "visible superficial venule," it is the sign of critical diseases.

Inspection of the Tongue

Inspection of the tongue is the tongue diagnosis, one of the most special diagnostic methods of TCM, which has an important status in TCM and plays a significant role in grasping the nature of diseases and guiding the syndrome differentiation and treatment.

1. Relations hip between the Tongue and the Viscera and Bowels

The tongue directly or indirectly connects the five viscera through meridians and collaterals, as defined "the tongue is the sprout of the heart and the external sign of the spleen." In addition, the spleen meridian, kidney meridian, liver meridian, and heart meridian all link with the tongue. The tongue fur, also called tongue coating, originates from the steaming stomach qi, so the tongue fur can reflect the condition of stomach qi. All these reveal that tongue fur has the close relation with the viscera and bowels, and meridians and collaterals. In the long clinical practice, doctors in the ancient time found that the different specific positions of the tongue link the different internal organs, like tip of the tongue pertaining to the heart and lung, central of the tongue pertaining to the spleen and stomach, root of the tongue pertaining to the kidney, and margins of the tongue pertaining to the liver and gallbladder (refer to figure 4-2). The occurrence of the pathological changes of a special internal organ can be reflected in the related position. This tongue diagnosis has certain reference values for judging the pathological changes of the internal organs.

2. Tongue Diagnostic Methods and Matters Needing Attention

Key points for inspection of the tongue: inspection of the tongue should be conducted in the environment where there is sufficient light, the natural and soft light in the room is the best. At the inspection, the tongue should naturally stretch out in a relaxed status so as to expose the tongue body fully. It should not overstretch the tongue or stretch the tongue for a long time; otherwise the tongue will become strained and curled. When observing the tongue, doctors should firstly inspect the tongue fur, and then the tongue body and make the inspection in the order of tongue tip, center of the tongue, root of the tongue and margins of the tongue. Meanwhile, they should pay attention to whether there is stained fur on it.

Normal tongue manifestation: pale red tongue and thin white fur. In another word, the tongue body is pale red, moderate in size and soft and flexible, coated evenly with thin and white, moderately moist, non-sticky and non-slimy fur, which cannot be removed.

3. Contents of Tongue Diagnosis

(1) Inspection of the Tongue Body

Inspection of the tongue color

Pale tongue refers to the tongue less red than normal, indicating deficiency syndrome and cold syndrome. In most cases, it indicates blood deficiency as the result of yang deficiency or qi and blood deficien-

3. 舌诊的内容

（1）望舌质

1）望舌色

淡白舌：舌色较正常浅淡。主虚证、寒证。多见于血虚，为阳气衰弱、气血不足。由于阳虚生化阴血的功能减退，推动血液运行之力亦减弱，以致血液不能营运于舌中，故舌色浅淡而白。色淡而胖嫩，为虚寒；胖嫩而边有齿痕，为气虚、阳虚。

红舌：舌色较正常深，呈鲜红色。主热证。因热盛致气血沸涌、舌体脉络充盈，则舌色鲜红。全舌红，甚有芒刺者，多为实热新病；伴有黄厚腻苔，多为湿热证；红而少苔或无苔，为阴虚火旺；舌红而舌心干燥，多为热灼胃津；舌尖红，是心火上炎；舌边红，为肝胆有热。

绛舌：舌色深红，较红舌颜色更深浓。主内热深重。所主之热病有外感与内伤之别：外感热病多为邪热深入营分、血分；内伤多为阴虚火旺。舌绛无苔，光亮如镜，称为"镜面舌"，为内热阴液亏耗。

青紫舌：舌质呈现青紫，或舌有青紫色之瘀点或斑点。所主其证或为热极，或为寒证，或为瘀血。舌质绛紫色深而干燥，为邪热炽盛；舌质淡紫或青紫而滑润者，为阴寒内盛。青紫兼有瘀斑或瘀点舌，多为内有瘀血蓄积。

2）望舌形

老嫩："老"即指舌质纹理粗糙，形色坚敛，多属实证、热证；"嫩"指舌质纹理细腻，形色浮嫩，多属虚证或虚寒证。

胖瘦："胖"指舌体胖大、肿胀。舌质淡而胖，舌边有齿痕者，多属脾虚或肾阳虚、水湿停留；舌质红而肿胀，多属湿热内蕴或热毒亢盛；舌胖嫩紫暗多为中毒证。"瘦"指舌体瘦小而薄。舌质淡而舌形瘦者，多为气血不足；舌质红绛而舌形瘦者，多属阴虚内热。

芒刺：舌乳头增生、肥大，突起如刺，多属热邪亢盛。芒刺越大、越多，热邪越重。根据芒刺出现的部位，可分辨病变部位。如舌尖有芒刺，多为心火亢盛；舌边有芒刺，多属肝胆火盛；舌中有芒刺，主胃肠热盛；芒刺紫绛而干多为热盛阴伤。

裂纹：舌体上有多种纵行或横行的裂沟，且裂沟中无舌苔覆盖，多由于黏膜萎缩而形成。舌质红绛而有裂纹者，多属热盛、津液耗伤；舌质淡而有裂纹者，多属精血亏损；舌生裂纹细碎，多见于老年阴虚。此外，裂纹舌也可出现在健康人中，称先天性舌裂，此不属病舌。

齿痕：舌体边缘有牙齿压印的痕迹，故称齿痕舌。常与胖大舌并见，多为脾虚或

cy. Pale tongue emerges as yang deficiency cannot engender sufficient yin blood and promote the blood circulation, which leads to the blood failing to nourish the tongue. The enlarged tongue with light color is the manifestation of deficiency-cold syndrome; while the enlarged tongue with teeth marks on the margins is the manifestation of qi deficiency or yang deficiency.

Red tongue refers to the tongue redder than normal, indicating the heat syndrome. It is the result of heat accelerating the qi and blood circulation to fill the vessels in the tongue body. The red tongue even with pricks presents the occurrence of new excessive heat. Red tongue with yellow thick slimy fur presents the dampness-heat syndrome. Red tongue with little or even no fur is the manifestation of yin deficiency with effulgent fire. Red tongue with dryness in the center of the tongue is the manifestation of heat injuring stomach fluid. Red tip of the tongue is the manifestation of heart fire flaming upward; and red margin of the tongue is the manifestation of liver-gallbladder heat.

Crimson tongue refers to the deep-red tongue, indicating the intense interior heat. The heat it indicates is composed of the one caused by exterior pathogens and the one caused by internal damages; with the former being the result of exterior pathogenic heat getting into the nutrient aspect or blood aspect, and the latter being the result of yin deficiency with effulgent fire. Mirror tongue, the crimson tongue with no fur and as bright as mirror, is the manifestation of interior heat leading to depletion of yin-fluid.

Bluish purple tongue refers to the cyanotic tongue or the tongue with bluish purple petechia or speckles. It indicates the extreme heat syndrome or extreme cold syndrome or blood stasis. The garnet and dry tongue is the manifestation of exuberant pathogenic heat. The pale purple or bluish purple tongue with moist slippery fur is the manifestation of interior yin-cold excess. The bluish purple tongue with ecchymosis or petechia is the manifestation of accumulation of blood stasis in the interior.

Inspection of the form of tongue

Tough and tender-soft: "tough" means the texture of the tongue is rough and its form is solid and color is dark, which indicates heat syndrome or excess syndrome. "Tender-soft" means the texture of the tongue is delicate and its form is large and color is light, which indicates deficiency syndrome or deficiency-cold syndrome.

Fat and thin: "fat" means the tongue body is enlarged and swollen. Pale and enlarged tongue with teeth marks on its margin indicates the spleen deficiency, kidney-yang deficiency, or water-dampness retention. Red and swollen tongue indicates interior dampness-heat coagulating or intense excessive heat toxin. And Enlarged, dark purple and tender tongue indicates intoxication. "Thin" means the tongue body is thinner than normal. Pale and thin tongue indicates qi and blood deficiency, and red or crimson thin tongue indicates yin deficiency with internal heat.

Prickly tongue refers to the tongue with proliferated and enlarged lingual papilla, which protrudes like thorns. It indicates intense excessive heat. The more and the larger the pricks are, the severer the heat is. The location of the pricks helps to differentiate the sick organs. Pricks on tip of tongue indicate heart fire flaming, pricks on margin of tongue indicate liver-gallbladder-fire flaming, pricks at the center of tongue indicate excessive stomach-intestine heat, and dark and dry pricks indicate heat injuring yin.

Fissured tongue refers to the tongue with vertical or horizontal fissures on its surface, in which there are no fur. It is the result of mucosa shrinking. Red and crimson tongue with fissures on it indicates excessive heat consuming fluid. Pale tongue with fissures on it indicates deficiency of the essence and blood. Tongue with thin and small fissures often appears on the elder who suffer from yin deficiency. In addition, fissured tongue also occurs in the healthy people as a normal phenomenon, which is also known as congenital tongue fissure.

气虚。伴舌质红胖嫩，为脾虚湿盛；伴舌质淡白，苔白湿润，多为寒湿困脾。

舌疮：疮形如粟粒，或为溃疡，局部红痛，多为心经热毒壅盛；若疮疼痛较轻，多为肝肾阴虚、虚火上炎。

舌下脉络：舌尖上卷，可见舌下静脉呈青紫色，若粗大迂曲，兼见舌有瘀斑、瘀点，多为有瘀之象。

3）望舌态

强硬：舌体僵硬强直，屈伸不利或运动不灵，以致语言謇涩不清，称为强硬舌。多因热扰心神、心无所主或高热伤阴、筋脉失养，或痰阻舌络所致。多见于热入心包、高热伤津、痰浊内阻以及中风或中风先兆等证。

痿软：舌体软弱、无力屈伸，痿废不灵，称为痿软舌。多因气血虚极，阴液失养筋脉所致。可见于气血俱虚、热灼津伤、阴亏已极等证。

舌纵：舌伸出口外，内收困难，或不能回缩，称为舌纵。可见于实热内盛、痰火扰心及气血两虚证。

卷缩：舌体卷缩而不能伸出，称为卷缩舌。舌卷缩淡白而润，属阳气暴脱、寒凝筋脉；舌卷缩而干红，属热盛伤津、筋脉拘挛；舌胖黏腻而卷缩，属痰浊内阻，引动肝风，风邪挟痰，舌根拘紧。无论因寒因热，皆属危重征候。

麻痹：舌有麻木感而运动不灵的，叫舌麻痹。多因营血不足，不能上荣于舌而致。若舌麻而时发颤动，属肝风内动之候。

颤动：舌体震颤抖动，不能自主，称为颤动舌。多因气血两虚、筋脉失养或血虚生风及热极生风等证。

歪斜：伸舌歪向一侧，舌体不正，称为歪斜舌。多因风邪中络或风痰阻络所致，多见于中风证或中风先兆。

吐弄：舌伸出口外，久不回缩为"吐舌"；舌不停舐上下左右口唇，或舌微出口外，立即收回，皆称为"弄舌"，二者合称为"吐弄舌"。此为心、脾二经有热所致。吐舌多见于疫毒攻心或正气已绝；弄舌常见于小儿智力发育不全或惊风先兆。

（2）望舌苔

1）苔质

厚薄：透过舌苔隐约可见舌质为薄苔，不能透过舌苔见到舌质为厚苔。苔质的厚薄反映病邪的深浅和重轻。薄苔亦属正常舌苔，患病时，亦多为疾病初起或病邪在表，病情较轻；厚苔多为病邪入里，病情较重，或有痰饮食积。舌苔由薄而增厚，多为病情由轻转重，病情进展；舌苔由厚变薄，多为正气恢复，病情由重转轻，病

Teeth-marked tongue refers to the tongue with dental indentation on its margin. It often appears in accompany with enlarge tongue, which indicates the spleen deficiency or qi deficiency. It is the manifestation of spleen deficiency with excessive dampness if the teeth marks appear on red, tender-soft and enlarged tongue; and the manifestation of cold dampness affecting spleen if the teeth marks appear on pale tongue with moist white fur.

Tongue sore refers to the millet-shaped red and swollen sore or ulcer on the tongue. It is the manifestation of intense excessive heat toxin of the heart-meridian. If the sore is achy slightly, it indicates deficiency-heat upcasting due to liver-kidney yin deficiency.

Sublingual vessels: it refers to bluish purple veins under the tongue, which are exposed when curling the tip of tongue. But if the vessels are thick and tortuous, together with ecchymosis or petechia on the tongue, it indicates blood stasis syndrome.

Inspection of motility of the tongue

Stiff tongue refers the tongue that is stiff, moves sluggishly, and inhibits speech. It is the manifestation of heat disturbing the heart spirit, or fever injuring yin, or phlegm obstructing the tongue vessels. It often occurs in the syndromes of heat entering the pericardium, fever injuring fluid, phlegm turbid obstructing in the interior, wind stroke or prodrome of wind.

Limp wilting tongue refers to the tongue that is flabby and cannot move easily. It indicates extreme deficiency of qi and blood or fluid failing to nourish sinews. It often occurs in the syndromes of qi and blood deficiency, heat injuring fluid and extreme yin debilitation.

Protracted tongue refers to the tongue that is habitually extended out of the mouth and cannot be retracted. It indicates intensive excessive heat in the interior, sputum heat disturbing the heart, or qi and blood deficiency.

Curled tongue refers to the tongue formed into a curved shape and drawn back, inhibiting speech. Pale moist curled tongue indicates collapse of yang or cold congealing the sinews. Red dry curled tongue manifests the syndrome of excessive heat injuring jin and leading to sinew spasm. Enlarged, sticky slimy curled tongue presents the syndrome of phlegm turbidity obstructing the interior and engendering liver wind. Curled tongue is always of the critical manifestation of diseases no matter they are cold syndrome or heat syndrome.

Paralyzed tongue refers that the numb tongue unable to move, indicating nutrient blood deficiency failing to nourish the tongue. Paralyzed and trembling tongue is the manifestation of liver wind engendering in the interior.

Trembling tongue refers that the tongue involuntarily trembles as it moves, indicating qi and blood deficiency in failing to nourish the sinews, blood deficiency engendering wind, or extreme heat engendering wind.

Deviated tongue refers that the tongue inclines to one side when extended, indicating wind-evil insulting collateral or wind phlegm obstructing collateral. It often occurs in the syndrome of wind stroke or prodrome of wind.

Protruded agitated tongue refers to both the "protruded tongue" hanging out of the mouth and unable to retract back into the mouth, and the "agitated tongue" moving in a circular motion whereby the tip is extended from and retracted back into the mouth, or licks the lips. It indicates heat in the heart meridian and spleen meridian. Protruded tongue often manifests epidemic toxin attacking the heart or exhaustion of the healthy qi; while agitated tongue manifests mental deficiency of infants or prodrome of infantile convulsion.

(2) Inspection of tongue fur

势退却。

润燥：反映体内津液的情况。舌苔润泽，干湿适中，为润苔。润苔为正常舌苔，患病时，亦表示津液未伤；水液过多，甚至伸舌涎流欲滴，为滑苔，多见于脾虚湿盛或阳虚水泛证；若干枯无津，为燥苔，多见于热盛伤津、阴液不足，或燥邪伤阴等证。舌苔由润变燥，多为燥邪伤津，或热甚耗津，表示病情加重；舌苔由燥变润，多为燥热渐退、津液渐复，说明病情好转。

腐腻：苔质疏松如豆腐渣，堆于舌面，易于擦去，为腐苔。多为实热蒸化脾胃湿浊，或为胃中宿食化腐所致；苔质致密、细腻如一层混浊光滑的黏液覆盖于舌面，为腻苔。多因脾失健运、湿浊内盛、阳气被遏所致；苔黄厚，为湿热或痰热；苔白而滑腻，为寒湿。

剥脱：舌苔全部或部分剥脱，剥处见底，称剥落苔。若全部剥脱，光洁如镜，称镜面舌、光舌，为胃阴枯竭、胃气大伤；舌苔剥脱不全，剥处光滑，称花剥苔，为胃之气阴两伤。舌苔从有到无，是胃之气阴不足、正气渐衰的表现；舌苔剥落之后，复生薄白之苔，为胃气渐复、邪去正胜之佳兆。此外，剥脱苔也可出现在健康人中，如若身体无其他不适，即不作为疾病依据。

2）苔色

白苔：常见于表证、寒证。苔薄白而润，为风寒表证；薄苔白而干、舌尖微红，为风热表证；苔白而厚腻，为寒湿证；苔白滑黏腻，为痰湿证。在特殊情况下白苔也主热证，若见舌上满布白苔，如白粉堆积称"积粉苔"，此为毒热内盛所致；若苔白燥裂称"糙裂苔"，此为湿温病邪热炽盛、内热暴起、津液暴伤。

黄苔：主里证、热证。黄苔有淡黄、嫩黄、深黄、焦黄等不同。一般说，黄苔的颜色越深，则热邪越重。苔薄黄而润，邪初入里，津液未伤；苔黄而干，为热伤津液；苔黄而腻，则为湿热内蕴。苔由白转黄，为表邪入里化热的征象；若苔薄淡黄，为外感风热表证或风寒化热。

灰苔：灰苔即浅黑色。主痰湿、里证。舌苔灰而润滑、舌质不红，为寒湿内蕴或痰饮内停；舌苔灰而干燥、舌质红，多属热炽伤津，常见于里热证或阴虚火旺。

黑苔：多主里证，见于病情较重者。舌苔黑而干，为实热内炽、伤及津液；苔黑燥裂、舌绛芒刺，为热极津枯；舌苔黑而湿润，多属阳虚寒盛；苔黑生刺，望之虽燥，但渴不喜饮，舌质淡白，多为假热真寒，多见于疾病比较严重的阶段。

（3）舌质与舌苔的关系：疾病的发生发展过程，是一个复杂的整体性变化过程，因此在分别掌握舌质、舌苔的基本变化及其主病时，还应同时分析舌质和舌苔的相

Texture of fur

Thick fur and thin fur: thin fur refers to the tongue coating through which the underlying tongue surface is faintly visible; while thick fur refers to the tongue coating through which the underlying tongue surface is invisible. Thickness or thinness of fur reflects the conditions of a disease. Thin fur, also the normal fur, indicates the beginning of a disease or the pathogens locating in the exterior, which is mild. While thick fur indicates the internal invasion of pathogens, a serious case, or phlegm, retained fluid or food accumulation. Tongue fur thickening indicates aggravation of a disease, while tongue fur thinning indicates recuperation of the healthy qi and relief of a disease.

Moist fur and dry fur: moisture and dryness of fur reflects the condition of body fluids. Moist fur refers to the moderately moistened tongue coating, indicating the normal condition of the body or the pathogens having not injured fluid. Slippery fur refers to the moist tongue coating with excessive fluid, which even flows out when the tongue stretches out, indicating spleen deficiency with overabundant dampness or yang deficiency with water flood. Dry fur refers to the tongue coating that looks dry and feels dry to the touch, indicating exuberant heat damaging fluid, deficiency of yin-fluid, or dryness damaging yin. Tongue fur drying indicates dryness damaging fluid or exuberant heat consuming fluid, and disease aggravating. While tongue fur gradually turning into moist often indicates dryness-heat withdrawing, fluid and humor recuperating, and disease improving.

Curdy fur and slimy fur: curdy fur refers to the tongue coating consisting of coarse granules like bean dregs, easy to wipe off, indicating excess heat steaming spleen-stomach dampness turbidity, or accumulating food in the stomach corrupting. Slimy fur refers to the dense, turbid, slimy tongue coating, sticking on the tongue, hard to wipe off, also known as greasy fur, indicating spleen failing in transportation and turbid dampness increasing in the exterior to obstruct yang. Yellow and thick fur is the sign of dampness-heat syndrome or phlegm heat syndrome; while white slippery and slimy fur is the sign of cold-dampness syndrome.

Peeling fur refers to the complete or partial peeling of the tongue coating. The complete peeling tongue as smooth as mirror is termed as mirror tongue, or smooth tongue, indicating debilitation of stomach-yin and exhaustion of stomach-qi; while partial peeling tongue with peeling place as smooth as mirror is termed as exfoliated fur, indicating stomach-qi and stomach-yin damaging. The tongue fur gradually disappearing indicates stomach-qi and stomach-yin deficiency and the healthy qi weakening; while the tongue fur gradually recuperating indicates stomach-qi recovering and the healthy qi defeating pathogens. In addition, peeling fur can also occur in the healthy people, and is not taken as basis of disease if one does not feel uncomfortable.

Fur color

White fur indicates exterior syndrome or cold syndrome. Thin, white and moist fur indicates exterior wind cold syndrome. Thin, white and dry fur with slight red tip of tongue indicates exterior wind heat syndrome. White, thick and slimy fur indicates cold-dampness syndrome. And white, slippery, sticky and slimy fur indicates phlegm-dampness syndrome. However, under some special circumstance, white fur also manifests heat syndrome. For example, white sandy fur, the white dry and thick tongue coating like a layer of sand, indicates exuberant heat toxin in the exterior; and dry and cracked fur, the tongue coating that lacks moisture and develops cracks, indicates exuberant dampness-warmth engendering the sudden extreme internal heat and seriously damaging fluid.

Yellow fur indicates interior syndrome or heat syndrome. Yellow fur can be divided into pale yellow fur, bright yellow fur, deep yellow fur, and dry yellow fur. Generally, the deeper the color means the heavier the heat. Thin yellow and moist fur indicates pathogens begin to invade interior and have not damaged the

互关系。在一般情况下，同一性质的疾病，其舌质与舌苔变化是一致的。如实热证，多见舌红苔黄而干；虚寒证多舌淡苔白而润；阴虚火旺证，多见舌红苔燥，或少苔，或无苔而少津；湿热蕴结证多舌红苔黄腻等。但由于疾病变化复杂，临床上也可出现舌苔与舌质二者变化不一致的情况。如苔白虽主寒主湿，但若红绛舌兼白干苔，则属燥热伤津；再如灰黑苔可属热证，亦可属寒证，须结合舌质润燥来辨。因此理论学习时可分别掌握，临床运用时必须二者合参，进行综合评判。

二、闻诊

闻诊是医生通过听声音和嗅气味来测知诊查疾病的一种方法。人体的声音和气味均由脏腑生理和病理活动产生，故而能够反应机体内在变化的情况。

（一）声音

1. 语言及语声　一般来说，语声高亢洪亮，多言而躁动，多属实证、热证；语声低微无力，少言而沉静，多属虚证、寒证或邪去正伤之证；声音重浊，多为感受风寒或风热犯肺，或湿浊阻滞、鼻气壅塞所致；哑音与失音，有外邪袭肺、肺失宣降之实证，亦有肺肾阴虚、津不上承之虚证或虚火灼肺所为；鼾声不绝、昏睡不醒，多见于高热神昏或中风入脏之危证；呻吟不止，为重病或身痛不适；小儿阵发惊呼，多是肝风内动、扰乱心神之惊风证。烦躁多言者，多属实证、热证；语声低微，时断时续者，多属虚证。

2. 呼吸与咳嗽

（1）呼吸：呼吸有力，声高气粗而急促，多为外感邪气有余，属实证和热证；呼吸声低气微而慢，气少不足以言，也称之为"少气"，多属虚证和寒证；呼吸急促而气息微弱，属元气大伤之危重证候；气粗而呼吸不匀，或时断时续，属久病肺肾之气欲绝之象。

呼吸急促困难，甚至张口抬肩、鼻翼煽动，称为"气喘"。发病急骤，呼吸困难，胸满声高气粗，呼出为快，甚则仰首目突，脉数有力，属实喘，多因外邪袭肺或痰浊阻肺所致；发病缓慢，呼吸短促，不相接续，吸入为快，活动后喘促更甚，气怯声低，形体虚弱，倦怠乏力，脉微弱，属虚喘，多因肺气不足或肾不纳气所致。呼吸时喉中痰鸣如哨，时发时止，称之为"哮"，多为痰饮内伏所致。遇冷而作，多发于冬春季节，称为"冷哮"；遇燥热易作，多发夏秋季节，称为热哮。哮必兼喘，但喘不一定兼哮。

（2）咳嗽："咳"是指有声无痰，"嗽"是指有痰无声，"咳嗽"为有声有痰。

fluid;dry and yellow fur indicates heat injuring the fluid;and yellow and slimy fur indicates dampness-heat generating in the interior.The fur turning from white to yellow is the sign of exterior pathogens entering the interior and transforming into heat;and thin and pale yellow fur is the sign of external contraction of wind heat syndrome or wind-cold transforming into heat.

Gray fur,pale black fur,indicates the phlegm-dampness or interior syndrome.The normal tongue with gray,moist and slippery fur indicates interior cold-dampness or stagnation of phlegm or retained fluid.Red tongue with gray and dry fur indicates heat blazing and damaging the fluid and manifests the interior heat syndrome or yin deficiency with effulgent fire.

Black fur often indicates the interior syndrome and severe disease.Black and dry fur indicates excess heat flaming inward and damaging the fluid;crimson and prickly tongue with black,dry and cracked fur indicates extreme heat depleting the fluid.Black and moist fur indicates yang deficiency with excess cold. Prickly and pale tongue with black and seemingly-dry fur together with the symptom of thirst without desire to drink indicates true cold with false heat.

(3)Relationship between the tongue body and tongue fur

The course of occurrence and development of a disease is a very complicated changing integrity,so when understanding the changes and indications of tongue body and tongue fur,doctors should analyze the interrelations between them.In the general circumstance,the change of tongue body is in line with that of tongue fur if the diseases are in the same nature.Excess heat syndrome often presents red tongue with yellow and dry fur,and deficiency-cold syndrome presents the pale tongue with white and moist fur.However,clinically there are also the circumstances that the change of tongue body is in discordance with that of tongue fur.For example,though white fur indicates cold and dampness,the red or crimson tongue with white and dry fur indicates dryness-heat damaging the fluid.Gray and black fur is the manifestation of both heat syndrome and cold syndrome,which syndrome it indicates should be analyzed in combination of the characteristics of tongue body.The theories of tongue body and tongue fur can be grasped separately,but they should be well(properly)combined in comprehensively analyzing the condition of a disease clinically.

Listening and Smelling Examination

Listening and smelling examination is a method of diagnosing a disease through listening to the patients and smelling the patients.As people's voice and odor are produced by physiological and pathological activities of the viscera and bowels,it can reflect the internal changes of the body.

Voice

1. Speech and voice

Generally,loud and sonorous voice,talkativeness and restlessness often indicate excess syndrome or heat syndrome;feeble voice,silence and quietness often indicate deficiency syndrome,cold syndrome or syndrome of the healthy qi being impaired though pathogenic factors being removed;heavy turbid voice indicates nasal qi congestion due to external contraction of wind-cold or wind-heat insulting the lung,or obstruction of dampness turbidity;muting and loss of voice indicate excess syndrome caused by exterior pathogens invading into the lung and leading it fail to diffuse,purify and descend,or deficiency syndrome caused by failure of deficient lung-kidney yin in carrying the fluid upward or deficiency-fire scorching the lung;continuous snoring with lethargy indicates high fever and loss of consciousness or wind stroking the viscera,all belonging to critical cases;unceasing moaning indicates heavy disease or generalized pain;paroxysm of exclamation in infants often indicates convulsion syndrome caused by live-wind disturbing the heart spirit;dysphoria and talkativeness indicates excess syndrome or heat syndrome;and intermittent

由于"咳"与"嗽"往往同时出现，因而临床应用中统称为"咳嗽"。咳嗽一症，首当鉴别外感与内伤。

外感咳嗽：起病较急，病程较短，必兼表证，多属实证；内伤咳嗽：起病缓慢，病程较长或反复发作，以虚证居多。如咳声紧闷，多属寒湿；咳声清脆多属燥热；如咳嗽昼甚夜轻者，常为热为燥；夜甚昼轻者，多为肺肾阴亏；若无力作咳、咳声低微者，多属肺气虚。此外，对咳嗽的诊断，还须参考痰的色、量等不同表现和兼见症状以鉴别寒热虚实。另有顿咳和犬吠样咳嗽，见于"百日咳"与"白喉"。

3．呕吐、嗳气与呃逆

（1）呕吐：呕是指欲吐而无物且有声，或仅呕出少量涎沫。有物无声称为吐，如吐酸水、吐苦水等。以上诸证临床统称为呕吐。吐势徐缓、声音微弱者，多属虚寒呕吐；而吐势较急、声音响亮者，多为实热呕吐。虚证呕吐，多因脾胃阳虚和胃阴不足所致；实证呕吐，多是邪气犯胃、浊气上逆所致。

（2）嗳气：是指气从胃中上逆出咽喉时发出的声音。声音低弱无力，多因脾胃虚弱所致；声音高亢有力、嗳后腹满得减，多为食滞胃脘，常因肝气犯胃或寒邪客胃所致。

（3）呃逆：为胃气上逆所致。呃声高亢、音响有力的，多属实、属热，多因寒邪直中脾胃或肝火犯胃所致，发病较急；呃声低沉、气弱无力的，多属虚、属寒，虚证多因脾肾阳衰或胃阴不足所致；久病呃逆不绝、声低气怯，多为胃气衰败之征。

weak and low voice mostly indicates deficiency syndrome.

2. Breathing and coughing

（1）Breathing

Strong,heavy,and rapid breathing indicates excess syndrome or heat syndrome caused by excessive pathogenic qi;low,slow,and weak breathing with less qi to speak mostly indicates deficiency syndrome or cold syndrome,also known as"shortage of qi";rapid and faint breathing indicates a critical case due to the collapse of source qi;and heavy,even and intermittent breathing indicates the exhaustion and forthcoming collapse of lung-kidney qi.

Rapid and labored breathing with mouth opening,shoulders rising and nasal flaring is termed as dyspnea.Dyspnea characterized by acute onset,labored breathing,chest fullness,loud voice,and coarse breathing,which can be relieved after exhalation,even head upward and eyeballs protruding,and rapid and powerful pulse belong to dyspnea of excess type,often caused by exogenic evil invading lung or phlegm turbidity obstructing lung.While dyspnea characterized by gradual onset,short and intermittent breathing,which is relieved after inhalation but aggravation exertion,low voice,feeble body,lack of strength,fatigue,and faint and weak pulse belong to dyspnea of deficiency type,often caused by lung qi deficiency or kidney failing to absorb qi.Difficult and labored breathing with a whistling sound is regarded as wheezing,mostly caused by internal retention of phlegm and retained fluid.It consists of cold wheezing often occurring in the colder seasons of spring and winter,and heat wheezing often occurring in the hotter and drier seasons of summer and autumn.Wheezing inevitably turns up with dyspnea,but dyspnea does not necessarily come up with wheezing.

（2）Coughing

It refers to the combination of Ke and Sou,characterized by voiced cough with sputum,as Ke and Sou often occurs concurrently.Ke means the voiced cough without sputum,and Sou means the unvoiced cough with sputum.Cough caused by external contraction or internal injuries should be identified first in clinical work.

Coughing caused by external contraction is characterized by rapid onset,short course,and concurrently with the manifestation of exterior syndrome,mostly indicating excess syndrome;while coughing caused by internal injuries is characterized by slowness on onset,long-lasting course and repeated relapse,mostly indicating deficiency syndrome.Tight and stuffy coughing indicates cold-dampness syndrome;clear coughing often indicates dryness-heat;coughing serious in daytime and light at night indicates dryness syndrome or heat syndrome;coughing light in daytime and serious at night indicates lung-kidney yin deficiency;and weak and faint coughing indicates lung-qi deficiency.Furthermore,diagnosis of coughing should be combined with the condition of sputum such as color and quantity,and other concurrent syndromes so as to differentiate its nature,namely cold,heat,deficiency or excess syndrome.There are still pertussis and barking-like cough,which often occur in whooping cough and diphtheria.

3. Vomiting,belching,and hiccup

（1）Vomiting:it is the combination of"throwing-up",voiced vomiting without vomitus or with little saliva,and"spitting",unvoiced vomiting with vomitus like acid dip and bitter water.Slow vomiting with faint voice often indicates deficiency-cold syndrome,mostly caused by spleen-stomach yang deficiency or stomach-yin deficiency;and acute vomiting with loud voice often indicates excess heat syndrome,mostly caused by pathogenic qi insulting stomach to lead to reverse flow of turbid qi.

（2）Belching:it refers to the sound when air casting up from the stomach.Weak and faint belching mostly indicates spleen-stomach deficiency.And powerful and loud belching characterized by abdominal

（二）嗅气味

1. 病体气味

（1）口气：酸馊者多见于胃有宿食；臭秽者多见于脾胃湿热或消化不良；腐臭者多见于口腔本身的病变如牙疳、龋齿或口腔不洁，或内有溃腐疮疡等。

（2）汗气：外感六淫邪气，如风邪袭表，或卫阳不足、肌表不固，汗出多无气味；实热壅盛，或久病阴虚火旺之人，汗出量多而有酸腐之气。

（3）身臭：身臭伴疮疡溃烂流脓水，为皮肤感染；腐臭或尸臭味，多见于是脏腑败坏；尿臊味多见于晚期尿毒症者。另外腋下汗臭为狐臭，非器质性疾病。

2. 排泄物与分泌物气味

各种排泄物与分泌物包括痰、涕、呕吐物、大小便、妇人经带等。异常气味可以反映疾病性质。

（1）痰、涕：痰浊腥臭，为肺痈；鼻涕黄稠腥臭，为肺热鼻渊。

（2）呕吐物：气味臭秽，多因胃热炽盛。若呕吐物气味酸腐，呈完谷不化之状，则为宿食内停；气味腥臭，挟有脓血，可见于胃痈；气味发腥，质地清稀，为脾胃有寒；气味酸腐，伴有嗳气，多因胃中热盛或宿食停滞于胃而化热；嗳气无臭，多因肝气犯胃或寒邪客胃所致。

（3）小便：气味臊臭，其色黄混浊，属实热证；若小便清长，微有腥臊或无特殊气味，属虚证、寒证。尿有"烂苹果味"，为消渴病。

（4）大便：气味恶臭，黄色稀便或赤白脓血，为大肠湿热内盛；气味发腥，大便溏泻，为脾胃虚寒；小儿大便酸臭，伴有不消化食物，为食积内停。

（5）经带：月经或产后恶露臭秽，因热邪侵袭胞宫；带下气臭秽，色黄，为湿热下注；带下气腥，色白，为寒湿下注。

三、问诊

问诊是医生向病人及其知情者询问疾病发生、发展、目前症状、治疗经过及其他与疾病有关的情况，是全面了解病情的主要方法。自明代张景岳以后，一般认为《十问歌》是比较全面而重点突出的问诊方法。十问之内容为："一问寒热二问汗，三问头身四问便，五问饮食六问胸，七聋八渴俱当辨，九问旧病十问因，再兼服药参机变；妇女尤必问经期，迟速闭崩皆可见；再添片语告儿科，天花麻疹全占验。"十问歌可供参考，现多归纳以下八问：

fullness which is relieved after belching mostly indicates food accumulated in the stomach,often caused by liver qi or cold evil invading the stomach.

(3)Hiccup:it is caused by stomach qi ascending counterflow.Powerful hiccup with loud voice and a-cute onset,often indicates excess syndrome or heat syndrome,mostly caused by cold directly attacking the spleen and stomach or liver fire insulting the stomach;faint hiccup with low voice often indicates deficien-cy syndrome or cold syndrome,mostly caused by spleen-stomach yang deficiency or stomach yin deficien-cy;and unceasing hiccup with low voice and insufficient qi in chronic disease often indicates the syndrome of stomach qi debilitation.

Smelling

1. Odor of the body

(1)Mouth odor:sour odor often indicates retained food in the stomach;fetid mouth odor often indi-cates spleen-stomach dampness-heat or indigestion;and rancid mouth odor often indicates oral diseases like ulcerative gingivitis,dental caries,uncleanness of the mouth,or sore and ulcer in the mouth.

(2)Sweat odor:external contraction like wind invading the exterior,or defensive yang deficiency,or insecurity of exterior qi often produce odorless sweat.But excessive heat or yin deficiency with effulgent fire in chronic diseases often generates sour and fetid sweat.

(3)Body smelliness:body smelliness accompanies with festered pus-flowing ulcer indicates skin in-fection;fetid or corrupted odor indicates the corruption of the internal organs;and urine-smelled odor often occurs in the later period of uremia.Sweat odor from oxter is bromhidrosis,not indicating any organic dis-ease.

2. Odor of excretion and secretion

Excretion and secretion include phlegm,snivel,vomitus,feces and urine,menses and vaginal dis-charge and etc.The abnormal odor can reflect the nature of disease.

(1)Phlegm and snivel:fishy and fetid turbid phlegm indicates lung abscess;and fishy and fetid yellow thick snivel indicates sinusitis caused by lung heat.

(2)Vomitus:fetid vomitus indicates excessive stomach heat;sour and spoiled vomitus with undigest-ed food indicates retained food;fishy and fetid vomitus with pus indicates stomach abscess;fishy clear vomitus indicates spleen-stomach cold;sour and spoiled vomitus accompanied with belching indicates exu-berant stomach heat or retained food in the stomach being transformed into heat;and belching without odor indicates liver qi invading the stomach or cold insulting the stomach.

(3)Urine:yellow turbid urine with fetid odor indicates excess heat syndrome.Clear abundant urine without fishy or fetid odor indicates deficiency syndrome or cold syndrome.Spoiled apple-smelled urine is the manifestation of wasting-thirst disease.

(4)Stool:yellow thin stool with stinking odor or reddish white stool with pus and blood indicates dampness-heat in the large intestine;loose and sloppy stool with fishy odor indicates deficiency-cold of spleen-stomach;and sour fetid feces of infant with undigested food indicates accumulating food.

(5)Menses and vaginal discharge:menses or postpartum lochia with stinking odor indicates heat at-tacking the uterus;yellow vaginal discharge with foul odor indicates dampness-heat pouring downward;and white vaginal discharge with fishy odor indicates cold-dampness pouring downward.

Inquiry

Inquiry is the method that doctors get to know the comprehensive conditions of a disease by asking the patient about the occurrence,development,current symptoms,treatment,and other information related

（一）问寒热

寒与热是病人常见的自觉症状。问寒热是询问患者有无冷与热的感觉。寒热感觉可为确定疾病的性质提供依据。

寒，有恶寒、畏寒之别。病人主观感觉怕冷，但覆加衣被或近火取暖仍不能缓解其寒冷的感觉，称之为恶寒，多为外感寒邪所致；病人身寒怕冷，覆加衣被或近火取暖则寒冷感觉缓解或消失，称之为畏寒，多为内伤阳虚而致。热，即发热，无论患者体温是否正常，只要全身或局部有发热的主观感觉，中医都称之为发热，多为阳盛或阴虚所致。寒热的产生，主要取决于病邪的性质和机体的阴阳盛衰两个方面。临床常见的寒热症状有以下四种情况：

1. 恶寒发热　恶寒与发热感觉并存称恶寒发热，是外感表证的主要症状之一。恶寒发热为外感表证初起，外邪与卫阳之气相争的反应。外邪束表，郁遏卫阳，肌表失于温煦，故恶寒；卫阳失宣，郁而发热。如恶寒重、发热轻，多属外感风寒的表寒证；发热重、恶寒轻，多属外感风热的表热证；恶寒发热，并有恶风、自汗、脉浮缓，是外感表虚证；恶寒发热，兼有头痛、身痛、无汗、脉浮紧，是外感表实证。

2. 但寒不热　患者只有怕冷的感觉而无发热者，即为但寒不热，多为里寒证。新病畏寒，可见于寒邪直中脏腑经络，或外感病初起尚未发热之时；久病畏寒，多为阳虚内寒证等。

3. 但热不寒　发热而不觉怕冷，称为但热不寒，多属于热证。临床上有壮热、潮热、低热之分。

（1）壮热：身发高热（体温超过39℃），持续不退，属里实热证。为风寒之邪入里化热或温热之邪直中于里，邪盛正实，交争剧烈，里热炽盛，蒸达于外所致。

（2）潮热：定时发热或定时热甚，有一定规律，如潮水之有定时。外感与内伤疾病中皆可见有潮热。由于潮热的热势高低、持续时间不同，临床上又有以下三种情况：

1）阳明潮热：其特点为热势较高，热退不净，多在日晡时（下午3~5时）热势加剧。

2）湿温潮热：此种潮热故称湿温潮热。其特点为初按肌肤多不甚热，扪之稍久才觉灼手。临床上又称之为"身热不扬"，多见于温病中的湿温病。

3）阴虚潮热：其特点为午后或夜间发热加重，热势较低或自觉发热而体温不高。多伴胸中烦热、手足心发热，故又称"五心烦热"、严重者有热自骨髓向外透发

with the disease.Since Zhang Jingyue of Ming Dynasty,Ten Inquires has been generally regarded as a best and most complete inquiry method,which says,"before making the prescription,doctors should inquire about:first,cold and heat;second,sweat;third,the head and body;fourth,stool and urine;fifth,diets;sixth, feeling in the chest;seventh,hearing condition;eighth,whether thirsty or not;ninth,the history of the disease;and tenth,the cause of the disease.With regards to the women patients,doctors should ask the menstruation status including delayed menorrhea,preceeded menorrhea,amenorrhea,metrorrhagia,and metrostaxis.As for the infant or child patients,doctors should additionally pay attention to whether they have smallpox or measles."

Inquiry about Cold and Heat

Cold and heat are the subjective symptoms that the patient can feel.Inquiry about cold and heat is to ask the patient whether she/he feels cold or hot.Such feeling provides basis for identifying the nature of the disease.

Cold is composed of aversion to cold and fear of cold.Aversion to cold refers to the sensation of cold which cannot be relieved by putting on more clothes or approaching the fire,which is caused by exogenic pathogenic cold.Fear of cold refers to the sensation of cold which can be relieved by putting on more clothes or approaching the fire,which is often caused by yang deficiency due to internal injuries.Heat here refers to fever.When the patient feels hot partially or overall even though he/she has the normal body temperature,it is called as fever in TCM,which is caused by excessive yang or yin deficiency.The occurrence of cold and heat mainly depends on the property of pathogens or conditions of yin and yang of the body. Clinically there are four common cold and heat syndromes as follows:

1. Aversion to cold with fever

Aversion to cold with fever refers to the combination of aversion to cold and fever and is one of the main symptoms of external contraction syndrome.It is caused by the struggle between the expathogens and defensive yang qi at the occurrence of external contraction syndrome.Aversion to cold is the result of external pathogens fettering the exterior and obstructing defensive yang from warming the skin surface.Fever arises from defensive yang failing to disperse and being blocked.Heavier aversion to cold with light fever indicates the exterior cold syndrome caused by wind cold,while heavier fever with light aversion to cold manifests the exterior heat syndrome caused by wind heat.Aversion to cold with fever,aversion to wind, spontaneous sweating,and floating moderate pulse are manifestations of the exterior deficiency syndrome. Headache,generalized pain,absence of sweating,and floating tight pulse are the indications of exterior excess syndrome.

2. Chills without fever

Chills without fever refer to the feeling of cold with no fever,mostly indicating the interior cold syndrome.Aversion to cold at the occurrence of a disease can be seen in such cases as the cold directly strike the visceral meridians,or at the beginning of external contract without fever.When it occurs in the patient with prolonged illness,it often indicates syndrome of yang deficiency with internal cold.

3. Fever without chills

Fever without chills refers to elevation of the body temperature with no feeling of cold,mostly indicating the heat syndrome.Clinically it is classified into high fever,tidal fever and mild fever.

(1)High fever:it will occur when the patient has a persistent high fever with body temperature above 39℃,belonging to interior excess heat syndrome.It is caused by either wind cold entering the interior and transforming into heat,or warm heat striking the interior directly,and then acute struggle between the excessive pathogenic factors and the abundant healthy qi bringing the effulgent internal heat to the exterior.

的感觉，则称为"骨蒸潮热"，潮热多见于阴虚证候之中。

（3）低热：即患者发热时间较长，热势较轻微，体温一般不超过38℃，又称长期低热。可见于温病后期、内伤气虚、阴虚以及小儿夏季热等病证中。

4. 寒热往来　恶寒与发热交替发作，寒时自觉寒而不热，热时自觉热而不寒。一日一发、隔日一发，也可一日数发，可见于少阳病、温病及疟疾。

（二）问汗

1. 自汗　日间汗出，活动尤甚，伴有气短、乏力、畏寒等症，为自汗，为气虚证或阳虚证。

2. 盗汗　入睡汗出，醒后汗止为盗汗，多伴有潮热、颧红、五心烦热、舌红脉细数等症状，多属阴虚。

3. 大汗　大汗不已，出汗量多，伴有面赤、口渴饮冷、脉洪大，属实热证。若汗出不止，渐伤正气，出现冷汗淋漓，或汗出如油，伴有呼吸喘促、面色苍白、四肢厥冷、脉微欲绝，此称为"脱汗"、"绝汗"，为久病、重病时正气大伤，阳气外脱，津液大泄，此为阳亡阴竭的危候，预后不良。

（三）问疼痛

1. 疼痛的性质

（1）胀痛：痛且有胀感，为胀痛。多因气机郁滞所致。

（2）刺痛：疼痛如针刺，部位固定不移。多因瘀血所致。

（3）窜痛：疼痛部位游走不定，或走窜攻痛。多为风邪留滞，阻滞气机所致。

（4）灼痛：痛处有烧灼感。多由火热之邪串之经络，或阴虚阳亢、虚热灼于经络所致。

（5）冷痛：痛处有冷感，或触之发凉，痛处喜温。多因寒凝筋脉或阳气不足而致。

（6）重痛：疼痛伴有沉重感。常见于头部、四肢及腰部。多因湿邪困阻气机而致。

（7）酸痛：疼痛并伴有酸楚感，喜揉喜按。多为精血不足、湿浊阻滞气机而致。

（8）隐痛：痛而隐隐，绵绵不休，痛势较轻，持续时间较长。多因气血不足，或阳气虚弱，导致经脉气血运行涩滞所致。

2. 疼痛部位

（1）头痛：外感内伤皆可引起头痛。外邪阻滞经络、气血郁滞不畅所致，属实；内伤多由脏腑虚弱、清阳不升、脑府失养，或肾精不足、髓海不充所致，属虚；痰

(2)Tidal fever:it refers to fever with periodic rise and fall of body temperature at fixed hours of the day like the morning and evening tides.It can occur both in the disease caused by the exogenic pathogens or the internal injuries.Tidal fever can be divided into three types according to its temperature and duration:

Yangming tidal fever refers to later afternoon tidal fever characterized by high fever which is difficult to leave and aggravates at 3-5 p.m.daily.

Dampness-warmth tidal fever refers to"unsurfaced fever"clinically,a persistent fever in which heat is not easily felt on the body surface and can be felt only by prolonged palpation,which often occurs in warm-dampness disease under the category of warm disease.

Yin-deficiency tidal fever is also termed as"five center heat"or vexing heat in the chest,palms and soles.It has the characteristics of the feeling of heat in the palms of hands,soles of feet and in the chest, which aggravates in the afternoon or at night with mild fever or mild body temperature even though the patient feel fever.Worse,it will develop into the bone-steaming tidal fever,a tidal fever in which the heat is felt to emanate from the bones.Tidal fever mostly occurs in yin-deficiency syndromes.

(3)Mild fever: it refers to persistent low-grade fever generally with the body temperature under 38℃ ,also known as long-term mild fever.It mostly occurs in the later period of warm disease,qi deficiency due to internal injuries,yin deficiency or infant summer fever.

4. Alternating chills and fever

Alternating chills and fever refers to chills without fever and fever without chills occurring in alternating succession.It occurs every day,or every other day or every several days,can be seen in shaoyang disease,warm disease,or malaria.

Inquiry about Sweating

1. Spontaneous sweating refers to excessive sweating during the daytime with no apparent cause, which aggravates during the activities and accompanies with shortness of breath,weakness,and fear of cold,indicating qi deficiency syndrome or yang deficiency syndrome.

2. Night sweating refers to sweating during sleep that ceases on awakening,often accompanied by tidal fever,red cheeks,vexing heat in the chest,palms and soles,red tongue,and thin rapid pulse,indicating yin deficiency.

3. Profuse sweating refers to abnormal continuous excessive sweating,accompanied by red face,thirst with desire to drink cold water,and surging pulse,indicating excess heat syndrome.Aggravation of profuse sweating will lead to"expiry sweating,"the incessant profuse sweating or oily sweating,accompanying with panting,pale complexion,cold limbs,and hardly perceivable pulse,indicating injury of healthy qi,external collapse of yang qi,depletion of fluid,moribund state of collapse of yang and yin,and poor prognosis.

4. Shiver sweating refers to sweating following shivering,the result of the struggle between the healthy qi and pathogenic factors.If heat retreats after sweating with static pulse and cool body,disappearance of the feeling of thirst and vexation,it indicates the healthy qi defeats the pathogenic factors and the disease tends to be recuperated.But if heat does not recede after sweating and still with dysphoria and racing pulse,it indicates debilitated healthy qi fails to defeat exuberant pathogenic factors,the further inward invasion of heat and deterioration,which often occurs in a critical case.

Inquiry about Pain

1. Property of pain

(1)Distending pain refers to pain accompanied by a distending sensation,mostly caused by qi stagnation.

饮及瘀血阻滞经络所致的疼痛，则属虚实夹杂。

头部不同部位的疼痛，一般与经络分布有关，如头项痛属太阳经病；前额或连及眉棱骨痛属阳明经病；两颞或太阳穴附近疼痛属少阳经病；头顶痛属厥阴经病，头痛连齿属少阴经病。

（2）胸痛：胸居上焦，为心肺之府，所以胸病以心肺病变居多。常见于热邪壅肺、肺阴不足、胸阳不振、痰浊内阻、气虚血瘀及气滞血瘀等证。如肺痈、肺痨、胸痹等。

（3）胁痛：多与肝胆病变有关。常见于肝气郁结、肝胆湿热、瘀血阻滞及水饮内停等病症。

（4）脘腹痛：多与脾胃疾病有关，有虚实寒热之别。拒按为实，喜按为虚，喜暖为寒，喜冷为热。可因寒凝、热结、食积、虫积、气滞、血瘀而发，也可由气虚、血虚、阳虚所致。

（5）腰背四肢痛：多为寒湿痹证、湿热痹阻、瘀血阻络、肾虚等证。风邪偏盛，疼痛游走者，多为风痹或行痹；疼痛伴周身困重，多为湿痹；疼痛剧烈，得热痛减，为寒痹；灼痛喜冷，或有红肿，多为热痹；腰膝或足跟冷痛，小便清长，属肾虚；痛如针刺，固定不移，属闪挫跌扑瘀血。

(2)Stabbing pain refers to a sharp pain in the fixed place as if caused by a stab,mostly caused by blood stasis.

(3)Scurrying pain refers to pain that repeatedly changes location,mostly caused by stagnant wind obstructing qi movement.

(4)Scorching pain refers to pain accompanied by a burning sensation,also called burning pain,mostly caused by fire heat crossing the meridians and collaterals,or yin deficiency with yang hyperactivity,or deficiency heat scorching the meridians and collaterals.

(5)Cold pain refers to pain accompanied by a cold sensation and relieved by warmth,mostly caused by cold congealing sinews or yang qi deficiency.

(6)Heavy pain refers to pain accompanied by heaviness sensation,often occurring in the head,limbs and waist,mostly caused by dampness obstructing qi movement.

(7)Aching pain refers to continuous dull pain as the sensation produced by prolonged physical exertion and lessened by pressing and rubbing,mostly caused by essence and blood deficiency or dampness turbidity obstructing qi movement.

(8)Dull pain refers to continuous long-lasting mild pain,mostly caused by qi and blood deficiency, or yang qi deficiency,both of which lead to stagnation of qi and blood in the meridians and collaterals.

2. Location of pain

(1)Headache:both external and internal injuries can cause headache.It belongs to excess syndrome if headache is caused by exopathogens obstructing the meridians and collaterals or stagnating qi and blood. It belongs to deficiency syndrome if headache is caused by internal injuries like weak internal organs failing to raise the clear yang to nourish the brain,or kidney essence deficiency failing to replenish the marrow sea.And it belongs to deficiency-excess complex if headache is caused by phlegm or retained fluid or blood stasis obstructing the meridians and collaterals.

Locations of headache are related to the meridians and collaterals on which the pain is located.Head and neck pain indicates bladder meridian(BL)disease;forehead pain or pain spreading from forehead to superciliary ridge indicates stomach meridian(ST)disease;pain in two temporos or pain surrounding temples indicates gallbladder meridian(GB)disease;pain on the top of the head indicates liver meridian (LR)disease;and headache spreading to teeth indicates kidney meridian(KI)disease.

(2)Chest pain:chest is located on the upper energizer,house of the lung and the heart,so most of the chest diseases are caused by lung disease and heart disease.Chest pain is often caused by heat obstructing in the lung,lung yin deficiency,devitalized chest yang,phlegm turbidity obstructing internally,qi deficiency and blood stasis,and qi stagnation and blood stasis.It often occurs in lung abscess,tuberculosis and chest impediment.

(3)Hypochondriac pain:it is mostly related with the liver or gallbladder diseases,often occurring in liver qi depression syndrome,liver-gallbladder dampness-heat syndrome,blood stasis syndrome,and syndrome of retained fluid retention.

(4)Stomachache and abdominal pain:they are mostly associated with the spleen or stomach diseases,and can be classified into excess syndrome characterized by refusal to be pressed,deficiency syndrome characterized by preference of being pressed;cold syndrome characterized by preference of warmth and heat syndrome characterized by preference of cold.They are often caused by cold coagulation,heat binding,food accumulation,warm accumulation,qi stagnation and blood stasis,or by qi deficiency,blood deficiency and yang deficiency.

(5)Back pain,lumbago pain and limbs pain:they mostly indicate syndrome of cold-dampness imped-

（四）问饮食与口味

1. 问食欲与食量

（1）食欲减退，食量减少：多见于脾胃气虚，或内伤食积，或湿邪困脾，或肝胆湿热等证。喜热饮或食后饱胀，多为脾胃虚寒；厌食饱胀，嗳腐吞酸，多为食滞胃脘；厌食油腻，胁胀气急，多为肝胆湿热；饥饿而又不想进食，或进食很少，可见于胃阴不足、虚火内扰证；喜进热食，多属寒证；喜进冷食，多属热证。进食后稍安，多属虚证；进食后加重，多属实证或虚中夹实证。疾病过程中，食欲渐复，表示胃气渐复，预后良好；反之，食欲渐退，食量渐减，表示胃气渐衰，预后多不良。若病重不能食，突然暴食，是脾胃之气将绝的危象，称"除中"，属"回光返照"的一种表现。

（2）多食易饥，食欲亢进：食量较多，又称为"消谷善饥"，可见于胃火亢盛、腐熟太过所致。常见于消渴病之中消证。

（3）偏嗜食物：嗜食某种食物或某种异物。其中偏嗜异物者，又称"异嗜"，若小儿异嗜，喜吃泥土、生米等异物，多属虫积；若妇女已婚停经而嗜食酸味，多为妊娠。

2. 问口渴与饮水

（1）口渴：口渴见于津液不足，湿热、痰饮、瘀血等证。若口渴喜冷饮，为热盛津伤，多见于热证；若口渴喜热饮，且饮水不多，常见于寒证；口渴不多饮，或水入即吐，见于痰饮水湿内停，或湿热阻滞、津不上承；若口干欲漱不欲咽，多为瘀血之象；若伴有多饮多尿，是为消渴。

（2）口不渴：为津液未伤，或见于寒证或无明显热邪之证。

3. 问口味 口味是指病人口中的异常味觉。口苦多见于肝胆湿热；口淡乏味，多因脾胃气虚而致；口甜，多见于脾胃湿热证；口黏腻，多属湿困脾胃；口中泛酸，可见于肝胆蕴热证，或肝胃不和；口中酸腐，多见于伤食；口咸多见于肾虚；口臭多见于胃火炽盛，或肠胃积滞；口腥伴有咳血呕血，或唾有血丝，多见于肺胃血络受伤；口中尿味可见于尿毒内蕴。

iment, dampness-heat impediment, blood stasis obstructing vessels and kidney deficiency syndrome. They can be classified into moving impediment, an impediment disease characterized by migratory joint pains, also called wind impediment; dampness impediment, an impediment disease with generalized heaviness sensation; cold impediment, an impediment disease with severe joint pain relieved by warmth; and heat impediment, an impediment disease with scorching pain, accompanied by local redness and swelling and cold preference. Such pains can also arise from kidney, with the manifestation of cold pain in the waist, knees or heels, clear and abundant urine; or from sudden sprain, tumbling or blood stasis, with the manifestations of pain as if stabbed in the fixed place.

Inquiry about Diet and Taste in the Mouth

1. Inquiry about appetite and food consumption

(1) Appetite decrease with decreasing intake of food often results from such syndromes as spleen-stomach qi deficiency, or food accumulation due to internal injuries, or dampness encumbering spleen, or dampness-heat of liver and gallbladder. Preference of warm or hot drink, or sensation of fullness and distention after meal indicates spleen-stomach cold-deficiency syndrome; fullness and distention, anorexia, belching and acid regurgitation indicates food stagnating in the stomach; hatred of greasy food and hypochondriac distention indicates liver-gallbladder dampness-heat; no desire to take food or just intake of little food at starvation indicates syndrome of stomach-yin deficiency or deficiency-heat disturbing interior; preference of hot food indicates cold syndrome; preference of cold food indicates heat syndrome; vexation relieved after meal indicates deficiency syndrome; and vexation aggravated after meal indicates excess syndrome or deficiency with excess complication. During the course of disease, recovery of appetite indicates recuperation of stomach-qi and favorable prognosis. On the contrary, appetite decreases with decreasing intake indicates stomach-qi weakening and unfavorable prognosis. Totally loss of appetite with sudden intake of massive food occurs in a critical case, indicating forthcoming collapse of spleen-stomach qi, also known as "collapse of spleen and stomach," a manifestation of "sudden spurt of vitality prior to collapse."

(2) Excessive appetite with increased food intake and recurrence of hunger sensation shortly after eating, also known as "swift digestion with rapid hungering," indicates stomach-fire overabundance decomposing the food too quickly, often occurring in middle wasting-thirst of wasting-thirst syndrome.

(3) Dietary predilection refers to a liking for particular flavors or specific foods, of which liking of specific foods is also known as "specific predilection," such as predilection of soil or unprocessed grain in children, indicating worm accumulation. The woman's predilection of sour food accompanied by menolipsis indicates she is pregnant.

2. Inquiry about thirst and water drinking

(1) Thirst: it often occurs in such syndromes as fluid-humor deficiency, dampness-heat, phlegm and retained fluid and blood stasis. Thirst with desire to drink cold water indicates heat syndrome; thirst with desire to drink warm or hot water but drinking little indicates cold syndrome; thirst but drinking little or vomit at drinking indicates internal retention of phlegm, retained fluid and dampness, or dampness-heat obstructing fluid from upbearing; thirst with desire to suck but not to drink indicates blood stasis; and polydipsia with polyuria indicates wasting-thirst.

(2) Hydroadipsia: it indicates undamaged fluid and humor, and often occurs in cold syndrome or unapparent heat syndrome.

3. Inquiry about taste in the mouth

Taste in the mouth refers to the abnormal taste in the mouth, including bitter taste in the mouth indicating liver-gallbladder dampness-heat, bland taste in the mouth indicating spleen-stomach qi deficiency,

（五）问睡眠

失眠，是指不易入睡，或睡而易醒、不易再睡，或睡而不酣、易于惊醒，甚至彻夜不眠的表现。其病机是阳不入阴，神不守舍。气血不足、神失所养，或阴虚阳亢、虚热内生，或肾水不足、心火亢盛等，皆可扰动心神，导致失眠，属虚证；痰火、食积、瘀血等邪气内扰，心神不宁，出现失眠，属实证。

嗜睡，是指时时思眠，眠而不醒，精神疲惫，头沉神倦者。实证多由湿邪困阻、清阳不升；虚证多因气血不足、精明之府失于荣养，或心肾阳衰、阴寒内盛、神气不振。

（六）问二便

1. 问大便

（1）便秘：即大便秘结。以大便次数减少，每周少于三次，质硬便难，或排便时间延长为特征。根据临床症状分热秘、燥秘、气秘、冷秘、虚秘等。

1）热秘：好发于素体阳盛、嗜酒、喜食辛辣或热病之后的人，表现为大便燥结，数日不通，脘腹胀满，疼痛拒按，苔黄厚腻或焦黄起芒刺，脉沉实或滑数。

2）燥秘：表现为大便干结如羊屎，排便异常困难，甚则十数日一次，舌红少津，脉细或细数无力。

3）气秘：多发于忧愁、思虑过度、情志不畅或久坐不动的人，表现为大便不通，欲便不得，甚则腹胀疼痛，嗳气频作，胸脘痞满，胁肋作胀，纳食减少，苔薄腻，脉弦。

4）冷秘（寒秘）：多发于年老体衰、久病或素体阳虚者，表现为大便秘结，面色青黑，腹中冷痛或腰脊冷乏，肢冷身凉，喜热畏寒，小便清长，舌淡苔白润，脉沉迟或反微涩。

5）虚秘：好发于劳倦过度、年高津衰或病后、产后及失血伤津过多者，表现为大便干结如羊屎，排便异常困难，甚则十数日一次，舌淡或舌红少津，脉细或细数无力。虚秘可分气虚便秘、血虚便秘、阴虚便秘三种，可根据临床中伴有的气虚证、血虚证及阴虚证加以区别。

（2）溏泻：又称便溏或泄泻。若发病急促，腹痛肠鸣，肛门灼热，或里急后重，大便臭秽，便有黏液、脓血，为湿热泄泻；若泻如稀水，大便腥臭，为寒湿泄泻；若吐泻交作，呕吐物气味酸臭，大便臭秽，为食积泄泻；若顽谷不化，便质溏薄，或肛门有重坠之感，甚则肛欲脱出，为脾虚泄泻；每日黎明前腹痛泄泻，泄后则安，亦称之为"五更泻"、"鸡鸣泄"，为脾肾阳虚。

sweat taste in the mouth indicating spleen-stomach dampness-heat syndrome, sticky slimy sensation in the mouth indicating dampness encumbering spleen-stomach, sour taste in the mouth indicating liver-gallbladder heat syndrome or syndrome of liver qi invading the stomach, sour and fetid taste in the mouth indicating food damage, salty taste in the mouth indicating kidney deficiency, fetid mouth odor indicating stomach heat syndrome or stomach-intestine accumulation syndrome, fishy taste in the mouth accompanied by hemoptysis and haematemesis or blood streak in spittle indicating the blood vessels of lung and stomach being injured, and urine odor in the mouth indicating uremic obstruction in the interior.

Inquiry about Sleep

Insomnia refers to inability to sleep, or easiness to be awakened up with a light sleep, or abnormal wakefulness throughout the night, caused by yang failing to well combine with yin and spirit failing to keep to its abode. Insomnia indicates deficiency syndrome if it is caused by qi and blood deficiency failing to nourish spirit, yin deficiency with yang hyperactivity engendering deficiency heat internally, or kidney-liquid deficiency failing to constrain effulgent heart fire, all of which can disturb the heart spirit. It indicates excess syndrome if it is caused by internal phlegm fire, food accumulation and blood stasis disturbing the heart spirit.

Somnolence refers to feeling of sleepiness and desire to sleep at any time accompanied by listlessness, heavy head and tiredness. Excess syndrome is caused by internal dampness encumbering the upward flow of clear yang, while deficiency syndrome is caused by qi and blood deficiency failing to nourish the head, or heart-kidney yang deficiency engendering internal cold and leading to downheartedness.

Inquiry about Stool and Urination

1. Inquiry about stool

(1) Constipation: it refers difficult evacuation of the feces characterized by decrease of evacuation times, less than three every week with feces too hard to be evacuated or prolonged evacuation time. Clinically, it can be classified into heat constipation, dryness constipation, qi constipation, cold constipation, and deficiency constipation.

Heat constipation: it often occurs in the patients with exuberant yang or often drinking wines or preferring hot and spicy food or suffering heat disease, with the manifestations of constipation, abdominal and stomach fullness and distention, pain but refusal to be pressed, yellow, thick and slimy fur or dry yellow prickly tongue, and sunken replete pulse, or slippery rapid pulse.

Dryness constipation: it manifests the extremely difficult evacuation of feces as dry as sheep shit, or even once evacuation of feces more than 10 days, red and dry tongue, thin pulse, or thin rapid weak pulse.

Qi constipation: it often occurs due to depression, pensiveness and sedentary life style, accompanied by the symptoms of dyschezia, abdominal distention and pain, frequent belching, stuffiness and fullness in the chest, hypochondriac distention, intake of little food, thin slimy fur, and string-like pulse.

Cold constipation: it often occurs in the weak aged patients, or the patients suffering a chronic disease or constitutional yang deficient, accompanied by the symptoms of constipation, bluish dark complexion, abdominal cold pain, lumbar vertebrae cold and lack of strength, generalized cold and cold limbs, preference of heat and fear cold, clear and abundant urine, pale tongue with white and moist fur, and sunken slow pulse or faint rough pulse.

Deficiency constipation: it often occurs due to excessive exertion, excessive loss of blood or fluid, or occurs in the aged, convalescent and postpartum patients, accompanied by the manifestations of extremely difficult evacuation of feces as dry as sheep shit, even once evacuation of feces more than 10 days, pale tongue or red and less moisten tongue, and thin pulse or thin weak pulse. Deficiency constipation can be

2. 问小便　小便清长量多，畏寒喜暖，为虚寒证；小便量少黄赤，为热盛伤津，或过用汗、吐、泻法后伤及阴液所致；尿量增多，伴有口渴多饮，体重下降，为消渴病；尿少，伴有浮肿，属水湿内停、气化不利；尿频尿急尿黄赤，甚则尿血尿痛，多为膀胱湿热；余沥不尽，或夜间遗尿或尿失禁，多为肾气不固、膀胱失约；小便频数不畅，或尿流中断，有沙石排出者，为石淋；老人膀胱胀满，小便不畅，或癃闭，多为肾气亏虚或血瘀湿热所致；重病癃闭无尿，或昏迷遗尿，为危证。

（七）问月经带

1. 问月经　正常周期为 28 天左右，行经 3~5 天，经量适中，经色红或暗红，经质不稀不稠，无血块或少量血块，无痛经或轻度腰腹部不适。若经色浅，质地稀，多为气血不足；经色红，质地稠，多为血热；经色紫暗，有血块，多为血瘀。月经异常见如下情况：

月经先期：月经周期提前八、九天以上，称为月经先期。多因血热妄行，或气虚不摄而致。

月经后期：月经周期错后八、九天以上，称月经后期。多因血寒、血虚、血瘀而致。

月经先后不定期：月经超前与错后不定，称为月经先后不定期，又称月经紊乱。多因情志不舒、肝气郁结、失于条达气机逆乱，或者脾肾虚衰气血不足冲任失调，或瘀血内阻气血不畅所致。

经量过多：超过正常血量，其色红而稠，多为热证、实证；若色淡质稀，多为气虚不摄而致。

月经量少：色淡质稀，多因精血亏虚；质稠色暗，为血瘀、行经不畅而致。

崩漏：指妇女不规则的阴道出血。临床以血热、气虚最为多见。经血不止，其势多急骤，为血热；经血不止，其势多缓和，为气虚统摄无权。此外，瘀血也可致崩漏。

闭经：停经三月以上，又未妊娠者，称闭经或经闭。多见于血之化源不足、血海空虚，或肝气郁结、血行不畅，或宫寒血瘀所致。

闭经应注意与妊娠期、哺乳期、绝经期等生理性闭经，或者青春期、更年期，因情绪、环境改变而致一时性闭经加以区别。

痛经：月经期或行经前后，出现小腹或腰部疼痛的症状称为痛经。多因气血运行不畅，或胞脉失养所致。可见于寒凝、气滞血瘀、气血亏虚等证。

2. 问带下　主要了解白带的量、色、质和气味等。凡带下色白而清稀、无臭，

further categorized into constipation due to qi deficiency,constipation due to blood deficiency,and consti-pation due to yin deficiency,which can be clinically distinguished according to the accompanying symp-toms of qi deficiency,blood deficiency,and yin deficiency.

(2)Sloppy stool and diarrhea:rapid onset,stomachache with borborigmus,scorching anus,tenesmus, fetid and foul stool,or stool containing mucus or pus and blood are the manifestations of dampness-heat di-arrhea;water-like stool with fishy stink are the symptoms of dampness-cold diarrhea;alternation of vomi-ting acid fetid vomitus and evacuating fetid and foul stool is the sign of diarrhea due to food accumulation; washy stool with undigested food or sensation of heaviness and falling in the anus,or even sensation of pro-lapse of rectum are the manifestations of diarrhea due to spleen deficiency;diarrhea with abdominal pain at dawn,which is relieved after diarrhea is the manifestation of spleen-kidney yang deficiency,also known "fifth-watch diarrhea"or"cock-crowing diarrhea."

2. Inquiry about urination

Clear and abundant urine and preference of warmth and fear of cold indicates deficiency-cold syn-drome;reddish yellow and scanty urine indicates excessive heat injuring body fluids or excessive applica-tion of sweating,vomiting,purgation methods damaging yin-fluid;increase of urination,thirst and drinking more and decline in weight indicates wasting-thirst;little urination with edema indicates internal dampness retention due to unfavorable transformation;frequent urination,urgent urination and reddish yellow urine, or even hematuria and dysuria is often caused by bladder dampness-heat;dribbling urination,enuresis,uri-nary incontinence is often caused by insecurity of kidney-qi and constraining dysfunction of bladder;fre-quent painful and difficult urination with calculi indicates stone strangury;urinary bladder distention and fullness,dribbling urination or dribbling urinary block indicates kidney-qi deficiency or blood stasis with dampness-heat if it occurs in the aged people;and dribbling urinary block even anuria,or coma with enu-resis is the manifestation of critical case.

Inquiry about Menstruation and Vaginal Discharge

1. Inquiry about menstruation

Under normal circumstance,menses is red or dark red and lasts for 3−5 days at every 28-day interval with moderate volume,with little or without coagula,without dysmenorrheal or with mild waist or abdomi-nal discomfort during the menstrual period.Light-colored and tenuous menses with large quantity indicates qi and blood deficiency;red and thick menses with large quantity indicates blood heat;and dark purple menses with coagula indicates blood stasis.Here are the abnormal menstruation conditions:

Advanced menstruation:it refers to menstrual periods that come 8 to 9 days or more ahead of due time,primarily caused by frenetic movement of blood due to heat or qi deficiency with failure to constrain

Delayed menstruation:it refers to menstrual periods that come 8 to 9 days or more after due time,pri-marily caused by blood cold,blood deficiency and blood stasis.

Menstruation at irregular intervals:it refers to menstrual periods that come with an irregular cycle,al-so known as menstrual disorder,mostly caused by emotional depression,liver-qi depression and inability to disperse,reverse flow of qi,or spleen-kidney debilitation,qi and blood deficiency,disharmony of the thor-oughfare and conception vessel,or internal obstruction of blood stasis and unsmooth circulation of qi and blood.

Profuse menstruation:it refers to excessive uterine bleeding occurring at regular intervals,the same as menorrhagia.Red,thick and excessive menses indicates heat syndrome or excess syndrome.While light-col-ored,tenuous,and excessive menses indicates qi deficiency with failure to constrain.

Scant menstruation:it refers to menstrual discharge of less than the normal amount occurring at regu-

多属虚证、寒证；带下色黄或赤，稠黏臭秽，多属实证、热证；若带下色白量多，淋漓不绝，清稀如涕，多属寒湿下注；带下色黄，黏稠臭秽，多属湿热下注；若白带中混有血液，为赤白带，多属肝经郁热。

（八）问小儿

若小儿不能诉说，可以询问其家长或保育员。除了一般的问诊内容外，还要注意询问出生前后情况、喂养情况、生长发育情况及预防接种情况、传染病史及传染病接触史。若孕期母体有病或早产，小儿则可先天禀赋不足、体质虚弱、抗病力低下，或发育障碍；若喂养不当、饥饱无度、饮食不节，均可损伤脾胃；若抚养失宜、冷热不均，易患外感疾患等。此外还要询问是否患过特殊疾病如麻疹、水痘等。

四、切诊

切诊，包括脉诊和按诊，是医生运用手的触觉，对病人寸口脉及体表特定的部位进行触摸、按压、体验，从而了解病情的一种诊断方法。

（一）脉诊

1. 诊脉的部位和方法

诊脉的常用部位：手腕部的寸口脉。寸口又称脉口、气口，其位置在腕后桡动脉搏动处。寸口脉分为寸、关、尺三部（图4-3），通常以腕后高骨处（桡骨茎突）为标记，高骨内侧为关脉位置，关前（近腕侧）为寸脉，关后（近肘侧）为尺脉。

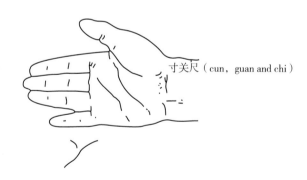

寸关尺（cun，guan and chi）

图 4-3 寸口脉诊图

（Figure 4-3 Wrist Pulse-based Diagnosis）

诊脉的方法：手臂放置位置和心脏近于同一水平。诊脉下指时，首先用中指按在关脉位置，然后示指按在寸脉位置，无名指按在尺脉位置。诊脉时用轻指力按在皮肤上叫举，又叫浮取或轻取；用重指力按在筋骨间，叫按，又称沉取或重取；指力不轻不重，还可亦轻亦重叫寻。因此诊脉必须注意举、按、寻之间的脉象变化。如此脉分三部，每部有轻、中、重取三法，共称三部九候。

lar intervals.Light-colored and tenuous menses indicates essence and blood deficiency;while dark and thick menses indicates blood stasis and dysmenorrheal.

Flooding and spotting refers to irregular vaginal bleeding.Clinically,it is primarily caused by blood heat characterized by urgent and incessant dripping of blood,and qi deficiency characterized by mild and incessant dripping of blood.In addition,blood stasis can also cause flooding and spotting.

Amenorrhea:it refers to cessation of menstruation for more than three months without being pregnant, primarily caused by insufficient source for blood transformation leading to vacuity of blood sea,or liver-qi depression giving rise to unsmooth blood circulation,or cold uterus with blood stasis.

Amenorrhea can be classified into physical amenorrhea occurring in gestation period,amenorrhea in lactation period and amenorrhea in menopause,and temporary amenorrhea occurring in puberty and climacterium or due to emotional and environmental changes,which should be clearly distinguished in diagnosis and differentiation.

Dysmenorrheal:it refers to the lower abdominal or lower back pain occurring around or during the menstrual period,mostly caused by unsmooth qi and blood circulation or de-nourishment of uterus vessel. It often takes place in the syndromes like cold coagulation,stagnation of qi and blood stasis,and qi and blood deficiency.

2. Inquiry about vaginal discharge

Inquiry about vaginal discharge is to get to know the quantity,color,nature and odor of leucorrhea. Clear white thin leucorrhea without abnormal odor indicates deficiency syndrome or cold syndrome;yellow or red sticky and thick vaginal discharge with foul odor indicates excess syndrome or heat syndrome;white and clear dripping vaginal discharge primarily indicates cold dampness pouring downward;yellow,sticky and thick vaginal discharge with foul odor primarily indicates dampness-heat pouring downward;and white vaginal discharge containing blood mostly indicates liver meridian heat.

Inquiry about the Conditions of Infant

If the child is too small to speak or cannot speak clearly,doctors can ask their parents for the condition of his/her disease.As for a child patient,besides the general inquiries,the doctors need to inquire about the prenatal and postnatal situation of the child,feeding patterns,growth and development and vaccination,contagion history,and contagion contact history.If the patient's mother is ill during pregnancy or makes a premature delivery,the child may be deficient in natural endowment and weak in constitution and resistance,or has some problems in development.If a child is improperly fed like excessive hunger or eating too much or improper diet,his/her spleen and stomach will be damaged;and if being taken care of improperly,the child will be easy to be affected by exopathogens.Besides all the above-mentioned,doctors also need to inquire about whether the child patient has caught the infectious diseases like measles and chickenpox.

Palpation

Palpation,composed of pulse diagnosis and body palpation,is a diagnostic method of knowing the conditions of a disease by touching and pressing the specific parts of the patient's body like wrist pulse.

Pulse Diagnosis

1. Locations of pulse and method of pulse diagnosis

Location of pulse:wrist pulse located at where the radial artery pulsates is the common one applied in feeling pulse,which is also known as Maikou or Qikou.It is composed of three sections of cun/inch,guan/ bar and chi/cubit(Figure 4-3) ,with the guan central to the radial styloid at the wrist,the cun next to it on

　　诊小儿脉可用"一指（拇指）定关法"，而不细分三部，因小儿寸口部短，不容三指定寸关尺。

　　诊脉时医者的呼吸要自然均匀，因医者以正常的一呼一吸（称一息）作为时间单位计算病人的脉搏至数。一般一息四、五至为正常。诊脉时要求有一个安静的内外环境。诊脉之前，先让患者休息片刻，使气血平静，医生也要平心静气，然后开始诊脉。

　　2. 正常脉象　　正常脉象古称平脉，其形态为三部有脉，一息四至五至，不浮不沉，不大不小，从容和缓，柔和有力，节律一致，尺脉沉取有一定力量，并随生理活动和气候环境的不同而有相应的正常变化。此外，少部分人脉不见于寸口，而从尺部斜向手背，称斜飞脉；若脉出现于寸口的背侧，则称反关脉，还有出现于腕部其他位置者，是桡动脉解剖位置的变异，不属病脉。

　　寸关尺分候脏腑，历代医家说法不一，目前多以下列为准（表4-1）：

　　左寸可候：心；右寸可候：肺。

　　左关可候：肝；右关可候：脾。

　　左尺可候：肾；右尺可候：肾（命门）。

表 4-1　寸口分部表

部位	左	右
寸	心	肺
关	肝	脾
尺	肾	肾（命门）

　　3. 脉象的分类与主病

　　（1）浮脉

　　【脉象】轻取即得，重按稍减而不空，举之泛泛而有余，如水上漂木。

　　【主病】表证、虚证。

　　（2）沉脉（附：伏脉）

　　【脉象】轻取不应，重按乃得，如石沉水底。

　　【主病】里证。

　　伏脉：比沉脉显现部位更深，重按推筋着骨始得。为邪气内闭或剧烈疼痛或厥证。

　　（3）迟脉

　　【脉象】脉来迟慢，一息不足四至。

　　【主病】寒证。迟而有力为寒痛冷积，迟而无力为虚寒。久经锻炼的运动员，脉迟而有力，则不属病脉。

the distal side, and the chi on the proximal side.

Methods of pulse diagnosis: the doctor needs to ask patient to place their arms at the same height with the heart in pulse diagnosis, and then place the tip of his/her middle finger on the guan, the tip of his index finger on the cun, and the tip of his ring finger on the chi. During pulse diagnosis, if the physician feels the pulse with light force on the skin, it is known as lifting; with moderate force, known as searching; and with heavy force pressed between sinews and bone, known as pressing. Therefore, the pulse is divided into three positions, and each position has three methods to study the superficial, medium and deep pulses, which is termed as three positions and nine indicators.

As for the infant patients, the physician can feel the wrist pulse only with his/her thumb rather than with three fingers as the wrist pulse of infant is very short and cannot be placed with three fingers.

When conducting pulse diagnosis, the physicians need to breathe naturally and evenly as they should count the patient's number of pulses within their own respiration. Generally, four to five pulses within one respiration is normal. Meanwhile, the doctor should also let the patients to rest for a while to tranquilize circulation of qi and blood before feeling the pulse of the patient.

2. Normal pulse condition

Normal pulse refers to the pulse felt superficially, medially and deeply, which gently and vigorously beats for four to five in one respiration at the same rhythm, with the deep position of the chi exhibiting certain strength. The normal pulse will vary with the physiological activities and climatic environment. In addition, instead of wrist pulse, some people have oblique-running pulse, the pulse beat felt running outwards from the chi to the back of the hand, or pulse on the back of the wrist, or pulse on other positions of the wrist, all of which are due to anatomical anomaly of the radial artery rather than as the morbid pulse.

The cun, guan, and chi positions reflect the conditions of different internal organs, with the details having been argued for centuries, but currently adopted as follows (Table 4-1):

The cun in the left wrist reflects the condition of the heart, and the cun in the right wrist reflects the condition of thelung.

The guan in the left wrist reflects the condition of the liver, and the guan in the right wrist reflects the condition of the spleen.

The chi in the left wrist reflects the condition of kidney, and the chi in the right wrist reflects the condition of the kidney (life gate).

Table 4-1   Details of the Wrist Pulse

Position	Left	Right
The cun	Heart	Lung
The guan	Liver	Spleen
The chi	Kidney	Kidney (Life Gate)

3. Categories of pulses and disease correspondences of the pulses

(1) Floating Pulse

Pulse condition: a superficially located pulse which can be felt by light touch and grows faint on hard pressure.

Disease correspondence: exterior syndrome, deficiency syndrome.

(2) Sunken pulse

（4）数脉（附：疾脉）

【脉象】脉搏次数多，一息六至以上。

【主病】热证。有力为实热，无力为虚热。

附 疾脉：一息七八至，多属阳气极盛、阴气欲竭，或元气将脱的重证。

（5）虚脉

【脉象】三部脉会之无力，按之空虚。

【主病】虚证。

（6）实脉

【脉象】三部脉举按均有力。

【主病】实证。

（7）滑脉

【脉象】脉来流利圆滑，如珠走盘，应指圆滑。

【主病】痰饮、食积、实热。

（8）涩脉

【脉象】脉来涩滞不畅，迟细而短，往来艰涩，极不流利，如轻刀刮竹。

【主病】精血亏少，气滞血瘀，挟痰，挟食。

（9）弦脉

【脉象】脉挺直而长，如按琴弦，有劲有弹力，脉管的硬度大。

【主病】肝胆病，痰饮，痛证，疟疾。

（10）紧脉

【脉象】脉来绷急，应指有力，如绳索绞转，脉的张力大，脉跳有力。

【主病】寒证、痛证。

（11）濡脉

【脉象】浮而细软，如帛在水中。

【主病】虚证，湿证

（12）洪脉（附：大脉）

【脉象】洪脉极大，状若波涛汹涌，来盛去衰。

【主病】里热证。常见于高热病人。

附 大脉：脉形大而无来盛去衰之势，多是病势进展之象，所谓"大则病进"（大而有力）；如脉大而无力则为正气不足。

（13）细脉（附：小脉）

【脉象】脉细如线，脉形窄，波动小，但应指明显。

【主病】气血两虚，诸虚劳损，湿证。

附 小脉也即细脉，主病与细脉同。

Pulse condition:a deeply located pulse which can only be felt when pressing hard.

Disease correspondence:interior syndrome.

Hidden pulse:a pulse which can only be felt upon pressing to the bone,located deeper than sunken pulse or even totally hidden,indicating internal block of pathogens or acute pain or syncope.

(3)Slow pulse

Pulse condition:a pulse with less than four beats to one cycle of the physician's respiration.

Disease correspondence:cold syndrome.Slow forceful pulse indicates cold pain and cold accumulation;and slow weak pulse indicates deficiency-cold.Athletes often exhibit a slow and powerful pulse,which is the normal one.

(4)Rapid pulse

Pulse condition:a pulse with more than five or six beats to one cycle of the physician's respiration.

Disease correspondence:heat syndrome.Rapid forceful pulse indicates excess heat,and weak rapid pulse indicates deficiency-heat.

Racing pulse:a pulse having more than seven beats per respiration,mostly indicating the seriousness of the disease like overabundant yang qi,or nearly exhaustion of yin qi,or collapse of original qi.

(5)Vacuous(feeble)pulse

Pulse condition:a feeble and void pulse.

Disease correspondence:deficiency syndrome.

(6)Replete pulse

Pulse condition:a pulse felt forceful at all the three sections,cun/inch,guan/bar and chi/cubit.

Pulse correspondence:excess syndrome.

(7)Slippery pulse

Pulse condition:a pulse coming and going smoothly like beads rolling on a plate.

Pulse correspondence:phlegm or retained fluid,food accumulation or excess heat.

(8)Rough pulse

Pulse condition:a pulse coming and going unsmoothly with small,fine,slow joggling tempo like scraping bamboo with a knife.

Pulse correspondence:deficiency of essence and blood,qi stagnation and blood stasis,complicated by phlegm or food.

(9)String-like(wiry)pulse

Pulse condition:a straight,long and taut pulse like a musical string to the touch.

Pulse correspondence:liver or gallbladder disease,phlegm and retained fluid,pain syndrome and diarrhea.

(10)Tight pulse

Pulse condition:a pulse feeling like a tightly stretched cord.

Pulse correspondence:cold syndrome,pain syndrome.

(11)Soggy pulse

Pulse condition:a thin and floating pulse which can be felt on light pressure,but growing faint upon hard pressure.

Pulse correspondence:deficiency syndrome,dampness syndrome.

(12)Surging pulse

Pulse condition:a pulse beating like dashing waves with forceful rising and gradual decline,also called flooding pulse.

（14）促脉

【脉象】脉来急数，时而一止，止无定数，即脉搏快有不规则的间歇。

【主病】阳热亢盛，气血痰食郁滞。

（15）结脉

【脉象】脉来缓慢，时而一止，止无定数。

【主病】阴盛气结，寒痰血瘀，气血虚弱，癥瘕积聚。

（16）代脉

【脉象】脉来时见一止，止有定数，良久方来。可见于心律失常的二联律、三联律等。

【主病】脏气衰微，风证，痛证。

4. 相兼脉与主病　相兼脉又称"复合脉"，是两种或两种以上单一脉象的综合表现。如浮紧、浮数、沉迟、沉细数等，其临床意义一般是组成相兼脉的各单一脉主病的总合。现将常见的相兼脉及主病列于下：

（1）浮紧脉：表寒证，或风寒痹证。

（2）浮缓脉：伤寒表虚证。

（3）浮数脉：表热证。

（4）浮滑脉：表证挟痰证，或有风痰。

（5）沉迟脉：里寒证。

（6）弦数脉：热证，或肝经有热。

（7）滑数脉：痰热证，或内热食积。

（8）洪数脉：气分热盛。

（9）沉弦脉：肝郁气滞，水饮内停。

（10）沉涩脉：血瘀证。

（11）弦细脉：肝肾阴虚，肝郁脾虚。

（12）沉缓脉：脾虚，水湿停留。

（13）沉细脉：阴虚或血虚证。

（14）弦滑数脉：肝火挟痰，痰火内蕴。

（15）沉细数脉：阴虚，血虚有热。

（16）弦紧脉：寒痛，寒滞肝脉。

Pulse correspondence:interior heat syndrome.It often occurs in patients with high fever.

Large pulse:a broad pulse with bigger amplitude than normal,indicating the development and aggravation of disease(large and forceful pulse).But the large weak pulse indicates deficiency of healthy qi.

(13)Fine pulse

Pulse condition:a pulse as thin as a silk thread,straight and soft,feeble yet always perceptible upon hard pressure,also called thin/thready pulse.

Pulse correspondence:deficiency of qi and blood,strain,and dampness syndrome.

Thin/thready pulse is also known as fine pulse,with its pulse correspondence in line with the fine pulse.

(14)Skipping(irregular-rapid)pulse

Pulse conditions:a rapid pulse with irregular intermittence.

Pulse correspondence:excessive yang heat,or stagnation of qi,blood,phlegm and food.

(15)Bound pulse(irregularly intermittent pulse)

Pulse condition:a moderate weak pulse,pausing at irregular intervals.

Pulse correspondence:excessive cold with binding qi,cold phlegm and blood stasis,deficiency of qi and blood,aggregation and accumulation.

(16)Intermittent pulse(regularly intermittent pulse)

Pulse condition:a moderate weak pulse,pausing at regular intervals,often indicating coupled rhythm or trigeminy caused by cardiac arrhythmia.

Pulse correspondence:visceral dysfunction,wind syndrome or pain syndrome.

4. Compound pulse and disease correspondences of the pulses

Compound pulse refers to the comprehensive pulse combining two or more than two single pulses, such as floating tight pulse,floating rapid pulse,sunken slow pulse,and sunken thin pulse,clinically manifesting the syndrome indicated by each component of the compound pulse.Here are the compound pulses and the disease correspondences of each of the compound pulses.

(1)Floating tight pulse:exterior cold syndrome,or syndrome of wind-cold impediment

(2)Floating moderate pulse:exterior deficiency syndrome

(3)Floating rapid pulse:exterior heat syndrome

(4)Floating slippery pulse:exterior syndrome complicated by phlegm or wind phlegm

(5)Sunken slow pulse:interior cold syndrome

(6)String-like rapid pulse:heat syndrome or heat in liver meridian

(7)Slippery rapid pulse:phlegm heat syndrome or syndrome of food accumulation with internal heat

(8)Surging rapid pulse:syndrome of excessive heat in qi aspect

(9)Sunken string-like pulse:liver depression and qi stagnation or fluid retention in the interior

(10)Sunken rough pulse:blood stasis syndrome

(11)String-like thin pulse:liver-kidney yin deficiency,or liver depression and spleen deficiency

(12)Sunken moderate pulse:spleen deficiency or water-dampness retention

(13)Sunken thin pulse:yin deficiency syndrome or blood deficiency syndrome

(14)Strong-like slippery rapid pulse:liver fire complicated by phlegm or phlegm fire engendering in the interior

(15)Sunken thin rapid pulse:yin deficiency or blood deficiency with heat

(16)String-like tight pulse:cold pain or cold stagnating liver meridian

三、按诊

（一）按肌肤

按肌肤是为了探明肌肤的寒热、润燥以及肿胀等情况。肌肤灼热为热证；肌肤清凉多为寒证；皮肤干燥者，多为无汗或津液不足；湿润者，为身汗出或津液未伤；皮肤甲错者，伤阴或内有瘀血；按之凹陷、举手即起的，为气肿；按之凹陷、不能即起的，为水肿。肌肤濡软而喜按者，为虚证；患处硬痛拒按者，为实证；轻按即痛者，病在表浅；重按方痛者，病在深部。

（二）按手足

按手足主要探明手足寒热，判断病证性质属虚属实，在内在外及预后。手足俱冷的，是阳虚寒盛，属寒证；手足俱热者，多为阳盛热炽，属热证；手足背部较热者，为外感发热；手足心较热者，为内伤发热。小儿手心热多为食积，手背热多为外感。此外按手足寒温可测知阳气存亡，四肢犹温，是阳气尚存，预后尚佳；若四肢厥冷，其病多凶，预后不良。

（三）按胸腹

1. 按虚里　虚里位于左乳下心尖搏动处，为诸脉所宗。探索虚里搏动的情况，可以了解宗气的强弱，其动微弱无力，是宗气内虚；若动而应衣，为太过，是宗气外泄之象；若按之弹手，洪大而搏，属于危重的证候。

2. 按胸胁　主要了解心、肺、肝的情况。前胸高起，按之气喘者，为肺脏证；胸胁按之胀痛者，多为痰热气结或水饮内停；若右胁下扪及肿大包块，或软或硬，多属气滞血瘀，若表面凹凸不平，则要警惕肝癌；摸之热感，按之疼痛，或为肝痈；左胁下扪及包块即肿大脾脏，则要警惕肝硬化、血吸虫病及某些血液病等；疟疾日久，胁下出现肿块，称为疟母。

3. 按腹部　按腹部主要了解凉热、软硬度、胀满、肿块、压痛等情况。腹壁冷，喜暖手按抚者，属虚寒证；腹壁灼热、喜冷指按抚者，属实热证。腹部有包块，按之柔软且聚散不定者，为瘕为聚，多属气机阻滞；按之坚硬，部位固定，为癥为积，多属血瘀痰阻。凡腹痛，喜按者属虚，拒按者属实；按之局部灼热，痛不可忍者，为内痈。腹部胀满，按之有充实感觉，有压痛，叩之声音重浊的，多为实满；腹部膨满，按之不实，无压痛，叩之作空声的，为气胀，多为虚满。如若左小腹作痛，按之累累有硬块者，为肠中有宿粪；右小腹作痛，按之疼痛，有包块应手者，为肠痈；如若腹部按之有条状物，凹凸不平，按之起伏聚散，多为虫积。

4. 按手足　手足冷暖，判别阳气之盛衰。冷凉为虚寒证，多为阳虚或阴盛；手足热为热证，多为阴虚或阳盛；手足心热为阴虚内热。

5. 按腧穴　通过按压特殊腧穴来判断脏腑病变。如肺俞、心俞、肝俞、肾俞、脾俞、大肠俞、小肠俞、膀胱俞、胆俞等等。相应的腧穴可以协助疾病判断。

Body Palpation

Palpation on the skin

Palpation on the skin is to detect the condition of the skin, cold or heat, moisture or dryness or swelling. Scorching heat of skin indicates heat syndrome; cold skin indicates cold syndrome; dry skin indicates absence of sweating or fluid deficiency; moist skin indicates sweating or undamaged fluid; encrusted skin indicates impairment of yin or blood stasis; sinking when pressed and recovering immediately after hands leave indicates emphysema; and sinking when pressed and recovering after a while after hands leave indicates edema. Soft skin which welcomes pressing indicates deficiency syndrome; the affected part with sensation of pain and refusing to be pressed indicates excess syndrome; pain felt when pressed lightly indicates superficial disease; and pain felt when pressed hardly indicates deep disease.

Examination of the hands and feet

Examination of the hands and feet is to explore the condition of hands and feet, cold or heat, then judge which syndrome it belongs to, excess one or deficiency one, exterior one or interior one and predict the prognosis. Cold hands and feet indicates cold syndrome-yang deficiency with excessive cold; hot hands and feet indicates heat syndrome of excessive yang with effulgent heat; hotter backs of hands and insteps indicates heat syndrome caused by external contraction; hotter palms and soles indicates heat caused by internal injuries; hotter infant palms often indicates food accumulation; and hotter infant backs of hands indicates internal contraction. In addition, it can predict the condition of yang qi, existence or collapse, from the cold or the heat of the hands and feet: warm limbs indicate yang qi exists and favorable prognosis, and cold limbs indicates the aggravation of the disease and unfavorable prognosis.

Palpation on the chest and abdomen

1. Apical impulse examination

It is also known as examination of Xuli, which is located at apical impulse under the left breast and where the ancestral qi is located. Examination of the apical pulsation is to know the conditions of apical impulse and ancestral qi. Weak and feeble apical impulse indicates internal deficiency of ancestral qi; apical impulse reflected from the motion of the clothes indicates excessive ancestral qi, which is escaping outside; and apical impulse beating hand on it indicates it is a critical disease.

2. Examination of the chest and hypochondrium

It is to understand the conditions of the heart, lung and liver. Protruding forechest with sensation of dyspnea when pressed indicates lung illness; distention and pain in chest and hypochondrium when pressed indicates phlegm heat and qi binding or retained fluid; swelling soft or hard mass under the right hypochondrium most indicates qi stagnation and blood stasis; uneven skin around the mass indicates possibility of liver cancer; sensation of heat when touched and pain when pressed indicates liver abscess; mass under the left hypochondrium indicates the possibility of cirrhosis, schistosomiasis or other kinds of blood illnesses; and lumps under the hypochondrium after long-lasting diarrhea indicates malaria.

3. Abdominal examination

It is to get such information as cold or heat, soft or hardness, fullness and distention, lump and tenderness. Cold abdomen preferring warm pressing indicates deficiency-cold syndrome, while scorching abdomen preferring cold pressing indicates excess heat syndrome. Aggregation, the soft abdominal mass gathering or scattering indicates obstruction of qi movement; and accumulation, the hard abdominal mass in the fixed place indicates blood stasis and phlegm blockage. Generally, abdominal pain relieved by pressing indicates deficiency syndrome, while abdominal pain aggravated by pressing indicates excess syndrome. Sen-

第二节 八纲及其辨证

八纲辨证是根据四诊取得的材料，进行综合分析，将疾病的性质、病变部位、病势的轻重、机体反应的强弱、正邪双方力量的对比等情况，归纳为阴、阳、表、里、寒、热、虚、实八类证候，即从疾病类别上，可分为阴证和阳证；从病位上，可分表证和里证；从病性上，可分为寒证和里证；从邪正盛衰上，又可分为实证和虚证。八纲辨证是中医辨证的基本方法，各种辨证的总纲，是从各种辨证方法的个性中概括出的共性，在诊断疾病过程中，起到执简驭繁、提纲挈领作用。

一、表里

表里是辨别病变部位深浅、病情轻重和病势趋向的两个纲领。

（一）表证

表证是病位浅在肌表的证候。六淫外邪从皮毛、口鼻侵入机体后，邪留肌表，具有起病急、病程短、病位浅和病情轻的特点，属外感病初起阶段。

证候：以发热恶寒（或恶风）、头痛、舌苔薄白、脉浮为基本证候，常兼见四肢关节及全身肌肉酸痛、鼻塞、咽痛、咳嗽等症状。

分析：外邪侵犯皮毛肌腠，正邪相争则发热；卫气受遏，肌表失于温煦，故而恶寒或恶风；邪气阻滞经脉，气血运行不畅故而头身疼痛；邪气在表，故舌苔薄白；正邪相争于表，故脉浮；肺主一身之表，鼻为肺之窍，咽喉为肺之通道，故外邪袭表，症为鼻塞、咽痛、咳嗽等。

此外，由于外邪有寒热之分，正气有强弱不同，所以表证又分为表寒、表热、表虚、表实证。表寒证：恶寒重发热轻，无汗，口不渴，舌淡红，苔薄白而润脉浮紧；表热证：恶寒轻发热重，有汗，口渴，舌质稍红，苔薄白不润，脉浮数；表虚证：恶风恶寒，有汗，舌质淡，舌苔薄白，脉浮而无力；表实证：恶寒，无汗，舌质淡，舌苔薄脉浮而有力。

sation of scorching heat and intolerable pain on the pressed place indicates internal abscess. Fullness and distention in the abdomen with pain when pressed and with turbid voice when tapped often indicates excess fullness, while fullness and distention in the abdomen without pain when pressed and with empty voice when tapped often indicates qi distention and deficiency fullness. Pain in the left lower abdomen with lump indicates retained stool in the large intestine, while pain in the right lower abdomen with lump indicates intestine abscess. And sensation of stick-like and uneven object in the abdomen when pressed indicates worm accumulation.

4. Examination of the hands and feet

The condition of hands and feet, hot or cold is used to judge the condition of yang qi. Cold hands and feet indicates deficiency-cold syndrome, often caused by yang deficiency or excessive yin; hot hands and feet indicates heat syndrome, often caused by yin deficiency or excessive yang; and hot palms and soles indicates yin deficiency with internal heat.

5. Palpation of the acupuncture point

It is to judge the pathological changes of internal organs by palpating special acupuncture points like lung shu, heart shu, liver shu, kidney shu, spleen shu, large intestine shu, small intestine shu, bladder shu and gallbladder shu, as the corresponding acupuncture point can help physicians to judge disease of the lung, heart, liver, kidney, spleen, large intestine, small intestine, bladder and gallbladder respectively.

Section 2   Eight Principal Syndromes and Their Differentiation

Eight principal syndrome differentiation refers to summarizing and categorizing diseases into eight syndromes (namely yin syndrome, yang syndrome, interior syndrome, exterior syndrome, cold syndrome, heat syndrome, deficiency syndrome and excess syndrome), according to the result of comprehensive analysis on the property, location and degree of the diseases, the reaction of the body, and contrast of powers of the healthy qi and pathogenic factors gathered through the four diagnostic methods. To be precise, from the aspect of category, diseases can be classified into yin syndrome and yang syndrome. From the aspect of location, they can be classified into interior syndrome and exterior syndrome. From the aspect of nature, diseases can be categorized as cold syndrome and heat syndrome. And from the aspect of struggle between the healthy qi and the pathogenic factors, diseases can be divided into excess syndrome and deficiency syndrome. Analysis and differentiation of pathological conditions in accordance with the eight principal syndromes is the basic differentiation method of TCM, the general principle of various syndrome differentiations, and the general character concluded from diverse syndrome differentiation methods. It allows the doctors to simplify the complex symptoms and concentrate on the main points of a disease in the course of diagnosing a disease.

Exterior Syndrome and Interior Syndrome

exterior syndrome and Interior syndrome are two principal syndromes used to differentiate the location, severity and prognosis of a disease.

Exterior Syndrome

Exterior syndrome refers to a general term for syndromes that occur chiefly at the early stage of external contractions affecting the exterior part of the body, characterized by sudden onset, short course, shallow location and light symptoms. It is often caused by the six excess invading the body through skins, mouth,

（二）里证

里证是与表证相对而言，表示病变部位在机体深层，是脏腑气血受病所反应的一系列证候的概括。

里证的成因，大致有三种情况：一是表证进一步发展，表邪不解，内传入里，侵犯脏腑而产生；二是外邪直接入侵脏腑而发病；三是其他原因如内伤七情、劳倦、饮食等因素，直接导致脏腑功能失调发生。

里证包括的证候范围很广，凡非表证的一切证候皆属里证。概括起来则以脏腑的证候为主，病程长，不恶寒，不恶风，脉不浮，多有舌质、舌苔的改变，其具体内容详见脏腑辨证部分。

（三）表证与里证的鉴别

辨别表证与里证是以病程、恶寒发热的轻重及舌象、脉象的变化依据。新病、病程短者，多见于表证；久病、病程长者，常见于里证。发热恶寒者，为表证；但热不寒或但寒不热者，均属里证。舌苔无变化，或仅见于舌边尖红属表证；舌苔有异常表现者多属里证；脉浮者为表证；脉沉者为里证。

（四）表证与里证的关系

1. 表里同病　表里同病是指在同一个人、同一个时期同时出现表证和里证。如病人既有恶寒、发热、头痛等表证，又有腹胀、尿黄、便秘等里证。常见的有三种情况：一是表证未解，邪已入里；二是病邪同时侵犯表里；三是旧病未愈，又感外邪。

2. 表里转化　在一定的条件下，表证和里证可以相互转化。这种转化取决于正邪双方相斗的状况。邪气过盛，或机体抵抗力下降，或护理不当，或失治、误治等，均可导致病邪入里，病情加重，此为"由表入里"；机体抗邪能力增强，病邪被驱，病势减轻，此为"由里出表"。

and nose.

Syndromes: with fever, aversion to cold (or aversion to wind), headache, thin and white fur and floating pulse as its basic manifestation, often concurrently with ache of joints of limbs and all the muscles, stuffy nose, sore throat, and cough.

Analysis: Fever occurs because the healthy qi struggles with the external pathogen which invades the skin, muscle, and interstices. Aversion to cold or aversion to wind turns up because the defense qi is obstructed from warming the skin and muscles. Headache and body pain emerge because the pathogenic factors block meridians and collaterals, which results in sluggish circulation of qi and blood. There is thin and white fur because the pathogenic factors still stay in the surface. Floating pulse turns up because the struggle between the healthy qi and the pathogenic factors takes place in the exterior. Stuffy nose, sore throat, and cough occur when the external pathogens invade the exterior as the lung is in charge of the body surface, with nose as its orifice and throat as its channel.

The exterior syndrome can be further divided into exterior cold, exterior heat, exterior deficiency, and exterior excess in accordance with the nature (cold or heat) of external pathogens and the status of healthy qi. Exterior cold syndrome manifests heavy aversion to cold with light fever, no sweat, no thirst, reddish tongue, thin and white fur and smooth, floating and tight pulse. Exterior heat syndrome shows light aversion to cold with high fever, sweat, thirst, red tongue, thin and white fur without moist, and weak, rapid and floating pulse. Exterior deficiency syndrome is characterized by aversion to cold and wind, sweat, light tongue, thin and white fur, and weak and floating pulse. Exterior excess syndrome features aversion to cold, no sweat, light tongue, thin fur, and strong floating pulse.

Interior Syndrome

Interior syndrome is a general term for syndromes that indicates the existence of disease in the interior of the body. It is the summary of series of syndromes caused by injury of qi and blood in the internal organs.

Generally, interior syndrome is caused by three circumstances: one is from further development of exterior syndrome, the exterior pathogen entering the interior and invades the internal organs; the second is the result that the exterior pathogen attacks the internal organs directly; and the third arises from the disfunctions of the internal organs, which is caused by seven emotions, overstrain and improper diet.

Interior syndrome covers a wide range of syndromes, including all those not categorized into exterior syndrome. In summary, all the syndromes reflecting the situation of the internal organs are classified into the interior syndrome, characterized by long course, no aversion to cold and wind, pulse not floated, and variation of tongue body and fur. Please refer to syndrome differentiation of the viscera and bowels for details.

Differentiation of Exterior Syndrome and Interior Syndrome

Differentiation of exterior syndrome and interior syndrome is based on the course of the disease, degree of aversion to cold and fever, and variation of tongue and pulse manifestations. Those newly occurring and with short course mostly belong to exterior syndrome; while those with long course of disease mostly belong to interior syndrome. Aversion to cold with fever is exterior syndrome; while fever without aversion to cold, and cold without aversion to heat are both interior syndrome. Fur unchanged, or only red tongue tip or red tongue edge is the embodiment of exterior syndrome; while abnormal fur is often the embodiment of interior syndrome. Floating pulse pertains to exterior syndrome, while sunken pulse pertains to interior syndrome.

Relations between Exterior Syndrome and Interior Syndrome

1. Disease involving both the exterior and interior

二、寒热

寒热是辨别疾病性质的两个纲领。

（一）寒证

寒证是感受阴寒之邪或阳虚阴盛，机体机能活动衰减所表现证候的概括。多由外感寒邪，或因内伤久病，耗伤阳气，阴寒偏盛所致。

主证：恶寒或畏寒喜暖，口不渴或喜热饮，面色苍白，肢冷蜷卧，小便清长，大便稀溏。舌质淡，苔白而润，脉沉迟或紧。

分析：外感寒邪，或阳气不足，机体不得温煦，故而恶寒或畏寒、肢冷蜷卧而喜暖；阴寒内盛，津液未伤，故口不渴或喜热饮；阳气不足，水液不得温化，故而小便清长、大便稀溏；阳虚不化，寒湿内生，故舌质淡、苔白而润；阳气不振，无力推动血脉运行，故而脉沉迟或沉紧。

（二）热证

热证是感受阳热之邪或阳盛阴虚，脏腑功能活动亢进所表现证候的概括。多由外感热邪，或寒邪入里化热，或素体阳盛，或情志内伤、郁而化火，或过食辛辣、郁积化热，致使机体阳热过盛。

主证：发热喜冷，口渴喜冷饮，烦躁不安，面红目赤，大便燥结，小便短赤。舌质红，苔黄，脉数。

分析：外感热邪，或阳热偏盛，故而发热喜凉；热伤津液，故而口渴喜冷饮、小便短赤、大便燥结；火性上炎，故而面红目赤；热扰心神，故而烦躁不安；舌质红、苔黄，属热象；邪热亢盛，鼓动血脉，故见脉数。

It means a patient reveals exterior syndrome and interior syndrome at the same time. For example, a patient manifests the exterior syndromes of aversion to cold, fever and headache, and concurrently with interior syndromes of abdominal distention, yellow urine and constipation. It occurs in three circumstances: one is from the exterior pathogen entering the interior before it being removed; the second arises from the pathogen invading the exterior and the interior concurrently; and the third is owed to invasion of new pathogen before the elimination of an old one.

2. Transformation between exterior syndrome and interior syndrome

It means that exterior syndrome and interior syndrome can be transformed mutually in certain conditions. Such transformation relies on the status of the struggle between the healthy qi and the pathogenic factors. Invasion of pathogenic factors from the exterior to the interior occurs when there are overabundant pathogens, or decline of the body resistance, or improper nursing, or lack of timely treatment or therapeutic error, which shows that the disease aggravates. Invasion of pathogenic factors from the interior to the exterior takes place when the resistance of the body improves, or pathogenic factors are eliminated, which indicates that the disease alleviates.

Cold Syndrome and Heat Syndrome

Cold syndrome and heat syndrome are two principal syndromes used to differentiate the nature of a disease.

Cold Syndrome

Cold syndrome is the summary of series of manifestations arising from body hypoactivity as the result of invasion of cold wind, or yang deficiency and yin excess. It is primarily caused by external contraction of cold, or impairment of yang qi due to chronic disease, or excess of yin and cold.

Principal syndromes: aversion to cold, or fear of cold, preference of warm, hydroadipsia or preference of warm drinks, pale complexion, cold limbs and cowering, clear abundant urine, sloppy stool, light tongue with moist and white fur, and sunken and slow pulse or sunken and tight pulse.

Analysis: Aversion to cold, fear of cold, cold limbs, cowering and preference of warm occur because the exterior cold or insufficient yang qi prevents the body from being warmed. Hydroadipsia and preference of warm or hot drinks take place because of inward overabundance of yin and cold and non-impairment of body fluids. Short abundant urine and sloppy stool come out because insufficient yang qi fails to warm and transform the water and fluids. Light tongue with moist and white fur turns up because yang deficiency fails to transform and cold-damp engenders inward. In addition sunken and slow pulse or sunken and tight pulse comes into being because devitalized yang fails to promote blood circulation.

Heat Syndrome

Heat syndrome is the summary of a series of manifestations arising from hyperactivity of the internal organs as the result of heat invasion or yang excess and yin deficiency. It is primarily caused by internal contraction of heat, or cold entering the interior and transforming into heat, or constitutional yang excess, or emotional depression transforming into heat, or heat produced from excessive pungent or hot food, all of which lead to excess of yang and heat in the body.

Principal syndromes: fever, preference of cold, thirst and preference of cold drinks, agitation, red face and eyes, constipation, scant red urine, red tongue with yellow fur and rapid pulse.

Analysis: fever and preference of cold occurs due to external contraction of heat, or excess of yang and heat. Thirst and preference of cold drinks, scanty dark urine and constipation turn up because heat injuries the body fluids. Red face and eyes come out as the result of fire flaming upward. Agitation is the re-

附：实热与虚热

中医临床之热证系指阳热过盛、正气未衰的实热证，与各种原因造成的机体阴液亏损、所谓阴虚阳越的虚热证，临床表现不同。实热证：发病急，病程短，发热，面红目赤，大汗出，烦渴喜冷饮，大便秘结，小便短赤，舌红，苔黄，脉洪数；虚热证：发病缓慢，病程长，两颧绯红，低热，盗汗，五心烦热，失眠多梦，口干但饮不多，大便量少，小便黄、量少舌红，少苔或无苔，脉细数。治疗原则为"虚则补之，实则泻之"，即清热泻火、滋阴清热。

（三）寒证与热证的鉴别

临床上多从病人的面色、寒热喜恶、口渴与否、二便情况以及舌脉变化等进行辨别表 4-2。

表 4-2　寒证、热证鉴别表

	面色	四肢	寒热	口渴	大便	小便	舌象	脉象
寒证	苍白	不温	怕冷	不渴或热饮不多	稀溏	清长	舌淡苔白润	迟或紧
热证	红赤	灼热	发热	口渴喜冷饮	秘结	短赤	舌红苔黄干	数

（四）寒证与热证的关系

1. 寒热错杂　寒证与热证交错同时出现，称之为寒热错杂。根据临床表现可分为表里与上下两部分。表里的寒热错杂表现为表寒里热、表热里寒；上下的寒热错杂表现为上热下寒、上寒下热等。如既见胸中烦热、频欲呕吐的上热证，又见腹痛喜暖、大便稀薄的下寒证，即属上热下寒证。又如，胃脘冷痛、呕吐清涎，同时又兼见尿频、尿痛、小便短赤，此为上寒在脾胃而下热在膀胱之证候。

2. 寒热转化　寒证与热证在一定条件下可以相互转化。病初为寒证，后出现热证，寒证消失，此属寒证转化为热证；病初为热证，后出现寒证，热证消失，此属热证转化为寒证。寒热转化反映了邪正盛衰的情况。

3. 寒热真假　在疾病过程中的一般情况下，疾病本质与临床表现是一致的，即寒证见寒象、热证见热象。但在疾病发展到寒极或热极的危重阶段，可以出现一些"热极似寒"、"寒极似热"的假象。

（1）真热假寒：内有真热而外见假寒的证候，又称之为"阳盛格阴"。如热性病

sult of heat disturbing the heart spirit. Red tongue with yellow fur presents the heat syndrome. And rapid pulse embodies that the excessive heat stirs and accelerates blood circulation.

Additional reading: excess heat and deficiency heat

Heat syndrome in TCM theory clinically refers to excess syndrome presenting excessive heat and unbated healthy qi. The deficiency heat syndrome arising from depletion of yin-fluid caused by various factors has different clinical manifestations. Excess heat syndrome is characterized by sudden onset, short course, fever, red face and eyes, excessive perspiration, polydipsia and preference of cold drinks, constipation, scanty dark urine, red tongue with yellow fur and surging and rapid pulse; while deficiency heat syndrome features slow onset, long course, scarlet cheeks, low fever and night sweating, vexing heat in chest, palms and soles, insomnia, dreaminess, thirst but little drinking, little stool, scanty yellow urine, red tongue with little or without fur, and thin and rapid pulse. In treating them, the doctors should follow the therapeutic principles of "treating deficiency by tonification" and "treating excess by purgation," the therapeutic methods are clearing heat to purge fire and enriching yin to clear heat.

Differentiation of Cold Syndrome and Heat Syndrome

Clinically, differentiation of cold syndrome and heat syndrome is based on the patient's complexion, preference of cold or warm, thirst or not, status of urine and excretion and variation of tongue and pulse. Please refer to the table 4-2 for details of cold syndrome and heat syndrome.

Table 4-2   Comparison of Cold Syndrome and Heat Symdrome

Syndrome	Complexion	Limbs	Chills or fever	Thirst	Feces	Urine	Tongue	Pulse
Cold	Pale	Not warm	Chills	Thirstless or drinking a little warm drink	Sloppy stool	Clear and much	Light tongue with moist and white fur	Slow or tight
Heat	Red or scarlet	Hot	Fever	Thirst and preference of cold drinks	Constipation	Scanty and dark	Red tongue with dry and yellow fur	Rapid

Relations between Cold Syndrome and Heat Syndrome

1. Cold-heat complex syndrome

It refers to the concurrent occurrence of cold syndrome and heat syndrome. It can be divided into two parts of exterior and interior, and upper and lower syndrome according to the clinical manifestations. With respect to the exterior and interior part, it manifests the syndrome of exterior cold and interior heat, or the syndrome of exterior heat and interior cold. With regard to the upper and lower part, it shows the upper heat and lower cold syndrome, or the upper cold and lower heat syndrome. For example, the patient must suffer from the upper heat and lower cold syndrome if he/she presents the upper heat symptoms of vexing heat in the chest and desire to vomit, concurrently with the lower cold symptoms of abdominal pain, preference of warm and sloppy stool. Cold pain in the stomach and vomiting of clear saliva, concurrently with frequent urination, dysuria and scant red urine is the embodiment of syndrome of cold in the upper spleen and stomach and heat in the lower bladder.

2. Transformation of cold and heat

It refers to the mutual transformation of cold syndrome and heat syndrome under certain conditions. Cold syndrome transforming into heat syndrome appears when the later occurrence of heat syndrome replaces the initial happened cold syndrome in a disease. And heat syndrome transforming into cold syndrome emerges when the later occurrence of cold syndrome substitutes for the initial happened heat syndrome during a disease.

3. True and false heat and cold

中毒较重时可见表情淡漠，困倦懒言，四肢厥冷，脉沉细等似为寒证；但其反见身寒恶热、不喜添加衣被、口渴喜冷饮、咽干口臭、谵语，并见小便短赤、大便秘结、舌红绛、苔黄干、脉虽沉细但数而有力等热象。其病机为阳热过盛，伏潜于里，阳气内郁不能外达四肢，就其本质仍属热证，故称"真热假寒"。治疗上应清泻里热、疏达阳气。

（2）真寒假热：内有真寒而外见假热的证候，又称之为"阴盛格阳"。如慢性消耗性疾病患者常见身热、面红、口渴，苔黑，脉浮大等似为热证；但身热欲加衣被、口渴而喜热饮且饮而不多、舌质淡白、苔黑而润，脉虽浮大但无力，并见小便清长、大便溏稀等寒象。其病机为阴盛于内，迫阳于外，虚阳外越，其本质仍是寒证，故称"真寒假热"。治疗上要用温里回阳、引火归原。

三、虚实

虚实是用以概括和辨别正气强弱和病邪盛衰的两个纲领。

（一）虚证

虚证是指正气虚弱、脏腑功能衰退所表现的证候。虚证的形成，多见于素体虚弱，先天不足，后天失养，或因久病、重病伤及正气，或七情劳倦，或因外伤出血等原因导致的气血阴阳亏虚。根据气血阴阳的不同虚损，临床上可分为气虚、血虚、阴虚、阳虚。

1. 阴虚证　阴虚证是阴液亏损所表现证候的概括。主症见午后潮热，夜间盗汗，两颧发红，五心烦热，口干咽燥，小便短黄，大便干结，舌红少苔、脉细或细数。

分析：阴虚内热生，故见午后潮热，两颧发红，五心烦热；阴虚阳越、逼津外泄，故见夜间盗汗；热伤津液，故见口干咽燥、小便短黄、大便干结；舌红少苔、脉细或细数，属阴虚内热的表现。

2. 阳虚证　阳虚证是体内阳气不足所表现证候的概括。主症见畏寒，形寒肢冷，面色㿠白，口淡不渴，小便清长，大便溏泄，舌淡苔白，脉沉或迟。

分析：阳虚内寒生，肌肤不得温煦，故见形寒肢冷；阳气不足、气血运行不畅，故见面色㿠白；阳气虚弱、阴寒内生，故见口淡不渴、小便清长、大便溏泄；舌淡苔白，脉沉或迟，为阳虚的表现。

Generally speaking, the nature of a disease is consistence with its clinical manifestations in the course of its development. In another word, cold syndrome exposes the cold signs, and heat syndrome appears the heat signs. However, when it develops to its extremity of cold or extremity of heat, the critical stage of a disease, there will emerge false images like extreme heat appearing with cold syndrome, and extreme cold appearing with heat syndrome.

True heat with false cold: it refers to the true heat in the exterior with false cold symptoms in the exterior, also known as "exuberant yang repelling yin". For example, when the heat disease develops to a severe stage, the false cold symptoms of indifferent expression, sleepiness and unwillingness to talk, cold limbs and sunken and thin pulse will occur. In spite of these, the patient still presents the heat syndrome of refusal to put on more clothes or quilt despite of feeling cold, thirst and preference of cold drinks, dry throat and mouth with fetid odor, delirium, scant red urine, constipation, scarlet tongue with dry and yellow fur, and sunken and thin, but rapid and strong pulse. The pathogenesis of the disease lies in extremely exuberant yang trapped in the interior prevents yang qi from diffusing outward to the limbs. So the disease naturally belongs to heat syndrome, also called "true heat with false cold." The therapeutic method of clearing and purging the interior heat to diffuse yang should be adopted in treatment.

True cold with false heat: it refers to true cold syndrome in the interior with false heat symptoms in the exterior, also known as "exuberant yin repelling yang." For example, those suffering from chronic wasting diseases often present the false heat syndrome of general fever, red complexion, thirst, black fur, and big and floating pulse. But meanwhile, the patients also manifest the cold syndrome of desire to put on more clothes or quilt, thirst and preference of warm and hot drinks but only with little, pale tongue with black and moist fur, large, floating but feeble pulse, clear abundant urine, and sloppy stool. The pathogenesis of the disease arises from extremely excessive yin entrenched in the interior forces the asthenic yang to float on the body surface. So the disease naturally belongs to cold syndrome, also called "true cold with false heat." The therapeutic method of warming the interior to save yang and conducting fire back to its origin should be adopted in treatment.

Deficiency Syndrome and Excess Syndrome

Deficiency syndrome and excess syndrome are two principal syndromes used to summarize and differentiate the status of the healthy qi and the pathogenic factors.

Deficiency Syndrome

Deficiency syndrome refers to the manifestations arising from dysfunction of the internal organs due to the deficiency of the healthy qi. It is primarily caused by the constitutional weakness, inadequate natural endowment, postnatal malnutrition, or impairment of the healthy qi due to chronic or serious disease, or qi, blood, yin and yang deficiency due to excessively intensive emotions, overexertion and traumatic hemorrhage, etc. According to the depletion ingredient, it can be clinically divided into qi deficiency, blood deficiency, yin deficiency, and yang deficiency. Please refer to the chapter on qi, blood, fluid and humor for the details of qi deficiency and blood deficiency.

1. Yin deficiency syndrome

It is the summary of manifestations of deficiency of yin fluid and essence. The principal syndrome includes postmeridian hectic fever, night sweat, red cheeks, vexing heat in chest, palms and soles, dry mouth and throat, scant and yellow urine, constipation, red tongue with little fur, and thin or thin and rapid pulse.

Analysis: postmeridian hectic fever, red cheeks, vexing heat in chest, palms and soles occur because yin deficiency generates interior heat. Night sweat is the result that deficient yin and floating yang dispels the fluid to escape. Dry mouth and throat, scant and yellow urine, and constipation arise from heat impairing the fluid. Red tongue with little fur, and thin or thin and rapid pulse are the manifestations of yin defi-

（二）实证

实证是邪气过盛，脏腑功能活动亢盛所表现证候的概括。

主症：由于病邪的性质及其侵犯的脏腑不同，临床表现不同，其特点是邪气盛，正气未衰，正邪相争处于激烈阶段。常见症状为高热，形体壮实，声高气粗，面红，烦躁谵妄，脘腹胀满疼痛而拒按，痰涎壅盛，大便秘结或下痢，小便不利或淋沥涩痛。舌苔厚腻，脉实有力。

分析：邪气过盛，正气与之抗争，阳热亢盛，故而发热；实邪扰心，故而烦躁谵妄；邪阻于肺，故而痰涎壅盛；邪积于肠胃，腑气不通，故而腹胀疼痛拒按、大便秘结；湿热下注大肠，则下痢；下注膀胱，则小便不利或淋沥涩痛；正盛邪实、气血壅盛，故而脉实有力、苔厚腻。

（三）虚证与实证的鉴别

新病：病程短，精神兴奋，声高气粗，疼痛拒按，大便秘结，小便短赤，苔厚腻，脉实而有力，多属实证；旧病、久病：病程长，精神萎靡，身倦乏力，气弱懒言，疼痛喜按，大便稀溏，小便清长，舌淡嫩少苔，脉细弱，多属虚证；外感多属实证，内伤多属虚证；从体质上，年青体壮者多属实证，年老体弱者多属虚证。

（四）虚证与实证的关系

疾病的变化是一个极其复杂的过程，经常受体质、治疗、护理等各种因素的影响致使虚证与实证之间发生虚实夹杂、虚实转化等相关变化。

1. 虚实夹杂　在同一病人身上虚证和实证同时出现，称之为虚实夹杂。虚实夹杂的证候表现不一，有以虚为主、夹有实证的；有以实为主、夹有虚证的；亦有虚实并重的。如肺心病患者，既有咳嗽、咯吐黄痰、下肢浮肿等实证，又有气短乏力、动则加剧、脉沉弱的虚证。

2. 虚实转化　在疾病发展过程中，由于正邪相争，故在一定条件下，虚证和实证可相互转化。实证转化为虚证，大多由于邪气过盛、损伤正气，或由于误治、失治而成。如病之初始为高热、汗出、口渴、脉洪大之实证，因未能及时治疗，日久不愈，导致津液耗伤，出现低热、形体消瘦、面色苍白、气短乏力、舌苔少或无苔、脉细无力等虚证，此为实证转化为虚证。虚证转化为实证，一般来讲，是由于正气本虚，脏腑生理功能低下，导致气、血、水等不能正常运行，产生了气滞、瘀血、痰饮、水湿等实邪，即病理产物停留体内，此为虚证转化为实证，而实际是虚实错杂证。如肾阳虚衰，气化不利，水液停滞，下肢浮肿，即阳虚水停之候。此证既有肾脏温化功能减退的虚象，又有水液停留于下肢的邪实之象，这种水湿泛滥乃由肾

ciency and interior heat.

2. Yang deficiency syndrome

It is the summary of the manifestations of yang qi deficiency in interior. The principal syndrome covers aversion to cold, cold limbs and body, bright pale complexion, bland taste in the mouth, hydroadipsia, clear and abundant urine, sloppy stool, light-colored tongue with white fur, and sunken or slow pulse.

Analysis: cold limbs and body emerge because yang deficiency engenders the interior cold and fails to warm the body. Bright pale complexion is the result of yang deficiency in failing to activate qi and blood circulation smoothly. Bland taste in the mouth, hydroadipsia, clear and abundant urine, and sloppy stool are the embodiment of yang deficiency engendering the interior yin cold. Light-colored tongue with white fur and sunken or slow pulse are the signs of yang deficiency.

Excess Syndrome

Excess syndrome is the summary of the manifestations of hyperactivity of the internal organs caused by excessive pathogenic factors. It is primarily caused by external contraction of the six excess invading into the body, or dysfunction of the internal organs, both of which will produce some pathological products like blood stasis, phlegm and retained fluid, water damp, worm accumulation and food accumulation.

Principal syndrome: the clinical manifestations vary with the nature of pathogenic factors and the internal organs they invade, characterized by fierce struggle between the flourishing pathogenic factors and unbated healthy qi. The principal syndrome includes high fever, strong physical shape, loud voice and heavy breath, red complexion, agitation and delirium, abdominal fullness, distention and pain, which aggravates when pressed, overabundant phlegm, constipation or diarrhea, difficult urination or dripping urination, thick and slimy fur, and powerful and full pulse.

Analysis: fever occurs because of intense struggle between the overabundant pathogenic yang heat and the healthy qi. Agitation and delirium are the result of the excessive pathogenic factors disturbing the heart. Overabundant phlegm is produced as the result of obstruction of the pathogenic factors in the lung. Abdominal full, distention and pains which aggravates when pressed, and constipation show that the pathogenic factors coagulate in the stomach and intestines and obstruct their qi from moving. Diarrhea is caused by damp-heat pouring down into the large intestine; and difficult and dripping urination is caused by damp-heat pouring down into the bladder. Powerful and full pulse and thick and greasy fur embody the vigorousness of healthy qi and over abundance of pathogenic factors, and the congestion and abundance of qi and blood.

Differentiation of Deficiency Syndrome and Excess Syndrome

Most of the syndromes and phenomena like newly onset diseases with short course, excited spirit, loud voice and heavy breath, pain which aggravates when pressed, constipation, scant dark urine, thick and slimy fur, and full and powerful pulse pertain to excess syndrome. While most of the syndromes and phenomena such as chronic disease with long-term course, listlessness, lack of strength, fatigue, weak breath, unwillingness to talk, pain which alleviates when pressed, sloppy stool, clear abundant urine, light-colored tongue with little fur and thin and weak pulse belong to deficiency syndrome. External contraction mostly belongs to excess syndrome, while internal injuries mostly belong to deficiency syndrome. In addition, excess syndrome often occurs in the strong and young patients, while deficiency syndrome often turns up in the old and weak patients.

Relations between Deficiency Syndrome and Excess Syndrome

Change of a disease is a very complicated course, which is affected by constitution, treatment, and nursing and etc. As the result of it, there are deficiency-excess complex, and conversion between deficiency and excess.

1. Deficiency-excess complex

阳不足、气化失常所致，可称之为因虚致实，也是一种虚实错杂的证候。

四、阴阳

阴阳是概括疾病类别的两个纲领。

疾病证候虽然复杂多变，但总不外阴阳两大类。阴阳又是八纲的总纲。它可以概括其他三对纲领，即表、实、热证属于阳证；里、虚、寒证属于阴证。临床上阴证多指里证的虚寒证，阳证多指里证的实热证。

（一）阴证与阳证

阴证是体内阳气虚衰或体内寒邪凝滞的证候。一般而言阴证必见寒象，属虚、属寒，机体反应呈衰退状态。主要临床症候：面色苍白，精神萎靡，畏寒肢冷，气短声微，口不渴，小便清长，大便溏泻，舌淡胖嫩，苔白，脉沉弱。

阳证是体内阳气亢盛或体内热邪壅盛的证候。一般而言阳证必见热象，属实、属热，机体反应呈亢奋状态。主要临床症候：身热面赤，精神烦躁，气壮声高，口渴喜饮，呼吸气粗，小便短赤，大便秘结，舌红绛，苔黄，脉洪滑实。

（二）亡阴与亡阳

亡阴与亡阳，是疾病过程中两种危险证候，多在高热、大汗不止、剧烈吐泻、失血过多、有阴液或阳气迅速亡失情况下出现。

亡阴证　是指体内阴液大量消耗或丢失后所出现阴液衰竭的证候。主要临床症候：汗出而黏，面色潮红，烦躁不安，身热，手足温，呼吸急促，渴喜冷饮，舌红而干，脉细数无力。

亡阳证　是指体内阳气严重耗损后所出现阳气虚脱的证候，主要临床症候：大汗淋漓，面色苍白，精神淡漠，身畏寒，手足厥冷，气息微弱，口不渴或喜饮热饮，舌淡，脉微欲绝。

由于阴阳是互根的，亡阴则阴液耗竭，阳气无所依附而散越；亡阳则阳气衰竭，阴液无以化生而枯竭。亡阴和亡阳的治疗都以扶正固脱为主。亡阴者，当益气敛阴、救阴生津；亡阳者，当益气固脱、回阳救逆。

It refers to the simultaneous occurrence of deficiency syndrome and excess syndrome in a patient.It exhibits different manifestations,including deficiency with excess complication(major deficiency syndrome concurrently with minor excess syndrome),excess with deficiency complication(major excess syndrome concurrently with minor deficiency syndrome),and equal scale of deficiency syndrome and excess syndrome.Take the patient with pulmonary heat disease as an example,who both manifests the excess syndrome of cough,spitting of yellow phlegm,and edema in the lower limbs;as well as the deficiency syndrome of shortness of breath,lack of strength and fatigue which aggravate on exertion,and sunken and weak pulse.

2.Conversion between deficiency and excess

It refers to the mutual transformation of deficiency syndrome and excess syndrome in certain conditions as the result of the struggle between the healthy qi and the pathogenic factors in the course of a disease.Conversion from excess syndrome into deficiency syndrome occurs mostly arising from the exuberant pathogenic factors impairing the healthy qi,or delay of treatment and therapeutic error.For example,the excess syndrome of high fever,perspiration,thirst,and surging and big pulse will turn into the deficiency syndrome of low fever,emaciation,pale complexion,shortness of breath,lack of strength and fatigue,little or no fur,and thin and weak pulse as the result of depletion of body fluids if they are not treated in time or not recuperated after a long time.Conversion from deficiency syndrome into excess syndrome turns up because the healthy qi and the internal organs cannot promote the circulation of qi,blood and water due to their deficiency and hypo-activities and therefore lead to qi stagnation,blood stasis,phlegm and retained fluid,dampness and other pathological products in the interior,which are actually the syndrome of deficiency-excess complex.For example,the syndrome of yang deficiency with fluid retention,caused by declined kidney yang failing to transforming and leading to stagnation and retention of water and fluid,and edema in the lower limbs,is a kind of deficiency-excess complication,manifesting not only the deficiency syndrome of kidney dysfunction in warming,but also the excess syndrome of fluid retention in the lower limbs which arising from failure of the insufficient kidney yang in transforming.Such deficiency-excess complex is the result of excess symptom caused by deficiency syndrome.

Yin Syndrome and Yang Syndrome

Yin syndrome and yang syndrome are two principal syndromes used to summarize the categories of diseases.

In spite of complex and variation,diseases can be all categorized as yin syndrome and yang syndrome,so yin syndrome and yang syndrome are the general ones among the eight principals.They sum up the other six principals,namely exterior syndrome,excess syndrome and heat syndrome,which belong to yang syndrome;and interior syndrome,deficiency syndrome and cold syndrome,which belong to yin syndrome.Clinically,yin syndrome often refers to the deficiency-cold syndrome in the interior,while yang syndrome often refers to the excess heat syndrome in the interior.

Yin Syndrome and Yang Syndrome

Yin syndrome refers to the syndrome of yang deficiency or cold stagnation in the body.Generally,yin syndrome gives rise to cold sign and belongs to deficiency and cold,with the hypoactivity manifestations such as pale complexion,listlessness,fear of cold,cold limbs,shortness breath and weak voice,hydroadipis,clear abundant urine,sloppy stool,enlarged light-colored tongue with white fur,and sunken and weak pulse.

Yang syndrome refers to the syndrome of hyperactivity of yang or excess of pathogenic heat in the body.Generally,yang syndrome leads to heat sign and belongs to excess and heat,with the hyperactivity manifestations like general fever,red complexion,agitation,heavy breath and loud voice,thirst,scant dark

五、八纲相互关系

表里、寒热、虚实、阴阳八纲的区分并不是单纯孤立、静止不变，而是互相联系、相互转化。归纳起来，八纲之间存在着"相兼"、"夹杂"、"转化"的关系。

（一）相兼关系

"相兼"即指两个纲以上的症状同时出现，如外感热病初期之表证，还可兼寒或兼热，故可分为表寒证和表热证；久病多虚证，还可有寒与热的相兼证出现，即虚寒与虚热。相兼证有主次和从属的区别，如表寒、表热证都是以表证为主，寒或热从属于表证；虚寒、虚热证都是以虚证为主，寒或热也从属于虚证。前者治法应解表为主，后者治法应补虚为主。

（二）夹杂关系

"夹杂"即指患者同时出现性质互相对立的两纲症状，如寒热夹杂、虚实夹杂、表里夹杂（习惯上叫表里同病）。另外，在疾病发展过程中，还会出现一些假象，如真热假寒、真寒假热等。所以，在辨证过程中，要细心观察，全面分析，去伪存真，抓住本质，以免造成误诊、误治，延误病情。

urine, constipation, scarlet tongue with yellow fur, and slippery, surging and full pulse.

Yin Collapse Syndrome and Yang Collapse Syndrome

Yin collapse syndrome and yang collapse syndrome are two serious syndromes and occur as the result of rapid depletion of body fluids or yang qi like high fever, incessant profuse sweating, acute vomiting and diarrhea, excessive hemorrhage.

Yin collapse syndrome refers to the syndrome of yin fluid exhaustion due to their excessive depletion or consumption, with the manifestations of sticky sweat, scarlet complexion, agitation, general fever, warm hands and feet, tachypnea, thirst and preference of cold drink, red and dry tongue, and thin, rapid and weak pulse.

Yang collapse syndrome refers to the syndrome of yang exhaustion as the result of its severe depletion, with the manifestations of great dripping sweat, pale complexion, indifferent expression, aversion to cold, cold hands and feet, weak breath, hydroadipsia or thirst with preference of warm or hot drink, light-colored tongue, and extreme weak pulse.

Yin and yang are interdependent with each other, so yin collapse will deprive yang of its carrier and lead to dissipation and depletion of yang, while yang collapse will deprive yin of its engendering source and lead to exhaustion of yin. Treatment of yin collapse and yang collapse both mainly follow the method of reinforcing the healthy qi to secure collapse. Replenishing qi and astringing yin fluid or saving yin and engendering fluid should be adopted for the yin collapse syndrome; while replenishing qi to secure collapse or restoring yang to save from collapse should be adopted for the yang collapse syndrome.

Relations between the Eight Principal Syndromes

Exterior syndrome and interior syndrome, cold syndrome and heat syndrome, excess syndrome and deficiency syndrome, and yin syndrome and yang syndrome are not isolated and static, but interrelated and interdependent. In a summary, they have the relations of concurrency, complex and transformation.

Relation of Concurrency

"Concurrency" refers to the occurrence of more than two syndromes at the same time. For example, the exterior syndrome of external contraction can be further divided into exterior cold syndrome and exterior heat syndrome on the basis of which syndrome emerges with it concurrently, the cold one or the heat one. The chronic diseases often give rise to deficiency syndrome, which can be further classified into deficiency-cold syndrome if the cold syndrome emerges concurrently and deficiency-heat syndrome if the heat syndrome emerges concurrently. In addition, there is the primary syndrome and the secondary syndrome in the concurrent syndrome. For example, in terms of exterior cold syndrome and exterior heat syndrome, the exterior syndrome is the primary one, while cold syndrome or heat syndrome is the secondary one subordinating to the exterior syndrome respectively. In terms of deficiency-cold syndrome and deficiency-heat syndrome, the deficiency syndrome is the primary one, while the cold syndrome or the heat syndrome is the secondary one subordinating to the deficiency syndrome respectively. As for the exterior cold syndrome and the exterior heat syndrome, the focus should be put on releasing the exterior; while with respect to the deficiency-cold syndrome and the deficiency-heat syndrome, the concentration should be made on tonifying the deficiency.

Relation of Complex

"Complex" refers to the occurrence of two syndromes at the same time, which are opposite in nature, like simultaneous cold-heat complication, simultaneous deficiency-excess complication and simultaneous exterior-interior complication(also known as disease involving both the exterior and interior). In addition, in the development of diseases, there are some false images like true heat with false cold symptoms, and true cold with false heat symptoms, so the doctors should make careful observations and all-around analysis

（三）转化关系

"转化"即指某一纲的症状向其对立的一方转化。表里之间、寒热之间、虚实之间、阴阳之间既是相互对立的，又可在一定条件下相互转化。如外感风寒，因病情发展或治疗不当，则病邪可由表入里，病变性质可由寒转热，最后由表寒证转化为里热证；实证可因误治、失治等原因，致病程迁延，虽邪气渐去，而正气亦伤，逐渐转化为虚证；虚证可由于正气不足，不能布化，以致产生痰饮或水湿、气滞或血瘀等实邪，而出现种种实证。转化是在一定条件下才能发生，辨证时必须随时审察病机的转变，及时诊断治疗，避免疾病向恶化方向发展，促进疾病向痊愈方向转化。

（徐慧媛）

so as to eliminate the false and grasp the intrinsic qualities of the diseases to make a timely and correct diagnosis and treatment.

Transformation

Transformation refers to transformation of one syndrome to its opposite side. Exterior syndrome and interior syndrome, cold syndrome and heat syndrome, deficiency syndrome and excess syndrome, and yin syndrome and yang syndrome can transform mutually in certain conditions. For instance, external contraction of wind cold, if aggravating or not treated properly, will transform from the exterior cold syndrome into the interior heat syndrome as the result of the pathogen entering the interior from the exterior, and turning from cold into heat in nature. Excess syndrome can gradually transform into deficiency syndrome due to delay of treatment or therapeutic error, which impairs the healthy qi although the pathogenic factors are eliminated during the long-term course of an illness. Whereas, deficiency syndrome can turn into excess syndrome as the result of healthy qi deficiency failing to transform and distribute, and leading to excess pathological products of phlegm, retained fluid, dampness, qi stagnation and blood stasis. Transformation takes place only in certain condition, so when differentiating the syndromes, the doctors should study the changes of pathology carefully and make a timely diagnosis and treatment so as to prevent the disease from aggravating and make the patient recuperate soon.

(Wu Qunli   Zhang Wen)

第五章 精、气、血、津液

第一节 精

中医学中精的概念有广义和狭义之分，广义的精泛指一切构成人体和维持人体生命活动的精微物质，包括脏腑之精、水谷之精等。狭义之精指的是肾所藏的"生殖之精"。肾藏之精禀受于父母，称为先天之精，需后天水谷之精微与自然界之清气的滋养。肾藏之精决定着人的生长、发育与生殖。肾精充盈，生长发育就正常，反之则会出现发育迟缓、智力低下或未老先衰、生殖功能障碍等。

第二节 气

气有两个含义：一是指构成人体和维持人体生命活动的基本物质，如水谷之气、呼吸之气等。二是指脏腑组织的生理功能活动，如脏腑之气、经络之气等。

一、气的生成

人体之气的生成来源有三：一为禀受于父母的先天之精气，亦称之为"元气"；二为饮食物中的营养物质，即水谷之精气；三为存在于自然界的清气。

二、气的运动形式

运动不息是气的基本特性，这种特性推动和激发人体的各种生理活动。气的运动形式可归纳为升、降、出、入四种基本运动形式，称为"气机"。升，是气由下向上的运动；降，是气由上向下的运动；出，是气由内向外的运动；入，是气由外向内的运动。

气的升降出入运动，体现在脏腑、经络等组织器官的生理活动中。例如，肺的呼

CHAPTER FIVE   ESSENCE,QI,BLOOD, FLUID,AND HUMOR

Section 1   Essence

In TCM, the concept of essence has both broad and narrow sense.In a broad sense, essence refers to all the fundamental substance that builds up the physical structure and maintains body function, including essence of the viscera and bowls and essence of water and food.In a narrow sense, it specifies "reproductive essence" stored in the kidney.The essence stored in the kidney originates from parents, also termed as innate essence, which needs to be nourished by the acquired nutrients from water and food and the air outside.The essence stored in the kidney plays a decisive role in growth, development and reproduction of human being.The full and vigorous kidney essence can promote the growth and development.On the contrary, the deficiency of kidney essence leads to growth retardation, hypophrenia, or geromorphism or dysgonesis.

Section 2   Qi

Qi consists of two aspects: one refers to the fundamental substance of that builds up the physical structure and maintains body function like the nutrients from water and food and air outside; the other refers to the physiological functions of the viscera and bowels such as the vital energy of the viscera and bowels, the energy of meridians and collaterals.

Generation of Qi

There are three sources for generation of qi: first, the innate essence endowed from parents, also known as "source qi;" second, the nutrients from the water and food, i.e. the essence of foodstuff; and third, the fresh air of the nature.

Movement of Qi

Perpetual movement is the basic characteristic of qi, which promotes and activates various physiological activities of human body.The basic forms of movement of qi can be summarized as ascending, descending, exiting and entering, which is also termed as "qi movement." Ascending refers to the upward movement of qi, descending refers to downward movement of qi, exiting refers to outward movement and entering refers to inward movement.

The movement of ascending, descending, exiting and entering of qi is embodied in the physiological activities of the viscera and bowels, meridians and collaterals, etc.For instance, the lung governs respiration which covers expiration(exiting) and inspiration(entering).In addition, its function of dispersion is the embodiment of movement of ascending and the function of descending is the embodiment of movement of descending.The spleen and the stomach govern transportation and transformation, with the spleen taking

吸功能，呼气是出，吸气为入；宣发是升，肃降为降。脾胃主运化，脾主升清，以升为健，胃主降浊，以降为和。

三、气的生理功能

人体之气的生理功能主要有以下五个方面：

1. 推动作用　气的推动作用是指气具有激发和推动功能。气是活力很强的精微物质，人体的生殖、生长、发育，以及脏腑、经络等组织器官的生理活动，血液的生成和运行，津液的生成、输布和排泄等，均由气的激发和推动作用来实现。

2. 温煦作用　气的温煦作用是指气具有温煦、温暖、熏蒸的作用。气通过运动变化能产生热量，温煦人体，保持体温相对恒定；各脏腑、经络等组织器官，也要在气的温煦作用下进行正常的生理活动；机体内的血和津液等液态物质，也需要依靠气的温煦、熏蒸，才能维持正常的循环运行。

3. 防御作用　气的防御作用是指气具有护卫全身肌表，抵御外邪入侵机体及驱邪外出的作用。《素问·评热病论篇》所说："邪之所凑，其气必虚"，则是说气的防御作用减弱，外邪则易于乘虚侵袭，从而使机体罹患疾病。

4. 固摄作用　气的固摄作用是指气对精、血、津液等具有固摄、控制和保护的作用。固摄血液，使之在脉管中循行，防止其逸出于脉外；固摄汗液、尿液、唾液、胃液、肠液等，控制和调节其分泌和排泄，以防止其无故流失；固摄肾精，使其不妄泄而耗损。

5. 气化作用　气的气化作用是指通过气的运动而产生的各种生理变化。具体地说，精、气、血、津液等物质各自的新陈代谢及其相互转化有赖于气的气化作用。例如，气将饮食物转化成水谷之精气，然后才能再化生成气、血、津液营养全身；同时津液经过代谢气化之后，转化成汗液和尿液排出体外；饮食物经过消化吸收之后，其残渣方能转化成糟粕等，这些都是气化作用的具体体现。

四、气的分类

1. 元气　元气，又称原气、真气，是人体生命活动的原动力。元气源于肾，由先天之精气化生，又赖于后天水谷精气的不断充养。故元气的盛衰强弱，与先天禀赋和后天充养，即肾、脾的功能密切相关。

2. 宗气　宗气由肺吸入的清气与脾胃化生的水谷精气结合而成，积聚于胸中。宗气的主要功能有二：一是上出喉咙走息道，以助肺司呼吸。人的语言、声音和呼吸的强弱均与宗气有关；二是贯通心脉，以推动心血的运行。凡心搏的强弱和节律、血脉的运行，皆与宗气的盛衰有关。

charge of ascending the clear,and the stomach in charge of descending the turbid.

Physiological Functions of Qi

Physiological functions of qi are in five aspects as follows:

1. Promoting function

Promoting function of qi refers to its motivation and promotion functions.Under this function,qi,as the vigorous subtle substance,can help achieve the reproduction,growth and development of human body; also,it triggers and promotes the physiological activities of the viscera and bowels,meridians and collaterals,the generation and circulation of blood,and the generation,distribution and metabolism of fluid and humor.

2. Warming function

Warming function of qi refers to its warming and steaming function.Qi produces heat during the movement to warm the body and keep body temperature at the normal level.All the viscera and bowels, meridians and collaterals conduct their physiological functions under this function.In addition,the blood, fluid,humor and other liquid materials maintain their normal circulation and flow with the help of warming and steaming function of qi.

3. Defending function

Defending function of qi refers to its function of defending the muscles and skin from being invaded by exogenic pathogenic factors and driving the pathogenic evil out,as described in *Plain Questions* "only when qi in the body is deficient can pathogenic factors invade the body,"which indicates when defending function of qi weakens,the exogenic pathogenic factors are apt to invade and cause diseases.

4. Securing function

Securing function of qi refers to its function of consolidating,controlling and protecting essence, blood,fluid and humor.It governs the blood so that it circulates in vessels rather than flowing out the vessels.It governs perspiration,urine,saliva,gastric and intestinal juice and other humor,controls and regulates their secretion and discharge so that they do not run off.In addition,it governs the kidney essence and protects it from being discharged too much and therefore consumed.

5. Transformation function

The transformation of qi refers to various physiological changes caused by qi movement.Concretely, essence,qi,blood,fluid and humor rely on qi transformation to accomplish the metabolism and interconversion.Qi converts water and food into essence and nutrients before turning them into qi,blood,fluid and humor to nourish the whole body.Fluid and humor are discharged and metabolized after converted to sweat and urine.And water and food are converted into dross after digested and absorbed.All of these are the embodiment of qi transformation.

Classification of Qi

1. Source qi

Source qi,also known as original qi and genuine qi,is the original motive power of life activities of the human body.Source qi derives from the kidney,is generated from the innate essence,and nourished by the acquired essence of food and water.So exuberance or debilitation of source qi is closely related with the natural endowment and the postnatal nourishment,which is the functions of the kidney and spleen.

2. Ancestral qi

Ancestral qi,stored in the chest,is the combination of the essential qi derived from the fresh air inhaled by the lung and the foodstuff engendered and transformed by the spleen and stomach.It has two main functions:one is to go upward to nourish the airway via the throat and help the lung govern respiration,is

3. 营气　营气由水谷精气化生。营气能化生血液，与血同行于脉中，是血液的组成部分，故常以"营血"并称。营气循环于脉中，随血液运行于机体各个部位，营养五脏六腑、四肢百骸，是脏腑经络生理活动的物质基础。

4. 卫气　卫气由水谷精微中最富有活力的部分化生，行于脉外，其主要功能有二：一是具有护卫肌表，抵御外邪的作用；二是温煦脏腑、肌肤、皮毛，调控腠理开合，启闭汗孔，调节汗液排泄，维持体温相对平衡。

营气与卫气都由水谷精气化生，但是营气行于脉中、卫气行于脉外，营主内守属于阴，卫主外卫属于阳，两者的运行必须协调，营卫调和才能维持腠理开合、体温以及防御外邪的能力。

除了上述最重要的四种气之外，还有脏腑之气、经络之气等，都是由元气所派生，是元气分布于某一脏腑或某一经络之气，属于元气的一部分。

第三节　血

血是循行于脉中的富有营养的红色液体，是构成人体和维持人体生命活动的基本物质之一。

一、血的生成

血，主要由营气和津液所组成，营气和津液均来自脾胃化生的水谷精微，故有"脾胃为气血生化之源"之说。另外精血互生，精藏于肾，血藏于肝。肾中精气充盛，则肝有所养，血有所充；肝血充盈，则肾有所藏，精有所资，故又有"精血同源"之说。

二、血的运行

血的正常运行，主要依赖于心气推动、肺朝百脉、脾气统摄和肝气疏泄等功能。心气推动是血液运行的主要动力；肺朝百脉和肝气疏泄等是推动和促进血液运行的重要因素；脾统血和肝藏血等是固摄和调节血液运行的重要因素。

associated with phonation and status of respiration; the other is to run through the heart and vessels to promote the circulation of heart blood.The status of ancestral qi is related with speed and rhythm of heart beat and the circulation of blood.

3. Nutrient qi

Nutrient qi is generated from the water and food essence.It can be converted into blood to flow in the vessels, so it is one of the components of the blood and they are together termed as "nutrient blood." Nutrient qi, the material base of the viscera and meridians to conduct their physiological activities, flows together with blood in the vessels to reach and nourish the viscera and meridians, limbs, bones and other parts of the body.

4. Defense qi

Defense qi, generated from the most vigorous part of the water and food essence and flowing outside the vessels, has two primary functions: firstly protecting the muscle and skin from being attacked by the exogenic pathogens, and secondly warming the viscera and bowels, muscles and skin, regulating the opening and closing of interstices and sweat pore, and controlling the discharge of perspiration to maintain the balance of body temperature.

Nutrient qi and defense qi are both generated from water and food essence, but the former flows in the vessels, and the latter flows outside the vessels, so nutrient qi belongs to yin guarding the interior and defense qi belongs to yang defending the exterior.They must coordinate and harmonize with each other to maintain the bodily functions of normal opening and closing of the interstices, body temperature and defense against the exogenic pathogens.

Besides the above-mentioned four kinds of qi, there are the visceral qi and meridian qi and etc., all of which derive from the source qi and located in certain viscera or meridians, so as the integral part of source qi.

Section 3   Blood

Blood is red and nourishing fluid circulating in the vessels.It is one of the fundamental substances that build up the physical structure and maintain body function.

Generation of Blood

Blood is made up of nutrient qi and fluid and humor, both of which come from the water and food essence engendered and transformed by the spleen and stomach, so there is the saying of "the spleen and stomach being the source of qi and blood." In addition, the essence and the blood are converted from each other, with the essence stored in the kidney and the blood stored in the liver.The abundance of kidney essence can nourish the liver and supply it with sufficient source of blood, whereas the sufficiency of liver blood can provide the kidney with the source of essence to be stored and replenish, so known as "homogeny of essence and blood."

Circulation of blood

The normal circulation of blood primarily depends on the promotion of the heart qi, the convergence of vessels in the lung, governance of the spleen qi and free coursing of the liver qi, and etc.Promotion of the heart qi is the primary impetus of blood circulation, convergence of vessels in the lung and free coursing of the liver qi are the important factors of propelling and motivating blood circulation, and governance of blood by the spleen and storing of blood by the liver are the key elements of constraining and regulating blood circulation.

三、血的生理功能

血的生理功能主要有两个方面：①营养和滋润全身；②为神志活动提供物质基础。

<h2 style="text-align:center">第四节 津 液</h2>

津液，是机体一切正常水液的总称，是构成人体和维持生命活动的基本物质之一。津与液同属水液，但二者性状、分布和功能等方面均有不同。津，质地清稀，流动性较大，布散于体表皮肤、肌肉和孔窍，并能渗入血脉之内，起滋润作用；液，质地浓稠，流动性较小，灌注于骨节、脏腑、脑、髓等部位，起濡养和润滑作用。津与液之间可以互相转化，病理过程中又可相互影响，故常常津液并称。

一、津液的生成、输布和排泄

1. 津液的生成 津液来源于饮食水谷。饮食物经过胃的消化转输，又经小肠的分清泌浊，吸收大部分的营养物质和水液；再由大肠将食物残渣中的剩余水液再度吸收。

2. 津液的输布 津液的输布主要靠脾、肺、肾、三焦等脏腑的功能协调来完成。脾通过运化水谷精微的功能，将津液上输于肺，由肺的宣发和肃降，也直接将津液向四周布散至全身，即脾之"灌溉四旁"功能；肾的气化功能是推动津液输布的动力，可将津液之清者蒸腾，经三焦上输于肺而布散于全身，浊者化为尿液注入膀胱，排出体外。

3. 津液的排泄 一部分通过肺气的宣发作用，转化为汗液，经汗孔排泄于体外。另一部分通过肾阳的气化作用，转化成尿液，下输膀胱并排出体外。另外，还有一少部分的残余水分通过大肠排出的水谷糟粕而带出体外。

二、津液的生理功能

1. 滋润濡养作用 津以滋润为主，液以濡养为主。分布于体表的津液，能滋润皮肤，温养肌肉，使肌肉丰润，毛发光泽；分布于体内的津液能滋养脏腑，维持各脏腑的正常功能；注入孔窍的津液，使口、眼、鼻等九窍滋润；流入关节的津液，能滑利关节；渗入骨髓的津液，能充养骨髓和脑髓。

2. 化生血液 津液是组成血液的基本物质之一。《脾胃论·用药宜忌论》中说："水入于经，其血乃成。"渗入于血脉的津液，具有充养和滑利血脉的作用。

Physiological functions of blood

The physiological functions of blood consists of two aspects: a) Nourish and moisture the body; and b) provide the material base for mental activities.

Section 4   Fluid and Humor

Fluid and humor, a general term for all kinds of normal fluid in the body except the blood, are one of the fundamental substances that build up the physical structure and maintain body function. Body fluids are composed of fluid and humor, which are different in shape and properties, distribution and functions. Fluid, clear and thin, with high flowability, spread over the skin, muscles and orifices, and penetrate into the vessels to nourish them. Humor, thick, with little flowability, gathers in joints, viscera and bowels, brain and marrow to moisten and nourish them. They can interconvert and affect each other during the pathological course, so they are often together called as body fluid.

Generation, Distribution and Discharge of Fluid and Humor

1. Generation of fluid and humor

Body fluids are originated from the water and food people eat, which are firstly digested through the stomach, then transported to the small intestine for separation of the clear and turbid and absorbing most of the nutrients and water, and finally passed to the large intestine for further extracting the rest water from the food residues.

2. Distribution of fluid and humor

It is completed primarily through the coordination of the spleen, lung, kidney and triple energizer. The spleen first transforms the water and food essence, and then transports the fluid and humor upward to the lung for diffusion, purification and down-sending and then distributing it directly around the whole body to realize the function of "transporting the body fluids to various parts of the body" of the spleen. The transformation function of the kidney is the impetus of distribution of fluid and humor. The kidney evaporates the clear part of body fluids and then transports it upward to the lung through the passage of triple energizer, while transforms the turbid one into urine and pour it into the bladder and finally excreted it out of body.

3. Discharge of fluid and humor

Part of the body fluids is converted into sweat through the dispersion of the lung and drained out through sweat pores. And the other part of them are converted into urine through the transformation of the kidney yang and discharged out by bladder. And the rest small part is excreted out with the dross by the large intestine.

Physiological Functions of Fluid and Humor

1. Moistening and nourishing function

Fluid is responsible for moistening the body and humor is in charge of nourishing the body. The fluid and humor spreading over the body surface can moisten the skin and nourish the muscle to enrich the muscles and luster the hair. The one distributing the interior can nourish the viscera and bowels to maintain their normal functions. The one flowing into the orifices can moisten the mouth, eyes, and noses and other orifices. The one going into the joints can lubricate them, and the one penetrating into the marrow can replenish and nourish bone marrow and brain marrow.

2. Generating and transforming into blood

Fluid and humor is one of the basic material bases for forming blood, as depicted in *Treatise on the*

3．排泄废物　津液在自身的代谢过程中，通过汗液与尿液将机体所产生的代谢废物排出体外，以维持脏腑组织器官正常的生理功能。

第五节　气血津液的关系

一、气与血的关系

1．气为血之帅

（1）气能生血：是指血液的化生过程离不开气的气化功能。脾胃之气将饮食物转化为水谷精微，进而化生为血。所以说，气能生血。

（2）气能行血：是指气能推动血液的运行。血液的运行有赖于心气、肺气的推动及肝气的疏泄调畅。气行则血行，气滞则血瘀。

（3）气能摄血：是指气固摄作用能使血液正常循行于脉中而不外溢。气能摄血主要体现在脾气统血的生理功能之中。

2．血为气之母

（1）血能养气：是指血为气的功能活动提供物质基础，不断地为气的功能活动补充营养，保证气的充盛及其功能正常发挥。血足则气旺，血虚则气衰。

（2）血能载气：是指血为气的载体，气依附于血而得以存在体内，并以血为载体而运行全身。若血不载气，可导致气浮无根，无所依托而涣散。临床可见大出血时，往往会发生气随血脱的危象。

二、气与津液的关系

1．气能生津　气是津液生成的动力。津液源于水谷精微，脾胃之气受气推动和激发发挥作用，将饮食水谷化生为津液而输布全身。脾胃之气充盛，所化生津液充足，气旺则津充，气弱则津亏。故临床上治疗气虚导致的津液不足时往往采用补气生津法。

2．气能行津　气的运动变化是津液输布、排泄的动力。津液依赖脾气的运化、肺气的宣降、肾气的蒸腾气化而输布于全身；同时津液代谢转化为汗液与尿液排出体外的过程也赖于气的气化作用。

3．气能摄津　气的固摄作用控制着津液的排泄，防止体内津液无故流失，维持体内津液量的相对恒定。若气的固摄作用减弱，则体内津液任意经汗、尿等途径外泄，出现多汗、漏汗、多尿、遗尿等病理现象。

Spleen and Stomach "blood comes into being when water infuses into the vessels."Body fluids penetrating into the vessels can nourish and fabricate them.

3. Discharging the metabolic waste

Body fluids can help discharge the metabolic waste out the body through sweat and urine in its course of metabolism to maintain the normal physiological functions of the viscera and bowels.

Section 5   Relation among Qi,Blood,Fluid and Humor

Relation between Qi and Blood

1. Qi is the commander of blood

(1) Qi is able to generate blood:it refers to the formation of blood relies on the transformation of qi. The spleen and stomach qi transforms the food and water into essence and then the blood.

(2) Qi is able to promote blood:it means qi can promote the circulation of blood,which is the result of the cooperation of the heart qi and the lung qi both responsible for promotion and the liver qi responsible for soothing and regulating.The free flow of qi boosts the circulation of blood,while stagnation of qi leads to blood stasis.

(3) Qi is able to control blood:it means qi can govern blood to flow in vessels rather than flowing out.This function is primarily embodied by the spleen qi controlling blood.

2. Blood is the mother of qi

(1) Blood is able to tonify qi:it means blood provides qi with material base,nutrients and replenishes qi to exert its normal functions.Sufficiency of blood leads to vigorousness of qi,while deficiency of blood gives rise to weakness of qi.

(2) Blood is able to carry qi:it means blood is qi's carrier,through which qi is able to stay in and flow through the body.The failure of blood in carrying qi brings about floating and slackness of qi,with the clinical manifestations of massive hemorrhoea leading to the crisis of qi collapse following bleeding.

Relation between Qi and Body Fluids

1. Qi is able to generate fluid

Qi is the motive power of forming body fluids,which stems from the essence of water and food.Then it promotes and motivates the spleen and stomach qi to transform water and food into body fluids and distribute it throughout the whole body.Sufficient spleen and stomach qi can generate plenty body fluids.Vigorousness of qi leads to sufficiency of body fluids,while weakness of qi brings about deficiency of body fluids.So tonifying qi to generate fluid is often adopted to treat deficiency of fluid caused by deficiency of qi clinically.

2. Qi is able to promote fluid

The movement change of qi is the impetus to distribute and discharge body fluids.The distribution of fluid and humor throughout the body rely on the transportation and transformation of spleen qi,diffusion and depurative downbearing of lung qi,and evaporation and transformation of kidney qi.Besides,the progress of body fluids metabolizing,turning into sweat and urine and discharging out of body also depends on the transformation of qi.

3. Qi is able to govern fluid

Qi controls the discharge of body fluids,prevents the interior fluids from flowing out and maintains body fluids at the normal level through its governing function.Weakening of governing function of qi can result in random discharge of body fluids in the forms of sweat and urine,manifesting the symptoms of hi-

三、血与津液的关系

血与津液均是液态物质，都有滋润和濡养作用，与气相对而言，二者均属于阴，在生理上相互补充，病理上相互影响。

血和津液的生成来源均为水谷精微。津液渗注于脉中则成为血的组成部分，而运行于脉中的血液，渗于脉外便化为有濡润作用的津液，故有"津血同源"之说。

在病理状态下，血和津液也相互影响，如失血过多时，脉外之津液渗入脉中以补偿血容量的不足，因之而导致脉外的津液不足，出现口渴、尿少、皮肤干燥等表现。

（尹德海 徐慧媛）

drosis, leaking sweat, profuse urine and enuresis, etc.

Relation between Blood and Body Fluids

Blood and body fluids are both liquid substance with moistening and nourishing functions. They, both belonging to yin relative to qi, complement each other physiologically and influence each other pathologically.

Blood and body fluids both originate from the essence of water and food. Body fluids will be the component of blood when they infuse into vessels, while blood will turn into nourishing body fluids when it flows out the vessels, so known as "homogeny of fluid and blood".

Blood and body fluids can affect each other pathologically. Losing too much blood will lead to body fluids deficiency as body fluids infusing into vessels to compensate for blood volume. It often accompanies the symptoms of thirst, scant urine and dry skin, etc.

(Wu Qunli   Zhang Wen)

第六章　脏腑功能及其辨证

　　脏腑学说通过对人体外部征象的观察，来研究内在脏腑的生理功能、病理变化及其相互关系和人体脏腑与自然界之间联系的学说。脏腑学说的主要内容是研究脏腑的生理功能、病理变化及其相互关系。脏腑是人体五脏、六腑和奇恒之府的总称。五脏是指心、肝、脾、肺、肾，多属实体性器官，其共同生理特点是化生和贮藏精气；六腑是指胆、胃、小肠、大肠、膀胱、三焦，多属管腔性器官，其共同生理特点是受盛和腐熟水谷。奇恒之府指脑、髓、骨、脉、胆、女子胞。奇恒之府不同于一般脏腑，其功能似五脏，而形态类六腑，故称"奇恒之府"。脏腑学说认为人体是以五脏为中心，以六腑相配合，以精气血津液为物质基础，通过经络内联五脏六腑，外联形体官窍所构成五个功能活动系统。

　　脏腑辨证是以脏腑学说为基础，根据脏腑的生理功能、病理表现，结合八纲、病因及气血等理论，综合四诊收集的数据，对疾病证候进行分析归纳，从而寻求病因，确定病位，了解病性，推究病机及正邪盛衰的一种辨证方法。它是其他各种辨证的基础，多用于内伤杂病的诊治。

第一节　心与小肠功能及其辨证

一、心的功能

心位于胸腔之内，五行属火，与小肠相表里，与四时之夏相通应。

（一）心主血脉

　　心主血脉，指心有主管血脉和推动血液循行于脉中的作用。心主血，血行于脉，心气有推动血液在脉管中运行以营养全身的功能。《素问·五脏生成篇》记载："诸血者皆属于心。"心主血脉的功能正常与否首先是依赖于心气的充沛，心气充沛，血液才

CHAPTER SIX   FUNCTIONS AND SYNDROMES OF VISCERS AND BOWELS

Theory of the viscera and bowels is to study the physiological functions, pathological changes and interrelationship of the internal organs and relations between the internal organs and the nature through observing the exterior signs of the human body. It primarily focuses on physiological functions, pathological changes and interrelationship of the internal organs, which cover the five viscera, six bowels and extraordinary organs. The five viscera are the heart, liver, spleen, lung and kidney, all of which are entity organs responsible for transforming and storing essential qi. The six bowels are the gallbladder, stomach, small intestine, large intestine, bladder, and triple energizers, all of which are lumen organs responsible for receiving, transporting and transforming water and food. The extraordinary organs are the brain, marrow, bones, vessels, gallbladder and uterus, which are similar as the five viscera in terms of function and as the six bowels in terms of form. The theory of viscera and bowels regards that the human body is composed of five functional systems, in which the five viscera are the core that coordinate and cooperate with the six bowels inside, as well as link with the body constituents and orifices of sense organs outside through meridians and collaterals, based on the materials of essence, qi, blood, fluid and humor.

Visceral syndrome differentiation is a study method of seeking for the cause of a disease, identifying its position, grasping its nature and studying its pathogenesis as well as exuberance and debilitation of the healthy qi and pathogenic qi, through analyzing and summarizing the disease's symptoms collected through the four examinations on the basis of the theory of the viscera and bowels, physiological functions and pathological conditions of the internal organs and in combination of the theories of eight principal syndrome, the cause of diseases and qi and blood. It is the basis of other differentiation methods and mostly used to diagnose and treat the miscellaneous internal injury diseases.

Section 1   Functions of the Heart and Small Intestine and Their Syndromes Differentiation

Functions of the Heart

The heart is situated in the thorax, pertains to fire in the five phases, corresponds to summer in the four seasons and stands in interior-exterior relationship with the small intestine.

Heart controls blood and vessels

Heart controlling blood and vessels means the heart takes charge of blood and vessels and promotes blood to circulate in vessels. The heart governs blood, which flows in the vessels, so heart qi can promote blood to circulate in the vessels and to nourish the whole body, as stated in *Plain Questions* "all blood are under the governance of the heart." Whether heart can control blood vessels firstly relies on whether heart qi is sufficient, as only with the sufficient heart qi, it can be promoted to circulate in the vessels and nourish the whole body. Otherwise, it cannot promote blood to circulate smoothly. It also requires sufficient heart

能在脉内正常地运行，营养全身。心气不足，推动无力，则血运不畅。其次有赖于心血的充盈，血液亏损则血脉空虚，心无所主。心主血脉的功能正常，则心搏动如常，节律调匀，脉象缓和有力。若心发生病变，则会通过心脏搏动、脉搏等方面反映出来。

（二）心主神志

中医学认为人的精神思维活动与脏腑有关，且主要是心的功能，即心主司意识、思维、等精神活动。《灵枢·邪客》说："心者，五脏六腑之大主也，精神之所舍也。"故有"心藏神"、"主神明"的说法。心主神志的功能发生异常时，可出现心神改变，如心悸不安、失眠多梦、健忘痴呆、狂妄躁动、哭笑无常、甚至昏迷不省人事等症。

心主神志与主血脉的关系：心具有主血脉的功能，能够运送血液以营养全身，也包括为自身提供生命活动必要的物质，所以血液是神的物质基础。因此，心主血脉的功能异常，亦必然出现神志的改变。

（三）心的连属关系

1. 在志为喜　心在志为喜，是指心的功能与精神情志活动的"喜"有关。喜乐愉悦，通常情况下对人体属于良性刺激，有益于心主血脉等功能。但是，喜乐过度，则又可使心神受伤，神志涣散而不能集中或内守。

2. 在液为汗　《素问·阴阳别论篇》说："阳加于阴谓之汗。"中医认为，汗液是人体津液经过阳气的蒸化，从汗孔排出之液体。由于汗为津液所化，津液与血又同出一源，因此又有"汗血同源"之说，而心主血，故汗与心有密切关系，有"汗乃心之液"的说法。

3. 在体合脉，其华在面　脉是指血脉。血脉内与心相连接，外则网络周身。心在体合脉，是指全身的血脉统属于心，即心主血脉。心气不仅推动血液在脉中运行，还充实于血脉之中，以使血脉充盈，血行流畅。华是荣华、光彩之意。中医学认为，五脏精气的盛衰，均可以显现于与之相应的某些体表组织器官上，称为五华。心其华在面，是说心的功能正常与否，反映于面部的色泽变化。若心气旺盛，血脉充盈，则面部红润有光泽；心血瘀阻，则可见面色青紫等。

4. 在窍为舌　心在窍为舌，即心开窍于舌，是指舌为心之外候，又称"舌为心之苗"。《灵枢·经脉》指出："手少阴之别……循经入于心中，系舌本。"因此心的气血上通于舌，而舌的功能要靠心的精气充养才能维持。同时，通过舌质的色泽可以直接察知气血的运行情况，并判断心主血脉的功能。心的功能正常，则舌体红活荣润，柔软灵活。而心血不足时舌质淡白；心火上炎时则舌尖红或舌体糜烂；心血瘀阻时则舌质紫暗或有瘀斑、瘀点；热入心包或痰迷心窍时，则舌强语謇。

blood.Without sufficient blood,the heart cannot exert its function.Only when the function of heart controlling blood and vessels is normal,the heart can beat with normal and harmonious rhythm and soft and powerful pulse.If there is something wrong with heart,it can be reflected from heart beat and pulse,etc.

Heart Governs Mental Activities

TCM regards that mental activities are related with the functions of the viscera and bowels,especially the function of heart—its function of governing spiritual activities like consciousness and thought,as defined in *Miraculous Pivot* "heart commands other internal organs and is where spirit lives."So there is the saying of"heart storing spirit"and"heart controls mental activities."Abnormality of heart's function of governing mental activities will lead to palpitation,sleepiness with dreams,amnesia and dementia,petulance and restlessness,weeping and laughing hysterically and even coma,etc.

Relations between heart governing mental activities and heart controlling blood and vessels:heart can promote blood circulation toprovide the necessary substances required in life activities to circulate in the vessels and nourish the whole body.Therefore,blood is the material basis of spirits.The mental activities will inevitably change when the heart fails to control blood and vessels.

Affiliations of Heart

1. Heart associates with joy in emotion

Heart associating with joy in emotion means the function of heart is influenced by the emotion of joy. Generally,joy and happiness can help the heart in controlling blood and vessels.But excessive joy can damage mental spirits and make people distracting.

2. Heart associates with sweat in humor

It is stated in *Plain Questions* "sweat is the result of addition of yang to yin."TCM deems that sweat is the body fluid which is steamed by yang qi and discharged from the sweat pores.Sweat is transformed from body fluids,and body fluids derives from the same source with blood,known as"homogeny of sweat and blood."In addition,as the heart controls blood,so,there is intimate connection of sweat and the heart, as statement of"sweat is the liquid of heart comes out."

3. Heart links with vessels,with its luster manifesting on the face

Vessels are connected with the heart inside and distributes all over the body outside.Heart linking with vessels means all blood vessels in the body are under governance of the heart,or heart controls blood and vessels.Heart qi not only motivates blood to circulate in vessels but also fill in vessels to make the vessels plentiful and blood flow smoothly.In TCM,the conditions(exuberance or debilitation)of five viscera can be reflected on the body surface organs which correspond with them respectively,also known as five lustres.The heart's luster being manifested on the face means whether the heart function is normal or not can be reflected by the luster changes of the face.For example,ruddy and lustrous face indicates exuberant heart qi with plentiful blood,while bluish purple face indicates stagnation of heart blood.

4. Heart opens at the tongue

Heart opening at the tongue,also known as"the tongue is the sprout of heart,"means the tongue's condition can reflect the status of the heart,as described in *Miraculous Pivot* "Heart meridian⋯links with the heart and connect with tongue."The heart blood and qi flow upward to nourish tongue and maintain its function.Meanwhile,the color and luster of tongue can directly reflect the condition of blood circulation and the heart's function of controlling blood and vessels.If heart exerts its function normally,the tongue is red,lustrous,soft,and flexible.Heart blood deficiency leads to pale tongue,heart fire flaming upward results in red tip of tongue or eroded tongue,stagnation of heart blood causes dark purple tongue with ecchymosis and petechia,and heat entering the pericardium or phlegm clouding the pericardium gives rise to stiff tongue and sluggish speech.

附：心包络

心包络，简称心包，亦称"膻中"，是心脏外面的包膜，其上附有通行气血的脉络，为心脏的外围组织，具有保护心脏的作用。心为君主之官，不得受邪，心包络既是心的外围，故邪气犯心，常先侵犯心包络。心主神志，如果外邪袭心，首先侵犯心包络，会出心神受扰的病症。如热病当中，温热之邪内陷，出现高热、神昏谵语等症，称之为"热入心包"。

二、小肠的功能

小肠与心之间有经脉相互络属，互为表里。小肠的功能是：

（一）受盛化物

受盛，即接受、以器盛物之意。化物，即变化、消化、化生之谓。小肠受盛化物的功能体现在两个方面：一是小肠接纳经胃初步消化的饮食物，起到容器的作用；二指经胃初步消化的饮食物，必须在小肠内停留一定的时间，由小肠对其进一步消化和吸收。所以《素问·灵兰秘典论篇》说："小肠者，受盛之官，化物出焉。"在病理上，小肠受盛功能失调，传化停止，则气机失于通调，滞而为痛，表现为腹部疼痛等。如化物功能失常，可以导致消化、吸收障碍，表现为腹胀、腹泻、便溏等。

（二）泌别清浊

泌，即分泌；别，指分别。清，指水谷之精微；浊，指食物之糟粕。泌清，就是将饮食物中的精华部分，包括饮料化生的津液和食物化生的精微，进行吸收，再通过脾之升清散精的作用，上输心肺，输布全身，供给营养。别浊，则体现为两个方面：其一，是将饮食物的残渣糟粕，传送到大肠，经肛门排出体外；其二，是将剩余的水分经肾脏气化作用渗入膀胱，经尿道排出体外。小肠在吸收水谷精微的同时，也吸收了大量的水液，参与了人体的水液代谢，故有"小肠主液"之说。若小肠泌别清浊功能失常，以致水走大肠，可见大便清泄，小便短少。

三、心和小肠病的辨证

（一）心气虚

【证候】心悸、胸闷气短，自汗，活动时加重，面白无华，体倦乏力，舌淡苔白，脉细弱或结代。

【辨证分析】本证多由禀赋不足，久病体虚，或年高气虚导致心气不足所致。心气不足，鼓动无力，故见心悸；胸中宗气运转无力则胸闷气短；气虚不固，心液外溢，则自汗出；劳累耗气，活动则心气益虚，故症状加重；心气不足，气血不得上

Additional reading: pericardium

Pericardium, also called "chest center", is the outer covering of the heart, on which there are collaterals allowing qi and blood flow in, and which can protect the heart from being damaged. The heart is the king (or monarch) organ and mustn't be attacked by the pathogenic factors. As pericardium is the peripheral tissue surrounding the heart, it is often attacked when the pathogenic qi invades the heart. Heart governs mental activities, so when pericardium substitutes the heart to be attacked by pathogens, then the syndrome of heart spirit being disturbed will occur. For instance, in epidemic febrile disease, symptoms like high fever, coma and delirium will be the result of inward invasion of warm and heat pathogens, which is also known as "heat entering the pericardium."

Functions of the Small Intestine

The small intestine stands in exterior-interior relationship with the heart, as there are meridians and collaterals linking with them. The functions of small intestine are as follows:

Receiving and Transforming Food

The function of small intestine in receiving and transforming food is embodied in two aspects: one is that the small intestine accepts and stores the foodstuff preliminarily digested by the stomach; and the second is that it makes further digestion and absorption of those food transmitted from the stomach, as defined by *Plain Questions* "the small intestine is the organ responsible for receiving, digesting and further transforming foodstuff." Pathologically, the dysfunction of small intestine in receiving and transmitting foodstuff will lead to qi stagnation, with the manifestation of abdominal pain. If it fails to transform foodstuff, indigestion and malabsorption will occur with the manifestation of abdominal distension, diarrhea, sloppy stool, etc.

Separating the Clear from the Turbid

The clear refers to the food essence and water, while the turbid refers to the waste matter. Secreting the clear means after absorbing the essence generated and transformed from drink and food, and transmitting it upward to the heart and lung, and then further spreading it all over and nourish the body through the spleen's function of upbearing the clear and spreading the essence. Separating the turbid is embodied in the following two aspects: the first one is the small intestine passes the residue and dross of foodstuff to the large intestine and discharges them via anus; the second one is it makes the remanent water infiltrate into the bladder with the transformation function of the kidney and then discharge it out via urethra. When absorbing food essence, the small intestine also absorbs a large quantity of water, which participates in metabolism of body fluids, so there is the saying of "the small intestine governing the fluids." If small intestine fails to separate the clear from the turbid, then the symptoms of clear and sloppy stool and short and little urine will occur as the result of fluid entering the large intestine.

Syndrome Differentiation of the Heart and Small Intestine

Heart qi deficiency

Syndrome: palpitation, oppression in the chest, breath shortness and spontaneous sweating, which aggravate on exertion, pale facial complexion without luster, tiredness, pale tongue with white fur, thin and weak pulse or intermittent and bound pulse.

Syndrome differentiation: it is often caused by heart qi deficiency due to constitutional insufficiency, weak physique, prolonged illness, or agedness qi deficiency. Palpitation occurs as the result of heart qi deficiency failing to promote heart beat powerfully. Chest oppression and breath shortness result from ancestral qi deficiency. Spontaneous sweating arises from qi deficiency failing to constrain heart fluid from overflowing. Aggravation of heart qi deficiency occurs because tiredness consumes qi. Pale complexion without luster is the result of heart qi deficiency failing to promote qi and blood upward to nourish the face. Tired-

荣，故面白无华；气虚则体倦乏力。舌淡苔白，脉细弱或结代均为心气不足的表现。

【治法】补益心气。

【代表方剂】炙甘草汤。

（二）心阳虚

【证候】心悸、气短，自汗，活动时加重，心胸憋闷，形寒肢冷，舌淡胖，脉细弱或结代。

【辨证分析】本证多由气虚日久，导致心之阳气受损所致。心气不足，鼓动无力，故见心悸、气短，脉细弱或结代；气虚卫外不固则自汗出；劳累耗气，活动时心气益虚，故症状加重；心阳不振，胸中阳气痹阻，故心胸憋闷；阳气不足，失于温煦，则形寒肢冷；舌淡胖为阳气不足之象。

【治法】温补心阳。

【代表方剂】桂枝人参汤。

（三）心血虚

【证候】心悸怔忡，头晕，健忘，失眠，多梦，面白无华，四肢无力，指甲苍白，唇舌色淡，苔白，脉细无力。

【辨证分析】本证多因阴血不足，或久病耗血，或失血过多，或情志不遂，耗伤心血所致。心血不足，心失所养，故心悸怔忡；血虚不能上荣清窍，故面白无华，头晕，健忘；心主神志，血不养心，神不守舍，故失眠多梦；血虚不能充实血脉，荣养四肢肌肉，故四肢无力；指甲苍白，唇舌色淡，脉细弱均为血虚之象。

【治法】补养心血。

【代表方剂】四物汤。

（四）心阴虚

【证候】心悸怔忡，失眠，多梦，颧红，潮热，盗汗，五心烦热，舌红少苔，脉细数。

【辨证分析】本证因素体阴虚或久病伤阴所致。心阴不足，心失所养，故心悸怔忡；心主神志，阴不敛阳，神不守舍，故失眠多梦；阴虚内热，则见颧红，潮热，盗汗，五心烦热。舌红少苔，脉细数为阴虚内热之象。

【治法】滋补心阴。

【代表方剂】天王补心丹。

（五）心火炽盛

【证候】心胸烦热，失眠多梦，口渴思饮，面赤；或口舌生疮，或见吐血衄血，甚或狂躁谵语，舌尖红赤，苔黄，脉数。

【辨证分析】本证常因七情郁久化火，或六淫内郁化火，或过食辛辣食物、温补药物所致。心火炽盛，内扰心神，轻者为心胸烦热，失眠多梦；重者见狂躁、谵语；

ness is due to qi deficiency.And pale tongue with white fur,thin weak pulse and bound intermittent pulse are all the manifestations of heart qi deficiency.

Method of treatment:tonify heart qi.

Formula:Prepared Gancao Decoction.

Heart yang deficiency

Syndrome:palpitation,breath shortness and spontaneous sweating,which aggravate on exertion,oppression in chest,cold body and limbs,pale and enlarged tongue,and thin weak pulse or bound intermittent pulse.

Syndrome differentiation:it is caused by prolonged qi deficiency damaging heart yang.Palpitation, breath shortness,and thin weak pulse or bound intermittent pulse occurs as the result of heart qi deficiency failing to promote heart beat powerfully.Spontaneous sweating arises from defense qi deficiency failing to exert its constraining function.Aggravation of heart qi deficiency occurs because tiredness consumes qi. Chest oppression results from heart-yang deficiency leading to yang obstruction in the chest.Cold body and limbs takes place because of yang qi deficiency failing to warm the body.And pale and enlarged tongue is the manifestation of yang qi deficiency.

Method of treatment:warm and tonify heart yang.

Formula:Guizhi Renshen Decoction.

Heart blood deficiency

Syndrome:palpitation,dizziness,amnesia,insomnia,dreaminess,pale complexion without luster,feeble limbs,pale finger nails,light-colored mouth lips and tongue with white fur and thin weak pulse.

Syndrome differentiation:it is caused by blood deficiency,or blood consumption due to prolonged illness,excessive hemorrhage,or injury of heart blood because of bad mood.Palpitation results from heart blood deficiency failing to nourish the heart.Pale complexion without luster,dizziness and amnesia arises from blood deficiency failing to flow upward to nourish the clear orifices,insomnia and dreaminess occurs because blood deficiency fails to nourish heart and lead to the heart failing to govern the mental activities. Feeble limbs take place as blood deficiency fails to replenish the vessels and nourish the muscles of limbs. And pale nails,pale mouth lips and tongue,and thin weak pulse are all the manifestations of blood deficiency.

Method of treatment:tonify heart blood.

Formula:Siwu Decoction.

Heart yin deficiency

Syndrome:palpitation,insomnia,dreaminess,red cheeks,tidal fever,night sweating,vexing heat in the chest,palms and soles,red tongue with little fur,and thin rapid pulse.

Syndrome differentiation:it is caused by yin deficiency or prolonged illness injuring yin fluid.Palpitation arises from heart yin deficiency failing to nourish the heart.Insomnia and dreaminess is the results of yin failing to constrain yang and spirit failing to keep to its abode.Red cheeks,tidal fever,night sweating and vexing heat in the chest,palms and soles are the result of yin deficiency with internal heat.And red tongue with little fur and thin rapid pulse are also the manifestations of yin deficiency with internal heat.

Method of treatment:nourish heart yin.

Formula:Tianwang Buxin Pill.

Intense heart fire

Syndrome:vexing heat in the chest,insomnia and dreaminess,thirst with desire to drink,red face,or mouth and tongue sore,hematemesis or epistaxis,and even mania and delirious speech,red tongue tip with yellow fur,and rapid pulse.

Syndrome differentiation:it is caused by depressed emotions transforming into fire,or six excesses de-

心火循经上炎则口渴思饮，面赤，或口舌生疮；火热迫血妄行，则有吐血衄血。舌尖红赤，苔黄，脉数均为心火亢盛的表现。

【治法】清心泻火。

【代表方剂】大黄黄连泻心汤。

（六）心血瘀阻

【证候】轻者心胸疼痛，憋闷或隐痛不适，痛处固定，时发时休。剧者可突然发作，心胸闷痛，或痛引肩背内臂，痛不可忍，面色唇甲青紫，舌质紫暗或有瘀斑，脉涩或结代。

【辨证分析】本病多因素体气虚，复加劳倦，致心气不充或心阳虚衰，气血运行不畅或阳虚无力温运血脉，致瘀血痹阻心脉而成。或由于劳倦感寒，寒凝心脉；或受精神刺激，气机郁结，或过食肥甘厚味，痰浊凝聚，气血运行不畅，而致心脉痹阻。心脉痹阻，气血运行不畅，故心胸憋闷疼痛，痛处固定；手少阴心经循肩臂而行，故痛引肩背内臂；瘀血内停则面色唇甲青紫，舌质紫暗、有瘀斑，脉涩、结代。

【治法】活血通脉。

【代表方剂】血府逐瘀汤。

（七）小肠实热

【证候】心烦口渴，口舌生疮，小便赤涩，尿道灼痛，尿频，尿急，甚至尿血，小腹拘痛，舌红，苔黄，脉数。

【辨证分析】本证多由心热下移，致小肠里热炽盛。心火内炽，热扰心神，则心烦；热灼津伤，则口渴；心火上炎，则口舌生疮；心热下移小肠，分清泌浊功能失常，热入膀胱，则小便赤涩，尿道灼痛，尿频，尿急，甚则小腹拘痛；若热伤血络，则出现尿血；舌红，苔黄，脉数均为里热之征。

【治法】清利实热。

【代表方剂】导赤散。

第二节 肺与大肠功能及其辨证

一、肺的功能

肺位于胸腔，五行属金，与大肠相表里，与四时之秋相应。

（一）肺主气、司呼吸

肺主气是肺主呼吸之气和肺主一身之气的总称。包括两个方面。

1. 主呼吸之气 肺具有主司呼吸的功能。肺是气体交换的场所，通过呼吸功能，不断吸进自然界的清气，呼出体内的浊气，进行体内外的气体交换，吐故纳新，以

pressed inward transforming into fire, or eating too much spicy or hot food or warm and tonic drugs. The light symptoms of vexing heat in chest, insomnia and dreaminess; or the heavier symptoms of mania and delirious speech occur as the result of intense heart fire disturbing heart spirit. Thirst with desire to drink, red complexion, or mouth and tongue sores result from heart fire flaming upward along with heart meridian. Hematemesis and epistaxis occurs because heart fire forces blood to move frenetically. Red tongue tip and yellow fur and rapid pulse are the manifestations of intense heart fire.

Method of treatment: clear the heart to purge fire.

Formula: Dahuang Huanglian Xiexin Decoction.

Heart blood stasis

Syndrome: as for the mild cases, chest pain, chest oppression or dull pain with the pain occurring intermittently in the fixed location. As for the severer cases, sudden breakout of chest oppressive pain which spread to the shoulders and cannot be tolerated in a company of signs of bluish purple complexion, nails and mouth lips, dark purple tongue or tongue with ecchymosis, and rough pulse or bound intermittent pulse.

Syndrome differentiation: it is caused by the prolonged qi deficiency and tiredness impairing heart qi or heart yang and retarding the circulation of blood, or yang deficiency failing to warm blood and promote blood circulation and leading to heart vessel obstruction. Or it is caused by exogenic pathogenic cold coagulating in heart meridian when overstraining; or by qi stagnation as the result of being stimulated emotionally; or by eating too much greasy, fat, or strong-flavored food, which engenders turbid phlegms and prevents against the smooth blood circulation. Chest pain and chest oppression with the pain occurring in the fixed place is due to heart Bessel obstruction and qi and blood failing to flow smoothly. The pain spreads to the insides of arms and shoulder because heart meridians go along with the arms and shoulders. Bluish purple complexion, nails and mouth lips, dark purple tongue or tongue with ecchymosis, and rough pulse or bound intermittent pulse are the manifestations of interior stagnation of blood stasis.

Method of treatment: activate blood circulation.

Formula: Xuefu Zhuyu Decoction.

Small intestine excess heat

Syndrome: vexation and thirst, mouth and tongue sores, deep and scanty urine, causalgia of urethra, frequent urination, urgent urination, even hematuria, lower abdominal pain, red tongue with yellow fur and rapid pulse.

Syndrome differentiation: it is caused by heart heat spreading to the small intestine with the interior intense heat. Vexation is due to heart fire flaming inside to harass the heart spirit. Thirst is the result of heat injuring body fluids. Mouth and tongue sores occur because of heart fire flaming upward. Deep and scanty urine, causalgia of urethra, frequent urination, urgent urination, and lower abdominal pain arise from heart heat transmitting downward into the small intestine to affect its function of separating the clear from the turbid and then descending to the bladder. Hematuria indicates that heat damages vessels. And red tongue with yellow fur and rapid pulse are all the manifestations of interior heat.

Method of treatment: remove excess heat.

Formula: Daochi Powder.

Section 2   Functions of the Lung and Large Intestine and their Syndrome Differentiation

Functions of the Lung

The lung locates in the thoracic cavitiy, pertains to metal in the five phases, corresponds to autumn in

保证人体新陈代谢的正常进行。肺的呼吸功能正常，则气道通畅、呼吸均匀；肺的呼吸功能减弱，则气短息微、声低乏力。

2. 主一身之气　肺主一身之气的生理功能具体体现在两个方面：一是宗气的生成，宗气是由水谷精气与肺所吸入的清气结合而成，又通过心肺布散到全身，以滋养各脏腑组织和维持它们的正常功能活动。二是肺对全身气机具有调节作用。气机，泛指气的运动，升降出入为其基本形式。呼吸运动，是气的升降出入运动的具体体现。肺通过有节律的一呼一吸，对全身之气的升降出入运动起着重要的调节作用。

（二）肺主宣发和肃降

肺主宣发即肺具有向上升宣和向外布散的作用。其一，通过气化作用，呼出体内的浊气；其二，将脾所转输的津液和水谷精微，布散到全身。其三，宣发卫气，调节腠理之开阖，并将代谢后的津液化为汗液，由汗孔排出体外。因此肺失宣发，则见呼气不利、胸闷、咳嗽、鼻塞、无汗等症。

肺主肃降，指肺气向下清肃通降，使呼吸道保持洁净。一是吸入自然界清气。二是将吸入的清气和由脾转输于肺的津液和水谷精微向下布散于全身。三是肃清肺和呼吸道内的异物，以保持呼吸道的洁净。因此，肺气失于肃降，则可现呼吸短促、喘息、咳痰等肺气上逆之候。

肺气的宣发和肃降，是相反相成的矛盾运动。生理情况下相互依存和相互制约；病理情况下又常常相互影响。没有正常的宣发，就不会有很好的肃降；没有正常的肃降，也不会有很好的宣发。

（三）肺主通调水道

通调水道，指肺通过宣发和肃降功能对体内水液代谢起到疏通调节作用。肺主宣发，将水液布散全身，调节汗液的排泄；肺又主肃降，将水液向下输送，经肾和膀胱排出体外，此即所谓的"肺为水之上源"。若肺失宣降，通调失职，则水液停聚，见小便不利、痰饮、水肿等。

（四）肺朝百脉、主治节

肺朝百脉，指全身的血脉都聚会于肺，经肺的呼吸，进行清气的交换；再通过肺的宣降作用，将富含清气的血液通过百脉布散到全身。肺主治节，是指肺气具有治理调节全身各脏腑组织生理功能的作用。

（五）肺的连属关系

1. 在志为忧　肺在志为忧，是指肺的功能与精神情志活动的"忧"有关。忧伤虽属不良情志刺激，但在一般情况下，并不都导致人体发病。只有在过度悲伤情况下，才能成为致病因素。若过忧则伤肺，出现呼吸气短、少气不足以吸等肺气不足的证候；反之，若肺气不足，机体耐受忧虑的机能降低，易于产生悲忧的负面情绪反应。

the four seasons and stands in interior-exterior relationship with the large intestine.

Lung dominates qi and control breathing

Lung dominating qi includes two aspects:one is that the lung governs respiration qi, and the other is that the lung governs the all of the bodily qi, with the details as follows:

1. The Lung governing respiration qi

The lung has the function of controlling breathing.The Lung is the place where natural clear and fresh air is inhaled and the turbid qi of human body exhaled so as to ensure the normal metabolism.Normal respiratory function of the lung keeps smooth airway and even breathing, while weakening respiratory function of lung will lead to weak and short breath with low voice.

2. Lung governing all of the bodily qi

Such physiological function embodies in two aspects:first, generation of ancestral qi, which is the combination derived from food essence and water and the clear fresh air inhaled, and dispersed throughout the body to nourish the internal organs and maintain their normal functions via the lung and heart; second, regulation on qi movement, which refers to the motion of qi, with ascending, descending, entering and exiting as its basic form.Respiration movement is the concrete embodiment of the four basic forms.The lung regulates qi movement of the body through the rhythmic respiration.

Lung governs diffusion and depurative downbearing

Lung governing diffusion refers to the function of lung qi in upward movement and outward dispersion, which includes three steps:first, the lung exhales the turbid qi through qi transformation, second, the lung disperses the body fluids and food essence transported and transformed by the spleen throughout the body, and third the lung diffuses the defensive qi, regulates the opening and closing of interstices, and transforms the metabolized fluids into sweat and then discharge it out through sweat pores.So there will be no unsmooth breathing, stuffy chest, coughing, nasal congestion and adiapheustia and so on if lung exerts its diffusing function abnormally.

Lung governing depurative downbearing refers to the downward movement and purifying action of the lung to keep the respiratory tract clean, which also includes three steps:first, the lung inhales fresh and clear air in the nature; second, the lung sends downward the fresh clear air together with the body fluids and food essence transported and transformed by the spleen throughout the body; and third, the lung purifies the foreign matters in lung and respiratory tract to keep them clean.As a result, failure of lung in purification and down-sending will lead to lung qi ascending counterflow syndrome like breathing shortness, panting, coughing up sputum.

Diffusion and depurative downbearing are both opposite and complementary movement forms to each other.Physiologically they are interdependent and inter-restrictive, and pathologically they often mutually affect.Without normal diffusion, there will be abnormal purification and vise verse.

Lung governs regulation of the waterway

It means the lung dredges and regulates the water and fluid metabolism through its functions of diffusion and depurative downbearing.Its diffusion function helps it spread water and fluid throughout the body and regulate the discharge of sweat; while its depurative downbearing function helps it transport water and fluid downward to the kidney and bladder, from which they drained, which is also known as"lung being as the upper source of water."The inability of lung to diffuse, purificate and downsend will cause fluid retention syndrome like inhibited urination, phlegm and retained fluid and edema, etc.

Lung connects all vessels and governs management and regulation

Lung connecting all vessels means all the blood vessels of human body converge in the lung, where realizes qi exchange through breathing, and then distributes blood rich in fresh air throughout the body through the vessels with lung's function of diffusion and depurative downbearing.Lung governing manage-

2．在液为涕 涕为鼻腔黏膜分泌的一种黏液，具有润泽鼻窍的功能。而鼻为肺窍，故涕与肺有密切的关系。此即《素问·宣明五气篇》中所说"五脏化液……肺为涕"，所以涕的状态可以反应肺的功能。

3．在体合皮，其华在毛 肺与皮毛在生理或病理上存在着十分密切的内在联系。皮毛为一身之表，依赖肺宣发的卫气和津液温养润泽，是机体抵御外邪的第一道屏障。肺的功能正常，则皮毛润泽，抵御外邪侵袭的能力较强。若肺气不足，卫表不固则多汗、易于感冒等。

4．在窍为鼻 鼻与喉相连而通于肺，故有"鼻为肺之窍"之说。鼻的功能有两方面：一是通气功能。二是嗅觉功能。鼻的通气和嗅觉功能都与肺气的作用有关，正如《灵枢·脉度》所说："肺气通于鼻，肺和则鼻能知香臭矣。"肺气和，则呼吸利，嗅觉灵敏；肺气不利则见鼻塞、流涕等症。

二、大肠的功能

大肠与肺之间有经脉相互络属，互为表里。

大肠的功能是传化糟粕。传，即传送；化，即变化。大肠把经过小肠泌别清浊后的食物残渣变化成粪便，向下传导，经肛门排出体外，并在这一过程中吸收多余的水液，故称大肠为"传导之官"。如大肠传导糟粕功能失常，则出现排便异常，常见便秘或泄泻。

三、肺与大肠病的辨证

（一）肺气虚

【证候】咳喘无力、气短，声音低微，动则益甚，痰液清稀，倦怠无力，面白无华，自汗畏风，舌淡白，脉虚弱。

【辨证分析】多由咳喘日久，耗伤正气，或气的生化不足所致。肺主气、司呼吸，肺气亏虚、宣降失职，则咳喘无力，气短，声低息微；动则耗气，故动则益甚；肺气虚，其输布水液功能减弱，水液停聚于肺，故见痰液清稀；肺气虚不能宣发卫气于肌表，卫外不固则自汗畏风；而倦怠无力、面白无华、舌淡白、脉虚弱均为气虚的表现。

【治法】补益肺气。

【代表方剂】补肺汤。

ment and regulation refers to its function of managing and regulating physiological functions of all the internal organs.

Affiliation of the Lung

1. Lung associates with sorrow in emotion

Lung associating with sorrow in emotion means lung's function is influenced by the motion of sorrow. In general case, sorrow cannot lead to disease. Only excessive sorrow can turn into the pathogenic factor. Excessive sorrow impairs lung and lead to lung-qi deficiency syndrome such as short breath and weakness of respiration, which vice verse will reduce the tolerance capacity of anxiety and result in the negative emotional reaction of sorrow.

2. Lung associates with snivel in humor

Snivel is a kind of mucus secreted by mucosa of nasal cavity with the function of moistening the nasal orifice. It has close relationship with the lung as nose is the orifice corresponding to the lung, as described in *Plain Questions* "five viscera produce different kinds of fluids···snivel as the fluid produced by lung," so snivel condition can reflect the function of lung.

3. Lung links with skin, with its luster manifesting on the hair

There is very close internal connection between the lung and skin and hair physiologically and pathologically. As the first protective screen to resist invasion by external evils, skin and hair, the surface of human body, is warmed and moistened by defense qi and body fluids diffused by the lung. So if the lung works normally, the skin and hair will be lustrous and has the strong disease resistance; and if lung qi is insufficient, the insecurity of defensive exterior will occur and make people apt to hidrosis and catch cold, etc.

4. Lung opens at nose

Both the nose and throat are connected with lung, so there is the saying of "lung opens at nose." The nose has two functions: breathing and smelling, both of which are related with lung qi, as depicted in *Miraculous Pivot* "lung qi connects with nose, so if lung works normally, then the nose can exert its function of smelling normally." If the lung functions normally, then people can breathe smoothly and distinguish different smells, otherwise, there will emerge such symptoms as stuffy nose and running nose, etc.

Functions of the Large Intestine

The large intestine stands in exterior-interior relationship with the lung, as there are meridians and collaterals linking with both of them.

Function of large intestine is to transport and transform feces

The large intestine transforms the food residue absorbed by the small intestine into feces and transports them downward to the anus to be discharged, during which the large intestine absorbs the surplus water. So it is called as "the organ in charge of transportation and transformation of the waste part of food into feces." If the large intestine dysfunctions, then abnormal defecation will occur such as constipation or diarrhea.

Syndrome Differentiation of the Lung and Large Intestine

Lung-qi deficiency

Syndrome: weak cough and pant, short breath, and low and feeble voice which aggravate on exertion, clear and thin phlegm, lack of strength and fatigue, pale and lustrous complexion, spontaneous sweating and fear of wind, pale tongue and weak and vacuous pulse.

Syndrome differentiation: it is often caused by prolonged cough and pant damaging healthy qi or insufficient generation of qi. Weak cough and pant, short breath, and low and feeble voice are due to lung-qi

（二）肺阴虚

【证候】干咳无痰，或痰少而黏，或痰中带血，口咽干燥，形体消瘦，颧红，潮热，盗汗，舌红少津，脉细数。

【辨证分析】本证多由痨虫袭肺，久咳伤阴，或热病后期阴津受损所致。肺主肃降，性喜柔润，肺阴不足，肃降无权，气机上逆发为咳嗽；虚热内生，灼伤津液，故无痰，或痰少而粘；阴虚火旺、灼伤脉络则痰中带血；肺阴亏虚，上不能滋润咽喉，则口咽干燥；外不能濡养肌肤，则形体消瘦。颧红、潮热、盗汗、舌红少津、脉细数均为阴虚内热之象。

【治法】滋阴润肺。

【代表方剂】百合固金汤。

（三）风寒束肺

【证候】咳嗽，咯痰稀薄色白，鼻塞流清涕，恶寒，轻度发热，无汗，头身疼痛，苔薄白，脉浮紧。

【辨证分析】本证为风寒之邪侵袭肺卫所致。肺主宣发肃降，外合皮毛，感受风寒，肺气被束不得宣发，逆而为咳；寒属阴，故痰液稀薄色白；肺开窍于鼻，风寒束肺，则鼻流清涕；而恶寒发热、无汗、头身疼痛、苔薄白、脉浮紧等均为风寒表证之象。

【治法】宣肺散寒。

【代表方剂】三拗汤。

（四）风热犯肺

【证候】咳嗽痰黄，鼻塞黄涕，口渴咽痛，恶风发热，舌尖红，苔薄黄，脉浮数。

【辨证分析】本证是由风热之邪侵犯肺卫所致。肺主宣发肃降，风热犯肺，肺失宣肃则咳嗽。热邪煎灼津液，炼液为痰，则痰黏稠色黄；肺开窍于鼻，风热犯肺则鼻塞黄涕；口渴咽痛、恶风发热、舌尖红、苔薄黄、脉浮数均为风热表证之象。

【治法】疏风清热，宣肺止咳。

【代表方剂】桑菊饮。

deficiency and lung failing to diffuse, purify and down-sent. Aggravation of the above phenomena on exertion is because exertion consumes qi. Clear and thin phlegm arises from water retention in lung, indicating its weakened function of distributing body fluids. Spontaneous sweating and fear of wind result from deficient lung-qi failing to diffuse defense qi around the skin. And pale tongue and weak and vacuous pulse are all the manifestations of lung-qi deficiency syndrome.

Method of treatment: tonify lung qi.

Formula: Bufei Decoction.

Lung-yin deficiency

Syndrome: dry cough without sputum, or cough with little sticky phlegm, or with phlegm containing blood, dry mouth and throat, emaciation, red cheeks, tidal fever, night sweating, red tongue with little fluid, and thin and rapid pulse.

Syndrome differentiation: it is primarily caused by tubercle bacillus attacking lung, or long-term cough impairing yin, or fluid being damaged in the later period of febrile diseases. Lung governs depurative downbearing and prefers soft and moist. Cough indicates lung-yin deficiency and lung-qi reversely flow upward rather than descending; cough without or with little sticky phlegm indicates internal deficiency-heat scorches body fluids; phlegm containing blood indicates yin deficiency with effulgent fire damages vessels; dry mouth and throat indicates lung-yin deficiency fails to moisten throat; emaciation indicates lung-yin fail to nourish the muscles and skin; red cheeks, tidal fever, nigh sweating, red tongue with little fluid, and thin and rapid pulse are all the manifestations of yin deficiency with internal heat.

Method of treatment: nourish yin to moisten lung.

Formula: Baihe Gujin Decoction.

Wind-cold fettering the lung

Syndrome: cough with thin and clear white phlegm, stuffy nose, running nose with clear snivel, aversion to cold, light fever, no sweat, headache and body pains, thin and white fur and floating and tight pulse.

Syndrome differentiation: it is caused by wind-cold invading the defense qi. Lung governs diffusion and depurative downbearing with its condition reflected from skin and hair. Cough indicates lung-qi is fettered and flows upward reversely rather than dispersing; and clear and thin white phlegm indicates it belongs to cold syndrome. In addition, lung opens at the nose, so wind-cold fettering lung will lead to running nose with clear snivel; and aversion to cold with fever, no sweat, headache and body pains, white and thin fur and floating and tight pulse are all manifestations of wind-cold exterior syndrome.

Method of treatment: diffuse the lung to remove coldness.

Formula: San'ao Decoction.

Wind-heat invading the lung

Syndrome: cough up yellow phlegm, running nose with yellow snivel, thirst, sore throat, aversion to wind with fever, red tough tip, thin and yellow fur and floating and rapid pulse.

Syndrome differentiation: it is caused by wind-heat invading defense qi. Lung governs diffusion and depurative downbearing, so wind-heat invading lung will lead to its dysfunction and then cough. Thick yellow sticky phlegm indicates heat scorches body fluids and turns it to phlegm. Lung opens at the nose, so wind-heat invading lung will result in running nose with yellow snivel. Thirst, sore throat, aversion to wind with fever, red tongue tip, thin yellow fur and floating and rapid pulse are all the manifestations of wind-heat exterior syndrome.

Method of treatment: disperse wind and clear heat, diffuse the lung to suppress cough.

Formula: Sangju Decoction.

（五）痰热壅肺

【证候】咳嗽喘促，咳痰黄稠，痰中带血，或咳吐脓血腥臭痰，胸痛，发热，口渴，烦躁，尿黄，便秘，舌红，苔黄腻，脉滑数。

【辨证分析】本证多因温热之邪从口鼻而入，或风寒入里化热，内壅于肺所致。肺主肃降，痰热壅肺、肃降无权，肺气上逆则咳嗽喘促；热邪炼液为痰，则痰稠色黄；热伤血络则痰中带血；热腐成脓则咳吐脓血腥臭痰；痰热阻滞肺络，致气机不畅，脉络不通，则胸痛；发热、口渴、烦躁、尿黄、便秘、舌红、苔黄腻、脉滑数均为痰热之象。

【治法】清化痰热。

【代表方剂】清金化痰丸。

（六）大肠湿热

【证候】腹痛，里急后重，泄泻秽浊，或下痢脓血，肛门灼热，小便短赤，发热口渴，舌红，苔黄腻，脉滑数。

【辨证分析】本证多因感受暑湿热毒，或饮食不节及饮食不洁，蕴湿生热，湿热侵犯大肠所致。湿热内蕴于大肠，气机阻滞故腹痛、里急后重，泄泻秽浊；湿热熏蒸，灼伤脉络，热腐为脓，故下痢脓血；热炽肠道，则肛门灼热；水液从大便外泄，故小便短赤；热盛伤津则发热口渴；舌红，苔黄腻、脉滑数亦为湿热之象。

【治法】清利湿热。

【代表方剂】白头翁汤。

第三节　脾与胃功能及其辨证

一、脾的功能

脾位于中焦，五行属土，与胃相表里，与四时之长夏相应。

（一）脾主运化

脾主运化，是指脾具有把水谷转化为精微，并将精微物质吸收转输至全身各脏腑，以维持其功能正常。包括运化水谷和运化水湿两个方面。

运化水谷：是指对饮食物的消化吸收和输布作用。饮食入胃后，经胃的受纳和腐熟作用，使其初步消化，并下送于小肠，经小肠"泌别清浊"作用，使之进一步消化分解成水谷精微和糟粕。水谷精微上输于肺，经肺之宣发肃降，使水谷精微得以输布全身。而水谷精微，是生成气血的主要物质基础，所以说脾为后天之本、气血生化之源。只有脾气健运，才能化生气血，以维持正常的生理活动；若脾失健运，可出现食后腹胀、便溏、食欲不振，以至于精神萎靡、四肢无力、肌肉消瘦和气血

Phlegm-heat obstructing the lung

Syndrome: cough, panting and tachypnea, cough up yellow and thick phlegm or phlegm containing blood, or coughing up fetid phlegm containing pus and blood, chest pain, fever, thirst, dysphoria, yellow urine, constipation, red tongue with yellow and slimy fur, and slippery and rapid pulse.

Syndrome differentiation: it is primarily caused by warm and heat pathogens entering the interior from the mouth and nose to obstruct the lung, or wind-cold transforming into heat in the interior to obstruct the lung. Cough, panting and tachypnea indicate phlegm-heat obstructs lung and cause the upward flow of lung-qi rather than descending; yellow and thick phlegm indicate heat turns body fluids into phlegm; phlegm containing blood indicates heat hurts vessels; fetid phlegm containing pus and blood indicates heat decays the muscles into pus; check pain indicates phlegm-heat obstructs lung meridian and unsmooth qi movement; and fever, thirst, dysphoria, yellow urine, constipation, red tongue with yellow slimy fur, and slippery and rapid pulse are all the manifestations of phlegm-heat.

Method of treatment: clear and resolve heat-phlegm.

Formula: Qingjin Huatan Pill.

Large intestinal dampness-heat

Syndrome: abdominal pain, tenesmus, diarrhea with turbid foul, or diarrhea with pus and blood, scorching anus, red and scanty urination, fever with thirst, red tongue with yellow and slimy fur, and slippery and rapid pulse.

Syndrome differentiation: it is primarily caused by dampness-heat invading the large intestine, which arising from infection of summer dampness and heat toxin, or improper diet or unclean diet. Abdominal pain, tenesmus and diarrhea with turbid foul indicate of dampness-heat accumulates in the large intestine and obstructs its qi movement. Diarrhea with pus and blood indicates dampness-heat damages vessels and muscles; scorching anus indicates intense heat burns the intestinal tract; red and scanty urination occurs as water is discharged with the stool; fever with thirst indicates excessive heat injures body fluids; and red tongue with yellow slimy fur and slippery and rapid pulse are all the manifestations of dampness-heat.

Method of treatment: clear and drain dampness-heat.

Formula: Pulsatilla decoction.

Section 3   Functions of the Spleen and Stomach and their Syndrome Differentiation

Functions of the Spleen

The spleen locates in the middle energizer, pertains to earth in the five phases, corresponds to late summer in the four seasons and stands in interior-exterior relationship with the stomach.

Spleen governs transportation and transformation

Spleen governing transportation and transformation refers to spleen's function of transforming food and water into essence and then transporting them to all the internal organs to maintain their normal functions, including transforming and transporting food, water, and dampness.

Transportation and transformation of food: it refers to the spleen's function of absorbing and digesting food and distributing the food essence. The food is received by the stomach for decomposition and preliminary digestion before being transported to the small intestine for further digestion and separating the food essence from the dross, and then the food essence is transported upward to the lung and then distributed throughout the body through lung's diffusing and depurative downbearing. The food essence is the main material base of generating qi and blood, so it is said that the spleen is the root of acquired constitution and

生化不足等病症。

运化水湿：又称运化水液，指脾对水液有吸收和转输，调节人体水液代谢的作用。人体所摄入的水液，经过脾的吸收和转化以布散全身而发挥滋养、濡润的作用；同时脾又把各组织器官利用后的多余水液，及时地转输于肺和肾，通过肺的宣发和肾的气化作用，化为汗和尿排出体外。当脾运化水液功能减退，可导致水液在体内停滞，产生湿、痰、饮等病理产物，甚则导致水肿。

（二）脾主升清

脾主升清，指水谷精微借脾气而上输于心、肺、头目，通过心肺的作用化生气血，以营养全身。与胃的降浊相对而言，降浊是指对水谷中的食物残渣，由胃至小肠、大肠的逐级下降，最后形成糟粕排出体外。此外，脾气的升清作用，可维持人体脏腑位置相对恒定，对防止人体内脏下垂具有一定的作用。若脾气虚不能升清，则水谷不能运化，气血生化无源，可出现神疲乏力、头目眩晕、腹胀、泄泻等症。脾气下陷，则可见久泻脱肛，甚或内脏下垂及子宫脱垂等病症。

（三）脾主统血

脾统血，是指脾有统摄、控制血液在脉中运行，而不溢出脉外的功能。脾统血的作用是通过气摄血来实现的。脾气健运，气血生化有源，则气固摄血液的功能得以正常发挥，血液不至于溢出脉外而发生出血；若脾不统血，脾气固摄血液的功能减弱，可使血溢出脉外而见各种出血证，如便血、尿血、崩漏、肌衄等。

（四）脾的连属关系

1. 在志为思 脾在志为思，是指脾的功能与精神情志活动的"思"有关。正常情况下，思考对于机体正常生理活动无不良影响，但若思虑过度，就会影响气的升降出入，导致气机郁结，升清功能失常，出现不思饮食、脘腹胀闷、眩晕健忘等症。

2. 在液为涎 涎为口腔分泌的液体，唾液中较清稀的部分，由脾气化生并转输布散，故说"脾在液为涎"。它具有保护口腔黏膜、润泽口腔的作用，在进食时分泌较多，有助于食物的吞咽与消化。

3. 在体合肌肉、主四肢 脾的运化功能与肌肉、四肢的丰满健壮及其功能发挥之间有着密切的联系。脾胃为气血生化之源，人体的肌肉四肢都需要脾所运化的水谷精微来营养，才能使肌肉发达，丰满健壮，四肢轻劲有力。若脾胃功能失常，必致肌肉消瘦，四肢痿软，甚至萎废不用。

4. 在窍为口，其华在唇 脾开窍于口，是指饮食口味与脾运化功能有密切关系，《灵枢·脉度》中记载"脾气通于口，脾和则口能知五谷矣"。如脾气健旺，则食欲、口味正常；若脾失健运，则食欲不振，口淡无味；脾有湿热，可觉口干、口腻；若脾有伏热伏火，可循经上蒸于口，发生口疮或口腔糜烂。

口唇的色泽，与全身的气血是否充足有关。如脾气健运，气血充足，营养良好，

the source of generating qi and blood. Vigorous spleen qi can help the spleen to generate qi and blood so as to maintain the normal physiological activities. The failure of spleen in transportation and transformation will lead to insufficiency of qi and blood syndrome like abdominal fullness after intake of food, sloppy stool and loss of appetite, and even listlessness, weak limbs, emaciation and etc.

Transportation and transformation of water and dampness: it refers to the spleen's function of absorbing and distributing water fluids and regulating the metabolism of them, also known as transportation and transformation of water fluids. The water and fluids people drink are absorbed, transformed and then distributed by the spleen to nourish and moisten the body; with the superfluous water transmitted to the lung and kidney by the spleen for being discharged out in the forms of sweat and urine under the functions of diffusing of the lung and transformation of the kidney. Hypoactivity of the spleen in transporting and transforming water and fluids will lead to retention of water in the body and produce dampness, phlegm and retained fluid, and other pathological products and even edema.

Spleen governs upbearing the clear

Spleen unbearing the clear means food and water essence is transported upward to the heart, lung, and head by spleen qi and then transformed into qi and blood through the heart and lung to nourish the body. It is in the relative terms to stomach downbearing the turbid, which means the residue of food is transmitted downward by the stomach to the small intestine and then the large intestine for being discharged in the form of feces. In addition, the spleen's function of upbearing the clear can maintain each of the internal organs at their fixed positions and prevent against visceroptosis. The spleen-qi deficiency depriving the spleen of upbearing the clear will lead to listlessness and fatigue, dizziness, abdominal distention and diarrhea as the food and water cannot be transformed into essence and transported to nourish the body. Sunken spleen qi can lead to prolonged diarrhea and prolapse of the rectum, or even visceroptosis and prolapse of uterus, etc.

Spleen controls blood circulation

Spleen controlling blood circulation refers to spleen's function of governing and controlling blood to circulate in the vessels rather than extravasation, which is achieved by qi commanding blood. As vigorous spleen qi provides sufficient source of generating qi and blood, the function of qi commanding blood can be normally exerted to prevent blood from flowing over the vessels and causing bleeding. Spleen fails to control the blood, and then it causes dysfunction of spleen qi commanding the blood and hemorrhagic diseases like hemafecia, hematuria, metrorrhagia and metrostaxis, and bleeding of muscles.

Affiliations of Spleen

1. Spleen associates with thought in emotion

Spleen associated with thought in emotion means the function of spleen is influenced by the motion of thinking. Generally thought will not produce negative effects on normal physiological activities, but excessive thought will affect upward, downward, inward and outward movements of qi and lead to qi stagnation and dysfunction of qi in upbearing the clear, which is characterized by poor appetite, abdominal fullness and distention, dizziness and forgetfulness, etc.

2. Spleen associates with drool in humor

Drool is the thinner saliva secreted by mouth cavity, and transformed, transported and distributed by the spleen qi, so it is said saliva is the fluid produced by the spleen. It has the functions of protecting mouth mucosa, moistening mouth, and helping ingestion and digestion of food as it is often secreted more with a meal.

3. Spleen links with muscles and dominates limbs

Spleen's function of transportation and transformation is closely related with the conditions of muscles and limbs and whether they can exert their functions normally. The spleen and stomach are the source for

则口唇红润有光泽。如《素问·五藏生成篇》说："脾之合肉也，其荣唇也。"若脾失健运，气血衰少，营养不良，则口唇淡白无华。

二、胃的功能

胃与脾之间有经脉相互络属，互为表里。胃的功能是：

（一）主受纳，腐熟水谷

受纳，是指接受和容纳。腐熟，是指饮食物经过胃的初步消化，变成食糜。饮食入口，容纳并储存于胃，经胃的初步消化，变成食糜。故胃有"水谷之海"、"太仓"和"仓廪之官"之称。水谷经胃的腐熟，下传于小肠，其精微物质由脾之运化而营养周身。如果胃的腐熟功能低下，就出现胃脘疼痛、嗳腐纳呆等食滞胃脘之症。

（二）主通降，以降为和

胃主通降与脾主升清相对。胃主通降是指胃气宜通畅、下降的特性。饮食物入胃，经胃的腐熟后，下行入小肠，再经过小肠的分清泌浊，其浊者下移于大肠，然后变为大便排出体外，以完成其通降传导作用。胃的通降是受纳的前提条件，若胃失通降，不仅影响食欲，而且因浊气上蒸可出现口臭；若胃气上逆，可见恶心、呕吐、呃逆、嗳气等症。

三、脾与胃病的辨证

（一）脾气虚

【证候】食少纳呆，腹胀，饭后尤甚，便溏，面色萎黄，少气懒言，四肢倦怠消瘦，舌淡，苔白，脉缓弱。

【辨证分析】本证多为过度劳倦，或饮食失调或饮食不节，损伤脾气所致。脾气虚弱，运化失常，故见食少纳呆、腹胀；脾失健运，消化无权，故食后腹胀愈甚；脾虚水湿不化，清浊不分，水谷齐下，故有便溏；脾气不足，精微不布，气血生化无源，气血不足不能上荣于面，则面色萎黄；不能荣润肌肤，则消瘦；少气懒言，四肢倦怠，舌淡，脉缓弱皆为脾气亏虚、气血不充之证。

【治法】健脾益气。

【代表方剂】六君子汤。

generating qi and blood, and the muscles and limbs are nourished by food and water essence transformed and transported by the spleen, so that the muscles are plump and strong and limbs are full of strength and flexible. Dysfunction of the spleen and stomach will lead to muscle emaciation as well as limbs wilting and paralyzing.

4. Spleen opening at the mouth, with its luster manifesting on the lip

Spleen opening at the mouth refers to the close relations between the appetite and the spleen's function of transportation and transformation, as described in *Miraculous Pivot* "As spleen opens at the mouth, people will have good appetite and can distinguish the tastes of food when spleen exerts its functions normally." With vigorous and sufficient spleen-qi, people will have the normal appetite and tastes. On the contrary, spleen failing to exert its function of transportation and transformation will lead to poor appetite and tastelessness; dampness-heat in the spleen will cause dry and greasy mouth; and the latent heat and fire in spleen will bring about aphtha or sore in the mouth as the heat and fire runs upward along the meridians to affect the mouth.

Color and luster of lip is related with the conditions of qi and blood of the whole body. The lip will be red and lustrous if the spleen exerts its function of transportation and transformation well to provide sufficient qi and blood to nourish the body, as depicted in *Plain Questions* "spleen nourishes the muscles and moistens lips." The failure of the spleen in transportation and transformation will lead to qi and blood deficiency and malnutrition characterized by pale lips.

Functions of the Stomach

The stomach stands in exterior-interior relationship with the spleen, as there are meridians and collaterals linking with both of them. The functions of stomach are as follows:

Stomach receives and decomposes food and drink

Stomach receiving and decomposing food and drink means the stomach receives and stores food and then preliminarily turns it into chime. So the stomach is also termed as "sea of food and water," "large depository" or "barn organ." After decomposed, drink and food are transmitted to the small intestine with its essence transported and transformed by the spleen to nourish the whole body. The hypoactivity of stomach in decomposing food and drink will lead to food stagnation in stomach syndrome like stomachache, belching with fetid odour and torpid intake, etc.

Stomach downbears the turbid

Stomach downbearing the turbid is opposite to spleen upbearing the clear. It refers stomach's property of sending food downward freely. The stomach decomposes food and drink and then transports them into the small intestine for separating the clear from the turbid, and transmits the turbid into the large intestine for being discharged out as stool. In this way, the stomach realizes its function of downbearing. Downbearing function of the stomach is the precondition of its function of receiving food. The failure of stomach in exerting its downbearing function will affect appetite and lead to fetid mouth odor as the result of turbid qi flowing upward. In addition, the stomach qi ascending counterflow will cause nausea, vomit, hiccup and belching, etc.

Syndrome Differentiation of the Spleen and Stomach

Spleen-qi deficiency

Syndrome: little and torpid intake, abdominal distention which aggravates after meal, sloppy stool, sallow complexion, weak breath and no desire to speak, weak and emaciated limbs, pale tongue with white fur, and weak moderate pulse.

Syndrome differentiation: it is often caused by excessive labor and improper diet which damage spleen

（二）脾阳虚

【证候】脘腹胀满，食少纳呆，腹痛，喜温喜按，畏寒肢冷，口淡不渴，或周身浮肿，大便溏薄，或白带量多质稀，舌质淡胖，苔白滑，脉沉迟无力。

【辨证分析】本证多因脾气虚日久，或因过食生冷、过用寒凉药物，损伤脾阳，或命门火衰，火不暖土所致。脾阳虚衰，运化失健，故见脘腹胀满，食少纳呆；中阳不振，虚寒内生，寒凝气滞，故腹中冷痛，喜温喜按；阳虚阴盛，失于温煦，故有畏寒肢冷；中阳不振，不能运化水湿，水湿内盛，则口淡不渴，流注肠中，故大便溏薄；水湿泛溢肌肤，则有周身浮肿；水湿下注，故白带清稀量多；舌淡胖、苔白滑、脉沉迟无力均为脾阳虚之征。

【治法】温中散寒。

【代表方剂】理中丸。

（三）脾气下陷

【证候】脘腹重坠作胀，食后加重，或便意频频，肛门重坠，或长期下痢不止，重则脱肛，或子宫脱垂，或小便混浊如米泔，少气无力，肢体倦怠，食少便溏，头晕目眩，舌淡，苔白，脉虚弱。

【辨证分析】本证多由过度劳倦，或久病伤脾，致脾气不升，或脾气虚弱进一步发展而来。脾气虚则升举无力，脏腑无托，故见便意频频，重则脱肛、子宫脱垂；食后气陷更甚，故脘腹重坠作胀，食后加重；脾气不足，固摄无权，故下痢不止；脾气虚致精微不能正常输布而反下流膀胱，则小便混浊如米泔；脾气不足，运化无权，则食少便溏；脾虚，清阳之气不能上升于头，头目失养，则头晕目眩。少气无力、肢体倦怠、舌淡、脉虚弱均为脾气虚弱之征。

【治法】健脾益气，升阳举陷。

【代表方剂】补中益气汤。

qi. Little and torpid intake and abdominal distention are due to spleen-qi deficiency failing to exert its transportation and transformation function; sloppy stool occurs because the spleen is too weak to transport water and dampness and separate the clear from the turbid and prevent them from flowing downward into the large intestine; sallow complexion results from spleen-qi deficiency failing to generate qi and blood and distribute essence to nourish the face; emaciated muscle occurs when qi and blood fail to nourish the skin; and weak breath, no desire to speak, weak limbs, pale tongue with white fur and weak moderate pulse are all the signs of spleen-qi deficiency failing to generate sufficient qi and blood.

Method of treatment: fortify the spleen to tonify qi.

Formula: Liu Junzi Decoction.

Spleen-yang deficiency

Syndrome: abdominal distention and fullness, little and torpid intake, abdominal pain with preference of being warmed and pressed, fear of cold with cold limbs, tastelessness and hydroadipsia, or general edema, sloppy stool, large quantity of thin leucorrhea, pale and enlarged tongue with white slippery fur, and sunken slow weak pulse.

Syndrome differentiation: it is often caused by long-term spleen-qi deficiency, or intake of too much raw or cold food, or excessive application of cool or cold drugs, which injures spleen-yang or lead to kidney life-gate fire deficiency failing to warm spleen earth. Abdominal distention and fullness, and little and torpid intake is the results of spleen-yang deficiency failing to transport and transform food and water; abdominal cold pain with preference of being warmed and pressed occurs because of devitalized spleen-yang leading to internal deficiency-cold and then both cold congealing and qi stagnation; fear of cold with cold limbs results from yang deficiency with excessive yin failing to warm the body; tastelessness and hydroadipsia indicate devitalized spleen yang failing to transport and transform the excessive internal water and dampness, which will lead to sloppy stool if they pouring into the intestine; general edema is due to water and dampness overflowing the skin; large quantity of thin leucorrhea is caused by the water and dampness pouring down to the lower energizer; and pale and enlarged tongue with white slippery fur, and sunken slow weak pulse are the manifestations of spleen-yang deficiency.

Method of treatment: warm the middle energizer to remove coldness.

Formula: Lizhong Pill.

Sunken spleen-qi

Syndrome: abdominal dropping and distention which aggravates after meal, or frequent desire to defecate, dropping anus, or prolonged diarrhea, even prolapse of anus or uterus, rice-swill-like turbid urine, weak breath and strength, weak body and limbs, little intake and sloppy stool, dizziness, pale tongue with white fur, and weak vacuous pulse.

Syndrome differentiation: it is often caused by spleen-qi failing to upbear due to overexertion or prolonged disease damaging the spleen, or further developed from spleen-qi deficiency. Frequent desire to defecate and prolapse of the anus or uterus are the result of spleen-qi deficiency failing to upbear the internal organs; abdominal dropping and distention which aggravates after meal is due to the aggravation of qi sinking after intake of food; diarrhea arsies from spleen-qi deficiency failing to exert its controlling function; rice-swill-like turbid urine occurs because spleen-qi deficiency fails to distribute the essence, which finally pour down into the bladder; little intake and sloppy stool turns up as spleen-qi deficiency fails to transport and transform the food and water; dizziness is due to spleen deficiency failing to upbear the clear to nourish the head and eyes; and weak qi and strength, weak body and limbs, pale tongue with white fur, and weak vacuous pulse are all the signs of spleen-qi deficiency.

Method of treatment: fortify the spleen to replenish qi and raise the sunken yang-qi.

Formula: Buzhong Yiqi Decoction.

（四）脾不统血

【证候】鼻衄，齿衄，肌衄，便血，尿血，或月经过多，崩漏，伴有纳少便溏，少气懒言，神疲乏力，面白无华，舌淡，脉细弱。

【辨证分析】本证多由久病或过度劳倦损伤脾气所致。脾主统血，脾气虚统血无权，血不能循经而行，溢于脉外，则有鼻衄，齿衄；如溢于肌肤，则见肌衄；溢于胃肠，则便血；溢于膀胱，则见尿血；脾虚统血无权，冲任不固，故月经过多，崩漏；纳少便溏、少气懒言、神疲乏力、舌质淡、脉细弱均为脾气虚弱之征。

【治法】补脾摄血。

【代表方剂】归脾汤。

（五）脾胃寒湿

【证候】脘腹痞闷胀痛，纳少便溏，恶心欲吐，口淡无味，头身困重，或肢体浮肿，小便短少，妇人白带过多，舌淡胖，苔白腻，脉濡。

【辨证分析】本证多由饮食不节，过食生冷，或淋雨涉水，久居湿处，或内湿素盛所致。脾为太阴湿土，喜燥而恶湿。今寒湿内侵，脾阳被困，升降失常，故见脘腹痞闷，重则作胀疼痛，纳少便溏，恶心欲吐，口淡无味；脾主四肢肌肉，湿性重着，阳气被困，故见头身困重；脾阳被寒湿所困，不能温化水湿，湿泛肌表，故见肢体浮肿，小便短少；寒湿渗注于下，故白带量多；舌淡胖、脉濡皆为寒湿内盛之征。

【治法】温中化湿。

【代表方剂】茵陈术附汤。

（六）脾胃湿热

【证候】腹部痞闷，纳呆呕恶，口粘，肢体困重，面目皮肤发黄，或身热起伏，汗出热不解，便溏不爽，小便色黄，舌红，苔黄腻，脉濡数或滑数。

【辨证分析】本证多由过食肥甘厚味，酿成湿热，内蕴脾胃，或感受湿热之邪所致。湿热之邪蕴于脾胃，受纳运化失职，升降失常，故见腹部痞闷，纳呆呕恶；湿热上泛于口，故口粘；脾主四肢肌肉，湿性重着，脾为湿困，故肢体困重；湿热蕴结，熏蒸肝胆，胆汁外溢肌肤眼目，则见面目皮肤发黄；湿遏热伏，热处湿中，湿热郁蒸，故身热起伏，汗出热不解；湿热蕴脾，交阻下迫，故见大便溏泄不爽，小便色黄；舌红、苔黄腻、脉濡数或滑数均为湿热内盛之征。

【治法】清热化湿，健脾和胃。

【代表方剂】三仁汤。

Spleen fails to control the blood

Syndrome: nosebleed, gum bleeding, muscle bleeding, hematochezia, hematuria, or hypermenorrhea, metrorrhagia and metrostaxis, little intake and sloppy stool, weak breath and no desire to speak, lassitude of spirit and lack of strength, pale complexion, pale tongue and thin weak pulse.

Syndrome differentiation: it is often caused by prolonged illness, or overexertion damaging spleen-qi. Nosebleed, gum and muscle bleeding are the results of blood spilling out the vessels or over the skin; hematochezia occurs when blood flows into the stomach and intestine; hematuria turns up when blood flows into the bladder; hypermenorrhea, metrorrhagia and metrostaxis occur owing to spleen deficiency failing to control the blood and unconsolidation of chong and conception channels; and little intake and sloppy stool, weak breath and no desire to speak, lassitude of spirit and lack of strength, pale complexion, pale tongue and thin weak pulse are all signs of spleen-qi deficiency.

Method of treatment: tonify the spleen to control the blood.

Formula: Guipi Decoction.

Spleen-stomach dampness and cold

Syndrome: abdominal stuffiness and fullness or distending pain, little intake and sloppy stool, nausea and vomiting, tastelessness, heavy head and body, edema, scant urine, profuse leukorrhagia, pale and enlarged tongue with white slimy fur and soggy pulse.

Syndrome differentiation: it is often caused by improper diet, or intake of too much cold and raw food, or exposure to rain, or living in moist place or constitutional excessive internal dampness in the body. The spleen belongs to greater yin earth, prefers dryness and dislikes dampness. Abdominal stuffiness and fullness, or even distending pain, little intake and sloppy stool, nausea and vomiting and tastelessness occur as the result of internal invasion of cold-dampness obstructing spleen-yang and leading to disturbance in ascending and descending of the spleen; heavy head and body is the result of heavy and turbid dampness obstructing yang qi as the spleen governs limbs; edema and scant urine arise from dampness overflowing in the skin as cold-dampness encumbers spleen-yang and prevents it to warm and transport water and dampness; profuse leukorrhagia comes when the cold-dampness pours downward to the low energizer; and pale and enlarged tongue with white slimy fur, and soggy pulse are all signs of overabundance of cold-dampness.

Method of treatment: warm the middle energizer to resolve dampness.

Formula: Yinchen Zhu Fu Decoction.

Spleen and stomach dampness-heat

Syndrome: abdominal stuffiness and fullness, torpid intake and vomiting and nausea, heavy limbs and body, yellow complexion, or fever which can not be relieved with sweating, sloppy stool, yellow urine, red tongue with yellow slimy fur, and soggy rapid pulse or slippery rapid pulse.

Syndrome differentiation: it is often caused by intake of too much greasy, sweat or strong-flavored food, which brings about dampness-heat in the spleen and stomach, or attack by the dampness-heat pathogens. Abdominal stuffiness and fullness, torpid intake and vomiting and nausea are due to dampness-heat in the spleen and stomach affecting their functions of receiving, transportation and transformation and leading to disturbance in ascending and descending; heavy limbs and body occurs as the heavy and turbid dampness encumbers the spleen; yellow complexion arises from dampness-heat affecting the liver and gallbladder and causing gall flowing over the skin and eyes; fever which cannot be relieved with sweating turns up because of mixing of dampness and heat depressed inward while struggling to evaporate outside; sloppy stool and yellow urine are the result of downward infusion of dampness-heat in the spleen; and red tongue with yellow slimy fur, and soggy rapid pulse or slippery rapid pulse are all the manifestations of excessive internal dampness-heat.

（七）胃火炽盛

【证候】胃脘灼痛，嘈杂吞酸，甚或食入即吐，消谷善饥，渴喜冷饮，或牙龈肿痛溃烂，齿衄，口臭，小便短赤，大便秘结，舌红，苔黄，脉滑数。

【辨证分析】本证多由情志不遂，肝气郁结，气郁化火，横逆侮土或邪热犯胃，或过食辛辣，化热生火所致。胃火内炽，胃腑络脉气血壅滞，故见胃脘灼热疼痛，肝经郁火横逆侮土，肝胃气火上逆，则嘈杂吞酸，甚或食入即吐；胃热炽盛，腐熟亢进，故消谷善饥；胃火灼伤津液，则渴喜冷饮；胃的经脉上络齿龈，胃热上蒸，故有口臭、齿龈肿痛或溃烂；热灼血络，迫血妄行，故见齿衄；大便秘结、小便短赤、舌红、苔黄、脉滑数皆为胃中热盛之征。

【治法】清胃泻火。

【代表方剂】清胃散。

（八）食滞胃脘

【证候】脘腹胀满，甚则疼痛，嗳气吞酸，或呕吐酸腐饮食，吐后胀痛得减，厌食，矢气酸臭，大便溏泄，泄下物酸腐臭秽，舌苔厚腻，脉滑。

【辨证分析】本证多由饮食不节，暴饮暴食，损伤脾胃，或脾胃素虚，食滞于胃脘，阻滞气机所致。食停胃脘，故见脘腹胀满，甚则疼痛；胃失和降而上逆，故见嗳气，胃中腐败谷物挟腐蚀之气上泛，则吞酸，或呕吐酸腐饮食，厌食；吐后食积减轻，故腹胀痛得减；若食积气滞，食浊下趋，积于肠道，则腹痛，腹泻，矢气酸臭，泻下物酸腐臭秽；苔厚腻、脉滑皆为食浊内阻之征。

【治法】健脾消食。

【代表方剂】保和丸。

第四节 肝与胆功能及其辨证

一、肝的功能

肝位于上腹部，五行属木，与胆相表里，与四时之春相应。

（一）肝主疏泄

肝主疏泄，是指肝具有疏通、舒畅、条达以保持全身气机疏通畅达，通而不滞，散而不郁的作用。肝的疏泄功能是以肝为刚脏，主升、主动、主散的生理特性为基础，其疏泄功能主要表现在五个方面：

调畅气机：肝的疏泄功能正常，则气机调畅，经络通利，脏腑器官的活动也就正常和调。肝的疏泄功能失常，一方面是肝的疏泄功能不足，即形成气机郁结的病证，

Method of treatment: clear heat and resolve dampness, fortify the spleen and harmonize the stomach.

Formula: San Ren Decoction.

Intense stomach fire

Syndrome: scorching stomachache, gastric upset and acid regurgitation, or even vomiting upon intake of food, swift digestion with rapid hungering, preference of cold drinks, gam pain and fester, gum bleeding, fetid mouth odor, scant and reddish urine, constipation, red tongue with yellow fur and slippery rapid pulse.

Syndrome differentiation: it is often caused by depressed mood leading to liver-qi depression and then stagnant qi transforming into fire to insult earth, or heat violating stomach, or intakes of too much spicy and hot food which is transformed into fire. Scorching stomachache occurs as the internal stomach fire flames to block the flow of qi and blood in the stomach vessels; gastric upset and acid regurgitation, or even vomiting upon intake of food turn up because stagnated fire ining liver meridians insulting earth and leading to upward movement of liver-stomach qi and fire; swift digestion with rapid hungering arises from effulgent stomach fire accelerating the decomposition of food; preference of cold drinks is the result of stomach fire scorching body fluids; fetid mouth odor and gum pain or fester result from stomach heat moving upward along the stomach meridians and collaterals which connect to the gum; and gum bleeding, scant and reddish urine, constipation, red tongue with yellow fur and slippery rapid pulse are all the manifestations of abundant stomach heat.

Method of treatment: clear the stomach to purge fire.

Formula: Qing Wei Powder.

Food stagnates in the stomach

Syndrome: abdominal fullness and distention and even pain, belching and acid regurgitation, or vomiting fetid and acid food, distending pain relieved after vomiting, anorexia, sour odor of flatus, sloppy and fetid stool, thick slimy fur, and slippery pulse.

Syndrome differentiation: it is often caused by improper diet especially overfeeding which damages the spleen and stomach, or constitutional spleen-stomach deficiency failing to digest the food stagnating in the stomach and then obstructing qi movement. Abdominal fullness and distention and even pain is the result of food stagnating in the stomach; belching indicates stomach ascending reversely rather than descending; acid regurgitation or vomiting fetid and acid food and anorexia turn up when undecomposed food moves upward with sour; distending pain relieved after vomit is because of food accumulated being reduced after vomiting; stomachache, diarrhea, fetid fecal qi and sloppy and fetid stool manifests food accumulation and qi stagnation leads to the food turbidity flowing downward to store in the intestine tract; and thick slimy fur, and slippery pulse are signs of the internal accumulation of turbid food.

Method of treatment: fortify the spleen to promote digestion.

Formula: Bao He Pill.

Section 4   Functions of the Liver and Gallbladder and their Syndrome Differentiation

Functions of the Liver

The liver locates in the upper abdomen, pertains to wood in the five phases, corresponds to spring in the four seasons and stands in interior-exterior relationship with the gallbladder.

Liver controls free coursing

Liver controlling free coursing means the liver has the function of ensuring the free movement of qi

出现胸肋、两乳或少腹等部位的胀满、疼痛等病症。另一方面是肝的疏泄功能太过，形成"肝气上逆"、"肝火上炎"等病证，出现头胀头痛，面红目赤，胸肋胀满，烦躁易怒等病症。

促进脾胃运化功能：肝的疏泄功能正常，全身气机疏通畅达，有助于脾升胃降和二者之间的协调以及脾胃对饮食物的消化、吸收。若肝的疏泄功能异常，影响脾的升清功能，在上则为眩晕，在下则为飧泄；影响胃的降浊功能，在上则为呕逆、嗳气，在中则为脘腹胀痛，在下则为便秘。

调畅情志：情志与肝的疏泄功能密切相关。肝的疏泄功能正常，气机调畅，则心情开朗；肝的疏泄功能减退，肝气郁结，则心情易于抑郁；肝的疏泄太过，阳气升腾而上则心情易急躁、发怒；若持久的情志异常，亦可影响肝的疏泄功能，导致肝气郁结，或疏泄不足的病证。

调节水液代谢：三焦为水液代谢的通道。肝主疏泄，能通过调节三焦的气机调节水液代谢。肝的疏泄正常，气机调畅，则三焦气治，水道通利；若肝失疏泄，三焦气机阻滞，气滞则水停，从而导致痰、饮、水肿等证。

（二）肝藏血

肝藏血，是指肝脏具有贮藏血液、防止出血和调节血量的功能。当人体处于安静状态时，部分血液就回流到肝脏并贮藏起来；当人体处于活动状态时，肝内的血液又被动员出来，运送到全身，供给各组织器官的需要。所以《素问·五脏生成篇》说："人卧血归于肝。"王冰注："肝藏血，心行之，人动则血运于诸经，人静则血归于肝脏。"若肝的藏血功能失常，不仅会引起血虚或出血，而且也能引起机体许多部分的血液濡养不足的病变。如肝血不足，不能濡养于目，则两目干涩昏花；不能濡养于筋，则见筋脉拘急，机体麻木，屈伸不利等。另外，肝不藏血还可发生血液妄行之证，如吐血、衄血、月经过多、崩漏等。

（三）肝的连属关系

1. 在志为怒　肝在志为怒，是指肝的功能与精神情志活动的"怒"有关。正常情况下，一般情绪的波动，不会导致人体发病。但若突然大怒，或经常发怒，则使肝主疏泄的功能失常，即所谓"怒伤肝"；而肝的阴血不足，阴不制阳，肝阳亢逆，则又急躁易怒。

2. 在液为泪　五脏六腑的精气、血脉皆注于目，目与肝脏有内在联系。即所谓"肝开窍于目"。所以肝的功能正常与否，常常表现在目的病变上。泪从目出，肝开窍于目，故泪为肝之液。泪有濡养、滋润和保护眼睛的功能。

3. 在体合筋，其华在爪　在五脏中，肝与筋关系最为密切。全身筋膜有赖于肝血的滋养。如肝血充盛、筋膜滋养充分，肢体活动正常；若肝血不足，血不养筋，

and preventing qi stagnation, also known as soothing. As unyielding viscus the liver is characterized by rising, moving and dispersing. The function of liver in smoothing is primarily embodied in five aspects as follows:

Smoothing and regulating qi movement: the normal function of the liver in smoothing will promote qi movement and harmonize the internal organs. Dysfunction of the liver's soothing includes two aspects: one is insufficient soothing, which leads to qi stagnation manifesting distention and fullness and pain of chest and hypochondrium, breasts and lower abdomen; the other is excessive soothing, which leads to liver-qi ascending counterflow and liver fire flaming upward manifesting headache and fullness of head, red face and hot eyes, distention and fullness in chest and hypochondrium, and agitation and aptness to be angry.

Promoting transportation and transformation of the spleen and stomach: the normal function of the liver in smoothing can ensure the fluent qi movement and conduce to the coordination between spleen upbearing and stomach downbearing to promote digesting and absorbing of food. Dysfunction of the liver will affect spleen's function of upbearing the clear, which gives rise to dizziness up and diarrhea down; and also affect the stomach's function of downbearing the turbid, which manifests vomiting and belching up, abdominal fullness, and distention in the middle and constipation down.

Regulating and smoothing emotions: emotions are closely related with the free coursing function of the liver. The normal function of the liver in free course can soothe qi movement and lead to happiness in mood. Hypofunction of the liver in smoothing will lead to liver-qi stagnation and depression in mood. And hyperactivity of the liver in smoothing will result in yang rising and agitation and anger in mood. Prolonged abnormal emotions also affect the free coursing function of the liver and lead to liver-qi stagnation syndrome.

Regulating water and fluid metabolization: the normal function of the liver in free coursing can adjust metabolization of water and fluid by regulating qi movement of the triple energizer. The normal smoothing function of the liver will contribute to free qi movement in the triple energizer. And failure of the liver in free course will leads to qi stagnation in the triple energizer and water retention, which finally results in the syndromes of phlegm, retained fluid and edema.

Liver stores blood

Liver storing blood refers to the function of the liver in depoting blood, preventing bleeding and regulating blood volume. When people are in rest, some of blood will flow back to the liver for storing; and when people do exercise, blood stored in the liver will be mobilized to spread around the body and cater for the needs of all the organs, as set forth in *Plain Questions* "blood flows back to be stored in the liver when prople are in rest," and annotated by Wang Bing, " blood is stored up in the liver when people are rest and circulates to supply all the meridians under the promotion and mobilization of heart when people are dynamic." Dysfunction of the liver in storing blood will lead to such pathological changes like blood deficiency, bleeding and blood failing to nourish the body. Blood deficiency will lead to dry and dim-sighted eyes as the result of blood failing to nourish the eyes; and contracture of sinews, numb and inflexible limbs as the result of blood failing to nourish the sinews. Still, failure of the liver in storing blood also results in frenetic movement of blood such as hematemesis, nosebleed, profuse menstruation, metrorrhagia and metrostaxis.

Affiliation of Liver

1. Liver associates with anger in the emotion

Liver associating with anger in emotion means the function of the liver is influenced by the motion of anger. In general case, anger cannot lead to disease. Only rage or frequent anger can lead to dysfunction of the liver, also known as "raging damages liver." Blood deficiency of the liver will lead to yin failing to constrain yang and liver-yang being hyperactive, which is apt to cause agitation and anger.

则可见手足震颤、肢体麻木、伸屈不利。爪，即爪甲，乃筋之延续，故称"爪为筋之余"。肝血充盛，则爪甲红润，坚韧明亮；肝血不足，则爪甲软薄，色泽枯槁，甚则变形、脆裂。

4. 开窍于目 中医认为目所以能视物，有赖于肝气之疏泄和肝血的濡养。故说"肝开窍于目"。如肝阴不足，见两目干涩；肝血不足，见夜盲、视物不清；肝经风热，见目赤肿痛；肝火上炎，见目赤生翳；肝阳上亢，见头晕目眩；肝风内动，见双目斜视、上吊等。

二、胆的功能

胆与肝之间有经脉相互络属，互为表里。胆的功能是：

（一）贮存和排泄胆汁

胆汁由肝分泌，进入胆腑贮藏、浓缩，并通过胆排入小肠，促进饮食物的消化和吸收。故《东医宝鉴》说"肝之余气，泄于胆，聚而成精"。《灵枢·本输》记载："胆者中精之腑。"

贮藏于胆腑的胆汁，由于肝的疏泄作用，使之排泄，注入肠中，以促进饮食物的消化。肝的疏泄功能正常，有助于胆汁的正常排泄。若肝失疏泄，肝气郁结，则胆汁排泄不利，从而出现胸胁胀满疼痛、食欲不振、厌食油腻、腹胀、便溏等症。

（二）主决断

决断是指胆在精神意识活动过程中具有判断、决定的作用。胆主决断对于防御和消除某些精神刺激的不良影响，以维持和控制气血的正常运行，确保脏器之间的协调关系有着重要的作用。因此《素问·灵兰秘典论篇》说："胆者，中正之官，决断出焉"。胆附于肝，肝胆相为表里，胆能助肝之疏泄以调畅情志。肝胆相济，则情志和调稳定。

三、肝与胆病的辨证

（一）肝气郁结

【证候】胸胁或少腹胀闷窜痛，胸闷，喜太息，情志抑郁或易怒，或咽有梗塞感，或颈部瘿瘤，或有癥瘕痞块，妇人见乳房胀痛，痛经，月经不调，甚至闭经，舌质紫或有瘀斑，脉沉弦涩。

【辨证分析】本证多因情志不遂，肝郁气滞，疏泄失常所致。情志不遂，肝失疏泄，气机郁滞，故见胸胁少腹胀闷窜痛；肝气不舒，则精神抑郁易怒、胸闷、善太息；气郁生痰，痰随气逆，痰气互结于喉，故咽喉有梗塞感；痰气积聚于颈项则为瘿瘤；肝郁日久不愈，气病及血，气滞血瘀，则成癥瘕痞块；肝气郁结，气血不畅，

2. Liver associates with tears in humor

Essence, qi, and blood of all the viscera and bowels flow upward to nourish the eyes, and the eyes have an internal connection with the liver, known as "liver opens at the eyes." So the function of the liver can be reflected from the eyes. Tears flows out from eyes, and eyes are the external orifice of the liver, so tears is the fluid of the liver, which can nourish, moisten and protect the eyes.

3. Liver links with sinews, with its luster manifesting on the nails

The liver has the closest relation with sinews among all the five viscera, as all the sinews are nourished by liver blood. With abundant liver blood, the sinews will be well-nourished and the body and limbs can move flexibly. Deficiency of liver blood leads to de-nourishment of sinews with the symptoms of trembling hands and feet, numb and inflexible limbs. The nails are the ends of the sinews, known as the "nails are associated with the sinews." Red, lustrous, bright and tenacious nails indicates sufficient liver blood; while withered, soft and thin nails or even deformed and cracked nails indicate deficiency of liver blood.

4. Liver opens at the eyes

TCM regards that the eyes can see because it is nourished by liver qi and blood, as said the "liver opens at the eyes." Liver-yin deficiency leads to dry eyes; liver blood deficiency brings about night blindness and invisibility; liver meridian wind-heat results in hot and pain eyes; liver fire flaming upward causes hot eyes with nebula; ascendant hyperactivity of liver yang causes light-headedness; and internal stirring of liver wind results in eyes looking awry or upward.

Functions of the Gallbladder

The gallbladder stands in exterior-interior relationship with the liver, as there are meridians and collaterals linking with both of them. The functions of gallbladder are as follows:

Gallbladder Stores and Discharges Bile

Bile, secreted by the liver and stored in and concentrated by the gallbladder, is discharged to the small intestine to help digest and absorb foodstuff, as described in Dong Yi Bao Jian "residual qi of the liver is discharged in the gallbladder and then concentrated to be essence" and recorded in *Miraculous Pivot* " the gallbladder is the bowel storing refined bile."

The bile stored in the gallbladder is discharged to the small intestine through free coursing function of the liver to promote the digestion of foodstuff. The normal soothing of liver is conducive to normal excretion of the bile, but dysfunction of the liver in soothing or liver-qi stagnation will lead to fullness and distention and pain in the chest and hypochondrium, poor appetite, dislike of greasy food, abdominal distention and sloppy stool as the result of inhibited excretion of the bile.

Gallbladder controls the power of decision

Power of decision refers to the gallbladder's function in making judgment and decision during the mental activities. Gallbladder controlling the power of decision plays a significant role in defending and removing the bad effects caused by mental stimulation so as to maintain and control the normal circulation of qi and blood and secure the coordination among all the viscera, as depicted in *Plain Questions* "the gallbladder is the just judge making the correct decision." The gallbladder attached to the liver, standing in exterior-interior relationship with the liver, can help the liver in free coursing and regulating mood. The harmony between the liver and gallbladder can stabilize people's mental status.

Syndrome Differentiation of the Liver and Gallbladder

Liver-qi depression and stagnation

Syndrome: oppressive and scurrying pain in the chest and hypochondrium or lower abdomen, oppression in the chest, sighing, depression or petulance, sensation of obstruction in the throat, or goiter and

冲任失调，故有月经不调、经前乳房胀痛、痛经或闭经；舌质紫或有瘀斑，脉沉弦涩，皆为肝郁血瘀之征。

【治法】疏肝理气。

【代表方剂】柴胡疏肝散。

（二）肝火上炎

【证候】头晕胀痛，面红目赤、或双目肿痛，耳鸣耳聋，口苦口干，急躁易怒，失眠或多梦，胁肋灼痛，或吐血，衄血，便秘，尿黄，舌红，苔黄，脉弦数。

【辨证分析】本证多由情志不遂，肝郁化火，或过食肥甘厚味，或因外感火热之邪所致。肝火上攻于头，故见头晕胀痛、面红目赤、甚或双目肿痛；肝火循经上扰于耳，则耳鸣耳聋；挟胆气上逆，则口苦；津为火热所伤，则口干；肝火内盛，急躁易怒；火热内扰，神魂不安，故失眠多梦；火热内炽，气血壅滞肝络，使胁肋部灼热疼痛；火热迫血妄行，则吐血、衄血；便秘、尿黄、舌红、苔黄、脉弦数均为肝火内盛之征。

【治法】清肝泻火。

【代表方剂】泻青丸。

（三）肝血虚

【证候】面白无华，眩晕耳鸣，夜眠多梦，视物模糊，双目干涩，夜盲，肢体麻木，筋脉拘挛，爪甲不荣，月经量少或闭经，舌质淡，脉细。

【辨证分析】本证多因脾气亏虚，生化之源不足，或慢性疾病耗伤肝血，或失血过多所致。肝血不足，不能上荣于头面耳窍，故面白无华、眩晕耳鸣；血不足以安魂定志，故夜眠多梦；肝血不足，不能上注于目，目失所养，故视物模糊、双目干涩、夜盲；肝血亏虚，血不荣筋，故肢体麻木、筋脉拘挛、爪甲不荣；肝血不足，血海空虚，故经少经闭；血虚，则舌淡；脉失充盈，故见脉细。

【治法】养血柔肝。

【代表方剂】四物汤。

tumors in the neck, or abdominal mass and lump, distending pain in the breast, dysmenorrhea, menstrual irregularities, and even amenorrhea for the women patients, purple tongue with ecchymosis, and sunken, rough and string-like pulse.

Syndrome differentiation: it is often caused by depression leading to liver-qi stagnation and dysfunction of the liver in free coursing. Depression in the mood, liver qi stagnation and dysfunction of the liver in soothing lead to oppressive and scurrying pain in the chest and hypochondrium; constrained liver qi gives rise to depression or petulance, oppression in the chest and sighing; qi depression engendering phlegm which obstructs in the throat together with the stagnated qi brings about sensation of obstruction in the throat; coagulation of phlegm and stagnated qi in the neck causes goiter and tumors; abdominal mass and lump occurs because prolonged liver-qi stagnation affects blood circulation and leads to qi stagnation and blood stasis; menstrual irregularities, breast distention and pain before menstruation, and dysmenorrheal or amenorrhea occurs due to liver qi depression and stagnation, and disharmony of thoroughfare and conception vessels; purple tongue with ecchymosis and sunken, string-like and rough pulse are all the manifestations of liver depression and blood stasis.

Method of treatment: soothe the liver and regulate qi.

Formula: Chaihu Shugan Powder.

Liver fire flaming upward

Syndrome: dizziness, distending pain of head, red face and eyes, or swelling and sore eyes, tinnitus, deafness, bitter taste in the mouth and dry mouth, agitation and petulance, insomnia often with nightmares, scorching pain in hypochondrium and rib, hematemesis, nosebleed, constipation, yellow urine, red tongue with yellow fur, and string-like and rapid pulse.

Syndrome differentiation: it is often caused by bad mood leading to depressed liver-qi transforming into fire, or by intake of too much strong-flavored, sweat and greasy food, or by infection of external fire evils. Dizziness, distending pain of head, red face and eyes, or swelling and sore eyes occur due to liver fire attacking head upward; tinnitus and deafness are attributed to liver fire disturbing ears through the meridians; bitter taste in the mouth occurs because of liver fire ascending counterflow with gallbladder qi; dry mouth comes out as the result of body fluids being damaged by liver fire; agitation and petulance indicates excessive internal liver fire; insomnia often with nightmares is owed to fire-heat disturbing the mental status; scorching pain in hypochondrium and rib arises from intense fire-heat flaming inside and qi and blood obstructing liver vessels; hematemesis and nosebleed is the result of frenetic movement of blood due to fire and heat; and constipation, yellow urine, red tongue with yellow fur, and string-like and rapid pulse are all the manifestations of exuberant internal liver fire.

Method of treatment: clear and purge the liver fire.

Formula: Xie Qing Pill.

Liver blood deficiency

Syndrome: pale complexion, dizziness and tinnitus, insomnia and dreaminess, blurred vision, dry eyes, night blindness, numb limbs, spasm of sinews; lusterless nails, scant menstruation or amenorrhea, light-colored tongue and thin pulse.

Syndrome differentiation: it is often caused by deficiency of spleen-qi, insufficiency of the source of qi and blood's transportation and transformation, or consumption of liver blood by chronic diseases or by excessive hemorrhage. Pale complexion, dizziness and tinnitus arise from liver blood deficiency which fails to flow upward to nourish the head, face and ears; insomnia and dreaminess is due to insufficient blood failing to tranquilize mental spirit; blurred vision, dry eyes and night blindness occur because of deficient liver blood failing to flow upward to nourish the eyes; numb limbs, spasm of sinews, and lusterless nail results from liver blood deficiency failing to nourish the sinews; scant menstruation and amenorrhea is attributed

（四）肝阴虚

【证候】头晕耳鸣，两目干涩，视物模糊，面部烘热，胁肋隐痛，烦躁失眠，五心烦热，潮热盗汗，咽干口燥，舌红少津，脉弦细数。

【辨证分析】本证多由情志不遂，气郁化火，或慢性疾病、温热病等耗伤肝阴引起。肝阴不足，不能上滋头目，则头晕耳鸣、两目干涩、视物模糊；虚热上蒸，则面部烘热；肝之经脉循行两胁，肝阴不足，不能濡养肝络，故有胁肋隐痛；阴虚内热，热扰心神，故见烦躁、失眠；五心烦热、潮热盗汗、咽干口燥、舌红少津、脉细数，均为阴虚内热之征。

【治法】滋阴柔肝。

【代表方剂】一贯煎。

（五）肝阳上亢

【证候】眩晕耳鸣，头目胀痛，面红目赤，急躁易怒，头胀痛，口苦，咽干，小便黄，大便秘结，舌红，苔黄，脉弦数。

【辨证分析】本证多因恼怒焦虑，气郁化火，耗伤阴液，致肝肾阴虚，阴不制阳，水不涵木而发病。肝肾之阴不足，肝阳亢逆无制，气血上冲，则眩晕耳鸣、头目胀痛、面红目赤；肝阳失潜，肝失疏泄，气郁化火，故见急躁易怒；阴不制阳，阴虚阳亢，挟胆气上逆，故口苦；气火内郁，耗伤阴津，则见咽干、小便黄、大便秘结、舌红苔黄、脉弦数。

【治法】平肝潜阳。

【代表方剂】镇肝熄风汤。

（六）肝胆湿热

【证候】胁肋部胀痛灼热，或有痞块，口苦，腹胀，纳呆，呕恶；或见身目发黄，发热，阴囊湿疹，睾丸肿大热痛，外阴瘙痒，带下黄臭，小便色黄，大便不爽，舌红，苔黄腻，脉弦数。

【辨证分析】本证多由感受湿热之邪，或偏嗜肥甘厚腻，生湿生热，或脾胃失健，湿邪内生，郁久化热所致。湿热蕴结肝胆，疏泄失常，气机郁滞，故见胁肋胀痛灼热，气滞血瘀，可致胁下痞块；湿热熏蒸，胆气上泛则口苦；肝气郁滞，肝木横逆侮土，脾胃运化失司，升降失常，故有腹胀、纳呆、呕恶；湿热熏蒸，胆汁不循常道而外溢，则面目周身发黄、发热、小便色黄；肝脉绕阴器，湿热下注，则阴囊湿疹或睾丸肿痛，妇人则见外阴瘙痒、带下黄臭；湿热内蕴，则大便不爽；舌红、苔黄腻、脉弦数，均为湿热之象。

【治法】清肝利胆。

【代表方剂】龙胆泻肝汤。

to liver blood deficiency and vacuity of sea of blood; light-colored tongue indicates blood deficiency; and thin pulse manifests vessel is not fully infused with blood.

Method of treatment: nourish the blood and emolliate the liver.

Formula: Si Wu Decoction.

Liver yin deficiency

Syndrome: dizziness and tinnitus, dry eyes, blurred vision, baking face, dull pain in hypochondrium and rib, insomnia and agitation, vexing heat in chest, palms and soles, tidal heat and night sweating, dry mouth and throat, red tongue with little fluid, and string-like, thin and rapid pulse.

Syndrome differentiation: it is often caused by bad mood leading to qi depression and then transforming into fire, or consumption of liver yin by chronic diseases and warm diseases. Dizziness and tinnitus, dry eyes and blurred vision result from liver-yin deficiency which fails to flow up to nourish the head and eyes; baking face is due to upward steaming of deficiency-heat; dull pain in hypochondrium and rib is attributed to liver yin deficiency failing to nourish the liver meridians and collaterals running along the hypochondriums; agitation and insomnia are the result of yin deficiency with internal heat disturbing the heart spirit; and vexing heat in the chest, palms and soles, tidal heat and night sweat, dry mouth and throat, red tongue with little fluid, and string-like, thin and rapid pulse are all the manifestations of yin deficiency with internal heat.

Method of treatment: nourish yin and emolliate the liver

Formula: Yi Guan Decoction

Ascendant hyperactivity of liver yang

Syndrome: dizziness and tinnitus, distending pain in the head and eyes, red face and eyes, agitation and petulance, bitter taste in the mouth, dry throat, yellow urine, constipation, red tongue with yellow fur, and string-like and rapid pulse.

Syndrome differentiation: it is often caused by anger and anxiety leading to stagnant qi transforming into fire and then impairs yin fluid, resulting in liver-kidney yin deficiency. Dizziness, tinnitus, distending pain in the head and eyes, red face and eyes occur due to liver-kidney yin deficiency failing to restrain hyperactive ascending liver yang and leads to upward rushing of qi and blood; agitation and petulance because failure of subdual of liver yang transforming into fire; bitter taste in the mouth occurs because yin fails to restrain yang, which flows upward with gallbladder qi; and dry throat, yellow urine, constipation, red tongue with yellow fur, and string-like and rapid pulse all indicates internal qi and fire stagnation injuring body fluids.

Method of treatment: pacify the liver to subdue yang.

Formula: Zhengan Xifeng Decoction.

Liver-gallbladder dampness-heat

Syndrome: distending pain, scorching heat, or lump in hypochondrim, bitter taste in the mouth, abdominal distention, torpid intake, vomiting, or yellow eyes and skin, fever, eczema in scrotum, swelling and hot pain testis, pruritus in vulva, yellow and fetid leucorrhea, yellow urine, sticky stool, red tongue with yellow and slimy fur, and string-like and rapid pulse.

Syndrome differentiation: it is often caused by infection of dampness-heat; or by predilection of strong-flavored, sweat and greasy food which produces dampness and heat; or by dysfunction of the spleen and stomach in transportation and transformation which results in internal dampness and heat transformed from prolonged dampness stagnation. Distending pain and scorching heat in the hypochondrim occur because dampness-heat coagulating in the liver and gallbladder leads to dysfunction of the liver and gallbladder in free coursing and qi stagnation; lumps in the hypochondrium is owed to qi stagnation and blood stasis; bitter taste in the mouth results from dampness-heat steaming upward; abdominal distention, torpid in-

（七） 胆郁痰扰

【证候】头晕目眩，耳鸣，惊悸不宁，烦躁不安，失眠多梦，口苦，恶心呕吐，胸闷胁胀，舌红，苔黄腻，脉弦滑。

【辨证分析】本证多由情志不遂，疏泄失职，气郁化火，炼液成痰而引起。胆脉络头目入耳，痰热循经上扰，故头晕目眩、耳鸣；痰热内扰，胆气不宁，故见惊悸不宁、烦躁不安、失眠多梦；胆气上逆则口苦；胆热犯胃，胃气上逆，故恶心呕吐；胆气郁滞，见胸闷胁胀；舌红、苔黄腻、脉滑，均为痰热内蕴之象。

【治法】清热涤痰。

【代表方剂】温胆汤。

第五节 肾与膀胱功能及辨证

一、肾的功能

肾位于腰部脊柱两侧，左右各一，五行属水，与膀胱相表里，与四时之冬相应。

（一） 肾藏精，主生长、发育与生殖

精，又称精气。肾藏精，是指肾对精气具有贮存、封藏的作用。精是构成人体的基本物质，也是人体生长、发育、生殖及脏腑组织器官功能活动的物质基础。根据其来源分为：①先天之精：秉受于父母，是人体生育繁殖的基本物质，故称"肾为先天之本"；②后天之精：来源于后天水谷精微，由脾胃化生，是维持人体生命活动的物质基础。先天之精和后天之精二者是相互依存、互相促进和相辅相成的。先天之精必须有后天之精的供养才能不断充实，后天之精又必须有赖先天之精的活动才能化生。

肾精所化之气称为肾气，肾气能够促进人体的生长、发育和生殖。从幼年开始，肾的精气逐渐充盛；到青春期肾气逐渐充盈，性机能成熟；到了老年，精气渐衰，性机能和生殖能力也随之减退而至消失。肾之精气不足可见生长发育迟缓、生殖功能减退等。

take and vomiting turn up because liver qi stagnation drives liver wood to insult the spleen and stomach earth and deprive them from normal transportation and transforming, and lead to their abnormality in ascending and descending; yellow face, eyes and skin, fever and yellow urine result from dampness-heat forcing the bile to overflow; eczema in scrotum, swelling and hot pain testis, pruritus in vulva, yellow and fetid vaginal discharge occur due to dampness-heat downflowing into the lower energizer since the liver meridian circling the genital; sticky stool indicates internal dampness-heat; and red tongue with yellow fur and string-like and rapid pulse are all the manifestations of dampness-heat.

Method of treatment: clear and drain the liver and gallbladder.

Formula: Longdan Xiegan Decoction.

Depressed gallbladder with harassing phlegm

Syndrome: dizziness, tinnitus, fright palpitation, agitation, insomnia and dreaminess, bitter taste in the mouth, nausea and vomiting, oppression in the chest, distention in the hypochondrium, red tongue with yellow slimy fur, and string-like and slippery pulse.

Syndrome: it is often caused by bad mood leading to dysfunction of the liver in free coursing, and then qi depression transforming into fire and finally fire makes body fluids into phlegm. Dizziness and tinnitus occur because the phlegum heat disturbs the head and ears along the gallbladder meridian running into the ears via the head and eyes; fright palpitation, insomnia and dreaminess turns up as the result of phlegm heat disturbing gallbladder qi; bitter taste in the mouth indicates gallbladder qi ascending counterflow; nausea and vomiting results from gallbladder heat insulting the stomach to make stomach qi reversely flow upward; oppression in the chest and distention in the hypochondrium indicate gallbladder qi stagnation; and red tongue with yellow slimy fur and slippery pulse are all the manifestations of internal phlegm-heat.

Method of treatment: clear heat and dispel phlegm.

Formula: Wen Dan Decoction.

Section 5   Functions of the Kidney and Bladder and their Syndrome Differentiation

Functions of the Kidney

The kidney is a pair of organs located in lumbar region, pertaining to water in the five phases, corresponding to winter in the four seasons and standing in interior-exterior relationship with the bladder.

Kidney stores vital essence and promotes growth, development, and reproduction

Essence, also known as essential qi, is the fundamental substance of building up the physical structure as well as the material base of promoting growth, development and reproduction and functions of the internal organs. Kidney storing essence refers to the kidney's function of storing and repositing essential qi. Essence is divided into innate essence and acquired essence according to the origins they derive from. The former inherits from parents, the basic material for reproduction, also referred as "Kidney is the root of innate endowment." The latter originates from food and water essence transformed and generated by the spleen and stomach, the material base for maintaining life activities. The innate essence and acquired essence are inter-dependent, inter-promoting and inter-supplementary as the former depends on the supply of the later to be replenished, while the later relies on the activities of the former to be transformed.

Kidney qi transformed by kidney essence can promote the growth, development and reproduction of human body. It gradually grows from the infancy to be full at puberty with gamomorphism and then to be deficient at senility with sexual function and reproductive capability weakening and withering. Deficiency of kidney essential qi leads to retardation of growth and development and reduction of reproductive func-

（二）肾主水

肾主水，指肾具有主司全身水液代谢、维持水液平衡的功能。人体水液代谢主要与肺、脾和肾有关，同时也和肝主疏泄的功能有关，其中与水液代谢关系最密切的是肾的气化作用。正常情况下，水液通过胃的受纳、脾的转输、肺的输布，通过三焦将水液中清的部分运送到全身各脏腑，浊的部分化为汗与尿液排出体外，使体内水液代谢维持着相对的平衡。而这些功能的正常发挥，都有赖于肾的气化作用才能实现。肾不主水、气化失常，则见尿少、水肿，或尿频、遗尿等。

（三）肾主纳气

指肾具有摄纳肺吸入之气而调节呼吸的功能。虽然人体的呼吸功能由肺所主，但肾具有摄纳肺气、调节肺呼吸深度的作用。此即所谓"肺主呼气、肾主纳气"。肾主纳气的功能正常则气道通畅、呼吸匀调，深度适中；肾不纳气则吸气困难、呼多吸少、动则气喘等。

（四）肾的连属关系

1. 在志为恐　肾在志为恐，是指肾的功能与精神情志活动的"恐"有关。恐为恐惧、害怕的精神状态，它对机体的生理活动产生不良的刺激。《素问·阴阳应象大论篇》中记载"恐伤肾"，《素问·举痛论篇》讲"恐则气下"，指突受惊恐可使肾气不固，气泄于下，见遗尿、滑精等症，甚至出现二便失禁。

2. 在液为唾　唾为口津，且为肾液，"五脏化液，……肾为唾"（《素问·宣明五气篇》）。唾液不仅润泽口腔，而且随食物下咽后能滋养肾中精气，故古代医家有主张"咽唾养精"者，方法是以舌抵上腭，唾溢则徐徐咽下，可养肾精。反之，多唾或久唾可伤肾精。

3. 在体为骨，主骨生髓、其华在发　肾藏精，精能生髓，髓藏于骨中，能充养骨骼。所以肾精充足，则骨髓的化生有源，骨骼得到滋养而坚强有力。肾中精气不足，不能生髓，可致骨软无力、小儿囟门迟闭、老人骨脆易折。齿为骨之余，也由肾中精气充养。肾精充足则牙齿坚固、质地致密；肾精不足则牙齿稀疏、松动易脱。

发赖血以滋养，故称"发为血之余"。肾精能化血，精血同源。精血充足，则发黑而健、润泽坚固；精血不足，则头发稀疏、枯槁脱落、须发早白等，所以肾其华在发。

4. 开窍于耳及二阴　肾开窍于耳，即肾之精气盛衰可反映于耳。耳的听觉功能依赖于肾之精气的充养，肾之精气充盈则听力灵敏；肾之精气不足则耳鸣耳聋、听力减退等。

二阴指前阴和后阴。前阴指尿道和外生殖器。尿液的贮留和排泄有赖于肾的气化功能完成。肾虚气化失常则小便不利；肾虚不固则见小便失禁或遗尿。后阴指肛门，大便的排泄也受肾气的影响与控制。肾阴不足失于濡润则大便秘结；肾阳不足则五更泄泻、下痢清谷；肾气不固则大便滑脱。

tion.

Kidney governs water

Kidney governing water refers to the kidney's function of regulating the general metabolism of water and maintaining the balance of fluids. Water metabolism of the body is related with the lung, spleen, kidney as well as the liver's soothing function. However, among all of them, the kidney plays the most important role in metabolizing water through its transformation. After received by the stomach, transformed and transported by the spleen and distributed by the lung, the water fluids is separated into clear and turbid, with the clear conveyed by the triple energizer to all over the internal organs and the turbid discharged in forms of sweat and urine. In this way, the water and fluids in the body can remain at a relative balance. However, the normal exertion of all these functions can be achieved only with the action of transformation of the kidney. Failure of the kidney in governing water and transformation will lead to scant urine and edema, or frequent urination and enuresis, etc.

Kidney governs qi absorption

It refers to the kidney's function of receiving and absorbing qi inhaled by the lung and then regulating respiration. The lung governs breathing, but the kidney governs the reception and absorption of qi and the regulation of respiratory depth, which is also termed as "the lung governs breathing qi and the kidney governs absorbing qi." The airway is free with smooth and moderate breathing ascribes to normal exertion of the kidney in absorbing qi. On the contrary, the failure of the kidney in absorbing qi will lead to inspiratory dyspnea, breathing out more than breathing in, and panting on exertion, etc.

Affiliation of the Kidney

1. Kidney associates with fear in emotion

It means the function of the kidney is influenced by the emotion of fear. Fear produces unfavorable stimulation on physiological activities, as described in *Plain Questions* "fear damages the kidney" and "fear leads to downward flowing of qi," which means sudden fear cause insecurity of kidney qi and qi discharging downside and therefore, results in enuresis, spermatorrhea and even urinary and fecal incontinence, etc.

2. Kidney associates with spittle in humor

Spittle is the thicker saliva and the humor of the kidney. It can not only moisten the mouth but also nourish the kidney qi after ingested with food, as put forth by ancient physicians "ingestion of spittle is able to nourish essence." The method is to place tip of tongue against the palate and then slowly ingest the overflowing spittle. While spitting spittle too much or for a long time will injury the kidney essence.

3. Kidney has a direct effect on the condition of the bone and marrow, and with its luster manifesting on the hair

The kidney stores essence and engenders marrow stored in the bone so as to fill and nourish bones. Sufficient kidney essence can transform and generate sufficient source of marrow to nourish and strengthen bones. Deficiency of essential qi for generating marrows leads to the weak bone lack of strength, retardation of fontanel closing and vulnerable bone inclined to be broken. The teeth, the sign of condition of the bone, are also nourished by kidney essential qi. Strong and compact teeth indicate kidney essence sufficiency, and sparse and flexible teeth indicate kidney essence deficiency.

The hair is nourished by the blood, termed as "the hair is the sign of condition of the blood." Kidney essence can be transformed into blood, so essence and blood share a common source. Black, healthy, bright and whippy hair indicates sufficiency of essence and blood; and sparse, dull, epilated and graying hair indicates deficiency of essence and blood, so it is said the condition of kidney can be reflected from the hair.

4. Kidney opens at the ears and two lower orifices

Kidney opening at the ears means that the condition of kidney essential qi can be reflected from the

二、膀胱的功能

膀胱与肾之间有经脉相互络属，互为表里。

津液经肾的气化作用生成尿液，下输于膀胱。尿液在膀胱内储留至一定程度时，通过肾的气化作用，使膀胱开合有度，则尿液可及时而自主地排出体外。如膀胱贮尿和排尿的功能失常，可见尿频、尿急、尿痛，或小便不利、尿少、尿闭，或尿失禁、遗尿等。

三、肾与膀胱病的辨证

（一）肾阳虚

【证候】腰膝酸软，畏寒肢冷，下肢为甚，面色黧黑，头晕耳鸣，男子阳痿，女子宫寒不孕，五更泄泻，完谷不化，或浮肿，腰以下为甚，按之凹陷不起，甚或腹部胀满，心悸咳喘，舌淡胖，脉沉弱。

【辨证分析】本证多由素体阳虚，或年高肾亏，或久病伤肾，以及房劳过度等因素引起。腰为肾之府，肾阳虚衰，不能温养腰府，则腰膝酸软；肾阳不能温煦肌肤，故畏寒肢冷，肾处下焦，阴寒盛于下，故畏寒肢冷下肢尤甚；肾水上泛，则面色黧黑；肾主骨生髓，肾阳不足、髓海空虚则头晕；肾开窍于耳，肾虚则耳鸣；肾主生殖，肾阳不足，命门火衰，生殖机能减退，男子则阳痿，女子则宫寒不孕。命门火衰，火不暖土，脾失健运，故见五更泄泻，完谷不化；肾阳不足，膀胱气化功能障碍，水液内停，溢于肌肤而为水肿；水湿下趋，故腰以下肿甚，按之凹陷不起；水势泛滥，阻滞气机，则腹部胀满；水气凌心，则心悸；水寒射肺，故见咳喘；舌淡胖、脉沉弱，为肾阳虚衰之象。

【治法】温补肾阳。

【代表方剂】金匮肾气丸。

ears.The ears depend on nourishment of kidney essential qi so that they can hear.Sufficiency of kidney essential qi leads to sensitive ears, and deficiency of kidney essential qi causes tinnitus and deafness, or hearing loss.

Two lower orifices refer to the frontal orifice, urethra and genitals; and the rear orifice, anus.Storing and discharge of urine is achieved with the transformation of the kidney.Kidney deficiency with abnormal transformation leads to difficult urination; and insecurity of kidney qi causes urinary incontinence or enuresis.In addition, discharge of feces is also affected and controlled by kidney qi.Kidney yin deficiency leads to constipation; kidney yang deficiency causes fifth-watch diarrhea (diarrhea occurring daily at dawn) and clear-food(undigested food diarrhea) ; and insecurity of kidney qi results in fecal incontinence.

Functions of the Bladder

The bladder stands in exterior-interior relationship with the kidney, as there are meridians and collaterals linking with both of them.The function of bladder is to store and discharge.

The body fluids are transformed into urine through transformation of the kidney and transmitted downward to the bladder, which is not discharged voluntarily outside until there is enough urine in the bladder. This is because the normal transformation of the kidney ensures the voluntary opening and closing of the bladder.Dysfunction of the bladder in storing and discharging urine brings about frequent urination, urgent urination, painful urination, or difficult urination, scant urine, anuresis, or uroclepsia and enuresis, etc.

Syndrome Differentiation of the Kidney and Bladder

Kidney-yang deficiency

Syndrome: aching and weak waist and knees, fear of cold and cold limbs especially legs, dark facial complexion, dizziness and tinnitus, erectile dysfunction of men, infertility of women due to cold uterus, fifth-watch diarrhea, undigested food in stool, edema particularly under the waist with deep dent when pressed, abdominal fullness and distention, palpitation, coughing and painting, light-colored tongue, and sunken weak pulse.

Syndrome differentiation: it is often caused by constitutional yang deficiency or kidney deficiency due to senility, or kidney injury due to prolonged illness or sexual overindulgence.The waist is as the abode of the kidney.Aching and weak waist and knees indicate kidney-yang deficiency failing to warm and nourish the waist; fear of cold and cold limbs indicate kidney-yang failing to warm the skin, and the colder legs is due to excessive cold yin arising from kidney yang deficiency accumulates in the lower energizer where the kidney is located; dark facial complexion indicates kidney water flooding upward; dizziness indicates kidney-yang deficiency failing to generate the marrow and replenish the sea of marrow; tinnitus indicates kidney deficiency as the kidney opens at the ears; erectile dysfunction of men and dysgenesis of women indicates life-gate fire deficiency(kidney-yang) leading to the hypofunction of reproduction; fifth-watch diarrhea and undigested food in stool indicate life-gate fire deficiency fails to warm the earth so that the spleen cannot transport and transform normally; edema indicates kidney-yang deficiency results in dysfunction of the bladder in transformation and then retained water-fluid overflows on the skin; edema especially under the waist with deep dent when pressed occurs because of dampness downward flow; abdominal fullness and distention indicates prevailing water obstructing qi movement; palpitation occurs due to water qi intimidating the heart; coughing and panting comes out due to cold water attacking the lung; and light-colored tongue and sunken weak pulse are the manifestations of kidney-yang deficiency.

Method of treatment: warm and tonify kidney-yang.

Formula: Jingui Shenqi Pill.

（二）肾气不固

【证候】腰膝酸软，耳鸣耳聋，神疲乏力，尿频清长，或尿后余沥不尽，或夜尿增多，小便失禁，男子滑精早泄，女子胎动易滑，白带清稀，舌淡，苔白，脉沉弱。

【辨证分析】多因年高肾气亏虚，或年幼肾气未充，或房事过度，或久病伤肾所致。腰为肾之府，肾主骨，开窍于耳，肾气亏虚，故腰膝酸软、耳鸣耳聋；肾气虚，固摄无权，膀胱失约，故小便清长而频数，尿后余沥不尽，或夜尿增多，甚则小便失禁；肾气不足，精关不固，精易外泄，故男子滑精早泄；肾虚而冲任亏损，下元不固，则女子胎动易滑、带下清稀；舌淡、苔白、脉沉弱，为肾气虚衰之象。

【治法】补肾固摄。

【代表方剂】五子衍宗丸。

（三）肾虚水泛

【证候】水肿，按之凹陷不起，腰以下尤甚，尿少，腰膝酸软，形寒肢冷，或心悸气短，喘咳痰鸣，舌淡胖嫩，苔白滑，脉沉细。

【辨证分析】本证多由素体虚弱，久病失调，肾阳虚衰不能温化水液，致水湿泛滥所致。肾主水，肾虚不能化气行水，水泛肌肤，则水肿、按之凹陷不起；肾处于下焦，水湿趋下，故腰以下肿甚；肾虚致膀胱气化无权，故尿少；腰为肾之府，肾虚则腰膝酸软；肾之阳气不足，失于温煦，则形寒肢冷；水气凌心则心悸气短；肾不纳气、水气射肺，则喘咳痰鸣；舌淡胖嫩、苔白滑、脉沉细，为肾之阳气不足的表现。

【治法】温肾助阳、化气行水。

【代表方剂】真武汤。

（四）肾阴虚

【证候】腰膝酸软，眩晕耳鸣，形体消瘦，口咽干燥，五心烦热，颧红盗汗，失眠多梦，男子遗精早泄，女子梦交，经少经闭，溲黄便干，舌红少津，脉细数。

【辨证分析】本证多由久病伤肾，或禀赋不足，房事过度，或急性热病，耗伤肾阴，或过服温燥劫阴之品所致。腰为肾之府，肾阴不足，骨骼失养，则腰膝酸软；肾能生髓，肾阴虚脑髓不足则眩晕；肾开窍于耳，肾阴虚则有耳鸣；阴虚形体失于濡养，则形体消瘦；阴虚生内热，故口咽干燥、五心烦热、颧红盗汗、溲黄便干；肾阴亏虚，水火失济，心火偏亢，致心神不宁，而见失眠多梦；相火妄动，则男子遗精早泄、女子梦交；女子以血为用，阴亏则经血来源不足，所以经量减少、甚至闭经；舌红少津、脉细数，为阴虚火旺的表现。

Insecurity of kidney-qi

Syndrome: aching and weak waist and knees, tinnitus and deafness, fatigue and lack of strength, frequent urination and clear and profuse urine, endless dripping urination, increase of nocturnal enuresis, urinary incontinence, spermatorrhea or premature ejaculation for men, habitual abortion for women, clear and thin leucorrhea, light-colored tongue with white fur, and sunken weak pulse.

Syndrome differentiation: it is often caused by kidney-qi deficiency due to senility or infant or sexual overindulgence, or kidney damage because of chronic diseases. Aching and weak waist and knees, tinnitus and deafness are the results of kidney qi deficiency because the waist is the abode of the kidney and the kidney governs the bones and opens at the ears; frequent urination and clear and profuse urine, endless dripping urination, increase of nocturnal enuresis and urinary incontinence indicate insecurity of kidney qi and unconstraint of the bladder due to kidney qi; spermatorrhea or premature ejaculation for men indicate kidney-qi deficiency fails to constrain the sperm from discharge; habitual abortion for women and clear and thin leucorrhea indicate kidney deficiency leading to deficiency and insecurity of thoroughfare and conception; and light-colored tongue with white fur and sunken weak pulse are signs of kidney-qi deficiency.

Method of treatment: tonify kidney to secure kidney qi.

Formula: Wuzi Yanzong Pill.

Kidney deficiency with water flood

Syndrome: edema particularly under the waist with deep dent when pressed, oliguria, aching and weak waist and knees, cold body and limbs, palpitation with shortness of breath, panting with phlegm rale, pale enlarged tongue with white slippery fur, and sunken thin pulse.

Syndrome differentiation: it is often caused by kidney-yang deficiency failing to warm and transform water fluid and then water flooding all over the body due to constitutional body weakness, or improper recuperation of chronic diseases. Edema with deep dent when pressed indicates kidney deficiency fails to transform and discharge water so that it overflows on the skin as the kidney governs water; edema particularly under the waist occurs as the kidney is located in the lower energizer and water dampness tends to flow downward; oliguria turns up as kidney deficiency results in the dysfunction of transformation of the bladder; aching and weak waist and knees is ascribe to "the waist is the abode of the kidney" and kidney deficiency; cold body and limbs occurs as the result of insufficient kidney yang failing to warm the body; palpitation arises from water qi intimidating the heart; coughing and panting with phlegm rale happens as the result of the kidney failing to absorbing qi and water qi attacking the lung; and pale enlarged tongue with white slippery fur and sunken thin pulse are signs of kidney-yang deficiency.

Method of treatment: warm the kidney and support yang to promote qi transformation and move water.

Formula: Zhenwu Decoction.

Kidney-yin deficiency

Syndrome: aching and weak waist and knees, dizziness and tinnitus, emaciation, dry mouth and throat, vexing heat in chest, palms and soles, red cheeks and night sweating, insomnia and dreaminess, spermatorrhea or premature ejaculation for men, dreaming of intercourse, scant menstruation or amenorrhea for women, yellow urine and dry stool, red tongue with little fluid, and thin rapid pulse.

Syndrome differentiation: it is often caused by chronic diseases damaging the kidney, or constitutional insufficiency, sexual overindulgence, or acute heat diseases or intake of too much warm and dry drugs or food injuring the kidney. Aching and weak waist and knees occurs due to kidney-yin deficiency failing to nourish the bones and the waist is the abode of the kidney; dizziness takes place as the result of kidney-yin deficiency failing to generate and replenish the brain marrow; tinnitus comes up due to kidney-yin deficiency and kidney opens at the ears; emaciation results from yin deficiency failing to nourish the body; dry mouth and throat, vexing heat in the chest, palms and soles, red cheeks and night sweat, yellow urine, and

【治法】补肾滋阴。

【代表方剂】六味地黄丸。

(五) 膀胱湿热

【证候】尿频尿急，尿涩而痛，小腹拘急胀痛，尿少黄赤、浑浊或有砂石，或尿血，或发热腰痛，舌红，苔黄腻，脉数。

【辨证分析】本证多由感受湿热，或饮食不节，湿热内生，下注膀胱所致。湿热蕴结膀胱，热迫尿道，故小便频急、排尿艰涩而痛、重者小腹拘急胀痛；湿热内蕴，膀胱气化失司，故尿液黄赤、浑浊；湿热久郁不解，煎熬尿中杂质而成砂石；热伤血络可见尿血；湿蕴郁蒸，热淫肌表，可见发热；波及肾脏，则见腰痛；舌红、苔黄腻、脉数，为湿热之象。

【治法】清利膀胱湿热。

【代表方剂】八正散。

第六节 脏腑之间的关系及其辨证

人体是一个有机的整体，必须从脏腑之间的相互关系上来研究整体的生命活动。这对于认识人体的生理功能、病理变化和辨证论治均具有重要意义。

一、脏腑之间的相互关系

1. **心与肺** 心主血而肺主气，心主行血而肺主呼吸。心和肺通过气与血的关系有机地联系在一起。血液的正常运行，必须依赖于心气的推动，亦有赖于肺气的辅助。肺朝百脉，助心行血，是血液正常运行的必要条件。心肺两脏互相配合才能完成气血的正常运行，维持机体各脏腑组织的新陈代谢。若肺气虚弱、宗气不足则推动心血无力、血运不畅，见心血瘀阻，出现胸闷、气短、心悸、唇青、舌紫等症；而心主血的功能减退则血液运行不畅，肺的宣降功能失调，症见咳嗽、喘息等。

2. **心与脾** 心与脾的关系，主要表现在血液生成方面的相互为用及血液运行方面的相互协同。一方面，心主一身之血，心血供养于脾以维持其正常的运化功能。脾健则血液化源充足、心血充盈；另一方面，血行脉中依赖心气的推动和脾气的统摄，心脾两脏互相配合保证血液的不断生成和正常运行。若脾虚化血不足则心血不足，脾不统血则出血；心血不足，脾失所养则脾气虚弱。最终形成心脾两虚，症见心悸健忘、失眠多梦、食少乏力、腹胀便溏、面色萎黄、眩晕、出血等。

dry stool indicate yin deficiency with internal heat; insomnia and dreaminess occur as kidney-yin deficiency fails to interact with the heart and leads to excessive heart fire disturbing the heart spirit; spermatorrhea or premature ejaculation for men and dreaming of intercourse for women are the results of frenetic stirring of the ministerial fire(fire of the liver and kidney); scant menstruation or even amenorrhea is owed to yin deficiency bringing about insufficient source of blood; and red tongue with little fluid and thin rapid pulse are signs of yin deficiency with effulgent fire.

Method of treatment: tonify the kidney and nourish yin.

Formula: Liu Wei Dihuang Pill.

Bladder dampness-heat

Syndrome: frequent and urgent urination, strangury, lower abdominal contracture and distending pain, scant reddish or turbid urine, urolithiasis or hematuria, or fever with lumbago, red tongue with yellow slimy fur and rapid pulse.

Syndrome differentiation: it is often caused by the attack of dampness-heat, or dampness-heat produced by the improper diet flowing downward to the bladder. Frequent and urgent urination, strangury, or lower abdominal contracture and distending pain occur as dampness-heat coagulates in the bladder and affects the urethra; scant reddish or turbid urine indicates the internal dampness-heat leads to dysfunction of transformation of the bladder; urolithiasis occurs as the dampness-heat boils impurities in the urine to be calculus; hematuria is the result of heat damaging vessels; fever takes place when dampness-heat invades skin and if it affects the kidney, then lumbago will emerge; and red tongue with yellow slimy fur and rapid pulse are signs of dampness-heat syndrome.

Method of treatment: clear away dampness-heat in the bladder.

Formula: Ba Zheng Powder.

Section 6 Relations among the Viscera and Bowels and Their Syndrome Differentiation

As an organic integrity, the life activities of human body must be studied through the interrelations of viscera and bowels, which has a significant meaning for understanding the physiological functions and pathological changes of the body and syndrome differentiation and treatment for diseases.

Relations among the Viscera and Bowels

The heart and lung

The heart governs blood and its circulation and the lung governs qi and respiration. The heart and lung are connected through qi and blood, as normal blood circulation must rely on the promotion of heart qi and assistance of lung qi. The lung connects all the vessels and assists the heart to circulate blood, so it is the prerequisite for blood circulation. Only when the heart and lung cooperate with each other, can they realize normal blood circulation and maintain the metabolism of all the internal organs. Deficiency of lung-qi and ancestral qi will lead to the heart blood stasis characterized by the symptoms of oppression in the chest, shortness of breath, palpitation, blue lips and purple tongue as they cannot promote the heart blood to circulate smoothly. Dysfunction of the heart in governing blood will lead to unsmooth blood circulation, and disorder of the lung in diffusing and depurative downbearing in company with the symptoms of coughing and panting, etc.

The heart and spleen

The interrelation between the heart and spleen lies in their coordination in generating and circulating blood. On one hand, the heart governs blood and provides blood for the spleen to maintain its functions of

3．心与肝 心与肝的关系主要表现在行血与藏血以及精神情志调节两个方面。在行血与藏血方面：心血充足，血脉充盈，肝有所藏，肝才能充分发挥其贮藏血液、调节血量的作用。而肝血充足，疏泄正常，气血通畅，有助于心主血脉。在精神情志调节方面：心肝两脏，相互为用，才能共同维持正常的精神情志活动。心、肝病变也都可表现为精神、心理活动的异常。如：肝阳上亢患者既可有头晕、目眩、烦躁易怒等肝病症状，又可兼有心悸、失眠等心病表现。

4．心与肾 心属火，肾属水。心与肾关系主要表现为"心肾相交"、"水火既济"。心位居上，心火（阳）必须下温于肾，使肾水不寒；肾位居下，肾水（阴）必须上济于心，使心火不亢。如此则心肾相交、水火既济。若肾水不足，心阳偏亢，上扰心神，会出现心悸、心烦、失眠等症；若心阳不振，心火不能下温肾水，可见腰膝酸软、遗精梦交；上凌于心，则会有心悸、水肿等症。

5．肺与脾 肺与脾的关系，主要表现在气的生成与水液代谢两个方面。在气的生成方面：肺吸入的自然界清气和脾化生的水谷之精气汇为宗气，宗气与元气再合为一身之气。在水液代谢方面，肺的宣发肃降和通调水道，使水液正常地输布与排泄，有助于脾的运化水液功能；而脾能转输津液，散精于肺，使水液正常地生成与输布，有助于肺的通调水道的功能。如果脾气虚损，会导致肺气不足，会出现疲乏倦怠，少气懒言等症。若脾虚运化失调，水湿内停，生成痰饮，也会影响肺的宣降功能，出现咳嗽、喘息等症，故有"脾为生痰之源，肺为贮痰之器"之说法。

transforming food essence into blood and transporting it to other organs. On the other hand, blood flowing in the vessels needs promotion of heart qi and governing of spleen qi. Only the cooperation and coordination of the heart and spleen can ensure the generation and circulation of blood. Spleen deficiency will lead to heart blood deficiency and bleeding as it can neither generate enough blood nor govern blood; and heart blood deficiency will lead to spleen-qi deficiency as heart blood fails to nourish the spleen. As a result, deficiency of both the heart and spleen will occur with the symptoms of palpitation, forgetfulness, insomnia and dreaminess, intake of little food and lack of strength, abdominal distention and sloppy stool, dull yellow facial complexion, dizziness, bleeding, etc.

The heart and liver

The interrelation between the heart and liver lies in promoting and storing blood and regulation of mental status. With regard to promoting and storing blood, the liver can exert its function of storing blood and regulating blood volume when there is sufficient heart blood flowing into the vessels. With sufficient liver blood, the liver can exert its function of free coursing and ensure smooth blood circulation and qi movement and therefore, help the heart govern blood vessels. As regards regulation of mental status, only when the liver and heart coordinate and cooperate with each other, can they maintain the normal mental activities. The pathological changes of the heart or liver can both present abnormalities of mental and psychological activities. Liver-yang flaming upward is often accompanied with the symptoms of liver diseases like dizziness, lightheadedness, agitation and petulance, and concurrently the symptoms of heart diseases such as palpitation and insomnia.

The heart and kidney

The heart corresponds with fire and the kidney corresponds with water in the five phases. The interrelation between the heart and kidney is embodied in "heart-kidney interaction" and "fire-water harmony." The heart located in the upper energizer shall drive heart fire(yang) to send downward to warm kidney and prevent the kidney water from being cold. While the kidney located in the lower energizer shall transmit water(yin) upward to replenish the heart and prevent hyperactive heart fire. Through the above-mentioned way, the heart-kidney interaction and fire-water harmony can be achieved. Kidney-water deficiency will lead to the symptoms of palpitation, vexation and insomnia as kidney-water fails to flow upward to constrain the effulgent heart fire from disturbing the heart spirit. Devitalized heart yang brings about the symptoms of aching and weak waist and knees, spermatorrhea and dreaming of intercourse as the heart fire fails to send downward to warm the kidney water. And kidney water intimidating the heart will result in palpitation, edema, etc.

The lung and spleen

The interrelation between the lung and spleen is primarily embodied in qi engendering and water metabolism. In regards to qi engendering, the clear air inhaled by the lung combines with the essential qi transformed from water and food by the spleen to form ancestral qi, which then mixes with original qi to compose the whole body qi. In terms of water metabolism, the lung distributes and discharges water through its function of diffusion, depurative downbearing and regulating the waterway, and therefore, helps the spleen to transport and transform water; while the spleen transports and diffuses the body fluids to the lung, and therefore, helps the lung to regulate the waterway. Spleen-qi deficiency leads to lung-qi deficiency characterized by fatigue and tiredness, weak breath, and no desire to speak. In addition, if spleen deficiency affects the spleen's function of transporting and transforming water and phlegm, it will affect the lung's function of diffusion and depurative downbearing, and therefore, lead to coughing and panting. So there is a statement that "the spleen is the source of phlegm formation and the lung is the receptacle that holds phlegm."

6. **肺与肝** 肺与肝的关系，主要体现在人体气机升降的调节方面。肺主肃降而肝主升发，肺气以肃降为顺，肝气以升发为宜。二者相互协调，对全身气机的调畅，气血的调和，起着重要的调节作用。如果肝升太过，或肺降不及，则会出现肝气上逆，表现为胁痛、易怒、咳逆、咯血等症，即所谓"肝火犯肺"。反之，如果肺失清肃，燥热内停，亦会导致肝失疏泄，气机郁结，出现咳嗽、胸胁胀满、头晕头痛等症。

7. **肺与肾** 肺与肾的关系，主要表现在水液代谢、呼吸运动两个方面。在水液代谢方面：肺气宣发肃降而行水的功能，有赖于肾气的促进；肾气所蒸化及升降的水液，有赖于肺气的肃降作用使之下归于肾或膀胱。在呼吸运动方面：人体的呼吸运动，虽由肺所主，但亦需肾的纳气功能协助，才能将吸入之气经肺的肃降下纳于肾，所以说："肺为气之主，肾为气之根。"肺气久虚，久病及肾，可致肾不纳气，出现气短喘息之症。

8. **肝与脾** 肝与脾的关系主要表现为疏泄与运化、藏血与统血之间的相互关系。肝主疏泄，调畅气机，协调脾胃升降，并疏利胆汁。肝主疏泄功能正常可促进脾的运化功能。脾气健旺，运化正常，水谷精微充足，气血生化有源，肝体得以濡养而使肝气冲和条达，有利于疏泄功能的发挥。肝主藏血，脾主生血、统血。肝血充足，疏泄正常，则脾气健运，生血、统血机能旺盛。而肝藏之血，又赖脾之化生，脾能生血、统血，则肝有所藏。肝血充足，方能根据人体生理活动的需要来调节血液。若肝失疏泄，影响脾胃功能，则可见抑郁、胸闷、腹胀、腹泻、便溏等肝脾不和之证。而脾失健运、水湿内停，日久蕴而化热，湿热郁蒸肝胆，则可形成黄疸。

9. **肝与肾** 肝肾之间的关系，有"肝肾同源"之称。肝藏血，肾藏精；精血皆由水谷之精化生和充养，且能相互资生，故曰肝肾同源（精血同源）。肝肾同源还表现在藏泄互用及肝肾阴阳之间的相互联系、相互制约，以保持着相对的平衡。肝气疏泄可使肾气闭藏而开合有度，肾气闭藏又可制约肝之疏泄太过，也可助其疏泄不及。另外，肝气由肝精肝血所化所养，可分为肝阴与肝阳；肾气由肾精化生，可分为肾阴与肾阳。它们在病理上也互相影响：一方不足可致另一方偏亢，如肾阴不足可致肝阴不足，导致肝阳偏亢；一方偏亢也可致另一方不足，如肝阳偏亢可下劫肾阴，致肾阴不足。同时，肾精亏损，可导致肝血不足；肝血不足，也常导致肾精的亏损，结果往往出现肝肾两虚的证候。

The lung and liver

The interrelation between the lung and liver is primarily presented at regulation of qi movement of ascending and descending. The lung governs depurative descending and the liver governs diffusing ascending. In this way, they cooperate and coordinate to regulate and harmonize the qi movements and blood circulation. Excessive ascending of the liver or deficient descending of the lung will both lead to liver-qi ascending counterflow characterized by pain in the hypochondrium, petulance, coughing and hemoptysis, also known as the"liver fire insulting the lung." On the contrary, the failure of the lung in depurative descending and ceasing of dryness-heat inward will lead to the failure of the liver in free coursing and qi stagnation characterized by fullness and distention in the chest and hypochondrium, dizziness, headache, etc.

The lung and kidney

The interrelation between the lung and kidney is primarily presented in water metabolism and respiratory movement. In respect of water metabolism, lung-qi function of distributing water based on its diffusing and depurative descending is promoted by kidney-qi; while the fluids processed by kidney-qi flows downward into the kidney or bladder relies on the lung's function of depurative descending. As for respiratory movement, though the lung governs respiration, the air inhaled by the lung can successfully descend to the kidney still required the kidney's coordination of absorbing qi, as stated"the lung is the governor of qi and the kidney is the root of qi." The prolonged lung-qi deficiency can affect the kidney and will lead to it incapable of absorbing qi, characterized by shortness of breath, panting, etc.

The liver and spleen

The interrelation between the liver and spleen is primarily presented in soothing and transportation and transformation, and storing blood and governing blood respectively. The liver governs free coursing and regulating qi movement to coordinate the ascending and descending of the spleen and stomach as well as to discharge the bile. So the normal performance of the liver's function of soothing can promote the spleen's function of transportation and transformation. With abundant spleen qi, the spleen can exert its normal function of transforming the food essence into blood to nourish the liver and harmonize liver-qi so that the liver can perform its function of free course. The liver governs storing of blood and the spleen governs generation and control of blood. With sufficient liver blood, the liver performs its function of soothing normally and with vigorous spleen-qi, the spleen performs its function of generation and control of blood. In addition, the blood stored in the liver is generated by the spleen, so only when the spleen generates enough blood, can the liver perform its function of storing blood. With enough liver blood, the liver can regulate the blood volume to cater for the need of human physiological activities. Dysfunction of the liver in free course will affect the functions of the spleen and stomach and lead to the syndrome of disharmony between the liver and spleen like depression, oppression in the chest, abdominal distention, diarrhea, and sloppy stool, etc. Failure of the spleen in transportation will bring about retained fluid, which is gradually transformed into dampness-heat and affects the liver and gallbladder to form jaundice.

The liver and kidney

The interrelation between the liver and kidney is explained by"the liver and kidney sharing the same source." The liver governs the storage of blood and the kidney governs the storage of essence. The liver and kidney shares the same source(also known as the essence and blood sharing the same source) as blood and essence are both generated and transformed from and nourished by food essence and can be mutually generated. Liver and kidney sharing the same source is also presented in mutual influence of storage and discharge, and mutual connection and restriction of the liver and kidney. In this way, they can maintain the relative balance between them. Free course of the liver qi can help closing and storage of the kidney, while the closing and storage of the kidney can restrict the liver from excessive soothing or inadequate soothing. In addition, liver-qi is transformed from and nourished by liver essence and liver blood, which can be fur-

10. 脾与肾 脾肾二者的关系首先是先后天相互滋养的关系。脾主运化水谷精微，化生气血，为后天之本；肾藏先天之精，是生命之本原，为先天之本。后天与先天，相互资生，相互促进。脾的运化功能需肾阳温煦，故有"脾阳根于肾阳"之说；肾之精气有赖水谷精微不断充养，才能保持充盛。另外，脾气运化水液功能的正常发挥，须赖肾气蒸化及肾阳温煦作用的支持。肾主水液输布代谢，又须赖脾气及脾阳的协助，即所谓"土能制水"。肾阳不足不能温旭脾阳，或脾阳久虚损及肾阳，终致脾肾阳虚，症见腹部冷痛、下痢清谷、五更泄泻、水肿等。

二、脏腑兼病辨证

凡两个以上脏腑相继或同时发病者，即为脏腑兼病。

（一）心脾两虚

心脾两虚证是指心血虚、脾气虚所表现的证候。

【证候】心悸健忘，失眠多梦，纳呆腹胀，乏力便溏，面色萎黄，皮下出血，月经量多色淡，崩漏，经少，闭经，舌淡，脉细弱。

【辨证分析】本证多由病久失调，或劳倦思虑过度，或慢性出血而致。心藏神，主神志，心血不足则心悸健忘、失眠多梦；脾主运化，脾虚运化失司则纳呆腹胀、便溏；脾虚运化不足，气血生化无源，气血亏虚则乏力、面色萎黄、月经量少、甚至闭经；脾主统血，脾虚统摄无权，血溢脉外，则皮下出血，女子可见月经量多色淡、甚或崩漏；舌淡、脉细弱，为气血不足的表现。

【治法】补益心脾。

【代表方剂】归脾汤。

（二）心肾不交

心肾不交证指心肾相交（水火既济）失调所表现的证候。

【证候】心烦失眠，心悸健忘，腰膝酸软，头晕耳鸣，遗精，潮热盗汗，溲黄便干，舌红，少苔，脉细数。

【辨证分析】本证多由五志化火，思虑过度，久病伤阴，或房事不节所致。心属火，肾属水，心火下温肾水使肾水不寒，而肾水又上滋心火使心火不亢，此即为心肾相交、水火既济。肾水不能上滋心火，使心火亢盛，火热扰心，心神不宁，则心烦失眠、心悸健忘；肾阴亏虚，骨髓不充，脑髓失养，则腰膝酸软、头晕耳鸣；阴虚内热，则有潮热盗汗、小便短黄，大便干燥；虚火内扰，精关不固，故见遗精；舌红、少苔、脉细数，为阴虚内热之象。

ther divided into liver yin and liver yang; while the kidney qi is engendered by kidney essence, which can be divided into kidney yin and kidney yang. They can affect each other pathologically: deficiency of one side leads to excess of the other side. For example, kidney-yin deficiency will lead to liver-yin deficiency and excessive liver-yang. On the contrary, excess of one side also cause deficiency of the other side. For instance, excessive liver-yang will consume kidney-yin and lead to kidney-yin deficiency. Meanwhile, insufficiency of kidney essence will lead to liver blood deficiency, which reversely results in deficiency of kidney essence. As a result, the deficiency of both the kidney and liver will occur.

The spleen and kidney

The interrelation between the spleen and kidney is primarily presented in innate endowment and the postnatal acquisition. The spleen governs transformation of food essence into qi and blood, known as the root of postnatal acquisition; and the kidney governs storage of innate essence, known as the root of innate endowment. The innate endowment and postnatal acquisition can be mutually generated, nourished and promoted. The spleen depends on the warming of kidney-yang to fulfill its function of transportation and transformation, so it is said that "the spleen yang roots in the kidney yang," while the kidney essential qi needs to be nourished and replenished by food essence. In addition, the spleen needs the evaporating of kidney qi and warming of kidney yang to exert its function of transporting and transforming water and fluids. The kidney also needs the coordination of spleen qi and spleen yang to exert its function of distributing and metabolizing water and fluids, which is called as "earth able to constrain water." Insufficient kidney yang failing to warm spleen yang or deficient spleen yang damaging kidney yang will finally lead to deficiency of spleen-kidney yang, characterized by abdominal cold pain, clear-food diarrhea, fifth-watch diarrhea and edema.

Combined Visceral Syndrome Differentiation

It refers to syndrome differentiation dealing with diseases in which two or more visceral organs are simultaneously involved.

Syndrome of dual deficiency of the heart and spleen

Syndrome of dual deficiency of the heart and spleen refers to the syndrome caused by heart blood deficiency and spleen qi deficiency.

Symptoms: palpitation, forgetfulness, insomnia and dreaminess, torpid intake and abdominal distention, lack of strength and sloppy stool, sallow complexion, subcutaneous bleeding, profuse and light-colored menstruation, metrorrhagia and metrostaxis, scant menstruation, amenorrhea, tastelessness, and thin weak pulse.

Syndrome differentiation: it is often caused by improper recuperation of chronic diseases, or excessive labor and thought, or chronic bleeding. Palpitation, forgetfulness, insomnia and dreaminess indicate heart blood deficiency as the heart stores spirit and governs mental status; torpid intake and abdominal distention and sloppy stool are owe to spleen deficiency depriving the spleen of exerting its function of transportation and transformation; lack of strength, swallow complexion, scant menstruation and amenorrhea occur due to spleen deficiency failing to fulfill its function of transportation and transformation of sufficient qi and blood; subcutaneous bleeding, profuse and light-colored menstruation, metrorrhagia, and metrostaxis are the results of spleen deficiency rendering spleen fail to control the blood flowing in the vessels; and tastelessness, and thin weak pulse are signs of deficiency of qi and blood.

Method of treatment: tonify the heart and spleen.

Formula: Guipi Decoction.

Non-interaction between the heart and kidney

It refers to a disorder of the normal relationship between the heart and kidney (interaction of water

【治法】滋阴降火、交通心肾。

【代表方剂】交泰丸。

（三）心肺气虚

心肺气虚证指心肺两脏气虚所表现的证候。

【证候】胸闷，心悸，咳喘，动则尤甚，咳痰清稀，乏力，气短，自汗，声低气怯，舌淡，苔薄白，脉沉细。

【辨证分析】本证多由久病咳喘，耗伤心肺之气，或禀赋不足，或年高体弱等因素引起。心气不足，不能养心，则胸闷心悸；肺主肃降，肺气虚肃降无权，气机上逆则咳喘，动则耗气，故咳喘尤甚；肺不能输布水液，停聚为痰，故痰液清稀；气虚则乏力、气短、自汗、声低气怯；舌淡苔薄白、脉沉细，为气虚之象。

【治法】补益心肺。

【代表方剂】升陷汤。

（四）肺脾气虚

肺脾气虚证指肺脾两脏气虚所表现的证候。

【证候】久咳不止，咳喘无力，痰多稀白，纳呆，腹胀，便溏，甚至面浮足肿，少气懒言，自汗乏力，舌淡，苔白，脉细弱。

【辨证分析】本证多由久病咳喘，肺虚及脾；或饮食，劳倦伤脾，脾虚不能散精于肺所致。肺气虚，肃降无权，气机上逆则咳喘，气虚则咳喘无力，且久咳不止；肺脾气虚，水津不布，聚湿生痰，故痰多稀白；脾气不足则纳呆、腹胀、便溏；少气懒言、自汗乏力；舌淡、苔白、脉细弱，为气虚之象。

【治法】补益脾肺。

【代表方剂】参苓白术散。

and fire).

Symptoms: vexation and insomnia, palpitation and forgetfulness, weak and feeble waist and knees, dizziness and tinnitus, spermatorrhea, tidal fever and night sweating, yellow urine and constipation, red tongue with little fur and thin rapid pulse.

Syndrome differentiation: it is often caused by transformation from the five minds into fire, excessive pensiveness, yin damaged by chronic disease or too frequent sexual intercourses. The heart pertains to fire, and the kidney pertains to water. The heart fire sends downward to warm the kidney water and prevent it being cold; and the kidney water flows upward to nourish the heart fire and prevent it from ascendant hyperactivity, which is termed as heart-kidney interaction or interaction of water and fire. Vexation and insomnia, palpitation and forgetfulness are ascribed to kidney water failing to flow upward to nourish heart fire, which is so effulgent to disturb the heart and heart spirit; weak and feeble waist and knees, dizziness and tinnitus are attributed to deficient kidney-yin failing to fill and nourish marrow; tidal fever and night sweating, yellow urine and constipation are the results of yin deficiency with internal heat; spermatorrhea results from deficiency-heat disturbing the security function of kidney; and red tongue with little fur and thin rapid pulse are all the signs of yin deficiency with internal heat.

Method of treatment: enrich yin to downbear fire, and coordinate the heart and kidney.

Formula: Jiao Tai Pill.

Heart-lung qi deficiency

It refers to the syndrome caused by heart qi deficiency and lung qi deficiency.

Symptoms: oppression in the chest, palpitation, coughing and painting which aggravate on exertion, coughing up clear and thin sputum, lack of strength, shortness of breath, spontaneous sweating, low voice and insufficient qi, pale tongue with thin white fur, and sunken thin pulse.

Syndrome differentiation: it is often caused by long-term coughing and panting injuring heart-lung qi, constitutional insufficiency, or weak constitution due to senility. Oppression in the chest and palpitation indicate deficient heart qi fails to nourish the hart; coughing and painting occur because the lung failing to depurative downbearing leads to qi flow upward rather than descending; aggravation of coughing and panting on exertion turns up as exertion impairs qi; clear and thin sputum indicates the lung fails to distribute fluids, which stops flowing and accumulates to be sputum; lack of strength, shortness of breath, spontaneous sweating, low voice and insufficient qi indicate qi deficiency; and pale tongue with thin white fur, and sunken thin pulse are the signs of qi deficiency.

Method of treatment: tonify the heart and lung.

Formula: Sheng Xian Decoction.

Lung-spleen qi deficiency

It refers to the syndrome caused by lung-qi deficiency and spleen-qi deficiency

Symptoms: continuous coughing, weak cough and panting, thin and white sputum, torpid intake, abdominal distention, sloppy stool, and even edema in face and feet, weak breath and no desire to speak, lack of strength and spontaneous sweating, pale tongue with white fur, and thin weak pulse.

Syndrome differentiation: it is often caused by continuous coughing or lung deficiency affecting the spleen, or the spleen damaged by improper diet or excessive labor, or deficient spleen failing to distribute essence to the lung. Continuous coughing and weak cough and panting occur as deficient lung qi deprives lung qi from depurative downbearing but to flow upward and finally leads to qi deficiency; thin and white sputum indicates lung-spleen qi deficiency failing to distribute fluids, which gathers to be sputum; torpid intake, abdominal distention and sloppy stool is owed to spleen-qi deficiency; weak breath and no desire to speak, lack of strength and spontaneous sweating, pale tongue with white fur, and thin weak pulse are the signs of qi deficiency.

（五）肝肾阴虚

肝肾阴虚证指肝肾两脏阴液亏虚所表现的证候。

【证候】头晕目眩，视物模糊，耳鸣耳聋，腰膝酸软，咽干胁痛，五心烦热，潮热盗汗，女子月经量少，男子遗精，舌红，少苔，脉细数。

【辨证分析】本证多由久病失调、房事不节、情志内伤等引起。肝肾阴虚，虚火上扰，则头晕目眩，肝开窍与目，肝阴不足，无以养目，则视物模糊；肾开窍于耳，肾阴不足，耳失所养，则耳鸣耳聋；腰为肾之府，肾虚则腰膝酸软；肝阴不足，肝脉失养，则胁痛；阴虚生内热，故咽干、五心烦热、潮热盗汗；冲任隶属肝肾，肝肾阴伤，则冲任空虚，而月经量少；肾主藏精，肾虚精关不固则遗精；舌红、少苔、脉细数为阴虚内热之象。

【治法】滋补肝肾。

【代表方剂】一贯煎。

（六）脾肾阳虚

脾肾阳虚证指脾肾两脏阳气亏虚所表现的证候。

【证候】面色㿠白，形寒肢冷，腰膝或少腹冷痛，下利清谷，或五更泄泻，尿少水肿，嫩舌淡，苔白滑，脉沉弱。

【辨证分析】本证多由久病、久泻或水邪久停，导致脾肾两脏阳气虚衰而成。阳气不足，不能温养形体，故见面色㿠白，形寒肢冷；腰为肾之府，肾阳虚则腰膝冷痛；阴寒内盛，气机凝滞，则少腹冷痛；脾肾阳虚，运化无权，则下痢清谷或五更泄泻；肾阳不足不能化气行水，则水肿尿少；水湿泛溢肌肤，则水肿；舌淡嫩、苔白滑、脉沉弱，为脾肾阳虚之象。

【治法】温补脾肾。

【代表方剂】实脾饮合四神丸。

（七）肝脾不调

肝脾不调证指肝失疏泄、脾失健运所表现的证候。

【证候】胸胁胀满或窜痛，喜太息，情志抑郁或急躁易怒，纳少，腹胀，便溏，或腹痛腹泻，泻后痛减，舌淡红，苔白，脉弦。

【辨证分析】本证常由情志不遂，郁怒伤肝，或饮食不节，劳倦伤脾，脾失健运所致。肝失疏泄，气郁气滞，则胸胁胀满或窜痛；肝失调达，故情志抑郁、喜太息；肝郁化火则急躁易怒；脾失健运，则纳少、腹胀、便溏；肝气乘脾，气机失调，清阳不升，则腹痛腹泻，排便后气滞得减，故泻后痛减；脉弦，为肝气郁

Method of treatment:tonify the spleen and lung.

Formula:Shen Ling Baizhu Powder.

Liver-kidney yin deficiency

It refers to the syndrome caused by liver-yin deficiency and kidney-yin deficiency.

Symptoms:dizziness, blurred vision, tinnitus and deafness, weak and feeble waist and knees, dry throat,pain in the hypochondrium,vexing heat in the chest,palms and soles,tidal fever and night sweating,scant menstruation;spermorrhea,red tongue with little fur,and thin rapid pulse.

Syndrome differentiation:it is often caused by improper recuperation of chronic diseases,too much sexual intercourses or internal injuries caused by emosions.Dizziness indicates liver-kidney yin deficiency and deficiency-fire disturbing the head;blurred vision occurs as the deficient liver yin cannot nourish the eyes;tinnitus and deafness turns up as deficient liver-yin fails to nourish the ears which link with the kidney;weak and feeble waist and knees indicates the deficiency of kidney,the abode of the waist;pain in the hypochondrium is ascribed to deficient liver-yin failing to nourshing the liver meridian;dry throat,vexing heat in the chest, palms and soles, tidal fever and night sweating indicate yin deficiency with internal heat;scant menstruation occurs as liver-yin deficiency leading to vacuity of thoroughfare and conception vessels affiliated to the liver;spermorrhea is the result of kidney failing to store essence due to its deficiency;and red tongue with little fur,and thin rapid pulse are signs of yin deficiency with internal heat.

Method of treatment:nourishi and tonify the liver and kidney.

Formula:Yi Guan Decoction.

Spleen-kidney yang deficiency

It refers to the syndrome caused by kidney-yang deficiency and spleen-yang deficiency.

Symptoms:bright pale complexion,cold body and limbs,cold pain in the waist and knees or in the lower abdomen, clear-food diarrhea, fifth-watch diarrhea, oliguria and edema, pale tender tongue with white slippery fur,and sunken weak pulse.

Syndrome differentiation:it is often caused by long-term illness like diarrhea, or water retention which leads to yang deficiency of the spleen and kidney.Bright pale complexion,cold body and limbs are due to insufficient yang failing to warm and nourish the body;cold pain in the waist and knees indicates kidney yang deficiency and waist is the abode of kidney;cold pain in the lower abdomen indicates excessive cold congealing and stagnating qi;clear-food diarrhea and fifth-watch diarrhea are attributed to the spleen failing to fulfill its function of transportation and transformation due to spleen-kidney yang deficiency;oliguria and edema indicate insufficient kidney yang failing to warm and transport water and leading to dampness flowing over the skin;and pale tender tongue with white slippery fur,and sunken weak pulse are the signs of spleen-kidney yang deficiency.

Method of treatment:warm and tonify the spleen and kidney.

Formula:Shi Pi Decoction combined with Si Shen Pill.

Liver depression and spleen deficiency

It refers to the syndrome caused by dysfunction of the liver in free coursing and failure of the spleen in transportation and transformation.

Symptoms:fullness and distention or scurrying pain in the chest and hypochondrium,sighing,depression or agitation and petulance,torpid intake,abdominal distention,sloppy stool,or abdominal pain and diarrhea with pain relieved after diarrhea,light-red tongue with white fur,and string-like pulse.

Syndrome differentiation:it is often caused by bad moods like depression and anger hurting the liver, or improper diet,or by excessive labor damaging the spleen resulting in its failure of transportation and transformation.Fullness and distention or scurrying pain in the chest and hypochondrium occurs due to the liver failing to soothing and leading to qi stagnation;depression and sighing are ascribed to the liver failing

结的表现。

【治法】疏肝健脾。

【代表方剂】逍遥散。

（田国庆　徐慧媛）

to exert its function of free coursing; agitation and petulance is the result of depressed liver qi transforming into fire; torpid intake, abdominal distention and sloppy stool indicate the spleen failing to transport and transform; abdominal pain and diarrhea result from depressed liver qi insulting the spleen and leading to inordinate qi movement like the spleen cannot upbear the clear yang; pain is relieved after diarrhea because qi stagnanion is reduced after defecation; light-red tongue with white fur, and string-like pulse are the signs of liver qi depression.

Method of treatment: soothe the liver and fortify the spleen.

Formula: Xiaoyao Powder.

(Wu Qunli   Zhang Wen)

第七章 防治原则与治疗方法

中医药学在长期的临床医疗实践过程中，积累了丰富的治疗经验，确立了临床治疗原则，创造了多种治疗方法，逐步形成了系统的中医治疗学。它包括了预防原则、治疗原则和治疗方法三个部分。预防原则体现了中医"治未病"的思想，包括了"未病先防"和"既病防变"两个方面。治疗原则是指导治疗方法的总的原则，治疗方法是治则的具体体现，任何具体的治法都是从属于治则的。"调节阴阳，以平为期"是中医治疗疾病的总的纲领；"治病求本"是中医治疗疾病的指导思想。在"治病求本"的思想指导下，审证求因，确定具体治疗原则，然后决定治疗方法。由于疾病的证候表现复杂多样，病变过程有轻重缓急；此外，不同时间、不同地点、个体差异对病情变化也会产生不同的影响。因此临床必须善于从复杂多变的疾病现象中，抓住病变的本质，根据邪正斗争所产生的虚实变化扶正祛邪；按脏腑、气血失调的病机调整脏腑功能、调理气血；按发病的不同的时间、地点和不同的病人，因时、因地、因人制宜。治疗方法一般归纳为汗、吐、下、和、温、清、补、消等八种方法，谓之"八法"。临床应用时在治则指导下可以使用一种治法，亦可以多种治法联合使用，以达到治疗疾病为目的。

第一节 预防原则

中医历来十分重视疾病的预防，早在《素问·四气调神大论》就有"圣人不治已病治未病，不治已乱治未乱，……夫病已成而后药之，乱已成而后治之，譬犹渴而穿井，斗而铸锥，不亦晚乎"的记载，体现了"治未病"的预防思想，强调"防患于未然"。所谓"治未病"包括未病先防和既病防变两个方面的内容。

一、未病先防

未病先防是指在疾病发生之前，充分调动人的主观能动性，增强体质，养护正

CHAPTER SEVEN   PREVENTIVE AND THERAPEUTIC PRINCIPLES AND METHODS OF TREATMENT

TCM has accumulated rich treatment experience, defined the clinical treatment principles, and created many treatment methods in the long course of clinical treatment practice, therefore, gradually forming systematic TCM therapeutics. It consists of preventive principles, treatment principles, and treatment methods. Preventive principles, the embodiment of TCM's philosophy of "preventive treatment of disease," include "prevention before disease onsets" and "preventing disease from exacerbating." Treatment principles refer to the general principles of treatment methods. Methods of treatment embody treatment principles, governing all the concrete therapeutic methods. "Regulating yin and yang until they meet balance" is the general principle of TCM in treating diseases. "Searching for the primary cause of disease in treatment" is the guiding ideology, under which doctors determine the etiologic factors based on differentiation, identify the concrete treatment principles and finally decide the treatment methods. Because the syndromes of diseases are diverse and complicated, their pathological changes can be minor or severe, slow or urgent, and the time, place and individual differences also have impacts on diseases, the doctors have to excel in finding and grasping the nature of diseases from the complicated symptoms, and then strengthen body resistance to eliminate pathogens in accordance of the excess and deficiency changes caused by the struggle of the healthy qi and pathogenic qi; regulate the functions of the internal organs and recuperate qi and blood according to their pathogenesis, and finally identify treatment methods suitable for the patients on the basis of where and when the disease occurs. Methods of treatment generally can be classified into eight methods, namely diaphoresis, emetic, purgation, mediation, warming, clearing, tonification, and elimination. To cure disease, doctors can clinically apply one or several methods simultaneously under the treatment principles.

Section 1   Preventive Principles

TCM attaches much importance to the prevention of disease. Dating back to several thousands of years, it was described in *Plain Questions* : "Wise man is always keen on performing the preventive treatment rather than treating the disease when it has already occurred··· To take treatment when the disease occurs, or to take measures when unrest takes place as if dig the well when one is thirsty, or to cast the weapons when the war almost starts. Isn't that too late?" which embodied the philosophy of prevention of disease and stressed "nip in the bud." Prevention of disease is composed of "prevention before disease onsets" and "preventing disease from exacerbating."

Prevention before Disease Onsets

Prevention before disease onsets means to fully mobilize people's subjective initiatives, invigorate health effectively, cultivate and maintain the healthy qi, raise the disease resistance, and adapt to the objective environments actively to avoid the invasion of pathogenic factors so as to prevent the occurrence of

气，提高机体抗病的能力，同时能动地适应客观环境，避免致病因素的侵袭，以防止疾病的发生。正如《素问·刺法论》所说："正气存内，邪不可干。"未病先防的措施主要有：

1. 调摄精神 做到"恬淡虚无，真气从之"，避免不良情绪的刺激，保持良好的心态。

2. 加强锻炼 增强体质，促进血脉流通，气机调畅；注重"形神合一"、"形动神静"，并应注意运动量要适度，要循序渐进、持之以恒。

3. 起居有节，劳逸适度 《素问·上古天真论》说："其知道者，法于阴阳，和于术数，饮食有节，起居有常，不妄作劳，故能形与神俱，而尽终其天年，度百岁乃去"。

4. 顺应自然 提高机体抗病的能力，同时还要注意防止病邪的侵袭，"虚邪贼风，避之有时"，"五疫之至，皆相染易"，应"避其毒气"。

5. 药物预防 我国很早就开始了药物预防的工作。16世纪的人痘接种预防天花，用苍术、雄黄等烟熏以消毒防病；贯众、板蓝根或大青叶预防流感；用茵陈、贯众等预防肝炎；用马齿苋等预防菌痢等。

二、既病防变

既病防变是指如果疾病已经发生，则应争取早期诊断，早期治疗以防止疾病的发展与传变。《素问·阴阳应象大论》说："故邪风之至，疾如风雨。故善治者治皮毛，其次治肌肤，其次治筋脉，其次治六腑，其次治五脏。治五脏者，半死半生也。"这说明外邪侵袭人体如果不及时诊治，病邪就有可能由表传里，步步深入，以致侵犯内脏。在防治疾病的过程中，一定要掌握疾病发生发展规律及其传变途径，做到早期诊断，有效地治疗才能防止其传变。根据疾病传变规律，先安未受邪之地。《难经·七十七难》说："上工治未病，中工治已病者，何谓也？然：所谓治未病者，见肝之病，则知肝当传之于脾，故先实其脾气，无令得受肝之邪。"肝属木，脾属土，肝木能乘脾，故临床上治疗肝病常配合健脾的方法，这是既病防变治则的具体应用。又如清代医家叶天士根据温热病易伤胃阴后进一步发展耗及肾阴，主张在甘寒养胃的方药中加入某些咸寒滋肾之品。

diseases, as depicted in *Plain Questions*: "with sufficiency of healthy qi inside, pathogenic factors have no way to invade the body." Here are the measures for preventing diseases:

1. Regulation of mental spirit

Avoid negative emotions and keep in good moods because "the genuine qi is generated when people live a plain and simple life with tranquil emotion."

2. Do more exercises

Invigorate health effectively through doing moderate exercises regularly to promote blood circulation and qi movement, with stress on "harmonization between soma and spirit" and "vigorous physique with tranquil mind."

3. Regular daily schedule with moderate labor and rest

According to *Plain Questions*, "those who know the natural law follow the principle of yin and yang and keep fit by living a regular life with moderate diet and labor. So they are able to acquire the harmonization between soma and spirit, and then fully live the natural span of their life."

4. Compliance with the natural rules

In order to raise the disease-resistance, people should also pay attention to preventing against the invasion of pathogenic factors by avoiding the evils in the nature.

5. Drug prophylaxis

In China, people began to prevent diseases with drugs in the very early time. In the 16th century, variolation was created to prevent smallpox, atractylodes lancea and realgar were burned for disinfection and preventing diseases; crytomium rhizome, radix isatidis and folium isatidis were used to prevent flu; virgate worm wood herb and crytomium rhizome were utilized to prevent hepatitis, and purslane was used o prevent bacillary dysentery, etc.

Preventing Disease from Exacerbating

Preventing disease from exacerbating means that early diagnosis and treatment should be taken to prevent the progress and aggravation of the already existing disease. According to *Plain Questions*, "the exogenic pathogens often invade from the exterior to the interior. At the beginning, they stay in and invade the skin and can be cured by expelling them from the skin; if they are not expelled at this stage, they will invade the muscles, then the meridians, then the six bowels and finally the five viscera. When they get to the interior and attack the five viscera, it is so serious that can affect people's lives." This indicates when the exogenic pathogens attack the body, if not cured promptly, it will turn from the exterior to the interior and even to affect the internal organs. In prevention and treatment of diseases, doctors should understand the occurrence and development principles of diseases and their transmission pathways, and then make early diagnosis and effective treatment to prevent exacerbating. In accordance with the regular pattern of invasion route, doctors should firstly protect and strengthen the organ that will be affected by the sick one, as represented in *Classic of Difficult Issues* : "the best doctors know to prevent diseases and the ordinary doctors just treat the existing diseases. For example, if there's something wrong with the liver, the best doctors will immediately be conscious that the spleen will be involved, so they meanwhile consolidate the spleen to prevent it being affected by the liver disease when they make treatment." According to the TCM theory, the liver corresponds to the wood and the spleen corresponds to the earth, so the liver wood can overwhelm the spleen earth. Clinically, doctors often fortify the spleen when treating the liver diseases, which is the application of preventing disease from exacerbating. Again, Ye Tianshi, a great physician of Qing Dynasty, advocated that the salty-cold kidney-enriching medicinals should be added into the sweat-cold prescription for nourishing the stomach because the warm-heat disease is apt to impair the stomach-yin and then further consume the kidney-yin.

第二节　治疗原则

一、调整阴阳（总纲）

疾病的发生，从根本上说就是阴阳的相对平衡遭到破坏，出现偏盛偏衰的结果。对于其治疗，《素问·至真要大论》指出："谨察阴阳所在而调之，以平为期。"因此调整阴阳，补偏救弊，恢复阴阳的相对平衡，促进阴平阳秘，是临床治疗的根本法则之一，也就是说是中医治疗疾病的总目标。

（一）损其所盛

《素问·阴阳应象大论》指出："阴胜则阳病，阳胜则阴病。"故对于阴阳偏盛应采用"损其有余"的治疗原则。如阳热亢盛的实热证，应"治热以寒"，即用"热者寒之"的方法以治其热盛；阴寒内盛的寒实证，则应"治寒以热"，即用"寒者热之"的方法以治其寒盛。

（二）补其不足

阴阳偏虚，或阴或阳的一方虚损不足，可致"阳虚则寒，阴虚则热"，应采用"补其不足"的治疗原则。如阴虚不能制阳，常表现为阴虚阳亢的虚热证，则应滋阴以制阳，"壮水之源，以制阳光"；因阳虚不能制阴而致阴寒偏盛应补阳以制阴，"益火之源，以消阴翳"。若阴阳两虚，则应阴阳双补。应当指出阴阳互根互用，故阴阳偏衰亦可互损。《景岳全书》中说："善补阳者必于阴中求阳，则阳得阴助而生化无穷；善补阴者必于阳中求阴，则阴得阳升而泉源不竭。"

二、治病求本（指导思想）

《素问·阴阳应象大论》曰："治病必求于本。"就是指治疗疾病要明确疾病的根本原因，针对其病因进行治疗。"治病求本"，"本"为疾病的根本，也就是发病的原因，疾病的发生、发展一般总是通过若干症状而显现出来，但这些症状只是疾病的现象，还不是疾病的本质。只有充分地收集、了解疾病的各个方面，包括症状在内的全部情况，在中医学基础理论的指导下，进行综合分析，才能透过现象看到本质，找出疾病的根本原因，从而确立恰当的治疗方法。比如头痛可由外感和内伤所引起。外感头痛又有风寒和风热之别：属于风寒，治宜辛温解表；属于风温，治当辛凉解表。而内伤头痛可由血虚、血瘀、痰湿、肝阳上亢等多种原因所致，故其治疗也应分别采用养血、活血、燥湿化痰、平肝潜阳等不同方法进行治疗。这就是"治病必求于本"。在治病求本思想的指导下，治则的基本内容包括正治与反治、治标与治

Section 2 Therapeutic Principle

Regulating Yin and Yang(General Principle)

Basically, the occurrence of diseases is owed to the breakdown of the relative balance between yin and yang, which leads to excess or deficiency of them. According to *Plain Question*, "doctors should find out in which part the imbalance of yin and yang occurs and then regulate it until they get balanced." So regulating yin and yang to reach their relative balance and keep them in equilibrium is one of the fundamental therapeutic principles and also the TCM's overall target of treating diseases.

Impairing the excess

Abnormal exuberance of yin or yang refers to the excess or hyperactivity of yin or yang, just as described in *Plain Questions* "predominance of yin leads to the disease of yang and predominance of yang results in the disease of yang." So the therapeutic principle of impairing the excessive one should be adopted. For instance, heat excess syndrome of hyperactivity of yang should be treated with cold drugs, while cold excess syndrome of hyperactivity of yin should be treated with hot drugs.

Complementing the deficiency

Abnormal debilitation of yin or yang refers to the deficiency of yin or yang. Deficiency of yang leads to cold, while deficiency of yin results in heat. So the therapeutic principle of complementing the deficient one should be adopted. Yin deficiency unable to restrain yang often leads to the deficient heat syndrome with yin deficiency and yang hyperactivity. In this case, doctors should adopt the methods of enriching yin to restrain yang. In case that deficient yang unable to restrain yin leads to cold yin exuberance, doctors should complement yang to control yin. In case of deficiency of both yin and yang, doctors should complement both of them. It is noticeable that as yin or yang are interdependent and mutually promoted, deficiency of either of them will injure the other, as specified in *Complete Works of Jingyue* "…those who excel in tonifying yang often applying nourishing yin together, so that yang can bring its function into full play with the help of yin; while those who are proficient in nourishing yin often applying tonifying yang meanwhile, so that yin can get refreshed with the help of yang."

Treating Disease Based on Its Root(Guiding Principle)

Plain Questions explicated "every treatment must be based on the root of disease," which definitely pointed out that, the first thing in disease treatment is to find out its primary cause, on the basis of which the treatment method should be made. Primary cause refers to the intrinsic reason of the occurrence of a disease, which can be finally found out through fully understanding all aspects of the disease, and comprehensively analyzing under the guidance of TCM theory all the data and symptoms. Finding out the intrinsic cause of a disease is the precondition of identifying the proper treatment method. For example, headache can be caused by exogenic pathogens, or internal injuries, with the former composed of wind cold and wind heat. Headache caused by wind cold should be treated by the method of relieving the exterior with pungent-warm, while headache caused by wind heat should be treated by the method of relieving the exterior with pungent-cool. Headache caused by the internal injuries including the causes of blood deficiency, blood stasis, damp phlegm, and liver-yang hyperactivity, should be treated by nourishing blood, activating blood, drying dampness to resolve phlegm, and pacifying the liver to subdue yang respectively. The above demonstrates the principle of "treating disease based on its root." Under the guidance of such principle, the therapeutic methods include routine treatment and paradoxical treatment, treating the root or tip, reinforcing the healthy qi and eliminating the pathogenic factors, adjusting the functions of viscera and bowels, regulation

本、扶正与祛邪、调整脏腑功能、调理气血、三因制宜等。

（一）正治与反治

《素问·至真要大论》提出"逆者正治，从者反治"两种方法，就其原则来说都是治病求本这一治疗原则的具体运用。其不同之处在于：正治适用于病变本质与其外在表现相一致的病证，而反治则适用于病变本质与临床征象不完全一致的病证。

1. 正治　是逆其证候性质而治的一种常用治疗原则，又称逆治。适用于疾病的现象与本质相一致的病证。如寒病见寒象、热病见热象、虚病见虚象、实病见实象等，采用与疾病的性质相反的方药进行治疗，如"寒者热之"、"热者寒之"、"虚则补之"、"实则泻之"等不同治疗方法。

2. 反治　是顺从疾病假象而治的一种治疗原则，又称从治。是指采用方药的性质顺从疾病的假象或与疾病的假象相一致而言，究其实质，还是在治病求本法则指导下，针对疾病根本而进行治疗的方法，故实质上仍是"治病求本"。主要有"热因热用"、"寒因寒用"、"塞因塞用"、"通因通用"等。

（1）"热因热用"：是以热治热，指用热性药物治疗具有假热症状的病证，适用于阴寒内盛、格阳于外、反见热象的真寒假热证，由于阳虚寒盛是其本质故仍用热药治其本质，而假热就自然会消失。

（2）"寒因寒用"：是以寒治寒，即用寒性药物治疗具有假寒症状的病证，适用于里热极盛、格阴于外、反见寒象的真热假寒证，因为热盛是其本质故须用寒凉药治其真热，而假寒方能消除。

（3）"塞因塞用"：是以补治塞，即用补益药治疗具有闭塞不通症状的病证，适用于因虚而闭阻的真虚假实证。例如脾虚病人常出现脘腹胀满时，用健脾益气的方法治疗；气虚血枯、冲任亏损引起的闭经，采用补气养血的方法治疗；老年人气虚便秘，采用补气以通便，这些治疗方法称为"塞因塞用"。

（4）"通因通用"：是以通治通，用通利的药物治疗具有实性通泄症状的病证。适用于食积腹泻、瘀血崩漏等病证。如食积导致的腹痛腹泻、瘀血引起的崩漏分别采用消导泻下、活血化瘀等方法治疗，这些方法称为通因通用。

（二）治标与治本

在复杂多变的病证中，常有标本主次的不同，因而在治疗上就应有先后缓急的区别。标本治法的临床应用，一般是"治病必求于本"。但在某些情况下，标病甚急，如不及时解决可危及患者生命或影响疾病的治疗，则应采取"急则治其标，缓则治其本"的法则，先治其标后治其本。若标本并重则应标本兼顾，标本兼治。

1. 急则治其标　是指标病甚急时可以采取急则治其标。如"鼓胀"的患者（相当于肝硬化、腹膜炎等引起的腹水）当腹水大量增加，出现腹部胀痛、呼吸喘急、

of qi and blood, and treatment in accordance with three specific factors.

Routine Treatment and Paradoxical Treatment

Plain Questions puts forward two methods of treatment, one is"routine treatment to treat the disease with medicines opposite in nature to the disease,"and the other is"paradoxical treatment to treat the disease with medicines similar in nature to the disease."Both of them are the application of the principle of treating disease based on its root, with the differences lies in the fact that routine treatment is applicable for the diseases whose nature of pathological change coincide with their manifestations, while paradoxical treatment is applicable for the diseases whose nature of pathological change are reverse to their clinical manifestations.

1. Routine treatment

It is a common therapeutic principle of using medicines opposite in nature to the disease, also known as reverse treatment.It is applicable for the diseases whose manifestations are in line with their natures, such as cold disease with cold symptoms, hot disease with heat symptoms, deficiency disease with deficiency symptoms, and excess disease with excess symptoms.It should be treated with medicines opposite in nature to the diseases, like"treating cold with heat,""treating heat with cold,""treating deficiency by tonification,"and"treating excess by purgation."

2. Paradoxical treatment

It is a therapeutic principle of treating a disease in compliance with its pseudomorphism, also termed as compliance treatment.It means to treat the disease with medicines whose nature are in compliance with or in coincidence with the pseudomorphism of the disease.But in principle and virtually, it is a therapeutic method of treating a disease based on its root under the guiding principle.It includes the methods of"treating heat with heat,""treating cold with cold,""treating the unstopped by unstopping,"and"treating the stopped by stopping."

Treating heat with heat: it refers to treating pseudo-heat symptoms with medicines warm or hot in nature.It is applicable for exuberant interior yin cold repelling yang exterior, which leads to true cold with false heat syndrome but with heat symptoms.Since it is essentially caused by yang deficiency and cold exuberance, heat medicals are used to treat its intrinsic cause to eliminate the false heat.

Treating cold with cold: it refers to treating pseudo-cold symptoms with medicines cool or cold in nature.It is applicable for exuberant interior heat repelling yin exterior, which leads to true heat with false cold syndrome but with clod symptoms.Since it is essentially caused by exuberant heat, cold medicals are used to treat its intrinsic cause to eliminate the false cold.

Treating the unstopped by unstopping: it refers to treating stopping conditions with tonics.It is applicable for true deficiency with false excess syndrome arising from obstruction due to deficiency.For example, the patients who suffering from abdominal fullness and distention due to spleen deficiency can be treated with the method of fortifying the spleen and replenishing qi.Those suffering from amenorrhea due to qi and blood deficiency and thoroughfare and conception vessels depletion can be treated with the method of tonifying qi and blood.The elderly have constipation due to qi deficiency are often treated with the method of tonifying qi to defecate.

Treating the stopped by stopping: it refers to treating the unstopped conditions with purgative medicals.It is applicable for abdominal pain and diarrhea caused by food stagnation, and metrorrhagia and metrostaxis caused by blood stasis.They can be treated with methods of promoting digestion and purgation, and activating blood and resolving stasis respectively.

Treat the Root and Treat the Tip

In the complex diseases, there are differences of root and tip or primary and secondary, so the treatments should be distinguished in order of urgency.Generally, doctors should treat a disease based on its

大小便不利的时候，应先治标病的水湿，当用利水、逐水法，待腹水减轻病情稳定后，再调理肝脾治其本病。又如大出血病，无论属于何种出血，均应采取应急措施先止血以治标，待血止病情缓和，再治本病。

2. 缓则治其本　对慢性病或急性病恢复期有重要指导意义。如肺痨咳嗽，其本多为肺肾阴虚，故治疗不应用一般的止咳法治其标，而应滋养肺肾之阴治其本。又如慢性咳喘，在缓解期，要以健脾补肾为主治疗，以除痰之源、固喘之根。

3. 标本同治　是指标病本病俱急，则应标本兼治，以提高疗效。如临床表现有身热、腹硬满痛、大便燥结、口干渴、舌苔焦黄，此属邪热内结、阴液受伤，为标本俱急的临床表现，治当标本兼顾，可用增液承气汤泻下与滋阴同用，泻其实热可以存阴，滋阴润燥则有利于通便，标本同治可收相辅相成之功。

（三）病治异同

所谓病治异同包括了"同病异治"和"异病同治"。临床治疗时必须遵循治病求本的原则，注意疾病的发生和发展及病机的变化以及疾病演变的阶段性，正确应用"同病异治"和"异病同治"的治疗原则。

1. 同病异治　是指同一种疾病，由于病邪的性质不同、个体反应性的差异，其病机和疾病的性质也不同，所以要根据辨证，给予不同的治疗方法。如同为感冒，病因有风寒、风热的不同，治疗就有辛温解表和辛凉解表之区别。

2. 异病同治　是指不同的疾病在发展的过程中可以看到同一性质的证候，可以采用相同的治疗方法。如久痢、久泻、脱肛、崩漏、子宫脱垂、胃下垂等几种不同的疾病，只要根据辨证属于中气下陷者，均可采用补脾升提的方法，用补中益气汤进行治疗。

root clinically.But in some cases,when the tip symptoms are so serious and acute that the principle of "treating the acute tip before the chronic root" should be applied,because the tip will affect the life of the patient or the treatment of the disease if it is not removed in time.If the tip is as serious as the root,then the consideration and treatment should be focused on both of them.

1. Treating the tip if it is urgent

It means in retreating an acute disease,doctors should resolve the symptoms first.For example,when the patient of tympanites(equal to ascites caused by liver cirrhosis or peritonitis)presents the symptoms of abdomenal distending pain,tachypnea and panting,and difficulty in defecation and urine,which is due to the mass increase of ascites,doctors should first treat the tip water and dampness through the method of draining or expelling water until the symptoms of ascites are alleviated before treating the root by regulating the liver and spleen.In case of occurrence of massive hemorrhoea,emergency measures should be taken immediately to stop bleeding,then the primary cause should be treated.

2. Treating the root if it is chronic

It has an important guiding significance for treating chronic disease and recovering from acute disease.For instance,the root of cough caused by tuberculosis is often ascribed to lung and kidney yin deficiency,so the treatment should be focused on enriching and nourishing the lung and kidney yin to treat its root rather than on suppressing cough.During the paracmasis of chronic cough and panting,the treatment should be concentrated on fortifying the spleen and tonifying the kidney to eliminate the phlegm from its generating source and to strengthen the function of absorbing qi of the kidney.

3. Treating both the root and the tip

It means when the root and tip are equally urgent,both of them should be treated to raise the curative effect.For instance,when treating a disease with the symptoms of fever,abdominal fullness and pain,constipation,dryness and thirst and dry yellow fur,which is the result of internal coagulation of pathogenic heat(the tip)and deficiency of body fluids(the root),methods of purgation and nourishing yin should be used simultaneously to cure it,because relieving the excessive heat can preserve yin and nourishing yin can moisten the dryness of the intestine and make smooth defecation.Zengye Chengqi Decoction can be adopted for this case.Treating both the root and the tip can supplement with each other.

Different Treatments for Different Diseases

It includes "different treatments for the same disease" and "same treatment for different diseases." When putting it into clinical practice,the principle of treating a disease based on its root must be obeyed. Doctors should pay attention to the changes of occurrence,development,pathogenesis and status of the disease for correct application of this therapeutic principle.

1. Different treatments for the same disease

It means on the basis of syndrome differentiation,different therapeutic methods are adopted and verified in accordance with the different nature and pathogenesis of the same disease as well as the different reactions of individuals.For example,different therapeutic methods are used to treat the common cold: method of releasing the exterior with pungent-warm is used to treat the cold caused by wind cold,while method of releasing the exterior with pungent-cool is used to treat the cold caused by wind heat.

2. Same treatment for different diseases

It means the same therapeutic method can be adopted into different diseases as long as they have the same nature during the course of development.For example,the method of tonifying the spleen to upraise the middle qi can be used to treat prolonged dysentery and diarrhea,rectocele,metrorrhagia and metrostaxis,prolapse of the uterus and stomach because they all belong to the sunken middle(spleen)qi syndrome. Buzhong Yiqi Decoction can be prescribed in this case.

（四）扶正与祛邪

疾病的演变过程，从邪正关系来说是正气与邪气双方互相斗争的过程，邪正斗争的胜负，决定着疾病的转归和预后。邪胜于正则病进，正胜于邪则病愈。通过扶正祛邪，改变邪正双方力量的对比，使其有利于疾病向痊愈方向转化。所以扶正祛邪是指导临床治疗的一个重要法则。

所谓扶正即扶助正气，提高机体的抗病能力。扶正多用"虚则补之"治法，包括药物、针灸、气功、体育锻炼及精神饮食调理等。所谓祛邪，即是祛除病邪，使邪去而正安。祛邪多用"实则泻之"的治法，临床疾病由于邪气的不同、部位的各异，其治法亦不一样，包括消食导滞、活血化瘀、除痰祛湿、软坚散结、利水消肿等。扶正与祛邪，虽然不同，但两者相互为用、相辅相成。运用扶正祛邪原则时要认真细致地观察和分析正邪双方消长盛衰，并根据正邪在矛盾斗争中的地位，决定扶正与祛邪的先后和主次。总之需权衡利弊，以"扶正而不留邪，祛邪而不伤正"为其原则。

1. 扶正　适用于以正气虚为主要矛盾，而邪气不盛的虚性病证。如气虚、血虚、阴虚、阳虚的病人，分别采用补气、养血、滋阴、壮阳的方法进行治疗。

2. 祛邪　适用于以邪实为主要矛盾，而正气未伤的实性病证，如血瘀、食积、痰郁、气滞、水肿等病证，分别采用活血化瘀、消食导滞、除痰祛湿、疏理气机、利水消肿等方法。

3. 扶正与祛邪兼用　适用于正虚邪实病证，而且两者同时兼用。但在具体应用还要分清以正虚为主还是以邪实为主。正虚较急较重者，应以扶正为主，兼顾祛邪；而邪实较急重，则以祛邪为主，兼顾扶正。

（五）调和脏腑

人体是一个有机整体，脏与脏、脏与腑、腑与腑之间在生理上是相互协调、相互为用，在病理上也相互影响。故在治疗脏病时，不能单纯考虑一个脏腑，而应注意调整各脏腑之间的关系。如肝的疏泄功能失常时，不仅肝脏本身出现病变，而且常影响到脾的运化功能而出现脘腹胀满、不思饮食、腹痛腹泻等症，也可影响肺气的宣发肃降而见喘咳，还可影响心神而见烦躁不安或抑郁不乐，影响心血的运行而见胸部疼痛。因此，五脏之中，一脏有病，可影响他脏。

Reinforcing the Healthy Qi and Eliminating the Pathogenic Factors

The development of a disease is the process of the struggle between the healthy qi and the pathogenic factors, and the result decides the prognosis of the disease. The disease will aggravate if the pathogenic factors defeat the healthy qi. On the contrary, the disease will recover if the healthy qi overcomes the pathogenic factors. The methods of reinforcing the healthy qi or eliminating the pathogenic factors aim to raise the healthy qi and weaken the pathogenic factors and therefore gradually get rid of disease. So they are the important therapeutic principles of guiding the clinical treatment.

Reinforcing the healthy qi can strengthen the body resistance. The method of "treating deficiency by tonification" is often used in this case, which covers drugs, acupuncture and moxibustion, qigong, physical exercises, and regulation of spirit and diets. Eliminating the pathogenic factors can insure the normal functions of the healthy qi. The method of "treating excess by purgation" is often adopted in this case, which includes such specific methods as promoting digestion and removing food stagnation, activating blood and resolving stasis, dispelling phlegm and eliminating dampness, softening hardness and dissipating binds, and inducing dieresis to alleviate edema, according to the different pathogens and locations of the diseases. Reinforcing the healthy qi and eliminating the pathogenic factors are interdependent and supplemented with each other. Careful observation and analysis of exuberance or debilitation in the healthy qi and the pathogenic factors should be made before applying this principle. Then the priority order of reinforcing the healthy qi and eliminating the pathogenic factors can be determined in line with their status in the struggling between the healthy qi and the pathogenic factors. In any case, doctors should weigh the pros and cons and abide by the principle of "reinforcing the healthy qi to totally remove the pathogens, and eliminating the pathogenic factors without injuring the healthy qi."

1. Reinforcing the healthy qi is applicable for such deficiency syndromes as qi deficiency, blood deficiency, yin deficiency, and yang deficiency, all of which are characterized by the healthy qi deficiency gives priority to the non-excessive pathogenic factors. So tonifying qi, nourishing blood, enriching yin, and invigorating yang can be applied to treat them respectively.

2. Eliminating the pathogenic factors is applicable for such the excess syndromes as blood stasis, food accumulation, phlegm stagnation, qi stagnation, and edema, all of which are characterized by excessive pathogenic factors gives priority to the uninjured healthy qi. So activating blood and resolving blood stasis, promoting digestion and removing food stagnation, dispelling phlegm and eliminating dampness, soothing qi movement, and inducing dieresis to alleviate edema can be used to treat them respectively.

3. Combination of reinforcing the healthy qi and eliminating the pathogenic factors is applicable for the syndrome of healthy qi deficiency and pathogenic factors excess. But the application of this method varies with the predominance of them. The focus should be put on reingforcing the healthy qi along with eliminating the pathogenic factors in case of acute and serious deficiency of the healthy qi; while in case of acute and serious excess of the pathogenic factors, the concentration should be put on eliminating the pathogenic factors along with reinforcing the healthy qi.

Harmonizing the Viscera and Bowels

Human body is an organic integrity, with the viscera and bowels coordinating with and depending on one another physiologically and affecting one another pathologically. So the treatment should not only be focused on the sick organ, but meanwhile on regulation of the relations among all the organs. For example, when the liver dysfunctions in free coursing, it can affect the function of the spleen in transportation and transformation and lead to abdominal fullness and distention, no appetite, stomachache and diarrhea; also affect the function of the lung in diffusing and depurative downbearing and lead to cough and panting; and affect the heart spirit and lead to dysphoria and depression as well as affect the heart blood circulation and lead to chest pain. It indicates that the illness of any organ can influence another one in the five viscera.

（六）调理气血

气血是各脏腑功能活动的主要物质基础。气血各有其功能，又相互为用。在生理上气能生血、气能行血、气能摄血，故称"气为血帅"。而血能为气的活动提供物质基础，血能载气、血能养气，故称"血为气母"。当气血相互为用及相互促进的关系失常时，就会出现各种气血失调病证。调理气血关系的原则为"有余泻之，不足补之"，从而促使气血关系恢复协调。

1. 气虚生血不足而致血虚者，宜补气为主、辅以补血，或气血双补。

2. 气虚行血无力而致血瘀者，宜补气为主，辅以活血化瘀。

3. 气滞致血瘀者，行气为主，辅以活血化瘀。

4. 气虚不能摄血者，补气为主，辅以收涩止血。

5. 血虚不足以养气，可致气虚，宜补血为主，辅以益气。

6. 气随血脱者，因"有形之血不能速生，无形之气所当急固"，故应先益气固脱以止血，待病势缓和后再进补血之品。

（七）三因制宜

三因制宜即因时制宜、因地制宜、因人制宜。疾病的发生、发展与转归是由多方面因素决定的，如时令气候、地理环境以及患者性别、年龄、体质等因素都会对疾病产生影响。因此在治疗疾病时必须考虑这些因素，因时、因地、因人制宜，实现治疗的个体化。

1. 因时制宜　是指根据不同季节气候特点来考虑治疗用药的原则。如春夏季节气候温热，人体腠理疏松，即使患外感风寒，也不宜过用辛温发散，以免开泄太过耗伤气阴；而秋冬季节，气候寒凉，人体腠理致密，阳气内敛，此时若非大热之证，当慎用寒凉药物，以防伤阳。如春季多风温、夏季多暑热、长夏多湿热、秋季多燥病、冬季多风寒，故春季要祛风清热，暑天要解暑化湿，秋天则宜辛凉润肺，冬季风寒应辛温解表。

2. 因地制宜　是指根据不同地域的地理特点来考虑治疗用药的原则。如我国西北高原地区，气候寒冷干燥少雨，病多寒多燥，治宜辛润，寒凉之剂必须慎用；东南地低气温高多雨，病多温热或湿热，治宜清化，温热及助湿之剂必须慎用。如同样是外感风寒，需要辛温解表，西北严寒地区常用麻黄、桂枝、细辛；东南温热地区多用荆芥、防风、苏叶。

3. 因人制宜　是指根据病人年龄、性别、体质、生活习惯等不同特点来考虑治疗用药的原则。如成人用药量较大，小儿用药量宜小；老年人脏腑机能减退，气血亏损，患病多虚证，或虚实夹杂，治疗多用补法，挟实者攻邪宜慎；小儿生机旺盛，但气血未充，脏腑娇嫩，易寒易热，易虚易实，病情变化较快，故治小儿忌投峻攻，

Regulation of Qi and Blood

Qi and blood are the primary material bases for the functional activities of the viscera and bowels. They are interdependent with each other and have the independent functions of their own.Physiologically, qi can generate, promote and govern blood, so it is called as the commander of blood; while blood provides material base for qi's activity and blood can carry and nourish qi, so blood is regarded as the mother of qi. A variety of syndromes caused by disorder of qi and blood will emerge when the normal relations between qi and blood is broken.The principle of"discharging the excess and tonifying the deficiency"should be followed by regulating qi and blood so as to recuperate the harmony of them.

1. Blood deficiency due to qi deficiency failing to generate blood should be treated mainly with the method of tonifying qi with supplement of tonifying blood, or tonifying both of them at the same time.

2. Blood stasis due to qi deficiency failing to promote blood circulation should be treated mainly with the method of tonifying qi with supplement of activating blood and resolving stasis.

3. Blood stasis due to stagnant qi failing to promote blood circulation should be treated mainly with the method of moving qi with supplement of activating blood and resolving stasis.

4. Qi deficiency failing to governing blood should be treated with the method of tonifying qi with supplement of inducing astringency to stop bleeding.

5. Qi deficiency due to blood deficiency failing to nourish qi should be treated mainly with the method of tonifying blood with supplement of tonifying qi.

6. Qi collapse following bleeding should be treated with tonifying qi to stop bleeding first and then follow with tonifying blood until the patient's condition is alleviated.This because the tangible blood cannot be generated in short time, while the qi collape is so serious and urgent that the intangible qi must be securing immediately.

Treatment in Accordance with Three Specific Factors

It refers to treatment in accordance with the time when a disease occurs, treatment in accordance with the place where a disease occurs and treatment in accordance with the situation of the patient.The occurrence, development and prognosis of a disease is determined by many aspects, such as seasonal climate, geographical environment, and the gender, age and constitution of the patient, all of which have impacts on the disease.So in treating diseases, all of these factors should be taken into account so as to realize the individualized treatment.

1. Treatment in accordance with the time

It refers to application of treatment methods and drugs on the basis of characteristics of different seasonal climates.For example, in warm spring and in hot summer, pungent-warming exterior-releasing medicinals should not be overused even if the patient suffering from external wind cold because the interstices are loose then, which can avoid excessive consuming of qi and yin from excessive diaphoresis.While in cool autumn and in cold winter, medicinals in cool and cold nature should be used with caution unless the patient suffering from the excessive heat syndrome because the interstices are compact and yang qi should be restrained inside then, so as not to impair yang.Wind warm often occurs in spring, summerheat often happens in summer, damp-heat often takes place in late summer, dryness often turns up in autumn, and wind cold often comes up in winter; so method of dispelling wind and clearing heat is used in spring, method of relieving summerheat and resolving dampness is used in summer, the method of moistening the lung with pungent-cool medicinals is applied in autumn, and method of pungent-warming exterior-releasing medicinals is adopted to wind cold in winter respectively.

2. Treatment in accordance with the place

It refers to application of treatment methods and drugs on the basis of geographical characteristics of different regions.In the northwest of China, the plateau region, where it is cold and dry with little rain and

少用补药。妇女病、带、胎、产等情况治疗用药应加以考虑。如在妊娠期，对峻下、破血、滑利、走窜伤胎或有毒药物当禁用或慎用。产后应考虑气血亏虚及恶露情况等等。再者体质的强弱，阴阳的盛衰，都应予以重视。

第三节　治疗方法

中医学的治疗方法一般归纳为汗、吐、下、和、温、清、补、消等八种治疗方法。治法是在治则指导下采取的治疗方法。历代医家创造了相当多的治法，清代程钟龄将其概括为八法。下面分别介绍。

一、汗法

汗法是使用辛散发汗作用的药物，以开泄腠理、调和营卫、逐邪外出的一种治疗方法。由于外邪侵袭人体大多始于皮毛，然后由表入里，故当邪在皮毛肌腠，尚未入里之时，即应采用汗法，使邪从汗解。

（一）汗法的适应证

外感六淫邪气之表证、麻疹初起、疹点隐隐不透，水肿病腰以上肿甚，疮疡初起而有寒热表证者。

（二）常用汗法

1. 辛温解表　适用于风寒表证，表现为恶寒重、发热轻、头身疼痛、舌苔薄白、脉浮紧等症。

2. 辛凉解表　适用于风热表证，表现为恶寒轻、发热重、咽痛口干、舌苔薄黄、脉浮数等症。

3. 解表透疹　适用于麻疹初期，疹出不透者。

4. 宣肺利水　适用于水肿兼有表证者。

cold and dry diseases are common, so pungent-moistening drugs are often prescribed, but the cool or cold drugs should be cautious to be applied. In the lower southeast of China, where it is hot and often rains and warm-heat or damp-heat diseases are common, so clearing and resolving drugs are often applied, but the warm, hot and moistening drugs should be cautious to be used. For example, pungent-warming exterior-releasing medicinals are often used to treat the common cold arising from exogenic wind cold, but the strong one like ephedra, cassia twig, and asarum are often utilized in the cold northwest regions, while the moderate one like schizonepeta, radices sileris, and Herba Periliae are often applied in the warm and hot southeast regions.

3. Treatment in accordance with the patient

It refers to application of treatment methods and drugs according to the age, gender, constitution, and life styles of the patients. For the adult patients, more dose can be prescribed; while for the child patients, only small dose can be prescribed. For the elderly who often have an deficiency syndrome or syndrome of mixing deficiency and excess as the functions of their internal organs decline, and qi and blood impair, tonifying method are often used, and it should be cautious to apply the method of eliminating the pathogenic factors when they present an excess syndrome. For the infant patient whose internal organs are tender, whose qi and blood has not grown sufficiently and whose qi activity is exuberant, they often present quick pathological changes of either cold or fever, or deficiency or exxess, so the method of eliminating the pathogenic factors with strong drugs should not be used and it should be cautious to use tonics. More consideration should be made when prescribing the drugs for women patients in treating the diseases related with the menses, leukorrhea, pregnancy and parturition. During the gestation period, drastic purgative medicinal, blood-breaking medicinal and the drugs easy to injure the fetus or poisonous drugs should not be utilized or should be used cautiously. For the postpartum patients, dual deficiency of qi and blood and lochia should be taken into account before deciding the treatment methods. Meanwhile, the constitution and exuberance or debilitation of yin and yang of the patients should also be considered.

Section 3   Methods of Treatment

The treatment methods of TCM can be categorized into eight methods, namely diaphoresis, emesis, purgation, mediation, warming, clearing, tonification and elimination. Therapeutic methods are under the guidance of treatment principles. A lot of therapeutic methods had been created along the history, which were summarized as the eight methods by Cheng Zhongling of Qing Dynasty. The details of the eight methods are as follows:

Diaphoresis

Diaphoresis is one of the principal therapeutic methods to open and discharge the interstices, harmonize the nutrient and defense, and expel the pathogenic evils out with pungent and sweating medicinals. It is adopted to expel the evils from the sweat when the exogenic pathogenic factors, which mostly invade the human body from the skin and then turn into the interior, still stays in skin or interstices.

Indications of Diaphoresis

Exterior syndromes caused by the six excesses, measles with the looming rash points at the beginning, edema emerging above the waist, and sore and ulcer with the exterior syndromes of cold or heat at the beginning.

Common Diaphoresis Methods

1. Releasing the exterior with pungent-warm

It is applicable for treating wind-cold exterior syndrome with manifestations of serious aversion to

（三）应用汗法的注意事项

1．汗法应以邪去为度，汗出不畅者可适当加衣被或服热粥汤等以助发汗。发汗太过，会耗伤津液，损失正气，甚至造成虚脱。汗后宜避风寒。

2．应用汗法要因人而异，对于虚人外感要根据患者体质等因素分别采用益气解表、滋阴解表等不同方法。

3．疮疡溃破，或麻疹已透，则不应再用汗法。

4．严重脱水、失血、热病后期均不宜使用汗法。

二、吐法

吐法是运用具有催吐作用的方药使有害物质排出体外的一种治疗方法。适应于误食毒物或食物中毒，胃内宿食停滞及痰涎阻塞咽喉者。

吐法是中医临床急救的一种方法。随着医学的发展在临床已经被洗胃所替代。

三、下法

下法是应用具有泻下作用的药物，通泻大便以攻逐邪实、荡涤肠胃、排除积滞的一种治疗方法。凡病邪结聚于里而形成的里实证，原则上都可用此法。但在临床运用时，必须仔细分辨病人正气的强弱和邪气的盛衰，选用适当的泻下方药，方能达到预期的效果。

（一）常用的下法及适应证

1．寒下　寒下法适用于热邪内结于肠道的里实热证，采用具有苦寒、泻下、通便、泻火作用的方药进行治疗。

2．温下　温下法适用于寒邪内结于肠道的里实寒证，采用辛热温里、泻下通便的方药进行治疗。

3．润下　润下法适用于阴血亏虚、大肠津亏之大便秘结证，采用养阴生津、润肠通便的方药进行治疗。

4．逐水　逐水法适用于水结于内的实证，采用峻下逐水的方药进行治疗。

5．攻下　攻下法适用于食积、虫积、瘀血、痰饮等积聚于胃肠的实证，采用化积导滞、破瘀除痰的方药进行治疗。

cold, light fever, body and head pain, thin and pale tongue coating, and floating and tight pulse.

2. Releasing the exterior with pungent-cool

It is applicable for treating wind-heat exterior syndrome with manifestations of light aversion to cold, high fever, sore throat and dry mouth, thin and yellow tongue coating, and floating and rapid pulse.

3. Releasing the exterior and outthrusting rashes

It is applicable for treating measles with looming rash on the skin at the beginning.

4. Diffusing the lung and inducing diuresis

It is applicable for edema with the exterior syndromes.

Cautions for Application of Diaphoresis

Doctors should stop using diaphoresis when it works. The patient can put more clothes or cover quilt, or eat the hot porridge or soup to promote sweating if it is not enough. Excessive sweating will consume the body fluids, impair the healthy qi and even lead to collapse. The patients should avoid the wind cold after sweating.

Application of diaphoresis should be varied with different patients. As for the asthenic patients suffering from the exterior syndrome, tonifying qi or enriching yin together with releasing the exterior should be adopted in accordance with their constitution factors.

Diaphoresis should not be used in case of diabrosis of sore and ulcer, or eruption of measles.

Diaphoresis also should not be used in such cases as serious dehydration, hemorrhage and the late stage of heat diseases.

Emesis

Emesis is one of the principal therapeutic methods to expel the harmful substance out with emetic medicinals. It is applicable for the patients eating toxins or with food poisoning, or with indigested food stagnating in the stomach or with phlegm obstructing the throat.

Emeis is a first aid method used by TCM doctors. It has been replaced by gastric lavage with the development of the medicine.

Purgation

Purgation is one of the principal therapeutic methods to expel the excessive pathogens, clean up the stomach and intestine and remove the accumulated stagnation by defecation with purgative medicinals. In principle, it can be used to treat the interior excess syndrome caused by internal coagulation of the pathogens. But clinically, doctors should carefully identify the situation of the healthy qi and the pathogenic factors before making the proper recipe so as to reach the effects as expected.

Common Purgation Methods and Their Indications

1. Cold purgation

It is used to treat the interior excessive heat syndrome caused by internal coagulation and stagnation of heat evil in the intestine with bitter-cold, purgative, relaxing the bowels and purging fire medicinals.

2. Warm purgation

It is used to treat the interior excessive cold syndrome caused by internal convergence and stagnation of cold evil in the intestines with pungent-warm the interior and purgative medicinals.

3. Lubricant laxation

It is used to treat constipation caused by yin and blood deficiency leading to large intestinal fluid deficiency. The medicinals with the functions of nourishing yin and engendering fluid to moisten the intestines and relax the bowels can be adopted.

4. Expelling water

（二）应用下法的注意事项

1. 邪在表者不宜用下法。

2. 下法以邪去为度，不宜久用。泻下太过易伤脾胃。

3. 老、幼、孕及体虚患者慎用。

四、和法

和法是运用和解或调和作用的方药，以达到祛除半表半里之邪、协调脏腑功能的一种治疗方法。

（一）常用的和法及适应证

1. 和解表里 和解表里法适应于少阳证，邪在半表半里，出现寒热往来、口苦咽干、心烦欲呕、胸胁苦满、不欲饮食等症。

2. 调和肝脾 调和肝脾法适用于肝气郁结并影响脾气运化之肝脾不和证，表现为心情郁闷、胁肋胀满、腹胀肠鸣、大便泄泻等症。

3. 疏肝和胃 疏肝和胃法适用于肝气犯胃之肝胃失和证，表现为胸胁胀痛、食欲不振、嗳腐吞酸等症。

4. 调和肠胃 调和肠胃法适用于邪犯肠胃、寒热互结、升降失常之肠胃不和证，表现为心下痞满、呕恶嗳气、肠鸣下利等症。

（二）应用和法注意事项

1. 邪在表或已入里者，均不宜用和法。

2. 阳明热盛、阴寒内结等亦不宜用和法。

五、温法

温法是运用温性或热性药物来补益阳气、祛除寒邪以治疗里寒证的一种治疗方法。里寒证有虚实之分，寒邪直中脏腑为里寒实证，而阳气不足寒自内生是里寒虚证。

It is used to treat the excessive syndrome caused by internal retention of water with drastic purgation to expel water medicinals.

5. Purgation

It is applied to treat the excessive syndrome caused by accumulation of food, parasites, blood stasis, and phlegm and retained fluid in the stomach and intestines with resolving accumulation, removing stagnation, dissipating stasis and dispelling phlegm medicinals.

Cautions of Application of Purgation

Purgation is not applicable for treating the disease having the pathogen in the exterior.

Purgation should not be used for a long time as soon as the pathogen is expelled, otherwise it will injure the spleen and stomach.

It should be cautious to use purgation on the old, the children, the pregnant and the weak patients.

Medication

Medication is one of the principal therapeutic methods to expel the pathogen located between the exterior and interior of the body and regulate the functions of the viscera and bowels with harmonizing medicinals.

Common Medication Methods and Their Indications

1. Harmonizing the exterior and interior

It is applicable for treating the Shaoyang syndrome, which is caused by the pathogen located between the exterior and interior of the body, with the symptoms of alternating chills and fever, bitterness in the mouth and dry throat, vexation and vomit, fullness and distention in the chest and hypochondrium and poor appetite.

2. Harmonizing the liver and spleen

It is applicable for treating the syndrome of incoordination between the liver and spleen, arising from liver qi depression affecting the spleen qi in transportation and transformation, with the manifestations of depression, fullness and distention in the hypochondriums, abdominal distention, borborygmus and diarrhea.

3. Soothing the liver and harmonizing the stomach

It is applicable for treating the syndrome of disharmony between the liver and stomach due to the liver qi invading the stomach, in company with the symptoms of fullness and pain of chest and hypochondrium, poor appetite, belching the turbid and acid regurgitation, etc.

4. Harmonizing the intestines and stomach

It is applicable for treating the syndrome of disharmony between the intestines and stomach arising from pathogens attacking the intestines and stomach leading to mutual binding of cold and heat and disorder of ascending and descending, with the manifestations of stuffiness and fullness below the heart, vomit and belching, borborygmus and diarrhea, etc.

Cautions of Application of Medication

1. Medication is not applicable for treating the disease having pathogen in the exterior or interior.

2. Medication is not applicable in case of the excessive heat in Yangming or the internal binding of yin and cold.

Warming

Warming is one of the principal therapeutic methods to treat the interior cold syndrome through tonifing yang qi and expelling the cold pathogen with warm or hot medicinals. The interior cold syndrome is divided into excess syndrome caused by the direct invasion of cold pathogen in the internal organs, and defi-

（一）常用的温法及适应证

1. 温中散寒　温中散寒法适用于寒邪直中脏腑或素体阳虚复感寒邪证。临床表现为腹部怕冷，腹痛、腹泻，得温痛减，舌苔白，脉沉迟等症。

2. 回阳救逆　回阳救逆法适用于元阳虚衰或亡阳证，临床表现为畏寒肢冷、大汗淋漓、面色苍白、脉微细欲绝等症。

3. 温阳利水　温阳利水法适用于肾阳虚衰、温煦不足、气化失司、水湿泛滥证，临床表现为全身或下肢水肿、小便量少、面色苍白、畏寒肢冷、舌淡苔白、脉沉细无力等症。

4. 温经散寒　温经散寒法适用于寒邪侵袭经络或寒凝血脉证。寒邪侵袭经络者表现为关节疼痛、屈伸不利、遇冷加重等症；寒凝血脉者表现为肢麻、肢冷、肢痛等症，寒凝胞宫表现为行经腹痛等症。

（二）应用温法注意事项

1. 素体阴虚者慎用。

2. 吐血、尿血、便血等患者及孕妇慎用。

3. 温热药多从小剂量开始，当中病即止，不可太过以损耗阴液。

六、清法

清法是运用寒凉的药物以治疗热性病证的一种治疗方法。清法具有清热、泻火、解毒、保津、凉血、祛暑及镇惊熄风等作用。热有表里虚实之不同，有在气、在营、在血之差别。根据热邪所在部位和性质的不同，可分为清热泻火、清热解毒、清热凉血、清热燥湿及清虚热等不同方法。

（一）常用的清法及适应证

1. 清热泻火　清热泻火法适用于各种里热证，如气分高热、肺热、心火、肝火等实热证，临床表现多为高热、口舌生疮、咳吐黄痰、面红目赤，大便秘结，甚至神昏谵语等症。

2. 清热解毒　清热解毒法适用于热毒所致的疮疡、痈疖、肿毒等证，临床表现为疮疡、痈疖等局部红、肿、热、痛、溢脓等症。

3. 清热凉血　清热凉血法适用于血热证，如热入营血阶段，出现神昏、发斑及出血等症。

4. 清热燥湿　清热燥湿法适用于湿热证，包括外感湿热、脾胃湿热、肝胆湿热等证。

5. 清虚热　清虚热法适用于阴血内热证或外感热病后期阴津受损所致的虚热证。

ciency syndrome caused by insufficient yang qi leading to the generation of internal cold.

Common Warming Methods and Their Indications

1. Warming the middle and dissipating cold

It is applicable for treating the syndromes arising from direct invasion of cold pathogen in the internal organs, or invasion of exogenic cold pathogen in the constitutional yang-deficient patients, with the manifestations of abdominal cold and pain, cold relief from warming, diarrhea, white fur and slow and sunken pulse.

2. Restoring yang to save from collapse

It is applicable for treating the syndromes arising from original yang debilitation or yang collapse, with the manifestations of fear of cold, cold limbs, great dripping sweat, pale complexion and extremely thin and weak pulse.

3. Warming yang to move water

It is applicable for treating the water-dampness flood syndrome arising from kidney yang debilitation leading to its failure to warm and transformation, with the manifestations of edema of the whole body or the lower limbs, little urine, pale complexion, fear of cold, cold limbs, pale tongue with white fur, and weak, sunken and thin pulse.

4. Warming the meridian to dissipate cold

It is applicable for treating the syndromes of invasion of cold in meridians and collaterals, or cold congealing in blood, with the former manifesting the sympoms of arthralgia, inflexibility to stretch the limbs, and aggravation in cold condition; while the latter presenting the symptoms of numb, cold and pain limbs, or dysmenorrhea as the result of cold congealing in the uterus

Cautions of Application of Warming

Doctors should be cautious to use it on the patients with constitutional yin deficiency.

Doctors should be cautious to use it on the patients with hematemesis, hematuria, and hemafecia and pregnant patients.

Doctors should gradually add the dose of such drugs and stop using it when it expels the cold diseases, otherwise, they will consume yin fluids.

Clearing

Clearing is one of the principal therapeutic methods to treat the heat syndromes with cold medicinals, as it can clear heat, discharge fire, detoxify, maintain fluid, cool the blood, release summerheat, and calm fright and extinguish wind. Heat covers interior heat, exterior heat, deficiency heat and excess heat, or heat in qi aspect, heat in nutrient aspect, and heat in blood aspect. Clearing heat to purge fire, detoxify, cool the blood, dry dampness, and clearing deficient heat can be adopted according to the locations and natures.

Common Clearing Methods and Their Indications

1. Clearing heat to purge fire

It is applicable for treating various interior heat syndromes like excessive heat in qi aspect, lung heat, heart fire, and liver fire, with the manifestations of high fever, sore tongue and mouth, red face and eyes, constipation, and even loss of consciousness and delirious speech.

2. Clearing to detoxify

It is applicable for treating sore and ulcer, abscess, furuncle and pyogenic infections, with the symptoms of redness, swelling, heat, ache and pyorrhea in the affected skin.

3. Clearing heat to cool the blood

It is applicable for treating blood heat syndromes such as the syndrome of heat entering nutrient-blood aspects, with manifestations of coma, petechiae and haemorrhagia, etc.

（二）应用清法的注意事项

1．清法多用苦寒药物，易伤脾胃、耗伤津液，热祛即止，不可久服。

2．脾胃虚寒者不宜使用清法。

七、补法

补法是运用补益的药物以治疗气、血、阴、阳虚损病证的一种治疗方法。

（一）常用的补法及适应证

1．补气　补气法适用于脏腑功能不足之气虚证，主要表现为乏力、气短、自汗、活动后加重、舌淡体胖有齿痕、脉沉弱等症。

2．补血　补血法适用于血虚及出血证，主要表现为面色苍白或萎黄、唇舌色淡、头晕心悸、月经量少或色淡、脉沉细等症。

3．补阳　补阳法适用于阳气虚弱证，主要表现为畏寒肢冷、腰脊酸软、阳痿早泄、小便清长、五更泻、舌淡、脉细弱或沉迟等症。

4．补阴　补阴法适用于阴津亏损证，主要表现为五心烦热、口干夜甚、盗汗、舌红少苔或光剥无苔、脉细数等症。

（二）应用补法的注意事项

1．脾胃虚弱者运用补法时，要首先健脾养胃，否则会出现"虚不受补"的状况。

2．滋阴补血药大多滋腻，在应用时可配合芳香理气健脾药，以免脾胃呆滞。补气助阳药性大多燥热可配合滋润敛阴药，以防化燥伤阴。

3．对于正虚邪盛者可采用攻补兼施法。

八、消法

消法是运用具有消导、消散、软坚、化积作用的药物以消除体内有害物质，使气血通畅、机能恢复的一种治疗方法。消法应用范围比较广泛，如癥瘕、积聚、痞块、结石、痰核、瘰疬等均可用消法治之。

4. Clearing heat to dry dampness

It is applicable for treating the damp-heat syndromes including external contraction of damp-heat, damp-heat in the spleen and stomach, and damp-heat in the liver and gallbladder, etc.

5. Clearing deficiency heat

It is applicable for treating the syndrome of endogenous heat in yin and blood, or deficiency heat syndrome due to impairment of yin and heat at the late stage of external contraction heat diseases.

Cautions of Application of Clearing

1. As clearing recipes are primarily made up of cold and bitter medicinals, which are apt to impair the functions of the spleen and stomach, and consume the fluid and humor, so they should not be used further when the heat is expelled.

2. The clearing methods are not suitable for the patients with syndrome of spleen and stomach deficiency cold.

Tonification

Tonification is one of the principal therapeutic methods to treat the deficiency syndromes of qi, blood, yin and yang with tonifying and replenishing medicinals.

Common Tonification Methods and Their Indications

1. Tonifying qi

It is applicable for treating the qi deficiency syndrome caused by dysfunction of the viscera and bowels, with the manifestations of debilitation, short breath, spontaneous perspiration, which aggravates after activities, pale and bulgy tongue with indentation, and weak and sunken pulse.

2. Tonifying blood

It is applicable for treating the syndromes of blood deficiency and haemorrhage, with the symptoms of pale or sallow complexion, pale lip and tongue, dizziness, palpitation, scant menstruation with light colour, and thin and sunken pulse.

3. Tonifying yang

It is applicable for treating the yang qi deficiency syndrome, with the manifestations of fear of cold, cold limbs, aching and limp waist, impotence, premature ejaculation, clear and abundant urine, fifth-watch diarrhoea, pale tongue, and thin and weak pulse or slow or sunken pulse.

4. Tonifying yin

It is applicable for treating the yin and fluid deficiency syndrome, with the manifestations of vexing heat in the chest, palms and soles, dry mouth especially during the night, night sweating, red tongue with little fur, or tongue without fur, and thin and rapid pulse.

Cautions of Application of Tonifying Methods

For the patients with dysfunction of the spleen and stomach, the method of fortifying the spleen and invigorating the stomach should be used first before applying the tonification methods. Otherwise, they cannot absorb the tonic drugs well, known as "the deficient are intolerance to the tonic."

The aromatic, qi-regulating and spleen-fortifing medicinals should be added into the recipes of enriching yin and tonifying blood, so as to activate the function of the spleen and stomach and avoid the stagnation and indigestion of them. While the nourishing and constraining yin medicinals are often added in the recipe of tonifying qi and assisting yang, which is dry and hot in nature, so as to avoid yin impairment.

Combination of tonification and purgation can be adopted on the patients with the syndrome of deficient healthy qi and excessive pathogenic factors.

Elimination

Elimination is one of the principal therapeutic methods to remove the harmful substances to promote

（一）常用消法及适应证

1. 消食导滞　消食导滞法适用于食积引起的脘腹胀满、食欲不振、嗳腐吞酸、恶心呕吐、腹痛腹泻等症。

2. 活血化瘀　活血化瘀法适用于由于血液郁滞引起的癥积、疼痛、痛经等症。

3. 软坚散结　软坚散结法适用于因痰湿郁滞引起的痰核、瘰疬等症。

4. 清热排石　清热排石法适用于因湿热壅结引起的痰核砂石内结之症。

（二）应用消法注意事项

1. 虚证不宜用。

2. 中病即止，不宜久用，以防伤正。

（梁晓春）

qi and blood circulation and recuperate the body functions with promoting digestion, dissipating, softening hardness and resolving accumulation medicinal. It can be extensively applied in such diseases as aggregation-accumulation, stuffy lumps, calculas, subcutaneous nodule and scrofula, etc.

Common Eliminating Methods and Their Indications

1. Promoting digestion and removing food stagnation

It is applicable for treating the food accumulation syndrome with the manifestations of abdominal fullness and distention, poor appetite, belching the turbid, acid regurgitation, nausea and vomit, abdominal pain and diarrhea, etc.

2. Activating blood and resolving stasis

It is applicable for treating the syndromes caused by blood stasis such as aggregation-accumulation, pain and dysmenorrhea, etc.

3. Softening hardness and dissipating masses

It is applicable for treating the syndromes caused by stagnation of phlegm and dampness such as subcutaneous nodule and scrofula, etc.

4. Clearing heat and removing calculus

It is applicable for treating the lithiasis caused by damp heat agglomeration and stagnation.

Cautions of Application of Eliminating

1. Eliminating method is not applicable for the deficiency syndromes.

2. Eliminating methods and drugs are not applicable for long use and should be stopped when they work, otherwise they will impair the healthy qi.

(Wu Qunli   Zhang Wen)

第八章 中 药

第一节 中药总论

中药包括中药材、中药饮片和中成药等。由于中药来源以植物类药材居多，所以历代将记载药物的专著称为"本草"，把药学叫做"本草学"。中药学就是专门研究中药基本理论和各种中药的来源、采制、性能、功效及配伍应用等知识的一门学科。

一、中药的性能

中药的性能是指中药与其疗效有关的性质和功能，即其具有的特性和作用，主要包括四气、五味、归经、升降浮沉及有毒、无毒等。它是中医学理论体系中一个重要的组成部分，是中医临床用药的理论基础。

（一）四气五味

1. 四气 四气也称四性，即寒、热、温、凉四种药性。寒凉和温热是对立的两种药性；寒和凉之间、热和温之间，仅在程度上有差别，温次于热、凉次于寒。

药性的寒、热、温、凉，是与所治疾病的寒、热性质相对而言，是从药物作用于机体所发生的反应或治疗效果归纳总结出来的。能够减轻或消除热证的药物，一般属于寒性或凉性，如黄芩、板蓝根可改善发热口渴、咽痛等热证，表明这两种药物具有寒凉药性。反之，能够减轻或消除寒证的药物，一般属于温性或热性，如干姜、吴茱萸可缓解脘腹冷痛、畏寒肢冷等寒证，表明这两种药物具有温热药性。

此外，还有一些药物的药性较为平和，寒热之性不甚显著、作用比较和缓，称为"平"性。其中也有微寒、微温的，但仍未超出四性的范围，所以平性是指相对的属性，而不是绝对性的概念。

2. 五味 五味就是辛、甘、酸、苦、咸五种药味。实际上不止五种，有些药物

CHAPTER EIGHT CHINESE MATERIA MEDICA

Section 1 Overview of Chinese Materia Medica

Chinese Materia Medica(CMM)is divided into Chinese medicinal plant,Chinese traditional medication decoction pieces,and ready-prepared Chinese medicine.Because most CMM comes from plants,they are called as"Bencao"in TCM literature,and the science of CMM are called"the science of Bencao".The science of CMM is a subject focusing on researching the basic theories of CMM and its source,collection, properties,functions,and clinical combination and application.

Characteristics of Chinese Materia Medica

The characteristics of CMM refer to the natures and properties of CMM related to their efficacies, which are comprised with the four natures(hot,warm,cool,cold),five flavors(pungent,sweet,sour,bitter,salty),meridian tropism,four directions(upbearing,downbearing,floating,and sinking),and toxicity. It is an important part of the theoretical systems of TCM,and is the theoretical basis of clinical pharmacy of TCM.

Four Natures and Five Flavors

1. Four natures

The four natures also named as the four properties,which are hot,warm,cool,and cold.Cold and cool and warm and hot are two kinds of opposite properties.Between cold and cool,or between hot or warm,are varieties in intensity.Warm is inferior to hot,and cool is inferior to cold.

The four natures(hot,warm,cool,and cold)correspond to cold or heat natures of diseases and syndromes that the medicinal treats,and are holistically summarized from the body responses to the treatment of different medicinal,and are based on the body's responses to the medicinal or the effects of the medicinal.Generally speaking,the medicinals that can alleviate or eliminate heat syndromes are of cold or cool nature.*Radix Scutellariae* and *Radix Isatidis*,for example,can ameliorate heat syndrome marked by fever, thirst and sore throat.This demonstrates that these two kinds of medicinals are of cool or cold nature.In contrast,those medicinals which can alleviate,or eliminate cold syndromes are of warm or hot nature.*Rhizoma Zingiberis* and *Fructus Evodiae*,for example,can ameliorate cold syndromes,manifested as cold pain in the abdomen,fear of cold and cold limbs,which illustrates these two medicinals are of warm or hot nature.

There are also Chinese medicinals of a neutral nature,whose medicinal preferences for cold or hot are inconspicuous,having a moderate efficacy,some of their natures are leaning toward slightly warm or cool; however,the natures are still in the parameter of the four natures.Thus,the neutral nature is a relative nature but not an absolute definition.

2. Five flavors

The five flavors refer to the five tastes of medicinals,pungency,sweetness,sourness,bitterness and saltiness.In addition to these five flavors,some medicinals also have bland flavor or astringent flavor.Be-

具有淡味或涩味。由于淡味，没有特殊的滋味，所以一般将它和甘味并列，称"淡附于甘"，而涩味的作用和酸味的作用相同，故五味是最基本的五种滋味，所以仍然称为五味。不同的味有不同的作用，味相同的药物，其作用也有相近或共同之处。各种味药物的作用如下：

（1）辛：有发散、行气、行血作用。发散解表的麻黄、薄荷，行气止痛的香附、木香和活血化瘀的川芎等都有辛味。

（2）甘：有补益、和中或缓急作用。常用于治疗虚证的滋补强壮药，如党参、熟地；缓和拘急疼痛、调和药性的药物，如饴糖、甘草等。

淡：有渗湿、利尿作用。多用于水肿、小便不利等证，如猪苓、茯苓等药物。

（3）酸：有收敛、固涩作用。一般用于治疗虚汗、泄泻、遗精等证，如五味子收敛止汗，乌梅涩肠止泻，山茱萸涩精止遗。

涩：与酸味作用相似。多用以治疗虚汗、泄泻、尿频、滑精、出血等证，如龙骨、牡蛎涩精，赤石脂能涩肠止泻。

（4）苦：能泄、能燥、能坚阴。泄的含义包括：①通泄，如大黄，适用于热结便秘；②降泄，如杏仁，适用于肺气上逆的喘咳；③清泄，如黄连、栀子适用于热盛心烦。至于燥，是指用于湿证。湿证有寒湿和湿热的不同，温性的苦味药如苍术，适用于前者；寒性的苦味药如黄连，适用于后者。

（5）咸：有软坚散结、泻下作用。常用于治疗瘰疬、痰核、痞块与便结等。如，芒硝泻下通便；瓦楞子、牡蛎软坚散结治疗瘰疬、痰核、痞块，均有咸味。

每种药物都具有气和味，气、味各有其作用。同性药物有五味之别，同味的药物亦各有四气之异。在辨识药性时，不能把药物的气与味孤立起来，而必须将气和味二者综合来看。

性味相同的药物，其主要作用也大致相同，例如，紫苏、荆芥均为辛温，它们都有发汗解表的作用，可用于外感风寒表证。性味不同的药物，功效亦不相同，例如，麻黄性味辛温，辛能发散，温能散寒，故其主要作用是发散风寒；芦根性味甘寒，甘能生津，寒能清热，故其主要作用为清热生津。

性同味不同、或味同性不同的药物在功效上也有共同之处和不同之点。

以寒性药物为例，性虽同，因味不同，其作用有差异：如栀子苦寒，清热泻火、凉血解毒；淡竹叶甘寒，清热利尿；浮萍辛寒，疏散风热、利尿退肿。共同之处是寒性均有清热作用。

以甘味药物为例，味虽同，因气不同，其作用亦不相同：如杜仲甘温以补肝肾、强筋骨、安胎；石斛甘微寒以养阴生津；甘草甘平，以补脾益气、润肺止咳、缓急

cause bland flavor has no specific flavor, it is always mentioned with sweet flavor, which is called the bland flavor pertains to the sweet flavor. The astringent flavor has the same functions as the sour flavor has. Thus, the five flavors are the fundamental flavors. Different flavor has different function, while the medicinals with the same flavor have the similar or same functions. The functions of the five flavors are discussed in detail as following:

The pungent flavor has the functions of dispersing and promoting the circulation of qi and blood. The medicinals have the functions of dispersing and resolving exterior evils, such as *Herba Ephedrae* and *Herba Menthae* ; and the medicinals have the functions of promoting qi and alleviating pain, such as *Rhizoma Cyperi* and *Radix Aucklandiae* ; and the medicinals have the functions of activating the blood and removing stasis, such as *Rhizoma Chuanxiong*, have pungent flavor.

The sweet flavor has the functions of nourishing, harmonizing the middle energizer and relieving spasm and pain. The medicinals have the functions of nourishing are used in the treatment of deficiency syndromes, such as *Radix Codonopsis* and *Radix Rehmanniae Praeparata* ; and the medicinals have the functions of relieving spasm and pain, hamorizing medicinal natures, such as *Extractum Malti* and *Radix Glycyrrhizae*, are all sweet medicinals.

The bland flavor has the functions of draining and promoting diuresis. The bland flavor medicinals are used for edema and dysuria, for example, *Polyporus* and *Poria*.

The sour flavor has the functions of absorbing, astringing and consolidating. The sour medicinals are generally used in the treatment of sweating due to weakness, diarrhea and nocturnal emission. For example, *Fructus Schisandrae* is used in securing essence and arresting sweating, *Fructus Mume* is used in astringe the intestines to stop diarrhea, and *Fructus Corni* is used in astringe essence and check emission.

The astringent flavor has the similar functions with the sour flavor. The astringent flavor medicinals are generally used in sweating due to weakness, diarrhea, frequent urination, seminal efflux and bleeding. For example, *Os Draconis* and *Concha Ostreae* astringe essence, and *Halloysitum Rubrum* astringes the intestine to stop diarrhea.

The bitter flavor has the functions of purging, drying and astringe essence. The concept of purgation refers to: ① discharing function, for example, *Radix et Rhizoma Rhei* is applicable to conspitation due to heat stagnation; ② lowering function, for example, *Semen Armeniacae Amarum* is used to treat cough due to the adcerse rising of lung qi; ③ clearing function, for example, *Rhizoma Coptidis* and *Fructus Gardeniae* are used in vexation due to excessive heat. As to the function of drying, it is utilized for dampness syn dromes, which are classified into cold-dampness syndrome and dampness-heat syndrome. The bitter medicinal of warm nature, such as *Rhizoma Atractylodis*, is applicable to the former; the bitter medicinal of cold nature, such as *Rhizoma Coptidis*, is applicable to the latter.

The salty flavor has the functions of softening hardness, dissipating binds, and purging. Salty medicinals are often used for scrofula, phlegm nodule, mass and conspitation. For example, *Natrii Sulfas* purges and relieves conspitation; and *Concha Arcae* and *Concha Ostreae* have the functions of softening and dispersing hardness and mass, and are used to treat scrofula, phlegm nodule and mass. All the medicinals as the above-mentioned examples are salty.

Every medicinal has its own flavor and nature, and the flavor and nature have their own functions. The medicinals with the same nature have diversity of the five flavors, while the medicinals with the same flavor have diversity of the four natures. During the process of distinguishing properties of the medicinals, we may not isolate the nature with flavor, but should combine the nature and flavor together.

The medicinals with the same nature and flavor have the similar functions. For example, both *Fructus Perillae* and *Herba Schizonepetae* are pungent in flavor and warm in nature, and they all have the functions of promoting sweating and releasing the exterior, and are applicable to the exterior syndromes due to wind-cold contraction. The medicinals with different natures and flavors have different functions. For example, *Herba Ephedrae* is pungent in flavor and warm in nature, and because the pungent can disperse and the

止痛、调和诸药。共同之处是味甘，故均有补益之功效。

（二）升降浮沉

升降浮沉，是指药物治疗人体疾病时的不同趋向性。升：就是上升、升提的意思，能治病势下陷的药物，都有升的作用；降：就是下降、降逆的意思，能治病势上逆的药物，都有降的作用；浮：就是轻浮、上行发散的意思，能治病位在表的药物，都有浮的作用；沉：就是重沉、下行泄利的意思，能治病位在里的药物，都有沉的作用。

升与浮、沉与降的趋向类似，升浮药物主上升而向外，有解表、散寒、祛风、升阳、催吐等作用；沉降药物主下行而向内，有清热、泻下、利水、平喘、降逆、潜阳、止呕等作用。

1. 升降浮沉与病位、病势的关系　凡病位在上在表，宜用升浮不用沉降。如外感风寒表证，当用麻黄、紫苏等升浮药以发散风寒；病位在下在里，宜用沉降不用升浮。如肠燥便秘里实证，当用大黄、枳实等沉降药以攻里通便。

病势上逆的宜降不宜升，如肝阳上亢之头痛、眩晕，当用石决明、生牡蛎等以潜阳降逆；病势下陷的宜升不宜降，如久泻、脱肛、阴挺等中气下陷，当用黄芪、升麻以补气升阳。

2. 升降浮沉与药物气味、质地轻重的关系　凡味属辛、甘，气属温热的药物，大多能升浮，如麻黄、黄芪等；味属酸、苦、咸，气属寒凉的药物，大多为沉降，如大黄、芒硝等。

凡植物的花、叶及质地轻的药物，大多能升浮，如辛夷、荷叶、苏叶、马勃等；凡种子、果实及质地重的药物，大多能沉降，如苏子、枳实、石决明、代赭石等。但也有例外：如旋覆花主降、蔓荆子主升。

3. 升降浮沉与炮制配伍的关系

炮制：酒炒则上升；醋炒则敛涩；姜汁炒则散；盐炒则下行入肾。

配伍：桔梗载药上浮；牛膝引药下行。此外，少数升浮药在大队沉降药中也能随之下降；少数沉降药在大队升浮药中也能随之上升。

warm can dispel cold, thus, its functions are dispersing wind and dispelling cold; *Rhizoma Phragmitis* is sweet in flavor and cold in nature, and because the sweet can engender fluid and the cold can clear heat, so its main functions are clearing heat and engendering fluid.

The medicinals with the same nature but different flavors, or the medicinals with the same flavor but different natures have the same or different efficacies.

Take the medicinals with the cold nature as an example, becaus the medicinals with the same nature have different flavors, they have different functions: *Fructus Gardeniae* is bitter in flavor and cold in nature, processing the functions of clearing heat and purging fire, cooling blood and resolving toxicity; *Herba Lophatheri* is sweet in flavor and cold in nature, processing the functions of clearing heat and promoting urine excretion; *Herba Spirodelae* is pungent in flavor and cold in nature, possessing the functions of dispersing wind and clearing heat, inducing diuresis to alleviate edema. Their same characteristics are that all of them are of the cold nature and having the function of clearing heat.

Take the medicinals with the sweet flavor as an example. The medicinals with the same flavor but different natures have different functions. For example, *Cortex Eucommiae* is sweet in flavor and warm in nature, possessing the functions of tonifying the liver and nourishing the kidney, strengthen the tendons and bones and quieting the fetus; *Herba Dendrobii* is sweet in flavor and slightly cold in nature, possessing the functions of nourishing yin and engendering body fluid; *Radix Glycyrrhizae* is sweet in flavor and neutral in nature, possessing the functions of nourishing the spleen and tonifying qi, nourishing the lung and stoping cough, alleviating spasm and pain, and mediating multiple medicinals. The common characteristic is that all the above-mentioned medicinals are sweet in flavor, thus, all have the functions of tonifying and nourishing.

Upbearing, downbearing, floating, and sinking

The four directions, upbearing, downbearing, floating and sinking, refer to the directional effect of Chinese materia medica on the human body. Upbearing means rising and arising, and all the medicinals used for falling downward conditions have the function of upbearing. Downbearing means dropping and declining, and all the medicinals used for inversing upward conditions have the function of downbearing. Floating means frivolous and dispersing upwards, and all the medicinals used for syndromes in the superficial part of the body have the function of floating. Sinking means heavy and relaxing the bowels and promoting diuresis and all the medicinals used for syndromes in the interior part of the body have the function of sinking.

Upbearing and floating, sinking and downbearing have the similar tendencies. Upbearing and floating medicinals move towards the upper and exterior part of the body, and have the functions of resolving exterior, dispersing cold, dispelling wind, upbearing yang and emeticing. Downbearing and sinking medicinals move towards the lower and interior part of the body, and have the functions of clearing heat, puring, draining urine, calming panting, downbearing counter flow, sunking yang and checking vomiting.

1. The relationship between the four directions of upbearing, downbearing, floating and sinking and syndrome location and pathogenic tendency

Generally, for syndromes in the upper and superficial part of the body, it is useful to employ medicinals of upbearing and floating nature. For example, *Herba Ephedrae* and *Fructus Perillae* of upbearing and floating narure are used for wind-cold external constraction to disperse wind and dispel cold. For syndromes in the lower and interior part of the body, it is better to utilize medicinals of downbearing or sinking nature. For example, *Radix et Rhizoma Rhei* and *Fructus Aurantii Immaturus* of downbearing and sinking narure are used for conspitation due to internal heat and dry intestine to purging heat and relaxing the bowels.

If the syndrome is of an upward tendency, medicinals of upbearing nature are superior to those of

（三）归经

药性的归经理论，是以脏腑经络理论为基础的。人体的脏腑各有特殊的生理功能和病理变化，经络则把人体内外各部分联系起来，构成一个整体。体表的外邪可以循经络内传脏腑，脏腑的病变也可由经络反映到体表。临床用药时，首先要审清证候病变所在的脏腑经络，然后再选用相应的药物进行治疗。

如咳喘属肺经病，杏仁、苏子平喘止咳归肺经；两胁胀痛属肝经病，柴胡、香附疏肝理气归肝经；心悸失眠属心经病，朱砂、茯神镇心安神归心经；食少便溏属脾经病，党参、白术健脾补中归脾经；腰酸遗精属肾经病，熟地、菟丝子补肾固精归肾经。归经理论有如下规律：

1. 一药归数经　一药归数经者，治疗范围则扩大，如杏仁归肺与大肠经，既平喘止咳又润肠通便；石膏归肺、胃经，既清肺热，又泻胃火。

2. 同归一经　同归一经的药物，作用有温、清、补、泻的区别。如同归肺经：黄芩清肺热，干姜温肺寒，百合补肺虚，葶苈子泻肺实。同归肝经：龙胆草泻肝火，香附理肝气，山茱萸敛肝精，阿胶补肝血。

3. 根据脏腑经络关系而选用药物　由于脏腑经络的病变是互相影响的，所以在用药时，往往不是单纯使用某一经药物。如：肺病而见脾虚的，可选用脾经药山药、茯苓等以补脾益肺；肝阳上亢而见肾阴不足的，可以选用肾经药熟地、玄参等以滋肾养肝。

4. 引经药　引经原称引经报使，或称诸经向导。指一种药可以引导其他药物的药力趋向某经或直达病所，这种作用称为引经。即指它除了对本经病证具有治疗作用外，还能把不归本经的药物引归到本经而发挥其治疗作用，以提高药物疗效。

downbearing nature. For example, for headache due to hyperactivity if liver yang, *Concha Haliotidis* and *Concha Ostreae* are used for downbearing yang and downbearing counterflow. While for syndromes of sinking tendency, medicinals of upbearing nature rather than downbearing nature are appropriate. For example, in treating middle qi collapse syndromes, such as chronic diarrhea and anal prolapse and vaginal protrusion, *Radix Astragali* and *Rhizoma Cimicifugae* are utilized to tonify qi and raise yang.

2. The relationship between the four directions of upbearing, downbearing, floating and sinking and natures, flavors and properties

There is a close relationship between natures, flavors and properties and the four directions of upbearing, downbearing, floating and sinking of CMM. Generally, CMM that are upbearing and floating, such as *Herba Ephedrae* and *Radix Astragali*, are mostly pungent and sweet in flavor, warm and hot in nature. The medicinals that are downbearing and sinking, such as *Radix et Rhizoma Rhei* and *Natrii Sulfas*, are mostly sour, bitter, salty and astringent in flavor and cool in nature. It is generally considered that flowers and leaves of herbal medicinals, and light medicinlas are mostly upbearing and floating, for example, *Flos Magnoliae*, *Folium Nelumbinis*, *Folium Perillae* and *Lasiosphaera seu Calvatia* ; those medicinlas of seeds or fruits, and heavy in property, are mostly downbearing and sinking, and *Fructus Perillae*, *Fructus Aurantii Immaturus*, *Concha Haliotidis*, and *Haematitum* are the examples. There is an exception: *Flos Inulae* is downbearing and sinking in nature, whereas *Fructus Viticis* is upbearing and floating.

3. The relationship between the four directions of upbearing, downbearing, floating and sinking and medicinal processing and combination

Medical processing: When stir-baked with liquor, medicinals may become upbearing; while, stir-baked with ginger extract, they may become astringent, stir-baked with vinegar, they may become dispersing, and if stir-baked with ginger extract, salty water, they may become descending to the kidney.

Combination: *Radix Platycodi* can load medicinals floating, and *Radix Achyranthis Bidentatae* can lead medicinals declining. In addition, when upbearing or floating medcinals are used in combination with more downbearing or sinking medicinals, they may also descend; when downbearing or sinking medicinals used in combination with more upbearing or floating medicinals, they may also upbearing.

Meridian Tropism

The theory of meridian tropism is based on the theories of viscera and bowels, and meridians and col laterals. The viscera and bowels have their own specific physiological functions and pathological changes, and the meridians and collaterals connect all the parts of body into a whole. The exterior evils contracted the superficial skin transfer into the viscera and bowels along with the meridians and collaterals, while the pathological changes of viscera and bowels are also with reflected in the superficial skin along the meridians and collaterals. In clinical practice, one should firstly dinstinguish the viscera and bowels and the meridians and collaterals where the pathological changes exist, and then apply relative medicinals to exert treatment.

For example, cough is a symptom relates to the lung meridian, *Semen Armeniacae Amarum* and *Fructus Perillae*, which have functions of calming panting and suppressing cough, belong to the lung meridian; swelling pain in the hypochondrium belongs to the liver meridian, *Radix Bupleuri* and *Rhizoma Cyperi*, which soothe the liver qi, belong to the liver meridian; palpitation is related to the heart meridian, *Cinnabaris* and *Poria cum Radice Pino* have the functions of settling the heart and quieting the spirit, belong to the heart meridian; the symptoms of decreased food intake and loose stool are related to the spleen meridian, *Radix Codonopsis* and *Rhizoma Atractylodis Macrocephalae* tonify the middle and nourish the spleen, and belong to the spleen meridian; the lower back pain and seminal emission are related to the kidney meridian, *Radix Rehmanniae Praeparata* and *Semen Cuscutae*, which nourish the kidney and consolidate essence, belong to the kidney meridian. The theory of meridian tropism has the following principles:

（四）有毒无毒

历代本草书籍中，常在每一味药物的性味之下，标明其"有毒"、"无毒"。如《神农本草经》将所载 365 种药分为上、中、下三品，上品无毒，中品无毒或有小毒，下品多毒，不可久服。又如《素问·五常政大论篇》云："大毒治病，十去其六；常毒治病，十去其七；小毒治病，十去其八；无毒治病，十去其九；谷肉果菜，食养尽之，无使过之，伤其正也。"把药物毒性强弱分为大毒、常毒、小毒三类。

对于中药的毒性必须正确对待。历代本草对药物毒性的记载由于受历史条件的限制，也出现了不少错误，如《本经》中把朱砂列为首药，视为上品无毒；《本草纲目》认为马钱子无毒；《中国药学大辞典》认为桃仁无毒等。这表明对药物毒性的认识是一个随着临床经验的积累逐步加深的过程。

二、中药的应用

应用中药，除了必须掌握每一药物的性能以外，对于它的配伍、用量以及炮制也必须有所了解。否则，药物配伍不当、用量不合适、炮制后药性变化等，可影响药效。

（一）配伍

配伍就是按照病情需要和药物性能，有选择地将两种以上的药物合在一起应用。有些药物配伍后因协同作用而增进疗效，但是也有些药物配伍后却可能互相对抗而抵消、削弱原有的功效；有些药物因为相互配用而减轻或消除了毒性或副作用，但是也有些药物反而因为相互作用而使作用减弱或发生不利人体的作用等。归纳为七种情况，叫做药性"七情"，内容如下：

1. 单行　就是单用一味药来治疗疾病。例如用一味马齿苋治疗痢疾；独参汤单用一味人参大补元气、治疗虚脱等。

2. 相须　就是功用相类似的药物，配合应用后可以起到协同作用，加强了药物的疗效，如石膏、知母都能清热泻火，配合应用作用更强；大黄、芒硝都能泻下通便，配用后作用更为明显等。

3. 相使　就是用一种药物作为主药，配合其他药物来提高主药的功效。如脾虚水肿，用黄芪配合茯苓，可加强益气健脾利水的作用；胃火牙痛，用石膏清胃火，再配合牛膝引火下行，促使胃火牙痛更快地消除。

4. 相畏　就是一种药物的毒性或其他有害作用能被另一种药抑制或消除。如生半夏有毒性，可以用生姜来消除它的毒性。

If a medicinal belongs to many meridians, the range of indications can be expanded. For example, *Semen Armeniacae Amarum* belongs to the lung and large intestine meridians, so it not only can calm panting and suppress cough, but also moisten the intestine and relax bowels; *Gypsum Fibrosum* belongs to the lung and stomach meridians, so it not only can clear heat of the lung, but also purge fire of the stomach.

The medicinals belongs to the same meridian, have the different functions, such as warm, clear, tonifying and eliminating. For example, all the medicinals below belong to the lung meridian: *Radix Scutellariae* clears the fire of the lung, *Rhizoma Zingiberis* warms the lung and dispels cold, *Bulbus Lilii* tonifies the deficiency of the lung, *Semen Lepidii seu Descurainiae* purges the excess of the lung; all the medicinals as below belong to the liver meridian: *Radix Gentianae* purges the liver fire, *Rhizoma Cyperi* soothes the liver qi, *Fructus Corni* astringes the essence of the liver, and *Colla Corii Asini* nourishes the blood of the liver.

Select medicinals according to the relationships between viscera and bowels and meridians. Because the pathological changes of viscera and bowels and meridians influence each other, using medicinals of a specific meridian is not common in clinical practice. For example, the lung diseases concurrent with the deficiency of the spleen, *Rhizoma Dioscoreae* and *Poria* may be chosen to tonify the lung and spleen; in case of hyperactivity of the liver-yang concurrent with deficiency of kidney yin, *Radix Rehmanniae Praeparata* and *Radix Scrophulariae* can be added to nourish yin of the liver and kidney.

Meridian conductor: meridian conductor is originally called as meridian courier, or meridian guide. It refers to certain medicinal that can lead the actions of the other medicinals to a certain meridian or directly to the location of the disease, and the action is named as meridian conduction. It means that the meridian conductor can not only treat diseases of the pertained meridian, but also lead the medicinals which do not belong to the certain meridian to the certain meridian, so as to reinforce the therapeutic effects.

Toxicity or no toxicity

In the ancient books on CMM, the items of "toxicity" and "no toxicity" are always tagged beneath the items of the nature and flavor of each medicinal. For example, *Shennong's Classic of Materia Medica* divided 365 medicinals into three kinds, the upper grade, the middle grade and the lower grade. The medicinals belonging to the upper grade has no toxicity, the middle grade has no toxicity or mild toxicity, and the lower grade has toxicity, and cannot be intaked for long time. The chapter 17 in *Plain Questions* says, " the medicinals with severe toxicity can reduce sixty percent of diseases, the medicinals with the nomal toxicity can reduce seventy percent of diseases, the mild toxicity can reduce the eighty percent of diseases, the medicinals with notoxicity can reduce the ninety percent of diseases, " which divides the degrees of toxicity into severe toxicity, nomal toxicity and mild toxicity.

We should properly deal with the toxicity of CMM. Due to historical limitation, many errors are found in the records of the toxicity of medicinals in the ancient books. For example, *Cinnabaris* was considered as the sovereign medicinal without toxicity in *Shennong's Classic of Materia Medica* ; *Semen Strychni* was considered of not oxicity in *Compendium of Materia Medica* ; *Semen Persicae* was considered of not oxicity in *Dictionary of Chinese Pharmaceutical*, and so on. These demonstrate that the acknowledgement of the toxicity of medicinals is a progressively process along with the accumulation of clinical practice.

Application of Chinese Materia Medica

When applying CMM, one should master its combination, dosage and medical processing, besides the nature and functions of each medicinal. Otherwise, changes after inappropriate combination, dosage, and medical processing will adversely affect therapeutic effects.

Combination

Combination is based on the specific need of syndromes and characteristics of medicinals. The combination refers to two or more medicinals are selectively combined together, to reach the purpose of reinfor-

5．相杀　就是一种药能消除另一种药物的毒性反应。如防风能解砒霜毒、绿豆能减轻巴豆毒性等。

6．相恶　就是两种药配合应用以后，一种药可以减弱另一种药物的药效。如人参能大补元气，配合莱菔子同用，就会减弱补气的功能等。

7．相反　就是两种药物配合应用后，可能发生剧烈的副作用。

相须、相使，是临床用药尽可能加以考虑的，以便使药物更好地发挥疗效。相畏、相杀，是临床使用毒性药物或具有副作用药物时要加以注意的。相恶、相反则是临床用药配伍禁忌。

（二）用药禁忌

用药禁忌包括以下四方面内容：

1．配伍禁忌　最早称"相恶"、"相反"，后世金元时期进一步总结为"十八反"和"十九畏"，影响较大，沿用至今。

十八反是在相反基础上形成的一组最为严格的配伍禁忌：

"本草明言十八反，半蒌贝蔹芨攻乌；藻戟遂芫俱战草，诸参辛芍叛藜芦。"

注：乌头（川乌、附子、草乌）反半夏、瓜蒌（全瓜蒌、瓜蒌皮、瓜蒌仁、天花粉）、贝母（川贝、浙贝、土贝母）、白蔹、白芨；甘草反海藻、大戟、甘遂、芫花；藜芦反人参、沙参、丹参、玄参、苦参、细辛、芍药（赤芍、白芍）。

十九畏是与十八反相仿的配伍禁忌，形成较晚，或可认为禁忌程度较十八反略轻。但不论十八反，还是十九畏，我国药典均列为不宜同用的配伍。

十九畏：硫磺原是火中精，朴硝一见便相争；水银莫与砒霜见，狼毒最怕密陀僧；巴豆性烈为最上，偏与牵牛不顺情；丁香莫与郁金见，牙硝难合荆三棱；川乌草乌不顺犀，人参最怕五灵脂；官桂善能调冷气，若逢石脂便相欺。大凡修合看顺逆，炮爁炙煿莫相依。

2．妊娠禁忌　妊娠期间服用某些药物，可引起胎动不安，甚至造成流产。根据药物对胎儿及母体影响程度大小，分禁用与慎用两类。

禁用药多为剧毒或药性峻猛，如水银、雄黄、砒霜、斑蝥、轻粉、马钱子、蟾酥、水蛭、虻虫、三棱、莪术、大戟、生附子、巴豆、牵牛子、藜芦、瓜蒂、芫花、甘遂、商陆、麝香、冰片、干漆、胆矾等。

慎用药常为辛热刺激之品，和/或具有活血祛瘀、破气行滞、攻下通便作用，如牛膝、川芎、桃仁、红花、姜黄、丹皮、王不留行、枳实、大黄、芒硝、番泻叶、芦荟、冬葵子、制附子、肉桂等。

凡禁用药都不能使用，慎用药则应根据孕妇病情酌情使用。可用可不用时，应尽

cing the therapeutic effects, or relatively neutralize or reduce efficacies, reducing or removing the toxicity or side-effect, or reinforcing the toxicity and side-effect. The combination relationships between medicinals are classified into seven groups, which are called "seven emotions" of medicinal natures. They are explained in details as follows:

1. Single usage

Single usage means using a single medicinal to treat diseases. For example, using the single medicinal *Herba Portulacae* to treat dysentery; using the single medicinal *Radix Ginseng* as "Single Ginseng Decoction" to replenish vigor qi and treat collapse.

2. Mutual reinforcement

Mutual reinforcement refers to the combination that medicinals with similar functions are used together to exert the cooperation and reinforce certain therapeutic effects. For example, both *Gypsum Fibrosum* and *Rhizoma Anemarrhenae* can clear heat and purge fire, the effects of the combination of these two medicinals are much more powerful; both *Radix et Rhizoma Rhei* and *Natrii Sulfas* can purge heat and relax the bowels, and when combined together the effects are much more significant.

3. Mutual assistance

Mutual assistance refers to taking one medicinal as the chief, and combined with other medicinals to enforce the chief's functions. For example, when treating edema due to the spleen deficiency, using *Poria* combined with *Radix Astragali* will reinforce the functions of tonifying spleen qi and inducing diuresis; when treating toothache due to stomach fire, *Gypsum Fibrosum* which is used to clearing fire, is combined with *Radix Achyranthis Bidentatae* which directs fire downwards, so as to relieve the toothache due to stomach fire faster.

4. Mutual restraint

Mutual restraint refers to the toxicity or side-effect of one medicinal can be reduced or removed by another medicinal. For example, the raw material of *Rhizoma Pinelliae* has toxicity, which can be reduced or be removed by *Rhizoma Zingiberis Recens*.

5. Mutual suppression

When one medicinal can reduce toxicity of another medicinal, it is called mutual suppression. For example, *Radix Saposhnikoviae* can remove the toxicity of *Arsenicum Trioxidum*, and *Semen Phaseoli Radiati* can reduce the toxicity of *Semen Crotonis*.

6. Mutual inhibition

Mutual inhibition means when two medicinals are combined together, one medicinal can reduce the efficacies of the other medicinal. For example, *Radix Ginseng* can replenish vigor qi, when combined with *Semen Raphani*, the function of replenishing qi will be weakened.

7. Mutual antagonism

Mutual antagonism refers to the combination that two medicinals used together might result in drastic side-effects.

Mutual reinforcement and mutual assistance should be considered during the process of clinical practice, in order that the medicinals achieve better therapeutic effects. Generally speaking, when using combination, mutual restraint and mutual suppression should be paid attention when using medicinals with toxicity and side-effects. Mutual inhibition and mutual antagonism should be prohibited and forbidden.

Precaution

Precaution includes the following three aspects:

1. Prohibited combination

The prohibited combinations mainly refer to medicinals which are in mutual inhibition and mutual antagonism. Presently, the commonly acknowledged and widely influential prohibited combinations in TCM

量避免使用，以免发生事故。

3. 饮食禁忌 饮食禁忌简称食忌，也就是通常所说的忌口。在服药期间，一般应忌食生冷、辛热、油腻及有刺激性的食物。具体应用时，要结合病情和治疗需要调整，如寒证忌生冷；热证忌辛热油腻；肝阳上亢者忌辣椒、胡椒、葱、蒜、酒等辛热上行之品；脾胃虚弱者忌油腻、生冷及不易消化食物等。

（三）中药的用量

中药确定用量的一般原则是：

1. 根据药物性能确定用量 凡有毒的、峻烈的药物用量宜小，如乌头、雄黄之类；质重的药物用量要大，如代赭石、牡蛎等；质轻的用量宜轻，如蝉蜕；芳香类药物用量宜轻，如丁香、檀香。

2. 根据病情确定用量 病情轻或慢性病，用量宜轻；病情深重顽固用量宜大；还有些药轻用、重用作用不同，如柴胡升阳宜轻用、疏肝宜重用。

3. 根据配伍、剂型确定用量 一味单用，用量宜重，复方配伍，用量宜轻。方中主药用量宜重，辅药用量宜轻；汤剂用药宜重，丸散剂用量宜轻。

4. 根据病人性别、年龄、体质确定用量 妇女、老年、体弱、儿童用量宜轻，男子、体壮、年轻者用量宜重。

5. 根据季节、自然环境因素确定用量 在夏季，发汗解表药用量宜小，苦寒泻火药适当加量；在寒冷地区温性药物比温热地区用量宜重。

are"the eighteen antagonisms"and"the nineteen incompatibilities,"proposed from the Jin and Yuan Dynasties.

The eighteen antagonisms are based on mutual antagonism, and are the strictest antagonisms:

Radix Aconiti antagonizes *Radix Phielliae*, *Fructus Trichosanthis*, *Bulbus Fritillariae Cirrhosae*, *Radix Ampelopsis*, and *Rhizoma Bletillae*; *Radix Glycyrrhizae* is antagnonistic to *Sargassum*, *Radix Euphorbiae Pekinensis*, *Radix Kansui*, and *Flos Genkwa*; *Rhizoma et Radix Veratri* antagonizes *Radix Ginseng*, *Radix Adenophorae*, *Radix Salviae Miltiorrhizae*, *Radix Scrophulariae*, *Herba Asari*, and *Radix Paeoniae Lactiflorae*.

The nineteen incompatibilities are the similar combination with eighteen antagonisms. Nineteen incompatibilities were formed later, and are considered milder than eighteen antagonisms. However, both of them are inadvisable combination in China Pharmacopoeia.

The nineteen incompatibilities are:

Sulfur is incompatible with *Natrii Sulfas*; Hydrargyrum is incompatible with Arsenicum; *Radix Euphorbiae Fischerianae* is incompatible with Lithargyrum; *Fructus Crotonis* is incompatible with *Semen Pharbitidis*; *Flos Caryophylli* is incompatible with *Radix Curcumae*; *Radix Aconiti* and *Radix Aconiti Kusnezoffii* are incompatible with *Cornu Rhinocerotis*; *Nitrum Depuratum* is incompatible with *Rhizoma Sparganii*; *Radix Ginseng* is incompatible with *Faeces Trogopterori*; and *Cortex Cinnamomi* is incompatible with *Halloysitum Rubrum*.

2. Contraindication during pregnancy

Certain medicinals may cause fetal irritability, even embryotocia, if they are used during the period of pregnancy. According to the degrees of these medicinals affecting fetus and pregnant women, such medicinals are divided into two types to be avoided completely or to be given cautiously.

Medicinals to be avoided during pregnancy are always with severe toxicity or strong efficacies, such as mercury, *Realgar*, *Arsenicum Trioxidum*, *Mylabris*, *Calomelas*, *Semen Strychni*, *Venenum*, *Hirudo*, *Tabanus*, *Rhizoma Sparganii*, *Rhizoma Curcumae Zedoariae*, *Radix Knoxiae*, *Radix Aconiti Lateralis*, *Semen Crotonis*, *Semen Pharbitidis*, *Veratrum nigrum Linn*, *Melon pedicle*, *Flos Genwa*, *Radix Kansui*, *Radix Phytolaccae*, *Moschus*, *Borneolum*, *Lacca Toxicodendri Verniciflne*, and *Alumen*.

Medicinals given cautiously during pregnence are mainly pungent in flavor and hot in nature, and/or with the functions of promoting circulation of blood and removing stasis, breaking qi and driving stagnation, purging conspitation, such as *Radix Achyranthis Bidentatae*, *Rhizoma Chuanxiong*, *Semen Persicae*, *Flos Carthami*, *Rhizoma Curcumae Longae*, *Cortex Moutan*, *Semen Vaccariae*, *Fructus Aurantii Immaturus*, *Radix et Rhizoma Rhei*, *Natrii Sulfas*, *Folium Sennae*, *Aloe*, *Fructus Malvae*, *Radix Aconiti Lateralis Praeparata*, and *Cortex Cinnamomi*.

3. Dietary incompatibility

Diatary incompatibility also known as"Jikou", and is the commonly known as forbidden food. During the period of taking CMM, raw and cold, spicy and hot, greasy, and pungent foods are forbidden. During the specific application, some adjustion should be taken according to the conditions and treatment. For example, raw and cold foods should be forbidden for cold syndromes; pungent, hot and fatty foods should be forbidden for heat syndromes; chili, pepper, onion, garlic and wine should be forbidden for hyperactivity of the liver yang; fatty, raw and cold foods, and foods hard to digest are forbidden for patients with weakeness of the spleen and stomatch.

Dosage

The dosage of a medicinal is decided by the following principles:

1. According to the properties of medicinals

Medicinals of toxicity and strong efficacies should be used in a relatively smaller dose, such as *Radix Aconiti* and *Realgar*; heavy medicinals should be used in a relatively larger dose, such as *Haematitum* and

第二节 中药各论

一、解表药

凡以发散表邪为主要功效，治疗表证为主的药物，称为解表药。解表药药味多辛，具辛散发汗作用。解表药可分为辛温解表药和辛凉解表药两类。使用解表药应注意以下几点：发汗过多可损耗阳气和津液，因此要注意中病即止，避免发汗太过；凡自汗、盗汗、热病后期或因吐泻津液亏耗、阴虚发热者忌用；久病体虚、阴血亏耗等，都应忌用；解表药多为辛散之品，入汤剂不宜久煎。

（一）辛温解表药

辛温解表药也称发散风寒药，性味辛温，主要具有发散风寒作用，发汗作用较强，适用于外感风寒表证，症见恶寒发热、无汗、鼻塞或流清涕、头痛、身痛、舌苔薄白、脉浮紧等。部分药物也应用于风寒湿痹、咳喘、水肿、风疹、麻疹等兼具表证者。

麻 黄

【药用】本品为麻黄科植物草麻黄（*Ephedra sinica Stapf*）、中麻黄（*Ephedra intermedia Schrenk et C. A. Mey.*）或木贼麻黄（*Ephedra equisetina Bge.*）的干燥草质茎。秋季采割绿色的草质茎，晒干。

【性味】辛、微苦，温。

【归经】归肺、膀胱经。

【功效】发汗散寒，宣肺平喘，利水消肿。

【临床应用】

1. 用于外感风寒表实证，常与桂枝相须为用，以增强发汗之力。

2. 用于肺气不宣导致的咳嗽、气喘，常与杏仁同用。

3. 用于水肿兼表证者，常与白术、生姜等同用。

【用量用法】2~9g，煎服。解表发汗宜生用；平喘止咳多炙用。

【使用注意】表虚自汗、阴虚盗汗及肾不纳气致喘咳者均忌用；失眠及高血压者慎用。

Concha Ostreae ; light medicinals should be used in a relatively smaller dose , such as *Periostracum Cicadae* ; and the medicinals with aroma should be used in a relatively smaller dose , such as *Flos Caryophylli* and *Lignum Santali Albi*.

2. According to the conditions

For mild diseases and chronic diseases , the dosage should be smaller ; for severe diseases and long lasting diseases , the dosage should be larger. As for certain medicinals , their functions between large dose and small dose are different , for example , when using *Radix Bupleuri* , a smaller dosage should be used with the purpose of ascending yang , while a larger dosage for the purpose of soothing the liver.

3. According to combination and form

If the medicinal is used alone then it should be used in large dose ; if the medicinal is used as compound formula , then it should be used in a small dose ; the chief medicinals should be used in large dose and the assistant medicinals should be used in small dose ; medicinals in docotion should be used in large dose , medicinals in pills or powders should be used in small dose.

4. According to gender , age and conditions of patients

For women , the elderly , the weak and children , the medicinals should be used in small dose ; for men , the strong and the young , the medicinals should be used in large dose.

5. According to the season and natural environment

In summer , the medicinals with the functions of exterior-releasing and promoting sweating should be used in small dose , while the medicinals with the functions of purging fire could be used in larger dose ; the medicinals of warm nature should be used in larger dose in cold regions than that in warm regions.

Section 2   Materia Medica

Exterior-Releasing Medicinals

Medicinals with the major efficacy to disperse exterior pathogens , and treat the exterior syndromes are known as exterior-releasing medicinals. Such medicinals are usually pungent in flavor , and have the functions of dispersing and promoting sweating. They are classified into two groups , pungent-warm exterior-releasing medicinals and pungent-cool exterior-releasing medicinals. Some precaution should be noted when using the exterior-releasing medicinals. Excessive sweating may consume yang qi and body fluid , thus , the treatment of sweating should be stopped as soon as the disease is cured to avoid excessive sweating. The medicinals are contraindicated for cases of spontaneous sweating , nocturnal sweating , the end stage of warm disease , and asthenic heat syndrome due to vomiting and diarrhea which result in consumption of body fluid ; in addition , the medicinals are contraindicate to the deficiency syndromes due to chronic diseases and depletion of yin and blood. Most of the exterior-releasing medicinals are pungent and dispersing , and should not be decocted for long time.

Pungent-warm exterior-releasing medicinals

Pungent-warm exterior-releasing medicinals are also called wind-cold dispersing medicinals , which are pungent in flavor and warm in nature , and have the functions of dispersing wind-cold and strongly promoting sweating , which are used to treat the exterior syndromes of wind-cold , manifested as aversion to cold , no sweating , nasal congestion , headache , pain in the whole body , white and thin tongue coating , floating and tense pulse. Some of the medicinals are also indicated for wind-cold-dampness impediment , cough and asthma , edema , roseolla and measles , which are concurrent with the exterior syndromes.

Herba Ephedrae (Ma Huang)

【 Source 】It is the dried stem or branch of herbal-like shrublets of *Ephedra sinica Stapf* , *E. intermedia*

桂 枝

【药用】本品为樟科植物肉桂（*Cinnamomum cassia Presl*）的干燥嫩枝。春夏两季采收，除去叶，晒干，或切片晒干。

【性味】辛、甘，温。

【归经】归心、肺、膀胱经。

【功效】发汗解表，祛风湿，温通经脉，通阳利水，温通胸阳。

【临床应用】

1. 用于风寒表证，不论有汗、无汗都可应用。如风寒表实证无汗，与麻黄相须配伍以助发汗；如风寒表虚证有汗，则配伍白芍以调和营卫。

2. 用于风寒湿痹，常配伍附子、羌活、防风等。

3. 用于经寒血滞导致的月经不调、经闭、痛经等证，常与当归、川芎、桃仁等配伍使用。

4. 用于阳虚兼水湿停滞导致的痰饮证，常与茯苓、白术等配伍。

5. 用于膀胱气化不利导致的小便不利、水肿等证，常与茯苓、猪苓、泽泻等同用。

6. 用于心阳不振导致的胸痹、胸痛，常与瓜蒌、薤白等配伍使用。

【用量用法】3～9g，煎服。

【使用注意】温热病及阴虚阳盛、血热妄行诸证均忌用，孕妇及月经过多者慎用。

本类药还有防风、紫苏、白芷、苍耳子、辛夷、生姜、藁本、香薷等。

Schrenk et C.A.Mey, or *Ephedra equisetina Bge*.The green herbal stem is collected and dried in autumn.

【Taste and Nature】Acrid, slightly bitter, warm.

【Meridian Entry】Lung and urinary bladder meridians.

【Function】Promote sweating and dispel cold, disffuse the lung and relieve asthma, promote diuresis and relieve edema.

【Indications】

1. It is indicated for excess syndrome due to exterior wind-cold, it is often used together with *Ramulus Cinnamomi*, to enforce the power of promoting sweating.

2. For cough and asthma due to dysfunction of the lung, it is often used together with *Semen Armeniacae Amarum*.

3. For edema with exterior syndrome, it is commonly used together with *Rhizoma Atractylodis Macrocephalae* and *Rhizoma Zingiberis Recens*.

【Preparation and Dosage】2-9g, decoct.Crude for promoting sweating and reliving the exterior; often prepared for relieving asthma and cough.

【Precaution】Contraindicated for patients with spontaneous sweating due to exterior deficiency or yin deficiency, and cough and asthma due to the syndrome of kidney failing to receive qi; and with caution for patients with insomnia or hypertension.

Ramulus Cinnamomi (Gui Zhi)

【Source】It is the dried tender twig of *Cinnamomum cassia Prsel*, it is collected in summer and autumn, leaves are cut off, and dried in the sun, or cut into small segments and dried in the sun.

【Taste and Nature】Acrid and sweet, warm.

【Meridian Entry】Heart, lung and urinary bladder meridians.

【Function】Promote sweating and dispel cold, dispel wind-dampness, warm the meridians, warm and invigorate yang to promote diuresis, warm and free yang in the chest.

【Indications】

1. It is indicated for exterior syndrome due to wind-cold, either with or without sweating.For exterior excess syndrome of wind-cold without sweating, it is often combined with *Herba Ephedrae*.For exterior dcfi ciency syndrome with sweating, it is often combined with *Radix Paeoniae Alba* in order to harmonize the nutrient and the defense.

2. For impediment caused by the invasion of wind, cold, dampness, it is often prescribed with *Radix Aconiti Lateralis Praeparata*, *Rhizoma et Radix Notopterygii*, and *Radix Ledebouriellae*.

3. For irregular menstruation, amenorrhea and menorrhalgia due to cold in the meridians and blood stasis, it is often used with *Radix Angelicae Sinensis*, *Rhizoma Chuanxiong*, and *Flos Carthami*.

4. For retention of phlegm and fluid due to deficiency and retention of fluid and dampness, it is often used together with *Poria* and *Rhizoma Atractylodis Macrocephalae*.

5. For dysfunction of the urinary baldder marked by dysuria and edema, it is often used togetther with *Poria*, *Polyporus Umbellatus*, and *Rhizoma Alismatis*.

6. For chest impediment and chest pain due to heart yang deficiency, it is often used together with *Fructus Trichosanthis* and *Bulbus Allii Macrostemonis*.

【Preparation and dosage】3-9g, decoct.

【Precaution】It is contraindicated for febrile diseases, cases of yin deficiency and yang excess, and bleeding due to blood heat; for pregnant women and women with menorrhagia, it should be used cautiously.

In this category, there are more medicinals such as *Radix Saposhnikoviae*, *Folium Perillae*, *Radix Angelicae Dahuricae*, *Fructus Xanthii*, *Flos Magnoliae*, *Rhizoma Zingiberis Recens*, *Rhizoma et Radix Ligusti-*

（二）辛凉解表药

辛凉解表药也称发散风热药，性味辛凉，主要具有疏散风热作用，发汗作用较缓和，适用于外感风热表证，症见发热、微恶风寒、咽干口渴、有汗或无汗，舌苔薄黄、脉浮数。部分药物配伍后也应用于风热咳嗽、麻疹不透及疮疡初起兼表证者。

柴　胡

【药用】本品为伞形科植物柴胡（*Bupleurum chinense DC.*）或狭叶柴胡（*Bupleurum scorzonerifolium Willd.*）的干燥根。春秋二季采挖，除去茎叶及泥沙，干燥。

【性味】苦，微寒。

【归经】入肝、胆经。

【功效】和解退热，疏肝解郁，升举阳气。

【临床应用】

1. 用于表证发热，常与葛根、羌活等同用。

2. 用于邪在半表半里，症见寒热往来的少阳证，常与黄芩同用；治疗疟疾可与青蒿、黄芩等同用。

3. 用于肝气郁结导致的胁肋胀痛、月经不调等，常与当归、白芍、郁金等药同用。

4. 用于气虚下陷导致的脱肛、胃下垂、子宫下垂等证，常配伍黄芪、升麻等。

【用量用法】3~9g，煎服。

薄　荷

【药用】本品为唇形科植物薄荷（*Mentha haplocalyx Briq.*）的干燥地上部分。夏秋二季分次采收，阴干。

【性味】辛，凉。

【归经】归肺、肝经。

【功效】疏散风热，清头目，利咽喉，透疹，疏肝解郁。

【临床应用】

1. 用于风热感冒、温病初起，常与荆芥、金银花、连翘等配伍应用。

2. 用于风热上扰导致的头痛、目赤、咽喉肿痛，常配伍菊花、荆芥、桑叶、桔梗等。

3. 用于小儿麻疹，常与荆芥、牛蒡子、蝉衣等同用。

ci , and *Herba Elsholtziae.*

Pungent-cool exterior releasing medicinals

Pungent-cool exterior releasing medicinals are also called wind-heat dispersing medicinals. The medicinals are pungent in flavor and cold , and have the functions of dispersing wind-heat and mildly promoting sweating , which are applicable to the exterior syndrome of wind-heat , manifested as fever , mildly aversion to cold , dry throat , thirst , sweating or without sweating , thin and yellow tongue coating , floating and rapid pulse. Some of the medicinals are also applicable for cough due to wind-heat , non-eruption of measles or early stage of sore and ulcer concurrent with the exterior syndromes.

Radix Bupleuri (Chai Hu)

【Source】It refers to the dried root of *Bupleurum chinense DC. Pr Bupleurum scorzonerifolium Willd.* It is collected in spring and autumn , and dried after cutting off the stem and the leaf , removing sands.

【Taste and Nature】Bitter , slightly cold.

【Meridian Entry】Liver and gallbladder meridians.

【Function】Relieve exterior syndrome and subdue fever , soothe the liver and relieve the qi stagnation , lift yang qi.

【Indications】

1. It is indicated for fever from exterior syndrome , and commonly used together with *Radix Perariae* and *Rhizoma seu Radix Notopterygii.*

2. It is indicated for shaoyang syndrome marked by alternating chills and fever , which pathogenic factor exists in half-exterior half-interior , and it is often prescribed with *Radix Scutellariae.* For malaria , it is often used with *Herba Artemisiae Annuae* and *Radix Scutellariae.*

3. For fullness in the chest and epigastrium , hypochondriac pain and irregular menstruation due to liver qi stagnation , it is often used with *Radix Angelicae Sinensis* , *Radix Paeoniae Alba* , and *Radix Curcumae.*

4. For gastroptosis , prolapse of the anus and uterus due to qi deficiency , it is often used with *Radix Astragali* , and *Rhizoma Cimicifugae.*

【Preparation and dosage】3–9 g , decoct.

Herba Menthae (Bo He)

【Source】*Herba Menthae* refers to the dried stem and leaf of the perennial herb *Mentha haplocalyx Briq.* , and it is collected twice yearly in summer and autumn , dried in shadow.

【Taste and Nature】Acrid , cool.

【Meridian Entry】Lung and liver meridians.

【Function】Dispel wind-heat , purge heat from the head and eye , soothe the throat , promote rash eruption , soothe the liver qi and relieve the qi stagnation.

【Indications】

1. For common cold due to wind-heat and the early stage of warm disease , it is often used with *Herba Schizonepetae* , *Flos Lonicerae* , and *Fructus Forsythiae.*

2. For headache , congested eyes and sore throat , it is often prescribed with *Flos Chrysanthemi* , *Herba Schizonepetae* , *Folium Mori* , and *Radix Platycodi.*

3. For infantile measles , it is often used together with *Herba Schizonepetae* , *Fructus Arctii* , and *Periostracum Cicadae.*

4. For syndromes due to liver qi stagnation marked by fullness in the chest and hypochondriac pain , it is often used with *Radix Paeoniae Alba* and *Radix Bupleuri.*

4. 用于肝气郁滞导致的胸闷、胁肋胀痛，常与白芍、柴胡等同用。

【用量用法】3~6g，煎服，宜后下。

本类药还有桑叶、菊花、牛蒡子、升麻、蔓荆子、蝉蜕等。

二、清热药

凡以清解里热为主要功效，治疗热性病证为主的药物，称为清热药。清热药药性多为寒凉或平而偏凉，可分为清热泻火药、清热凉血药、清热解毒药、清热燥湿药、清虚热药等类。清热药性多寒凉，易伤脾胃阳气，脾胃虚弱者慎用，忌用于真寒假热证。

（一）清热泻火药

清热泻火药，性味多甘寒或苦寒，主要具有清火泻热作用，适用于外感热病之气分实热证，症见高热、汗出、烦渴、谵语、小便短赤、舌苔黄燥、脉洪实有力等，也应用于肺热、胃火、肝火、心火等脏腑实热证。

石　膏

【药用】本品为硫酸盐类矿物硬石膏族石膏，主含含水硫酸钙（$CaSO_4 \cdot 2H_2O$），采挖后，除去泥沙及杂石。

【性味与归经】甘、辛，大寒。

【归经】归肺、胃经。

【功效】清热泻火，除烦止渴。

【临床应用】

1. 用于温病气分热证，症见高热不退、大汗、口渴、烦躁、脉洪大等，常与知母相须为用。

2. 用于胃火亢盛导致的头痛、齿痛、牙龈肿痛等证，常配合知母、黄连、生地等同用。

3. 用于肺热咳喘，常与麻黄、杏仁、黄芩等同用。

4. 肺胃燥热导致口渴多饮，常与知母、天花粉等同用。

【用量与用法】15~60g，打碎，先煎。

【使用注意】脾胃虚寒和阴虚内热者忌用。

知　母

【药用】本品为百合科植物知母（*Anemarrhena asphodeloides Bge.*）的干燥根茎。春秋二季采挖，除去须根及泥沙，晒干。

【Preparation and dosage】3-9g, decoct later.

Other medicinals in this catergory include *Folium Mori*, *Flos Chrysanthemi*, *Fructus Arctii*, *Rhizoma Cimicifugae*, and *Periostracum Cicadae*.

Heat-Clearing Medicinals

Heat-clearing medicinals refer to the medicinals which major function is clearing interior heat, and are mainly indicated for heat syndromes. Heat-clearing medicinals are usually cold, cool or neutral in nature, and can be classified into five categories as follows: heat-clearing and fire-purging medicinal, heat-clearing and blood-cooling medicinal, heat-clearing and toxicity-relieving medicinal, heat-clearing and dampness-drying medicinal, deficiency heat-clearing medicinal. These medicinals usually are cold or cool in nature, therefore, they tend to consume the yang qi of the spleen and stomach, and should be cautiously used in patients with the deficiency of the spleen and stomach, and are contraindicated for the syndromes of true cold with false heat.

Heat-clearing and fire-purging medicinals

Heat-clearing and fire-purging medicinals are usually cold in nature and sweet or bitter in flavor, and have the functions of clearing heat and purging fire. These medicinals are applicable for the excessive syndrome of qi aspect heat, manifested as high fever, sweating, thirst, dysthesia, short voidings of reddish urine, dry and yellow tongue coating, surging, full and forceful pulse. These medicinals are also applicable for excessive heat syndromes of viscera and bowels, such as lung heat, stomach fire, liver fire and heart fire.

Gypsum Fibrosum (Shi Gao)

【Source】It refers to calcium sulfate mineral anhydrite that contains $CaSO_4 \cdot 2H_2O$. It can be mined anytime with muds and sands removed.

【Taste and Nature】Sweet and acrid, cold.

【Meridian Entry】Lung and stomach meridians.

【Function】Purge heat and fire, relieve restlessness and thirst.

【Indications】

1. For qi aspect heat syndrome of febrile diseases, marked by high fever, profuse sweating, thirst, restlessness, and bounding and large pulse, it is often used in combination with *Rhizoma Anemarrhenae*.

2. For heahache, toothache, and swelling and pain in the gum due to excessive stomach fire, it is often used together with *Rhizoma Anemarrhenae*, *Rhizoma Coptidis*, and *Radix Rehmanniae*.

3. For cough and ashma due to excessive lung heat, it is often used together with *Herba Ephedrae*, *Semen Armeniacae Amarum*, and *Radix Scutellariae*.

4. It is indicated for thirst and polydipsia due to dryness-heat of the lung and stomach, and it is often used with *Rhizoma Anemarrhenae* and *Radix Trichosanthis*.

【Preparation and dosage】15-60 g, smash to pieces, decoct first.

【Caution】Contraindicated for deficiency of the spleen and stamoch and internal fever due to yin deficiency.

Rhizoma Anemarrhenae (Zhi Mu)

【Source】It refers to the dried root of perennial herb *Anemarrhena asphodeloides Bge*. It is collected in spring and autumn, and dried in the sun with the fibrous roots and foreign matters removed.

【Taste and Nature】Bitter, sweet, cold.

【Meridian Entry】Lung, stomach and kidney meridians.

【性味与归经】苦，甘，寒。

【归经】归肺、胃、肾经。

【功效】清热泻火，滋阴润燥。

【临床应用】

1. 用于外感热病、高热烦渴及肺热喘咳、痰黄而稠，常和石膏相须配伍。

2. 用于阴虚导致的潮热盗汗、骨蒸等，常与生地、丹皮同用。

3. 用于肺虚燥咳、虚劳久咳，常配伍沙参、麦冬。

4. 用于内热伤津或消渴病，症见口渴多饮，常配伍天花粉、麦冬、葛根。

【用量用法】6~12g，煎服。

【使用注意】脾虚便溏者不宜使用。

本类药还有栀子、龙胆草、芦根、天花粉、淡竹叶、谷精草、夏枯草等。

（二）清热凉血药

清热凉血药性味多苦寒或咸寒，多归心、肝经，主要具有清热凉血作用，适用于血分实热证，外感热病热入营血，血热妄行，症见各种出血（如吐血、齿衄、便血、尿血等）、斑疹、心烦、舌绛甚或神昏谵语等。

生地黄

【药用】本品为玄参科植物地黄（*Rehmannia glutinosa Libosch.*）的干燥块根。秋季采挖，除去芦头、须根及泥沙，晒干或烘焙至约八成干。又称干地黄。

【性味】甘，寒。

【归经】归心、肝、肾经。

【功效】清热凉血，养阴生津。

【临床应用】

1. 用于温病热入营血，症见身热、口干、舌红绛、或身发斑疹、咽喉肿痛，常配伍玄参、丹皮、赤芍、水牛角等。

2. 用于血热妄行导致的吐血、衄血、尿血、崩漏等证，常配合丹皮、赤芍等。

3. 用于热病后期伤阴、阴虚内热或消渴病，症见骨蒸潮热、盗汗、口渴、咽干等，可与青蒿、鳖甲、知母等同用。

4. 用于肠燥便秘，常与麦冬、玄参、玉竹等同用。

【用量与用法】9~15g，煎服。

【使用注意】脾虚及湿阻中焦者慎用。

牡丹皮

【药用】本品为毛茛科植物牡丹（*Paeonia suffruticosa Andr.*）的干燥根皮。秋季采挖根部，除去细根，剥取根皮，晒干。

【Function】Purge heat and fire, nourish yin and moisten dryness.

【Indications】

1. For qi aspect heat syndrome of febrile diseases, marked by high fever and restlessness, it is used in combination with *Gypsum Fibrosum*.

2. It is often prescribed for tidal fever, nocturnal sweating and bone sweating due to yin deficiency, together with *Radix Rehmanniae* and *Cortex Moutan*.

3. For dry cough due to lung deficiency and chronic cough due to deficiency syndrome, it is often used together with *Radix Glehniae* and *Radix Ophiopogonis*.

4. For fluid consumption due to interior heat or diabetes, marked by thirst and polydipsia, it is often used with *Radix Trichosanthis*, *Radix Ophiopogonis*, and *Radix Scrophulariae*.

【Preparation and dosage】6−12 g, decoct.

【Caution】It should not be used in cases with loose stool due to spleen deficiency.

There are more medicinals in this catergory such as *Fructus Gardeniae*, *Radix Gentianae*, *Rhizoma Phragmitis*, *Radix Trichosanthis*, *Herba Lophatheri*, *Flos Eriocauli*, and *Spica Prunellae*.

Heat-clearing and blood-cooling medicinals

Heat-clearing and blood-cooling medicinals are usually cold in nature with bitter or salty flavor, and mainly enter the heart and liver meridians. These medicinals mainly have the functions of clearing heat and cooling blood, and are applicable for excessive heat of the blood aspect, heat entering the nutrient and blood aspect due to exterior pathogenic factors, bleeding due to blood heat, manifested as various symptomes of bleeding (such as, hematemesis, teeth bleeding, hemafecia, and hematuria), maculae, vexation, purple tongue, even clouded spirit and dilirious speech.

Radix Rehmanniae (Sheng Di Huang)

【Source】It is the dried root of perennial herb *Rehmannia glutinosa Libosch*. It is collected in autumn, and dried in the sun or baked with mild heat till it is 80% dry with the fibrous roots and foreign matters removed. Known as "Gan Di Huang" as well.

【Taste and Nature】Sweet, bitter.

【Meridian Entry】Heart, liver, and kidney meridians.

【Function】Purge heat and cool the blood, nourish yin and promote fluid secretion.

【Indications】

1. For heat in the nutrient aspect and/or blood aspect of febrile diseases, marked by fever, thirst, red tongue, or hematemesis, extravasation, swelling or pain in the throat, it is often used together with *Radix Scrophulariae*, *Cortex Moutan Radicis*, *Radix Paeoniae Rubra*, and *Cornu Bubali*.

2. For hematemesis, epistaxis, hematuria, and metrorrhagia due to heat in blood, it is often used with *Cortex Moutan Radicis* and *Radix Paeoniae Rubra*.

3. It is indicated for the end stage of febrile disease, interior heat due to yin deficiency or diabetes, which are marked by steaming bone, nocturnal sweating, thirst and dry throat; and it is often used together with *Herba Artemisiae Annuae*, *Carapax Trionycis*, and *Rhinzoma Anemarrhenae*.

4. For constipation due to dryness in the intestines, it is often used together with *Radix Ophiopogonis*, *Radix Scrophulariae*, and *Rhizoma Polygonati Odorati*.

【Preparation and dosage】9−15 g, decoct.

Cortex Moutan Radicis (Mu Dan Pi)

【Source】It is the dried root bark of deciduous shrublet *Paeonia suffruticosa Andr*. (*Fam Ranunculaceae*). The root is dug in autumn, the rootlets are removed and the bark is peeled, and then dried in the

【性味】苦、辛，微寒。

【归经】归心、肝、肾经。

【功效】清热凉血，活血散瘀。

【临床应用】

1. 用于温病热入营血而发斑疹以及血热妄行导致吐血、衄血、尿血等，常与水牛角、生地黄、赤芍等同用。

2. 用于血瘀导致经闭、痛经、癥瘕积聚，常与赤芍、桃仁、红花等同用。

3. 用于跌扑损伤、瘀滞疼痛，可与乳香、没药等配伍。

4. 用于疮痈肿毒、肠痈等证。治疗疮痈可配合大黄、金银花、连翘等。

【用量用法】6~12g，煎服。

【使用注意】血虚有寒及孕妇忌用；月经过多慎用。

本类药还有赤芍、玄参、紫草、水牛角、龙胆草等。

（三）清热解毒药

清热解毒药性味多苦寒，或辛寒、甘寒，主要具有清热解毒作用，适用于各种热毒病证，包括痈疮肿毒、丹毒、斑疹、痄腮、咽喉肿痛、肺痈、肠痈、热毒痢疾、水火烫伤和蛇虫咬伤等。

金银花

【药用】本品为忍冬科植物忍冬（*Lonicera japonica Thunb.*）、红腺忍冬（*Lonicera hypoglauca Miq.*）、山银花（*Lonicera confusa DC.*）或毛花桂忍冬（*Lonicera dasystyla Rehd.*）的干燥花蕾或带初开的花。夏初花开放前采收，干燥。

【性味】甘，寒。

【归经】归肺、心、胃经。

【功效】清热解毒，疏散风热。

【临床应用】

1. 用于外感风热表证或温病初起，常与连翘相须为用，并配伍薄荷、荆芥等。

2. 用于疮疡肿毒、咽喉肿痛、肠痈、乳痈、肺痈等，可与蒲公英、连翘、牡丹皮、赤芍等同用。

3. 用于热毒引起的泻痢便血、里急后重，可配伍黄连、赤芍、白头翁等。

【用量用法】6~15g，煎服。

【使用注意】脾胃虚寒及气虚疮疡不宜使用。

sun.

【Taste and Nature】Bitter, acrid, slightly cold.

【Meridian Entry】Heart, liver, and kidney meridians.

【Function】Purge heat and cool the blood, activate blood circulation, and remove stasis.

【Indications】

1. For macula due to heat invading the nutrient aspect or blood aspect in febrile diseases, hematemesis, epistaxis and hematuria due to blood heat, it is often used together with *Cornu Bubali*, *Radix Rehmanniae*, and *Radix Paeoniae Rubra*.

2. It is indicated for amenorrhea, dysmenorrhea, hard or soft masses in the abdomen due to boold stasis; and it is often used together with *Radix Paeoniae Rubra*, *Semen Persicae*, and *Flos Carthami*.

3. For contusions, sprain, and pain due to blood stasis, it is often used with *Oblibanum*, and *Myrrha*.

4. For carbuncle, abscess, swelling due to toxin and appendicitis, it is often used with *Radix et Rhizoma Rhei*, *Flos Lonicerae*, and *Fructus Forsythiae*.

【Preparation and dosage】6–12 g, decoct.

【Caution】The drug is contraindicated for cold syndrome due to blood deficiency, and preganent patients; it should be cautiously used in menorrhagia.

There are more medicinals in this catergory such as *Radix Paeoniae Rubra*, *Radix Scrophulariae*, *Radix Arnebiae seu Lithospermi*, *Cornu Bubali*, and *Radix Gentianae*.

Heat-clearing and toxicity-removing medicinals

Heat-clearing and toxicity-removing medicinals are usually cold in nature, and bitter, pungent or sweet in flavor. These medicinals have the functions of cleating heat and removing toxicity, and are applicable for ulcers and swelling, erysipelas, maculae, mumps, sore throat, lung abscess, intestinal abscess, dysentery due to heat toxin, burns and scalds, and worm and snake bites.

Flos Lonicerae (Jin Yin Hua)

【Source】*Flos Lonicerae* is the bud or early flower of the semi-evergreen twining shrub *Lonicera japonica Thunb.*, *Lonicera hypoglauca Miq.*, *Lonicera confusa DC.*, or *Lonicera dasystyla Rehd.* It is collected and dried in early summer before it blossoms.

【Taste and Nature】Sweet, cold.

【Meridian Entry】Lung, heart, stomach meridians.

【Function】Eliminate heat and toxicins and dispel wind-heat.

【Indications】

1. For exterior syndrome of wind-heat and early stage of febrile diseases, it is often prescribed in combination with *Fructus Forsythiae*, together with *Herba Menthae* and *Herba Schizonepetae*.

2. For carbuncles or swellings due to toxic heat, swelling and pain in throat, appendicitis, mastitis and lung abscess, it is used together with *Heba Taraxaci*, *Fructus Forsythiae*, *Cortex Moutan*, and *Radix Paeoniae*.

3. For dysentery with bloody discharge and tenesmus due to toxic heat, it is used together with *Rhizoma Coptidis*, *Radix Paeoniae Rubra*, and *Radix Pulsatillae*.

【Preparation and dosage】6–15 g, decoct.

【Caution】The drug is contraindicated for deficiency cold of the spleen and stomach and abscess due to qi dificiency.

连　翘

【药用】本品为木樨科植物连翘［*Forsythia suspensa*（*Thunb.*）*Vahl*］的干燥果实。秋季采收，晒干。

【性味】苦，微寒。

【归经】归肺、心、小肠经。

【功效】清热解毒，消肿散结。

【临床应用】

1. 用于外感风热表证或温病初起，常与金银花相须为用，并配伍薄荷、荆芥等。

2. 用于温病热入心包，症见高热神昏、烦躁，常与水牛角、黄连、莲子心、淡竹叶等同用。

3. 用于疮疡肿毒、瘰疬、丹毒、乳痈等证，常和金银花、玄参、夏枯草、蒲公英、贝母等同用。

【用量用法】6~15g，煎服。

【使用注意】脾胃虚寒及气虚疮疡不宜使用。

本类药还有蒲公英、大青叶、板蓝根、鱼腥草、败酱草、穿心莲、白花蛇舌草、射干、山豆根、蚤休、青黛、绿豆等。

（四）清热燥湿药

清热燥湿药性味多苦寒，主要具有清热燥湿作用，适用于湿热证，如湿温、暑湿以及痢疾、黄疸、湿疮、湿疹、带下、淋证、耳肿疼痛流脓等属湿热证者。清热燥湿药多兼泻火解毒作用，可用于各种脏腑实热证。

黄　连

【药用】本品为毛茛科植物黄连（*Coptis chinensis Franch.*）、三角叶黄连（*Coptis deltoidea C. Y. Cheng et Hsiao*）或云连［*Coptis teeta Wall.*）的干燥根茎。秋季采收，除去苗叶、须根，干燥。

【性味】苦，寒。

【归经】归心、脾、胃、肝、胆、大肠经。

【功效】清热燥湿，泻火解毒。

【临床应用】

1. 用于湿热阻滞中焦所致胸脘痞满、恶心呕吐、黄疸，常与黄芩、木香、半夏等同用；湿热泻痢，常配伍黄芩、葛根等。

2. 用于三焦热盛，症见高热、口渴烦躁、甚至神昏谵语，常与栀子、黄芩、黄柏、石膏等同用。

3. 用于热毒疮疡等证，可与赤芍、丹皮、玄参、金银花等同用。

Fructus Forsythiae (Lian Qiao)

【Source】It is the dried fruit of the deciduous shrublet *Forsythia suspensa(Thunb.) Vahl*.It is collected in autumn and dried in the sun.

【Taste and Nature】Acrid,slightly cold.

【Meridian Entry】Lung,heart and small intestine meridians.

【Function】Eliminate heat and toxicins and disperse swelling and binds.

【Indications】

1. For exterior syndrome of wind-heat and early stage of febrile diseases,it is often prescribed in combination with *Flos Lonicerae*,together with *Herba Menthae*,and *Herba Schizonepetae*.

2. For heat invading the pericardium syndrome of febrile disease,marked with high fever,coma and restlessness,it is used together with *Cornu Bubali*,*Rhizoma Coptidis*,*Plumula Nelumbinis*,and *Herba Lophatheri*.

3. For carbuncles or swellings due to toxic heat,scrofula,erysipelas,and acute mastitis,it is used together with *Flos Lonicerae*,*Radix Scrophulariae*,*Spica Prunellae*,*Herba Taraxaci*,and *Bulbus Fritillariae*.

【Preparation and dosage】6–15 g,decoct.

【Caution】The drug is contraindicated for deficiency cold of the spleen and stomach and abscess due to qi dificiency.

Other medicinals in this category, include *Herba Taraxaci*, *Folium Isatidis*, *Radix Isatidis*, *Herba Houttuyniae*,*Herba Patriniae*, *Herba Andrographitis*, *Herba Oldenlandiae*, *Rhizoma Belamcandae*, *Radix Sophorae Tonkinensis*,*Rhizoma Paridis*,*Indigo Naturalis*,and *Semen Phaseoli Radiati*.

Heat-clearing and dampness-drying medicinals

Heat-clearing and dampness-drying medicinals are usually cold in nature and bitter in flavor,mainly have the functions of clearing heat and drying dampness,and are applicable for syndromes of dampness-heat,such as dampness-warmth and summerheat-dampness, or dysentery,jaundice,dampness sore,eczema,leukorrhagia,strangury diseases,and pain and swelling in ears which pertain to dampness-heat syndrome.Most of the medicinals also have the functions of clearing heat and relieving toxicity,and are applicable for various excessive heat syndromes of viscera and bowels.

Rhizoma Coptidis (Huang Lian)

【Source】It is the dried rhizome of the perennial herb *Coptis chinensis Franch.* ,*Coptis deltoidea C.Y. Cheng et Hsiao*,or *Coptis teeta Wall*.It is collected in autumn and dried with the fibrous roots and foreign matters removed.

【Taste and Nature】Bitter,cold.

【Meridian Entry】Heart,spleen,stomach,liver,gallbladder,large intestine meridians.

【Function】Eliminate heat and dampness,purge fire and detoxicate toxin.

【Indications】

1. For fullness in chest and abdomen,nausea,vomiting,jaundice due to dampness-heat in the middle enerziger,it is often prescribed with *Radix Scutellariae*,*Radix Aucklandiae*,and *Rhizoma Pinelliae* ;for diarrhea and dysentery due to dampness-heat,it is often used with *Radix Scutellariae* and *Radix Puerariae*.

2. For excessive heat in three enerzigers,manifested with high fever,thirst,restlessness,or even coma and delirium,it is often used with *Fructus Gardeniae*,*Radix Scutellariae*,*Cortex Phellodendri*,and *Gypsum Fibrosum*.

4. 用于血热妄行导致的吐血、衄血等，可配伍黄芩、大黄等。

【用量用法】2~5g，煎服。

【使用注意】脾胃虚寒及阴虚津亏者慎用。

黄 芩

【药用】本品为唇形科植物黄芩（*Scutellaria baicalensis Georgi*）的干燥根。春秋二季采挖，除去残茎、须根，晒干。

【性味】苦，寒。

【归经】归肺、胆、脾、大肠、小肠经。

【功效】清热燥湿，泻火解毒，凉血安胎。

【临床应用】

1. 用于湿热病邪导致的多种病证。湿温证，症见发热、胸闷、口渴不欲饮，可与滑石、通草、茯苓等同用；湿热泻痢，常与黄连、葛根、白头翁同用；湿热黄疸，可配伍茵陈、栀子等；下焦湿热，可配伍生地黄、泽泻、瞿麦等。

2. 用于热病高热烦渴及热毒疮疡等证，常与黄连、栀子等配伍。

3. 用于肺热咳嗽，可与知母、桑白皮等同用。

4. 用于血热妄行导致的吐血、衄血、便血、崩漏等证，可与生地黄、牡丹皮、侧柏叶等同用。对热毒疮疡，可与银花、连翘等药同用。

此外，本品又有清热安胎作用，可用于胎动不安，常与白术、竹茹等配伍应用。

【用量用法】3~9g，煎服。

【使用注意】脾胃虚寒及阴虚津亏者慎用。

黄 柏

【药用】本品为芸香科植物黄皮树（*Phellodendron chinense Schneid.*）或黄檗（*Phellodendron amurense Rupr.*）的干燥树皮。

【性味】苦，寒。

【归经】归肾、膀胱经。

【功效】清热燥湿，泻火解毒，清虚热。

【临床应用】

1. 用于湿热下注导致的小便淋沥涩痛、赤白带下、阴部肿痛、足膝肿痛等证，可配伍黄芩、黄连、苍术、知母、泽泻、龙胆草等。

2. 用于湿热之邪导致的湿热黄疸、湿热泻痢、湿疹等证，内服配黄芩、黄连、栀子、茵陈等药同用，外用可配大黄、滑石等。

3. 用于阴虚发热、梦遗滑精等证，常与知母、生地黄等同用。

【用量用法】3~12g，煎服。

3. For carbuncles or swellings due to toxic heat, it can be used together with *Radix Paeoniae Rubra*, *Cortex Moutan*, *Radix Scrophulariae*, and *Flos Lonicerae*.

4. For hematemesis and bleeding due to heat in the blood, it is often used with *Radix Scutellariae*, and *Radix et Rhizoma Rhei*.

【Preparation and dosage】2-5 g, decoct.

【Caution】The drug is contraindicated for deficiency cold of the spleen and stomach, fluid consumption, and yin deficiency.

Radix Scutellariae (Huang Qin)

【Source】It is the dried root of the perennial herb *Scutellaria baicalensis Georgi*. It is collected in spring and autumn, dried in the sun with the fibrous roots and foreign matters removed.

【Taste and Nature】Bitter, cold.

【Meridian Entry】Lung, gallbladder, spleen, large intestine, small intestine meridians.

【Function】Eliminate heat and dampness, purge fire and detoxicate toxin, cool the blood, and prevent abortion.

【Indications】

1. It is indicated for various symptoms due to dampness-heat. In case of dampness-warmth syndrome, marked by fever, oppression in the chest, thirst with no desire of drinking water, it is prescribed with *Talcum*, *Medulla Tetrapanacis*, and *Poria* ; it is often prescribed with *Rhizoma Coptidis*, *Radix Puerariae*, and *Radix Pulsatillae* for dysentery due to dampness-heat; for jaundice due to dampness-heat, it is often prescribed with *Herba Artemisiae Scopariae*, and *Fructus Gardeniae* ; in case of lower energizer dampness-heat syndrome, it is often used with *Radix Rehmanniae*, *Rhizoma Alismatis*, and *Herba Dianthi*.

2. For febrile diseases marked by high fever, restlessness and thirst, and sore and ulcer due to heat toxin, it is often used with *Rhizoma Coptidis* and *Fructus Gardeniae*.

3. For cough due to lung heat, it is used together with *Rhizoma Anemarrhenae*, and *Cortex Mori*.

4. For hematemesis, hemorrhinia, hematochezia, metrorrhagia and metrostaxia due to frenetic blood heat, it is often used with *Radix Rehmanniae*, *Cortex Moutan*, and *Cacumen Platycladi*. In case of sore and ulcer due to heat toxin, it is often used with *Flos Lonicerae*, and *Fructus Forsythiae*.

In addition, it has functions of clearing heat and preventing abortion, and is applicable for threatened abortion in combination with *Rhizoma Atractylodis Macrocephalae*, and *Caulis Bambusae in Taeniam*.

【Preparation and dosage】3-9 g, decoct.

【Caution】It should be cautiously used in case of deficiency cold of the spleen and stomach, fluid consumption, and yin deficiency.

Cortex Phellodendri (Huang Bai)

【Source】It refers to the dried bark of the deciduous tree *Phellodendron chinense Schneid*. or *Phellodendron amurense Rupr*.

【Taste and Nature】Bitter and cold.

【Meridian Entry】Kidney and gallbladder meridians.

【Function】Eliminate heat and dampness, purge fire and detoxicate toxin, clear deficiency heat.

【Indications】

1. For dribbling urination, leukorrhagia, pain and swelling in the genitals, feet and knees, it is prescribed with *Radix Scutellariae*, *Rhizoma Coptidis*, *Rhizoma Atractylodis*, *Rhizoma Anemarrhenae*, *Rhizoma Alismatis*, and *Radix Gentianae*.

【使用注意】脾胃虚寒者慎用。

本类药还有苦参、白鲜皮、秦皮等。

（五）清虚热药

清虚热药性寒味苦咸甘，多归肝、肾经，主要具有清虚热作用，适用于阴虚内热证，症见潮热、低热不退、盗汗、五心烦热、失眠、舌红少苔、脉细数等。本类药物应用时要注意配伍养阴药以标本兼治。

青 蒿

【药用】本品为菊科植物黄花蒿（*Attemisia annua L.*）的干燥地上部分。秋季花盛开时采割，除去老茎，阴干。

【性味】苦、辛，寒。

【归经】归肝、胆经。

【功效】清热解暑，退虚热，截疟。

【临床应用】

1. 用于暑热外感、症见发热、无汗或有汗、头昏头痛、脉数等，可与藿香、佩兰、荷叶、西瓜翠衣等同用。

2. 用于热病后期，症见夜热早凉、热退无汗或低热不退，可与牡丹皮、生地黄、鳖甲等同用。

3. 用于阴虚发热，症见潮热、盗汗、骨蒸、手足心热等证，常和秦艽、鳖甲、地骨皮等同用。

4. 用于疟疾，可用鲜品，剂量要比平时大。

【用量用法】6~12g，煎服，入煎剂宜后下。

本类药还有地骨皮、胡黄连、白薇等。

三、泻下药

凡以通利大便或攻逐水饮为主要功效，治疗便秘及水肿的药物，称为泻下药。本类药物分为攻下药、润下药和逐水药三类。其中攻下药和逐水药攻下峻猛，易伤正气，适用于邪实而正气未虚之证；久病正虚、年老体弱者慎用；妇女胎前产后以及月经期忌用。

2. For jaundice, dysentery, and eczema due to dampness-heat, it is often used with *Radix Scutellariae*, *Rhizoma Coptidis*, *Fructus Gardeniae*, and *Herba Artemisiae Scopariae* for internal treatment. For exteranl treatment, it can be used together with *Radix et Rhizoma Rhei*, and *Talcum*.

3. For fever, spermatorrhea and seminal efflux due to deficiency of yin, it is often used together with *Rhizoma Anemarrhenae* and *Radix Rehmanniae*.

【Preparation and dosage】3－12 g, decoct.

【Caution】The drug is contraindicated for deficiency cold of the spleen and stomach.

Other medicinals in this category include *Radix Sophorae Flavescentis*, *Cortex Dictamni*, and *Cortex Fraxini*.

Deficiency-heat clearing medicinals

Deficiency-heat clearing medicinals are cold in nature and bitter, salty and sweet in flavor, and mainly enter the liver and kidney meridians. They mainly have the functions of clearing deficiency heat, and are applicable for yin deficiency heat syndrome, manifested as tidal fever, prolonged low fever, nocturnal sweating, heat sensation in chest, palms and soles, insomnia, red tongue with slim tongue coating, fine and rapid pulse. When using these medicinals, one should pay attention to the clinical combination with nourishing yin medicinals to treat both the tip and the root.

Herba Artemisiae Annuae (Qing Hao)

【Source】It is the aerial part of *Attemisia annua L.* of *Compositae*. It is cut and collected in the period of blossoms in autumn, dried in the shade with the tough stems removed.

【Taste and Nature】Bitter, acrid, and cold.

【Meridian Entry】Liver and gallbladder meridians.

【Function】Eliminate heat and release summerheat, purge fire and detoxicate toxin, interrupt malaria.

【Indications】

1. For external contraction of summer-heat, manifested as fever, with sweating or without sweating, dizziness, headache and rapid pulse, it is prescribed with *Herba Agastachis*, *Herba Eupatorii*, *Folium Nelumbinis*, and *Exocarpium Citrulli*.

2. For the late stage of febrile diseases, manifested as night fever relieved in the morning, no sweating after fever relieved and long lasting lower fever, it is often used with *Cortex Moutan*, *Radix Rehmanniae*, and *Carapax Trionycis*.

3. For yin deficiency with internal heat, manifested as tidal fever, night sweating, steaming bone and heat in the heart of the palms and soles, it is often used together with *Radix Gentianae Macrophyllae*, *Carapax Trionycis*, and *Cortex Lycii*.

4. Fresh *Herba Artemisiae Annuae* is used to treat malaria in higher dose than usual.

【Preparation and dosage】6－12 g, decoct. Decoct later.

Other medicinals in this category include *Cortex Lycii*, *Rhizoma Picrorhizae*, and *Radix Cynanchi Atrati*.

Precipitating Medicinals

All the medicinals that have the functions of clearing stool or expelling water and are used for treating constipation and edema are called precipitating medicinals. Precipitating medicinals are classified into three categories: offensive precipitating medicinals, laxative medicinals and drastic water-expelling medicinals. Among them, the offensive precipitating medicinals and drastic water-expelling medicinals strongly expel stool and water and are apt to consume healthy qi, so they are applicable for the syndromes of exces-

（一）攻下药

攻下药多味苦性寒，主要具有通便和泻火作用，适用于热结便秘、食积化热及实热证等。部分药物配伍温里药可应用于寒结便秘。

大 黄

【药用】本品为蓼科植物掌叶大黄（*Rheum palmatum L.*）、唐古特大黄（*Rheum tanguticum Maxim. ex Balf.*）或药用大黄（*Rheum officinale Baill.*）的干燥根及根茎。

【性味】苦，寒。

【归经】归脾、胃、大肠、肝、心包经。

【功效】泻热通便，凉血解毒，逐瘀通经。

【临床应用】

1．用于热结便秘、胃肠积滞、湿热泻痢等，常与芒硝、厚朴、枳实等配伍。

2．用于火热之邪导致的目赤、咽喉肿痛、口舌生疮、牙龈肿痛、热毒疮疖等，可配黄连、黄芩、丹皮、赤芍等同用。

3．血热妄行导致各种出血证，如吐血、咯血、便血等，可配伍侧柏叶、仙鹤草、大蓟、小蓟等。

4．用于瘀血导致的产后瘀滞腹痛、瘀血凝滞、月经不通以及跌打损伤等，可配伍桃仁、赤芍、红花等。

5．用于湿热黄疸，常与茵陈、栀子等药配伍。

【用量用法】3～30g，煎服，不宜久煎。

【使用注意】脾胃虚寒者慎用。孕妇及哺乳期忌用。

芒 硝

【药用】本品为硫酸盐类矿物芒硝族芒硝，经加工精制而成的结晶体。主含含水硫酸钠（$Na_2SO_4 \cdot 10H_2O$）。

【性味与归经】咸、苦，寒。归胃、大肠经。

【功效】泻下通便，清热解毒，软坚回乳。

【临床应用】

1．用于实热积滞、大便燥结，常与大黄相须为用。

2．用于火热毒邪导致的咽喉肿痛、口疮、目赤、痔疮、乳痈等，可外用本品。

3．用于断奶，外敷乳房可回乳。

【用量与用法】6～12g，冲入药汁内或开水中溶化后服，不入煎。

【使用注意】孕妇忌用。不可与三棱同用。

本类药还有番泻叶、芦荟等。

sive pathogenic qi without deficiency of healthy qi. The medicinals should be used cautiously in the patients with deficiency of healthy qi due to chronic diseases, and the senile or patients of weak physique. The medicinals are contraindicated for women during pregnancy or menstruation.

Offensive precipitating medicinals

Most of the offensive precipitating medicinals are bitter in flavor and cold in nature. They have main functions of discharging stools and purging fire, and are applicable for constipation due to heat stagnation, fever due to food accumulation, and excess heat syndromes. Some of the medicinals can be applicable for constipation due to cold accumulation, with combination of interior-warming medicinals.

Radix et Rhizoma Rhei (Da Huang)

【Source】It is dried root and rhizome of *Rheum palmatum L, R. Decoctionuticum Maxim. ex Balf.* or *R. officinale Baill.* of *Polygonaceae.*

【Taste and Nature】Bitter, cold.

【Meridian Entry】Spleen, stomach, large instestine, liver and heart meridians.

【Function】Discharge stools and clear fire, cool blood and remove toxin, activate blood and remove stasis.

【Indications】

1. For constipation due to heat stagnation, stagnation in the stomach and intestine, dysentery due to dampness-heat, it is often prescribed with *Natrii Sulfas, Cortex Magnoliae Officinalis,* and *Fructus Aurantii Immaturus.*

2. For red eyes, sore throat, mouth and tongue sores, pain and swelling in the teeth, and sores and boils due to heat toxin, it is often prescribed with *Rhizoma Coptidis, Radix Scutellariae, Cortex Moutan,* and *Radix Paeoniae Rubra.*

3. For hematemesis, epistaxis, and hematuria due to heat in the blood, it is prescribed with *Cacumen Platycladi, Herba Agrimoniae, Herba seu Radix Cirsii Japonici,* and *Herba Cephalanoploris.*

4. For post partum abdominal pain, absence of menses, and bruises due to blood stasis, it is often used with *Semen Persicae, Radix Paeoniae Rubra,* and *Flos Carthami.*

5. For jaundice due to dampness-heat, it is often used with *Herba Artemisiae Scopariae* and *Fructus Gardeniae.*

【Preparation and dosage】3-30 g, decoct. It is not advisable to be decocted for long time.

【Caution】It should be used cautiously in patients with spleen-stomach deficiency cold syndrome. It is prohibited for women during pregnancy and lactation period.

Natrii Sulfas (Mang Xiao)

【Source】It refers to the refined crystalline sodium sulphate obtained from processing sulfate mineral, and its chief component is $Na_2SO_4 \cdot 10H_2O$.

【Taste and Nature】Salty, bitter, cold.

【Meridian Entry】Stomach and large intestine meridians.

【Function】Relieve conspitation with purgation, clear heat and remove toxin, soften hardness and terminate lactation.

【Indications】

1. For constipation and stagnation due to excess heat, it is often prescribed with combination of *Radix et Rhizoma Rhei.*

2. For sore throat, mouth sores, red eyes, hemorrhoids and mammary welling-abscess due to fire and heat toxin, it is externally used.

（二）润下药

润下药大多为植物的种仁，富含油脂，具有润燥滑肠作用，可使大便易于排出，适用于年老、体虚、久病、产后所致阴虚津亏、血虚便秘。临床应用还应酌情配伍其他药物，如热盛伤津而便秘者，可与清热养阴药配伍；兼血虚者，可与补血药配伍；兼气滞者，须与理气药配伍。

火麻仁

【药用】本品为桑科植物大麻（*Cannabis sativa L.*）的干燥成熟果实。秋季果实成熟时采收，除去杂质，晒干。

【性味】甘，平。

【归经】归脾、胃、大肠经。

【功效】润肠通便。

【临床应用】

用于老人、产妇及体虚之津枯肠燥便秘，可与郁李仁同用。

【用量与用法】9~15g，煎服。

郁李仁

【药用】本品为蔷薇科植物欧李（*Prunus humilis Bge.*）、郁李（*Prunus Thunb.*）或长柄扁桃（*Prunus pedunculata Maxim.*）的干燥成熟种子。夏秋二季采收成熟果实，取出种子，干燥。

【性味】辛、苦、甘，平。

【归经】归脾、大肠、小肠经。

【功效】润肠通便，利水消肿。

【临床应用】

1. 用于肠燥便秘，常配合火麻仁、瓜蒌仁同用。

2. 用于小便不利、水肿、脚气等证，常与茯苓、泽泻等同用。

【用量与用法】6~9g，煎服。

（三）逐水药

逐水药也称峻下逐水药，味多苦，性或温或寒，均有毒，可引起剧烈腹泻，使体内潴留的水液从大便排出，适用于水肿、臌胀、胸胁停饮等。部分药物还兼有利水作用。本类药物不可久服，临床应用要注意用量、炮制方法及配伍禁忌等。

3. It is used to terminate lactation, applying externally to the breast.

【Preparation and dosage】6-12 g. It is dissovled in a decoction or in boiling water to use orally. Do not decoct.

【Caution】It is contraindicated for women in pregnancy. Do not combine with *Rhizoma Sparganii*.

Medicinals in this category also include *Folium Sennae* and *Aloe*.

Laxative medicinals

Most of the laxative medicinals are seeds of herbs that are rich in oil. The medicinals have the functions moistening dryness and lubricating the intestines, so as to make the stools easy to discharge, and they are indicated to constipation of dryness, blood deficiency and depletion of body fluid syndromes, which are due to aging, weak physique, long lasting diseases or post partum. In clinical practice, it should be combined with other medicinals, for example, in case of constipation due to excess heat and depletion of body fluid, it is used with heat-clearing and yin-tonifying medicinals; for cases concurrent with blood deficiency, it is combined with blood-tonifying medicinals; and for cases concurrent with qi deficiency, it is combined with qi-regulating medicinals.

Semen Cannabis (Huo Ma Ren)

【Source】It is dried ripe fruit of *Cannabis sativa L.* of *Moraceae*. It is collected in autumn when the fruits are ripe, removed foreign substance, and dried in the sun.

【Taste and Nature】Sweet and neutral.

【Meridian Entry】Spleen, stomach and large intestine meridians.

【Function】Moisten the intestine to relax the bowels.

【Indications】For constipation of the elderly or pregnant women or the weak with depletion of body fluid and dryness in the intestines, it is often used with with *Semen Pruni*.

【Preparation and dosage】9-15 g, decoct.

Semen Pruni (Yu Li Ren)

【Source】The medicinals are dried ripe seeds of *Prunus Humilis* Bge., *Prunus Japonica Thumb.* or *Prunus Pedunculata Maxim*. The ripe fruits are collected in the summer and autumn, and seeds are taken out and dried.

【Taste and Nature】Pungent, bitter, sweet, and neutral.

【Function】Moisten the intestine to relieve conspitation, promote diuresis, and relieve edema.

【Meridian Entry】Spleen, large intestine, and small intestine meridians.

【Indications】

1. For constipation due to dryness of untestine, it is often used together with *Semen Cannabis*, and *Fructus Trichosanthis*.

2. For dysuria, edema and beriberi, it is often used with *Poria* and *Rhizoma Alismatis*.

【Preparation and dosage】6-9 g, decoct.

Drastic water-expelling medicinals

Drastic water-expelling medicinals are also named as drastic water-expelling precipitating medicinals, all of them are of toxicity, most of them are bitter in flavor and warm or cold in nature. The medicinals cause drastic diarrhea and induce expelling retention of fluid by purgation, and are applicable for edema, tympanitis and fluid retention in the chest and abdomen. Some of them also have the function of inducing diuresis. In clinical practice, the medicinals should not be used for long time, and one should pay attention to the dosage, processing and prohibited combination of the medicinals.

甘 遂

【药用】本品为大戟科植物甘遂（*Euphorbia kansui T. N. Liou ex T. P. Wang*）的干燥块根。春季开花前或秋末茎叶枯萎后采挖，撞去外皮，晒干。

【性味】苦，寒；有毒。

【归经】归肺、肾、大肠经。

【功效】泻水逐饮，消肿散结。

【临床应用】

1. 水肿胀满，胸胁停饮，可与牵牛子、泽泻等同用。

2. 湿热肿毒，热结便秘，可与大黄、芒硝等同用。

【用量与用法】0.5~1.5g，炮制后入丸散。

【使用注意】孕妇忌用。反甘草。

本类药还有大戟、牵牛子。

四、利水渗湿药

凡以通利小便、渗泄水湿为主要功效，治疗水湿内停病证的药物，称为利水渗湿药。利水渗湿药的药味多甘淡或苦，性多寒凉或平，有利水消肿、通淋、退黄等功效。本类药物易耗伤津液，阴虚津液不足者慎用。

茯 苓

【药用】本品为多孔菌科真菌茯苓［*Poria cocos （Schw.） Wolf*］的干燥菌核。

【性味】甘、淡，平。

【归经】归心、肺、脾、肾经。

【功效】利水渗湿，健脾，宁心安神

【临床应用】

1. 用于小便不利、水肿、痰饮等证，常与猪苓、泽泻、白术等配伍。

2. 用于脾虚证，兼便溏泄泻更佳，常与党参、白术、山药等配伍。

3. 用于心悸、失眠等证，常与龙眼肉、远志、酸枣仁等配伍。

【用量用法】9~15g，煎服。

泽 泻

【药用】本品为泽泻科沼泽植物泽泻［*Alisma orientalis （Sam.） Juzep.*］的干燥块茎。

【性味】甘，寒。

【归经】归肾、膀胱经。

Radix Kansui (Gan Sui)

【Source】It is the root tuber of *Euphorbia kansui T.N.Liou ex T.P.Wang* (*Euphorbiaceae*).It is collected either when the stem and leaves wither in the end of autumn or before bloom next spring.It is skinned and dried for use.

【Taste and Nature】Bitter,cold,and toxic.

【Meridian Entry】Lung,kidney,and large intestine meridians.

【Function】Purge water and expel fluid,resolve the swelling and disperse the mass.

【Indications】

1. For edema,tympanites and fluid retention in the chest and hypochondrium,it is often used together with *Semen Pharbitidis*,and *Rhizoma Alismatis*.

2. For swelling due to dampness-heat toxin and constipation due to heat stagnation,it is often used with *Radix et Rhizoma Rhei*,and *Natrii Sulfas*.

【Preparation and dosage】0.5－1.5g.It is applied in the form of pill or powder after preparation.

【Caution】It is contraindicated in pregnant women.It is imcompatible with *Radix Glycyrrhizae*. *Herba seu Radix Cirsii Japonici* and *Semen Pharbitidis* are also in this category.

Dampness-Draining Diuretic Medicinals

All the medicinals that have the main functions of inducing diuresis,draining water and dampness, and are applicable for internal retention of water and dampness,are called dampness-draining diuretic medicinals.The dampness-draining diuretic medicinals are usually sweet,bland or bitter in flavor,and cold, cool or neutral in nature,and have the functions of inducing diuresis,removing swelling,freeing strangury, and relieving jaundice.The medicinals are apt to consume the body fluid,and should be used cautiously in patients with yin deficiency and fluid deficiency.

Poria (Fu Ling)

【Source】It is the dried sclerotium of *Poria cocos(Schw.) Wolf* of *Polyporaceae*.

【Taste and Nature】Sweet,bland,and neutral.

【Meridian Entry】Heart,lung,spleen,and kidney meridians.

【Function】Induce diuresis to drain dampness,invigorate the spleen,and quiet the heart to tranquilize.

【Indications】

1. For dysuria,edema and phlegm-rheum,it is often used with *Polyporus*,*Rhizoma Alismatis*,and *Rhizoma Atractylodis Macrocephalae*.

2. For spleen deficiency syndrome,and has a better efficacy in case of concurrent with loose stool and diarrhea,it is often used with *Radix Codonopsis*,*Rhizoma Atractylodis Macrocephalae*,and *Rhizoma Dioscoreae*.

3. For palpitation and insomnia,it is often used with *Arillus Longan*,*Radix Polygalae* and *Semen Ziziphi Spinosae*.

【Preparation and dosage】9－15 g,decoct.

Rhizoma Alismatis (Ze Xie)

【Source】It is dried stem tuber of *Alisma orientalis(Sam.) Juzep.*of *Alismataceae*.

【Taste and Nature】Sweet and cold.

【Meridian Entry】Kidney and bladder meridians.

【功效】利水渗湿，清湿热。

【临床应用】

1. 用于小便不利、水肿、痰饮停聚等证，常与茯苓、猪苓、车前子、白术等配伍。

2. 用于下焦湿热之泄泻、淋浊、带下，可与茯苓、猪苓、黄柏等同用。

【用量用法】6~9g，煎服。

本类药还有金钱草、茵陈、车前子、薏苡仁、萆薢、赤小豆、滑石、海金沙、萹蓄、石韦、瞿麦等。

五、化湿药

凡以化湿运脾为主要作用，治疗湿邪困脾证为主的药物，称为化湿药。本类药物气味芳香，故又称为"芳香化湿药"。因多辛香温燥，易耗气伤津，故阴虚血燥气虚者慎用。化湿药多含挥发油成分，入汤剂不宜久煎。

广藿香

【药用】本品为唇形科植物广藿香 ［*Pogostemon cablin（Blanco）Benth.*］ 的干燥地上部分。

【性味】辛，微温。

【归经】归脾、胃、肺经。

【功效】醒脾化湿，和中止呕，解暑，发表。

【临床应用】

1. 用于湿阻中焦证，症见脘闷纳呆，在临床上常与佩兰等同用。

2. 用于呕吐。湿阻中焦所致可配苏叶、半夏、厚朴、陈皮等同用；胃寒呕吐可配半夏同用；湿热所致可配黄连、竹茹。

3. 用于暑湿证及湿温初起，常与佩兰、薄荷、茵陈、黄芩同用。

4. 用于外感风寒兼有湿阻中焦的证候，症见发热恶寒、胸脘满闷，常配伍紫苏、陈皮。

【用量用法】3~9g，煎服。鲜品加倍。

本类药还有苍术、佩兰、砂仁、白豆蔻、草豆蔻、草果、厚朴等。

六、祛风湿药

凡以祛风除湿为主要功效，治疗风湿痹证为主的药物，称为祛风湿药。祛风湿药多辛散苦燥，具有祛除肌表、经络及筋骨间风湿的作用，有些药物还兼有散寒或清热、活血舒筋、通络止痛、解表以及补肝肾强筋骨作用。本类药物可制成酒剂或丸散常服。部分祛风湿药辛温香燥，易耗伤阴血，故阴虚血亏者慎用。

【Function】Promote diuresis to drain dampness, clear heat, and expel dampness.

【Indications】

1. For dysuria, edema and phlegm-rheum, it is often used with *Poria*, *Semen Plantaginis*, and *Rhizoma Atractylodis Macrocephalae*.

2. For diarrhea, strangury and leucorrhea due to dampness-heat in the lower energizer, it is often used with *Poria*, *Polyporus*, and *Cortex Phellodendri*.

【Preparation and dosage】6−9 g, decoct.

There are more medicinals in this category, such as *Herba Lysimachiae*, *Herba Artemisiae Scopariae*, *Semen Plantaginis*, *Semen Coicis*, *Rhizoma Dioscoreae Hypoglaucae*, *Semen Phaseoli*, *Talcum*, *Spora Lygodii*, *Herba Polygoni Avicularis*, *Folium Pyrrosiae*, and *Herba Dianthi*.

Dampness-Resolving Medicinals

All the medicinals with the functions of resolving dampness and improving the spleen's transportation and transmation, which are used for dampness harassment of the spleen, are called dampness-resolving medicinals. Because most of these medicinals are of fragrance in flavor, they are also called frangrant dampresolving medicinals. Because most of the medicinals are pungent and fragrant in flavor, and are apt to consume qi and body fluid, they should be cautiously used for blood dryness and qi deficiency. In addition, most of the medicinals contains volatile oil with fragrance, and should not be decocted for long time.

Herba Agastaches (Huo Xiang)

【Source】It refers to the dried aerial parts of the perennial herb *Pogostemon cablin*(*Blanco*)*Benth*.

【Taste and Nature】Pungent and slightly warm.

【Meridian Entry】Spleen, stomatch, and lung meridians.

【Function】Arouse the spleen and resolve dampness, harmonize the center and stop vomiting, and disperse exterior pathogens.

【Indications】

1. For retention of dampness in the middle energizer, manifested as epigastric fullness and stiffness and poor appetite, it is often used with *Herba Eupatorii*.

2. It is indicated for vomiting. For vomiting due to retention of dampness in the middle energizer, it is often used with *Folium Perillae*, *Rhizoma Pinelliae*, *Cortex Magnoliae Officinalis* and *Pericarpium Citri Reticulatae*; for vomiting due to stomatch cold, it is prescribed with *Rhizoma Pinelliae*; for vomiting due to dampness-heat, it is used with *Rhizoma Coptidis* and *Caulis Bambusae in Taeniam*.

3. For the early stage of summer-dampness and dampness-warmth syndromes, it is usually used with *Herba Eupatorii*, *Herba Menthae*, *Herba Artemisiae Scopariae*, and *Radix Scutellariae*.

4. For affection of exogenous wind-cold with dampness in the middle energizer, manifested as fever, aversion to cold, fullness and oppression in the chest and stomach duct, it is used with combination of *Fructus Perillae*, and *Pericarpium Citri Reticulatae*.

【Preparation and dosage】3−9 g, decoct. The amount of the fresh is doubled.

There are more medicinals in this category, such as *Rhizoma Atractylodis*, *Herba Eupatorii*, *Fructus Amomi*, *Fructus Amomi Rotundus*, *Semen Alpiniae Katsumadai*, and *Cortex Magnoliae Officinalis*.

Removing Wind-Dampness Medicinals

All the medicinals with the main functions of expelling wind and removing dampness, and are applied for treating arthralgia syndromes due to wind-dampness, are called as removing wind-dampness medicinals. These medicinals are usually pungent to disperse and bitter to dry, and have the functions of removing

独　活

【药用】本品为伞形科植物重齿毛当归（*Angelica pubescens Maxim. f. biserrata Shan et Yuan*）的干燥根。

【性味】辛、苦，微温。

【归经】归肾、膀胱经。

【功效】祛风除湿，通痹止痛，解表。

【临床应用】

1．用于风寒湿痹，症见腰膝酸痛、两足痿痹、屈伸不利等，常与桑寄生、秦艽、牛膝等同用。

2．用于风寒表证有湿邪者，常与羌活、麻黄等同用。

【用量用法】3~9g，煎服。

【使用注意】阴虚及气血不足者慎用。

本类药还有威灵仙、秦艽、五加皮、海风藤、桑寄生、木瓜、豨莶草、伸筋草、防己、马钱子、桑枝、络石藤、乌梢蛇。

七、理气药

凡以疏通调畅气机为主要功效，治疗气滞或气逆证为主的药物，称为理气药。理气药味多苦辛芳香，性多温，主要归脾、胃、肺、肝经。本类药物多辛温香燥，易耗气伤阴，故气虚阴虚者慎用。

陈　皮

【药用】本品为芸香科植物橘（*Citrus reticulate Blanco*）及其栽培变种的干燥成熟果皮。采摘成熟果实，剥取果皮，晒干或低温干燥。

【性味】苦、辛，温。

【归经】归肺、脾经。

【功效】理气健脾，燥湿化痰。

【临床应用】

1．用于脾胃气滞导致的胸腹胀满、消化不良，常与木香、枳壳等配伍。

2．用于脾胃虚弱，症见纳差、消化不良及恶心呕吐等，可与党参、白术、茯苓等应用。

3．用于湿阻中焦，症见脘腹痞胀、便溏泄泻等，可配伍苍术、厚朴等。

4．用于痰湿阻肺、咳嗽痰多，可配伍半夏、茯苓等。

【用量用法】3~9g，煎服。

【使用注意】实热证及阴虚证不宜用。

wind-dampness in the skin, meridians, collaterals, tendons and bones. Some of these medicinals also have the functions of expelling cold or clearing heat, activating blood and relaxing tendons, relieving pain, dispersing exterior pathogens, nourishing the liver and kidney, and strengthening tendons and bones. The medicinals can be prepared to medicinal wine, pill or powder for long time oral application. Some of the removing wind-dampness medicinals are pungent in flavor, and warm and dry in nature, and are apt to consume the blood and yin, and should be cautiously used in cases of yin deficiency and blood deficiency.

Radix Angelicae Pubescentis (Du Huo)

【Source】It is the dried root of *Angelica pubescens Maxim.f.biserrata Shan et Yuan of Umbelliferae*.

【Taste and Nature】Pungent, bitter, and slightly warm.

【Meridian Entry】Kidney and bladder meridians.

【Function】Expel wind-dampness, resolve arthralgia syndrome, alleviate pain, and disperse exterior pathogens.

【Indications】

1. For arthralgia syndrome of wind-cold-dampness, manifested as sore and pain in the lower back and knee, wilting and impediment of feet, inhibited bend and stretch, it is often used together with *Ramulus Taxilli*, *Radix Gentianae Macrophyllae*, and *Radix Achyranthis Bidentatae*.

2. For the exterior syndrome of wind-cold concurrent with dampness, it is used with *Rhizoma seu Radix Notopterygii*, and *Herba Ephedrae*.

【Preparation and dosage】3-9 g, decoct.

There are more medicinals in this category, such as *Radix Clematidis*, *Radix Gentianae Macrophyllae*, *Cortex Acanthopanacis*, *Caulis Piperis Kadsurae*, *Ramulus Taxilli*, *Fructus Chaenomelis*, *Herba Siegesbeckiae*, *Herba Lycopodii*, *Radix Stephaniae*, *Semen Strychni*, *Ramulus Mori*, *Caulis Trachelospermi*, and *Zaocys*.

Qi Regulating Medicinals

All the medicinals that have the main functions of regulating qi, treating qi stagnation and qi counterflow, are called qi-regulating medicinals. These medicinals are usually bitter, pungent, and fragrant in flavor, warm in nature, enter the spleen, stomatch, lung, and liver meridians. These medicinals are pungent, warm, fragnant, and dry, and are apt to damage qi and yin; thus, they should be used with caution in case of yin or qi deficiency.

Pericarpium Citri Reticulatae (Chen Pi)

【Source】It is the dried pericarp of mature fruit if *Citrus reticulate Blanco* and its cultivated varieties of *Rutaceae*. The mature fruits are collected in late autumn and early winter. They are peeled to dry in the sunshine or in low temperature.

【Taste and Nature】Bitter, pungent, and warm.

【Meridian Entry】Lung and spleen meridians.

【Function】Regulate qi and invigorate spleen, dry dampness and resolve phlegm.

【Indications】

1. For spleen-stomach qi stagnation, manifested as fullness of chest and abdomen, indigestion, it is often prescribed with *Radix Aucklandiae* and *Fructus Aurantii*.

2. For spleen-stomach weakness syndrome, manifested as torpid intake, indigestion, nausea and vomiting, it is often used with *Radix Codonopsis*, *Rhizoma Atractylodis Macrocephalae* and *Poria*.

3. For retention of dampness in the middle energizer, manifested as fullness and distention in the stomach and abdomen, loose stool or diarrhea, it is prescribed with *Rhizoma Atractylodis* and *Cortex Mag-*

木　香

【药用】本品为菊科植物木香（*Aucklandia lappa Decne.*）的干燥根。

【性味】辛、苦，温。

【归经】归脾、胃、大肠、三焦、胆经。

【功效】行气止痛，健脾消食。

【临床应用】

1. 用于脾胃气滞、肝气不舒导致的胸腹胀痛、胁肋疼痛等，可与枳壳、川楝子、柴胡、延胡索同用。

2. 用于气滞大肠，泻痢腹痛、里急后重，可与枳实、大黄等同用。

3. 用于食积不消、不思饮食，可与白术、枳实等合用。

【用量用法】1.5~6g，煎服。

【使用注意】阴虚火旺者慎用。

本类药还有香附、青皮、沉香、檀香、乌药、川楝子、大腹皮、佛手。

八、活血药

凡以通利血脉、促进血行、消散瘀血为主要功效，治疗血瘀证为主的药物，称为活血药，也称为活血祛瘀药或活血化瘀药。其中活血祛瘀作用较强者，又称破血药。活血药药味多辛苦，归心、肝经，入血分，多耗血动血，故出血无瘀者、月经过多、血虚经闭及孕妇忌用。

川　芎

【药用】本品为伞形科植物川芎（*Ligusticum chuanxiong Hort.*）的干燥根茎。夏季采挖，除去泥沙，晒干后除去须根。

【性味】辛，温。

【归经】归肝、胆、心包经。

【功效】活血行气，祛风止痛。

【临床应用】

1. 用于月经不调、痛经、闭经、产后瘀阻腹痛等，常配当归、白芍、赤芍等。

2. 用于癥瘕腹痛、胸胁刺痛等，可配伍柴胡、香附等同用。

3. 用于外伤、疮疡肿痛等，可配伍三棱、莪术、乳香、没药等。

4. 用于感冒头痛、偏正头痛，可配荆芥、细辛、白芷、菊花、防风等同用。

5. 风湿痹痛，可配羌活、独活等同用。

6. 用于真心痛，常与丹参、红花、赤芍等同用。

【用量用法】3~9g，煎服。

noliae Officinalis.

4. For productive cough due to retention of phlegm-dampness in the lung, it is often prescribed with *Rhizoma Pinelliae*, and *Poria.*

【Preparation and dosage】3–9 g, decoct.

【Caution】This drug is not advisable for excess heat syndrome and yin deficiency syndrome.

Radix Aucklandiae (Mu Xiang)

【Source】It is the dried root of *Aucklandia lappa Decne.* of *Compositae.*

【Taste and Nature】Pungent, bitter, and warm.

【Meridian Entry】Spleen, stomach, large instestine, triple energizer, and gallbladder meridian.

【Function】Promote qi flow to relieve pain, invigorate spleen, and promote digestion.

【Indications】

1. For fullness in the chest and abdomen, pain in rib-sides due to spleen-stomach qi stagnation and/ or constrained liver qi, it is often prescribed with *Fructus Aurantii*, *Fructus Toosendan*, *Radix Bupleuri*, and *Rhizoma Corydalis.*

2. For dysentery with pain in the abdomen and tenesmus due to large intestine qi stagnation, it is often prescribed with *Fructus Aurantii Immaturus* and *Radix et Rhizoma Rhei.*

3. For food accumulation marked by aversion to food, it is prescribed with *Rhizoma Atractylodis Macrocephalae*, and *Fructus Aurantii Immaturus.*

【Preparation and dosage】1. 5–6 g, decoct.

【Caution】It is used with caution for cases with yin deficiency and effulgent fire.

There are more medicinals in this category, such as *Rhizoma Cyperi*, *Pericarpium Citri Reticulatae Viride*, *Lignum Aquilariae Resinatum*, *Radix Linderae*, *Fructus Toosendan*, *Pericarpium Arecae*, and *Fructus Citri Sarcodactylis.*

Blood-Activating Medicinals

Blood-activating medicinals refer to the medicinals that have the main functions of facilitating blood vessels, promoting blood circulation, and removing blood stasis, also named as blood activating and stasis-resolving medicinals. The medicinals in the category which have stronger efficacy of activating the blood and removing stasis, are called blood-breaking medicinals. Most of the blood-activating medicinals are pungent and bitter in flavor, and enter the heart and liver meridians; the medicinals are related to the blood aspect, most of them activate and consume the blood, thus, the medicinals are contraindicated for bleeding without stasis, menorrhagia, amenorrhea due to blood deficiency, and women during pregnancy.

Rhizoma Chuanxiong (Chuan Xiong)

【Source】It is the dried rhizome of *Ligusticum Chuanxiong Hort.* of *umbrelliferae.* It is collected in summer and washed clean. It is then dried in the sunshine and removed fibrous roots.

【Taste and Nature】Pungent and warm.

【Meridian Entry】Liver, gallbladder, and pericardium meridians.

【Function】Activate blood and move qi, expel wind, and alleviate pain.

【Indications】

1. For irregular menstruation, dysmenorrheal, amenorrhea, and postpartum abdominal pain due to blood-stasis, this medicinal is usually combined with *Radix Angelicae Sinensis*, *Radix Paeoniae Alba*, *Radix Paeoniae Rubra.*

2. For abdominal pain caused by mass, and epigastric and hypochondriac stabbing pain, it is com-

【使用注意】本品辛温升散，凡阴虚阳亢及肝阳上亢者不宜应用；月经过多、孕妇亦忌用。

丹 参

【药用】本品为唇形科植物丹参（*Salvia miltiorrhiza Bge.*）的干燥根及根茎。春秋二季采挖，除去泥沙，干燥。

【性味】苦，微寒。

【归经】归心、肝经。

【功效】祛瘀止痛，活血调经，清心除烦。

【临床应用】

1. 用于月经不调、经闭、痛经、产后瘀痛等证，常与川芎、红花、桃仁、益母草等配伍使用。

2. 用于胸胁刺痛、热痹疼痛、癥瘕结块、跌仆伤痛。气滞血瘀之心、腹、胃脘疼痛，可配合砂仁、檀香等药同用；癥瘕结块，可与三棱、莪术、泽兰、鳖甲等配伍；热痹，关节红肿疼痛，配合清热消肿、祛风通络之忍冬藤、赤芍、桑枝、秦艽等。跌仆伤痛属瘀滞作痛者，常与当归、红花、川芎、三七活血祛瘀止痛药物同用。

3. 用于疮痈肿毒，常与清热解毒药金银花、连翘等配伍。

4. 用于温病热入营血、身发斑疹、神昏烦躁等，常与生地、玄参、黄连等药同用。

5. 用于心悸怔忡、失眠等。常与酸枣仁、柏子仁、夜交藤等药配合同用。

【用量用法】9~15g，煎服。

【使用注意】反藜芦。孕妇慎用。

本类药还有桃仁、红花、益母草、延胡索、郁金、姜黄、乳香、没药、五灵脂、牛膝、王不留行、莪术、三棱、水蛭。

bined with *Radix Bupleuri*, and *Rhizoma Cyperi*.

3. For physical trauma, sores and ulcers, abscess and swelling, it is combined with *Rhizoma Sparganii*, *Rhizoma Curcumae Zedoariae*, *Olibanum*, and *Myrrha*.

4. For headache due to cold and migraine, it is used in combination with *Herba Schizonepetae*, *Herba Asari*, *Radix Angelicae Dahuricae*, *Flos Chrysanthemi*, and *Radix Saposhnikoviae*.

5. For pain of impediment diseases due to wind-cold-dampness, it is used in combination with *Rhizoma seu Radix Notopterygii*, and *Radix Angelicae Pubescentis*.

6. For angina pectoris, it is combined with *Radix Salviae Miltiorrhizae*, *Flos Carthami*, and *Radix Paeoniae Rubra*.

【Preparation and dosage】3-9 g, decoct.

【Caution】It is pungent, warm, upbearing and dispersing, so it is contraindicated for cases of yin dificiency with effulgent-fire and hyperactivity of liver yang. It is contraindicated for menorrhagia, and for women during pregnancy.

Radix Salviae Miltiorrhizag (Dan Shen)

【Source】It is the root and rhizome of *Salvia miltiorrhiza Bge.* of *Labiatae.* It is dug and collected in spring and winter, washed clean and then dried in the sun.

【Taste and Nature】Bitter and slightly cold.

【Meridian Entry】Heart and liver meridians.

【Function】Remove blood stasis and alleviate pain, promote blood circulation to promote menstruation, remove annoyance, and tranquilize the mind.

【Indications】

1. For irregular menstruation, amenorrhea, dysmenorrheal and postpartum abdominal pain, it can be combined with *Rhizoma Chuanxiong*, *Flos Carthami*, *Semen Persicae*, and *Herba Leonuri*.

2. It is indicated for epigastric and hypochondriac pain, pain of heat impediment, abdominal masses and physical trauma. For angina pectoris and epigastric pain caused by blood-stasis and stagnation of qi, it is combined with *Fructus Amomi* and *Lignum Santali Albi.* In cases of abdominal masses, it is used in combination with *Rhizoma Sparganii*, *Rhizoma Curcumae Zedoariae*, *Herba Lycopi*, and *Carapax Trionycis*. For heat impediment marked by reddish, swelling and painful joints, it should be combined with *Caulis Lonicerae*, *Radix Paeoniae Rubra*, *Ramulus Mori*, and *Radix Gentianae Macrophyllae.* For physical trauma due to blood-stasis, combined with *Radix Angelicae Sinensis*, *Flos Carthami*, *Rhizoma Chuanxiong*, and *Radix Notoginseng*.

3. For sores and ulcers, abscess and swelling, it is combined with *Flos Lonicerae* and *Fructus Forsythiae*.

4. For heat invading the nutrient and blood systems in the seasonal febrile disease, it is usually combined with *Radix Rehmanniae*, *Radix Scrophulariae*, and *Rhizoma Coptidis*.

5. For palpitation and insomnia, it is usually combined with *Semen Ziziphi Spinosae*, *Semen Platycladi*, and *Caulis Polygoni Multiflori*.

【Preparation and dosage】3-9 g, decoct.

【Caution】It is incompatible with *Rhizoma et Radix Veratri.* It should be used with caution in pregnancy.

There are other blood-activating medicinals such as *Semen Persicae*, *Flos Carthami*, *Herba Leonuri*, *Rhizoma Corydalis*, *Radix Curcumae*, *Rhizoma Curcumae Longae*, *Olibanum*, *Myrrha*, *Faeces Trogopterorum*, *Radix Achyranthis Bidentatae*, *Semen Vaccariae*, *Rhizoma Curcumae Zedoariae*, *Rhizoma Sparganii*, and *Hirudo*.

九、止血药

凡以制止体内外出血为主要功效，治疗各种出血病证的药物，称为止血药。止血药是治标之品，临床应用需配合相应的药物如清热药、温里药、活血药以及补益药，以标本兼治。使用止血药要注意以下几点：大量出血可致气随血脱，应急予大补元气以益气固脱；使用凉血止血药和收敛止血药时，要注意有无瘀血，如有瘀血未尽，应酌加活血药，以免留瘀。

仙鹤草

【药用】本品为蔷薇科植物龙牙草（*Agrimonia pilosa Ledeb.*）的干燥地上部分。夏、秋二季茎叶茂盛时采割，除去杂质，日光下干燥。

【性味】苦、涩，平。

【归经】归心、肝经。

【功效】收敛止血，止痢，解毒疗疮。

【临床应用】

1. 用于多种出血病证，如咳血、吐血、崩漏下血、便血、尿血、鼻衄等。血热妄行可配合生地黄、小蓟、白茅根、牡丹皮、侧柏叶等；虚寒性出血可配伍党参、黄芪、灶心土、艾叶。

2. 用于泻痢。虚寒久泻，常与肉桂、诃子等配伍；湿热泻痢，常与黄连、白头翁、地榆等配伍。

3. 用于痈肿疮毒，常与清热解毒之金银花、蒲公英、紫花地丁等同用。

【用量用法】6~12g，煎服。

三 七

【药用】本品为五加科植物三七［*Panax notoginseng*（*Burk*）*F. H. Chen.*］的干燥根。秋季花开前采挖。

【性味】甘、微苦，温。

【归经】入肝、胃经。

【功效】散瘀止血，消肿定痛。

【临床应用】

1. 用于各种出血之证，如咯血、吐血、衄血、便血、崩漏、外伤出血等证，出血而有瘀滞者尤宜。单用或者配合其他止血药，如花蕊石、血余炭等。

2. 用于各种瘀滞疼痛与跌打伤痛等证，单用或配合活血、理气等药同用。

【用量用法】3~9g，煎服。如研粉吞服，一次1~3g，每天2~3次。外用适量。孕妇慎用。

Hemostatic Medicinals

All the medicinals that have the functions of stopping various types of bleeding, internally or externally, are called hemostatic medicinals. Hemostatic medicinals are the medicinals which treat the tip, so they should be combined with heat-clearing medicinals, interior-warming medicinals, blood-activating medicinals and tonics to treat with both the root and the tip. Attentions when using the medicinals are as below: in case of excessive bleeding followed by exhaustion of qi, one should supplement source qi urgently, so as to secure qi and avoid shock; when using blood-cooling hemostatic medicinals and astringent hemostatic medicinals, one should cautiously distinguish the existence of stasis; if there is the unremoved stasis, one should add activating blood medicinals to avoid the retention of the stasis.

Herba Agrimoniae (Xian He Cao)

【Source】It is the dried plant of *Agrimonia pilosa Ledeb.* of *Rosaceae*. Collected during summer and autumn when the plants are flourishing, the impurities removed, dried in the sun.

【Taste and Nature】Bitter, astringent, and neutral.

【Meridian Entry】Heart and liver meridians.

【Function】Stop bleeding by astringing, relieve dysentery, detoxicify, and cure sores.

【Indications】

1. It is indicated for various bleedings, such as hemoptysis, hematemesis, hematochezia, hematuria, nasal bleeding, matrorrhagia and metrostaxis, etc. For bleeding due to blood-heat, it is used in combination with *Radix Rehmanniae*, *Herba Cephalanoploris*, *Rhizoma Imperatae*, *Cortex Moutan*, and *Cacumen Platycladi*. For bleeding due to deficiency cold, it is used with *Radix Codonopsis*, *Radix Astragali*, *Terra Flava Usta*, and *Folium Artemisiae*.

2. It is used for dysentery. For dysentery due to deficiency cold, it is often used with *Cortex Cinnamomi*, and *Fructus Chebulae*. For dysentery due to dampness-heat, it is often used with *Rhizoma Coptidis*, *Radix Pulsatillae*, and *Radix Sanguisorbae*.

3. For abscess, swelling, sores and toxin, it is often used in combination with *Flos Lonicerae*, *Herba Taraxaci*, and *Herba Violae*.

【Preparation and dosage】6-12 g, decoct.

Radix Notoginseng (San Qi)

【Source】It is the dried root of *Panax notoginseng(Burk.) F.H.Chen.* of *Araliaceae*. Dug and collected before it blossoms in early autumn.

【Taste and Nature】Sweet, slightly bitter, and warm.

【Meridian Entry】Liver and stomach meridians.

【Function】Remove blood stasis to stop bleeding, remove swelling, and relieve pain.

【Indications】

1. It is used for all kinds of bleedings, such as hemoptysis, hematemesis, hematochezia, epistaxis, atrorrhagia and metrostaxis, especially for bleeding with blood stasis. It can be used alone or combined with *Ophicalcitum*, *Crinis Carbonisatus*.

2. For trauma and pain due to blood stasis, it can be used alone or together with blood-activating medicinals and qi-regulating medicinals.

【Preparation and dosage】3-9 g, decoct. One to three grams of the powder to be taken orally two or three times per day. It should be used with caution in pregnant women.

There are other hemostatic medicinals such as *Herba seu Radix Cirsii Japonici*, *Radix Sanguisorbae*,

本类药还有大蓟、地榆、槐花、侧柏叶、白茅根、茜草、艾叶。

十、消导药

凡以消食导滞、促进消化为主要功效，治疗食积不化、消化不良为主的药物，称为消导药。本类药物多味甘，性平或微温，主要归脾胃经。临床应用时，应根据不同证候，适当配伍其他药物，如有气滞则配伍理气药，如有脾胃虚弱则配伍健脾益胃药等。

山 楂

【药用】蔷薇科植物山里红（*Crataegus pinnatifida Bge. var. major N. E. Br.*）或山楂（*Crataegus pinnatifida Bge.*）的干燥成熟果实。秋季果实成熟时采收，切片，干燥。

【性味】酸、甘、微温。

【归经】归脾、胃、肝经。

【功效】消食化积，行气散瘀。

【临床应用】

1. 本药为消化食积停滞常用要药，尤能消化油腻肉积，常与麦芽、神曲等配伍应用。

2. 用于瘀血闭经及产后瘀滞腹痛、恶露不尽，常与当归、川芎、益母草等配伍。

【用量与用法】9～12g，煎服。

本类药还有莱菔子、鸡内金、六神曲、麦芽。

十一、化痰止咳平喘药

凡以祛痰或消痰为主要功效，治疗痰邪导致病证为主的药物，称为化痰药；以减轻或者抑制咳嗽和喘息为主要功效的药物称为止咳平喘药。化痰药和止咳平喘药临床常配伍同用，故合称为化痰止咳平喘药。本类药物或辛或苦，或温或凉，多归肺经。根据药性和功效不同，可分为温化寒痰、清化热痰和止咳平喘药三类。使用化痰止咳平喘药应注意：肺阴不足所致干咳少痰或咳嗽兼咯血者，忌用药性温燥之品；外感咳喘初起或痰多咳喘者，忌用具有收敛作用的止咳平喘药。

（一）温化寒痰药

温化寒痰药药性多温燥，主要具有温肺祛寒、燥湿化痰作用，适用于寒痰、湿痰导致的咳嗽、气喘、痰多以及痰湿阻滞经络导致的肢节酸痛、阴疽流注、瘰疬等。

Flos Sophorae,*Cacumen Platycladi*,*Rhizoma Imperatae*,*Radix Rubiae*, and *Folium Artemisiae*.

Digestant Medicinals

All the medicinals that take promoting digestion and relieving dyspepsia as the dominant actions are considered as the digestant medicinals.Most digestant medicinals are sweet and slightly warm in flavor, neutral in nature,and enter the spleen and stomach meridians.In clinical practice,it should be combined with other medicinals according to the different syndromes,for example,combined with qi-regulating medicinals in case of qi stagnation syndrome;combined with spleen-stomach qi tonifying medicinals in case of spleen-stomach deficiency syndrome.

Fructus crataegi (Shan Zha)

〖Source〗It is the dried ripe fruit of *Crataegus pinnaifida Ege.Var.major.N.E.Br.*or *Crataegus pinnatidida Bge.of Rosaceae.*It is collected in autumn when the fruit is ripe,cut into pieces and dried.

〖Taste and Nature〗Sour,sweet,and slightly warm.

〖Meridian Entry〗Spleen,stomach,and liver merdians.

〖Function〗Promote digestion,relieve dyspepsia,move qi,and disperse blood-stasis.

〖Indications〗

1. It is the essential medicinal for food accumulation,especially good for indigestion caused by improperly eating meat and fat.It is usually used together with *Fructus Hordei Germinatus*,and *Massa Fermentata Medicinalis*.

2. For amenorrhea due to blood-stasis,postpartum lochiorrhea and abdominal pain,it is often used with *Radix Angelicae Sinensis*,*Rhizoma Chuanxiong*,and *Herba Leonuri*.

〖Preparation and dosage〗9–12 g,decoct.

There are other digestant medicinals,such as *Semen Raphani*,*Endothelium Corneum Gigeriae Galli*, *Massa Fermentata Medicinalis*,and *Fructus Hordei Germinatus*.

Phlegm-Resolving Cough-Suppressing and Panting-Calming Medicinals

All the medicinals that have main functions of resolving phlegm and are applied to treat phlegm syndromes are called phlegm-resolving medicinals.All the medicinals that have the functions of suppressing cough and calming panting are called cough-suppressing and panting-calming medicinals.The phlegm-resolving medicinals and the cough-suppressing and panting-calming medicinals are usually used in combination in clinical practice,so they are collectively named as phlegm-resolving,cough-suppressing,and panting-calming medicinals.These medicinals are pungent or bitter,warm or cold,and mainly enter the lung meridian.According to their different properties and efficacies,they are categorized into three groups: warming and resolving cold-phlegm medicinals,clearing and resolving heat-phlegm medicinals,and cough-suppressing and panting-calming medicinals.

It should be noted when using these medicinals:the medicinals with warm and dry nature are contraindicated for dry cough caused by lung yin deficiency or cough concurrent with hemoptysis;cough-suppressing and panting-calming medicinals with astringent efficacy are contraindicated for cough at the early stage caused by external contraction or productive cough with panting.

Warming and resolving cold-phlegm medicinals

Most of the warming and resolving cold-phlegm medicinals are warm and dry,and have main functions of warming the lung to dispel cold and drying dampness to resolve phlegm,and they are indicated for cough,asthma and profuse sputum due to cold-phlegm or dampness-phlegm,and syndromes such as arthrodynia of the extremities,yin carbuncles and suppruative tissue diseases and sceofula due to phlegm-damp-

半 夏

【药用】本品为天南星科草本植物半夏［*Pinellia ternata*（*Thunb.*）*Breit.*］的干燥块茎。夏、秋采挖，洗净，除去外皮及须根，晒干。

【性味】辛，温；有毒。

【归经】归脾、胃、肺经。

【功效】温化寒痰，燥湿化痰，消痞散结，降逆止呕。

【临床应用】

1. 用于痰证。湿痰常与陈皮、茯苓等配伍；寒痰可与白芥子、生姜等同用；痰多咳嗽，可与贝母配伍；热痰可与瓜蒌、黄芩等配伍；风痰可与天南星等同用。

2. 用于胸脘痞闷、胸痹、结胸等证。胸脘痞闷常配伍陈皮、茯苓等；胸痹疼痛可配伍瓜蒌、薤白等；结胸证可与瓜蒌、黄连等同用。

3. 用于痰湿结聚所致的瘿瘤瘰疬、痈疽肿毒、梅核气等证，常与贝母、厚朴、紫苏等同用。

4. 用于胃气上逆、恶心呕吐。胃寒呕吐可配伍高良姜、丁香等；胃热呕吐可配伍黄连、竹茹等；胃虚呕吐，可与党参、生姜同用。

【用量与用法】3~9g，煎服。

【使用注意】阴虚燥咳者忌用。反乌头。

本类药还有天南星、白前、白芥子等。

（二）清化热痰药

清化热痰药药性多寒性，主要具有清热化痰作用，适用于热痰导致的咳喘、癫痫惊厥、瘰疬、瘿瘤等。

贝 母

【药用】贝母有川贝母、浙贝母之分。川贝母为百合科植物川贝母（*Fritillaria cirrhosa D. Don*）、暗紫贝母（*Fritillaria unibracteata Hsiao et K. C. Hsia*）、甘肃贝母（*Fritillaria przewalskii Maxim.*）或梭砂贝母（*Fritillaria delavayi Franch.*）的干燥鳞茎。夏、秋二季或积雪融化时采挖，除去须根、粗皮及泥沙，晒干或低温干燥。

浙贝母为百合科植物浙贝母（*Fritillaria thunbergii Miq.*）的干燥鳞茎。初夏植株枯萎时采挖，洗净，干燥。

【性味】川贝母：苦、甘，微寒；浙贝母：苦，寒。

【归经】归肺、心经。

【功效】清热化痰，解毒散结。

ness blocking the meridians.

Rhizoma Pineliae (Ban Xia)

【Source】It is the dried tuber of *Pinellia ternate*(*Thunb*) *Breit.* of *Araceae.* The tubers are dug and collected in summer and autumn. After they are peeled and fibrous roots are removed, they are washed clean and dried in the sunshine.

【Taste and Nature】Pungent, warm, and toxic.

【Meridian Entry】Spleen, stomach, and lung meridians.

【Function】Warm and resolve cold-phlegm, dry dampness and resolve phlegm, relieve stuffiness and dissipate binds, and suppress adverse ascending qi to stop vomiting.

【Indications】

1. For various syndromes of phlegm. For damp-phlegm, it is combined with *Pericarpium Citri Reticulatae* and *Poria.* For cold-phlegm, it is used together with *Semen Sinapis Albae* and *Rhizoma Zingiberis Recens.* For cough and profuse sputum, it is usually combined with *Bulbus Fritillariae.* For heat-phlegm, it is used in combination with *Fructus Trichosanthis* and *Radix Scutellariae.* For wind-phlegm, it is combined with *Rhizoma Arisaematis.*

2. It is indicated for chest and epigastric fullness, chest impediment and chest bind. For chest and epigastric fullness, it is combined with *Pericarpium Citri Reticulatae* and *Poria.* For chest impediment, it is usually combined with *Fructus Trichosanthis* and *Bulbus Allii Macrostemonis.* For chest bind, it is used together with *Fructus Trichosanthis*, and *Rhizoma Coptidis.*

3. For goiter, scrofula, large carbuncle and globus hystericus due to damp-phlegm, it is usually used together with *Bulbus Fritillariae*, the raw *Rhizoma Pinelliae* can combined with *Rhizoma Arisaematis*, *Cortex Magnoliae Officinalis*, and *Fructus Perillae.*

4. It is indicated for nausea and vomiting due to stomach qi ascending counterflow. For vomiting due to stomach cold, it is combined with *Rhizoma Alpiniae Officinarum* and *Flos Caryophylli.* For vomiting due to stomach heat, it is combined with *Rhizoma Coptidis* and *Caulis Bambusae in Taeniam.* For vomiting due to stomach deficiency, it is used together with *Radix Codonopsis*, and *Rhizoma Zingiberis Recens.*

【Preparation and dosage】3–9 g, decoct.

【Caution】It is contraindicated for dry cough due to yin deficiency. It is incompatible with *Radix Aconiti.*

There are other warming and resolving cold-phlegm medicinals, such as *Rhizoma Arisaematis*, *Rhizoma Cynanchi Stauntonii*, and *Semen Sinapis Albae.*

Clearing and resolving heat-phlegm medicinals

Clearing and resolving heat-phlegm medicinals are mainly cold in nature, and have functions of clearing and resolving heat-phlegm. They are mainly indicated for heat-phlegm syndrome, which is manifested as cough and asthma, epilepsy, infantile convulsion, goiter, and scrofula.

Bulbus Fritillariae (Bei Mu)

【Source】There are two kinds of *Bulbus Fritillariae*: *Bulbus Fritillariae Cirrhosae* and *Bulbus Fritillariae Thunbergii.* *Bulbus Fritillariae Cirrhosae* is the dried bulb of *Fritillaria cirrhosa D. Don*, *Fritillaria unibracteata Hsiao et K. C. Hisa*, *Fritillaria przewalskii Maxim.*, or *Fritillaria delavayi Franch.* of family *Liliaceae.* The bulbs are dug and collected in summer and winter or when snow melts. After the fibrous roots, balk, mud and sand are removed, they are dried in the sunshine or in low temperature.

Bulbus Fritillariae Thunbergii is the dried bulb of *Fritillaria thunbergii Miq.* of family *Liliaceae.* The bulbs are dug and collected after the plants are withered in early summer. They are washed clean and then

【临床应用】

1. 用于肺热咳喘、外感咳嗽，常用川贝母，常与桑叶、杏仁、牛蒡子、前胡等同用。

2. 用于肺阴虚燥咳、肺虚久咳，常用川贝母，可与沙参、麦冬、天冬等品配伍。

3. 用于瘰疬、疮痈肿毒、肺痈、乳痈等证。常用浙贝母，可与玄参、连翘、蒲公英等同用。

【用量与用法】川贝母3~9g，煎服。浙贝母4.5~9g，煎服。川贝母研粉冲服，一次1~2g。

【使用注意】寒痰、湿痰忌用。反乌头。

本类药还有前胡、瓜蒌、竹茹、天竺黄、胖大海、枇杷叶等。

（三）止咳平喘药

止咳平喘药药性或寒、或温、或平，主要具有止咳平喘作用，适用于外感或内伤导致的咳嗽、喘息病证。

杏 仁

【药用】本品为蔷薇科植物山杏（*Prunus armeniaca L. var. ansu Maxim.*）、西伯利亚杏（*Prunus sibirica L.*）、东北杏［*Prunus mandshuica*（*Maxim.*）*Koehne*］或杏（*Prunus armeniaca L.*）的干燥成熟种子。夏季采收成熟果实，取出种子，晒干。

【性味】苦，微温。有小毒。

【归经】归肺、大肠经。

【功效】止咳平喘，润肠通便。

【临床应用】

1. 用于咳嗽气喘，风寒、风热都可配伍使用。风寒咳喘可与麻黄、甘草等配伍；风热咳嗽可与桑叶、浙贝等配伍。

2. 用于肠燥便秘，可与火麻仁、瓜蒌仁等同用。

【用量与用法】4.5~9g，煎服。生品入煎剂宜后下。

本类药还有旋覆花、百部、桑白皮、葶苈子、白果等。

十二、温里药

凡以温里散寒为主要功效，治疗里寒证为主的药物，称为温里药，又称祛寒药。温里药药味多辛性温热，主要归脾、胃、肾、心经，兼归肝、肺经。温里药易耗伤津液，凡热证、阴虚证忌用，孕妇慎用。

dried.

〖Taste and Nature〗*Bulbus Fritillariae Cirrhosae*：bitter，sweet，and slightly cold；*Bulbus Fritillariae Thunbergii*：bitter and cold.

〖Meridian Entry〗Lung and heart meridians.

〖Function〗Clear heat and resolve phlegm，detoxify and dissipate binds.

〖Indications〗

1. For cough caused by lung heat or external contration，*Bulbus Fritillariae Cirrhosae* is often used and combined with *Folium Mori*，*Semen Armeniacae Amarum*，*Fructus Arctii*，and *Radix Peucedani*.

2. For dry cough caused by lung yin deficiency and chronic cough due to lung deficiency，*Bulbus Fritillariae Cirrhosae* is often used and combined with *Radix Glehniae*，*Radix Ophiopogonis*，and *Radix Asparagi*.

3. For scrofula，carbuncle，pulmonary abscess and mammary abscess，*Bulbus Fritillariae Thunbergii* is often used，and combined with *Radix Scrophulariae*，*Fructus Forsythiae*，and *Herba Taraxaci*.

〖Preparation and dosage〗*Bulbus Fritillariae Cirrhosae*，3－9 g，decoct；*Bulbus Fritillariae Thunbergii*，4. 5－9 g，decoct.*Bulbus Fritillariae Cirrhosae* is ground into powder and taken 1－2 g orally for each time.

〖Caution〗It is contraindicated for cold-phlegm and dampness-phlegm.It is incompatible with *Radix Aconiti*.

There are other clearing and resolving heat-phlegm medicinals，such as *Radix Peucedani*，*Fructus Trichosanthis*，*Caulis Bambusae in Taeniam*，*Concretio Silicea Bambusae*，*Pangdahai*，and *Pibaye*.

Cough-suppressing and panting-calming medicinals

Cough-suppressing and panting-calming medicinals are cold，warm or neutral in nature，and mainly have functions of suppressing cough and calming panting，and are indicated for cough and asthma caused by external contration or internal damage.

Semen Armeniacae Amarum (Xing Ren)

〖Source〗It is the dried ripe seed of *Prumus armeniace L.var.ansu Maxim.* ，*Prunus sibirica L.* ，*Prunus mandshurica(Maxim.) Koehne*，or *Pruns armeniace L.* of *Rosaceae*. The seeds are collected from the ripe fruits in summer，and dried in the sunshine.

〖Taste and Nature〗Bitter，slightly warm，and mildly toxic.

〖Meridian Entry〗Lung and large intestine meridians.

〖Function〗Suppress cough and calm panting，moisten the intestines，and free the bowels.

〖Indications〗

1. It is indicated for cough and asthma.In case of cough due to wind-cold，it is used in combination with *Herba Ephedrae* and *Radix Glycyrrhizae* ；in case of cough caused by wind-heat，it is used together with *Folium Mori*，and *Bulbus Fritillariae Thunbergii*.

2. For constipation due to intestinal dryness，it is usuallty used together with *Fructus Cannabis*，and *Fructus Trichosanthis*.

〖Preparation and dosage〗4. 5－9 g.The raw medicinal is decocted later.

There are other cough-suppressing and panting-calming medicinals，such as *Flos Inulae*，*Radix Stemonae*，*Cortex Mori*，*Semen Lepidii seu Descurainiae*，and *Semen Ginkgo*.

Interior-Warming Medicinals

All the medicinals with the main functions of warming the interior and dispelling cold，that are mainly indicated for interior cold syndrome，are called interior-warming medicinals，also named dispelling cold

附　子

【药用】本品为毛茛科植物乌头（*Aconitum carmichaeli Debx.*）的子根的加工品。6月下旬至8月上旬采挖，除去母根、须根及泥沙。

【性味】辛、甘，大热；有毒。

【归经】归心、肾、脾经。

【功效】回阳救逆，补火助阳，散寒止痛。

【临床应用】

1. 用于亡阳证，症见冷汗自出、四肢厥逆、脉微弱，常配合人参、干姜、炙甘草等同用。

2. 用于肾阳不足、命门火衰，症见畏寒肢冷、腰酸腿软、阳痿水肿等，常配伍肉桂、熟地、菟丝子、山萸肉等同用。

3. 用于脾阳不振，症见脘腹冷痛、大便溏薄、完谷不化等，常配伍合党参、白术、干姜、砂仁等。

4. 用于风寒湿痹、阳虚外感等证，常与桂枝等合用。

【用量与用法】3~15g，煎服，先煎30~60分钟以减弱其毒性。

【使用注意】孕妇忌用。不宜与半夏、瓜蒌、天花粉、贝母、白蔹、白芨同用。本类药还有肉桂、干姜、吴茱萸、丁香等。

十三、开窍药

凡以开窍醒神为主要功效，治疗神志昏迷之闭证为主的药物，称为开窍药。开窍药药味芳香，善于走窜行散、通窍开闭，均归心经。开窍药为救急、治标药物，不宜久服，以免耗伤正气；忌用于脱证；药味辛香，易挥发，内服多入丸散。

麝　香

【药用】本品为鹿科动物林麝（*Moschus berezovskii Flerov*）、马麝（*Moschus sifanicus Przewalski*）或原麝（*Moschus moschiferus Linnaeus*）成熟雄体香囊中的干燥分泌物。将香囊割下，阴干。

【性味】辛，温。

【归经】归心、脾经。

【功效】醒神开窍，消肿定痛，活血通经。

【临床应用】

1. 用于高热神昏、中风痰厥，惊痫等闭证。常与冰片、牛黄配伍使用。

medicinals. Mostly of the medicinals are pungent in flavor, warm and hot in nature, and mainly enter the spleen, stomach, kidney, and heart meridians, some of them enter the lung and liver meridians. This kind of mdicinals consume body fluids, thus, they are contraindicated for excess-heat syndrome, yin deficiency syndrome, and pregnant women.

Radix Aconiti (Fu Zi)

【Source】It is the processed daughter root of *Aconitum carmichaeli Debx*. of *Ranunculaceae*. It is mostly harvested and collected from the last 10 days of June to the first 10 days of August. The main-root, fibrous roots, mud, and sand are removed.

【Taste and Nature】Pungent, sweet, extremely hot, and toxic.

【Meridian Entry】Heart, kidney, and spleen meridians.

【Function】Restore yang from collapse, reinforce fire and strengthen yang, disperse cold to relieve pain.

【Indications】

1. For yang collapse syndrome, manifested as spontaneous cold sweating, cold clammy limbs, indistinct and faint pulse, it is used together with *Radix Ginseng*.

2. For kidney yang deficiency syndrome and debilitation of the life gate fire, manifested as coldness, cold extremeties, weakness of lumbar region and knees, impotence, and edema, it is often used together with *Cortex Cinnamomi*, *Radix Rehmanniae Praeparata*, *Semen Cuscutae*, and *Fructus Corni*.

3. For spleen yang deficiency syndrome, manifested as cold pain in epigastric and abdomen, loose stools, undigested food in stools, it is used with *Radix Codonopsis*, *Rhizoma Atractylodis Macrocephalae*, *Rhizoma Zingiberis*, and *Fructus Amomi*.

4. For impediment due to wind-cold-dampness and external syndrome due to yang deficiency, it is used together with *Ramulus Cinnamomi*.

【Preparation and dosage】3-15 g, decoct. Decoct first for 30-60 min in order to reduce its toxicity.

【Caution】It is contraindicated in pregnant women. It is incompatible with *Rhizoma Pinelliae*, *Fructus Trichosanthis*, *Radix Trichosanthis*, *Bulbus Fritillariae*, *Bailian*, and *Rhizoma Bletillae*.

There are other interior-warming medicinals, such as *Cortex Cinnamomi*, *Rhizoma Zingiberis*, *Fructus Evodiae*, and *Flos Caryophylli*.

Orifice-Opening Medicinals

All the medicinals that have main functions of opening the orifices to regain consciousness, and mainly indicated for sthenia-syndrome of coma, are called orifice-opening medicinals. The medicinals are aromatic in flavor, and are good at opening the orifices and freeing the blocking, and all the medicinals enter the heart meridian. The medicinals are used to treat emergent conditions and the tips of the diseases, and should not be used for a long period to avoid consumption of healthy-qi. This medicinal is contraindicated for collapse syndromes. Their active ingredients are easily volatilized, so when used orally, they always are applied in form of pill or powder.

Moschus (She Xiang)

【Source】It is the dry substance secreted by the gland in the sub-umbilical sac of the mature male *Moschus berezovskii Flerov*, *Moschus sifanicus Przewalski* or *Mochus moschiferus Linnaeus*. of *Cervidae*. The musk gland is cut-off and dried in shade.

【Taste and Nature】Pungent and warm.

【Meridian Entry】Heart and spleen meridians.

2. 用于痈疽肿毒，内服外用均可，可与乳香、雄黄等配伍。

3. 用于胸痹、跌扑损伤及风湿痹等证。胸痹可配伍木香、桃仁等；跌扑损伤，可配伍苏木、没药等；风湿痹可配伍祛风湿药。

4. 用于瘀郁内阻导致的经闭、月经不调等证，可配伍川芎、益母草、桃仁、红花等。

【用量与用法】0.03~0.1g，入丸散用。

【使用注意】孕妇忌用。

本类药还有石菖蒲、苏合香、冰片、安息香、樟脑等。

十四、平肝息风药

凡以平降肝阳、止息肝风为主要功效，治疗肝阳上亢证或肝风内动证为主的药物，称为平肝息风药。本类药物均归肝经，多为贝壳类或者虫类药。平肝息风药性不尽相同，或寒、或温、或平，临床应用要注意：药性寒凉者，脾虚所致的慢惊风忌用；药性温燥者，阴血亏虚者慎用。

天　麻

【药用】本品为兰科植物天麻（*Gastrodia elata Bl.*）的干燥块茎。立冬后至次年清明前采挖，立即洗净，蒸透，敞开低温干燥。

【性味】甘，平。

【归经】归肝经。

【功效】平肝息风，祛风通络。

【临床应用】

1. 用于肝阳上亢导致的头晕目眩，可与钩藤、石决明等配伍。

2. 用于肝风内动导致的惊痫抽搐、角弓反张等，常与钩藤、全蝎等配伍。

3. 用于风湿痹，症见肢体疼痛或麻木，常与当归、牛膝等、全蝎、乳香等配伍。

【用量与用法】3~9g，煎服。

本类药还有钩藤、珍珠母、石决明、牡蛎、赭石、牛黄、地龙、僵蚕、蜈蚣等。

【Function】Open the orifices to regain consciousness, relieve swelling, alleviate pain, activate blood and merdians.

【Indications】

1. For cases of heat type of sthenia-syndrome of coma, wind-stroke, phlegm-syncope and fright epilepsy, it is often used together with *Calculus Bovis* and *Borneolum*.

2. For abscess, carbuncle, swelling, and toxin, it can be used together with *Olibanum* and *Realgar* orally or externally.

3. It is indicated for chest impediment, physical trauma and wind-cold-dampness arthralgia syndrome. For chest impediment, it is combined with *Radix Aucklandiae* and *Semen Persicae*. In cases of trauma, it is used with *Lignum Sappan* and *Resina Myrrhae*. For wind-cold-dampness arthralgia syndrome, it is combined with wind-dampness-dispelling medicinals.

4. For amenorrhea and irregular mensturation due to blood stasis, it is used in combination with *Rhizoma Chuanxiong*, *Herba Leonuri*, *Semen Persicae*, and *Flos Carthami*.

【Preparation and dosage】0. 03−0. 1 g, applied in the form of powder or pill.

【Caution】It is contraindicated in pregnant women.

There are other orifice-opening medicinals such as *Rhizoma Acori Tatarinowii*, *Styrax Liquidus*, *Borneolum*, and *Benzoinum*.

Liver-Pacifying and Wind-Extinguishing Medicinals

All the medicinals with the major efficacy of pacifying the liver and subduing yang or exitinguishing wind and stopping spasms, and are mainly used for hyperactivity of liver yang and stirring of liver wind syndromes, are called liver-pacifying and wind-extinguishing medicinals. All the medicinals in this category enter the liver meridian, most of them are from shells or animals. The medicinals have different properties in nature, either cold, or warm, or neutral. In clinical practice, the medicinals with cold or cool nature should not be used for chronic infantile convulsions due to spleen deficiency; the medicinals with warm and dryness nature should not be used in yin and blood deficiency.

Rhizoma Gastrodiae (Tian Ma)

【Source】It is dried rhizome of *Gastrodia elate Bi.*, pertaining to *Orchidaceae*. It is collected from early winter to early spring. After dug out, it is washed, completely steamed, and then dried in low temperature and open space.

【Taste and Nature】Sweet and neutral.

【Meridian Entry】Liver meridian.

【Function】Pacify the liver and extinguish wind, expel wind and unblock collaterals.

【Indications】

1. For dizziness and dizzy vision caused by hyperactivity of liver yang, it can be used with *Ramulus Uncariae cum Uncis*, and *Concha Haliotidis*.

2. For fright epilepsy, convulsion, opisthotonos-in tetanus, due to stirring of liver, it may be used in combination with *Ramulus Uncariae cum Uncis*, and *Scorpio*.

3. For wind-dampness impediment, manifested as pain and/or numbness in the extremities, it is used together with *Radix Angelicae Sinensis*, *Radix Achyranthis Bidentatae*, *Scorpio*, and *Olibanum*.

【Preparation and dosage】3−9 g, decoct.

There are other liver-pacifying and wind-extinguishing medicinals such as *Ramulus Uncariae cum Uncis*, *Zhenzhumu*, *Concha Haliotidis*, *Concha Ostreae*, *Haematitum*, *Calculus Bovis*, *Lumbricus*, *Bombyx Batryticatus*, and *Scolopendra*.

十五、安神药

凡以安定神志为主要功效，治疗神志不安病证为主的药物，称为安神药。本类药物多为矿物药或种子类植物药，多入心、肝经。安神药分为重镇安神药和养心安神药两类。矿石类药物易伤胃气，不宜久服，应酌情配伍健脾养胃药物；部分矿石类药物有毒，须慎用。

（一）重镇安神药

重镇安神药多为矿石、贝壳、化石类药物，具有重镇安神作用，适用于心火亢盛、痰火扰心证，症见心悸、失眠、惊风、癫狂、躁动不安等。部分药物还有平肝潜阳作用，可用于肝阳上亢证。

磁　石

【药用】本品为氧化物类矿物尖晶石族磁铁矿，主含四氧化三铁（Fe_3O_4）。采挖后，除去杂石。

【性味】咸、寒。

【归经】归肝、心、肾经。

【功效】重镇安神，纳气平喘，益肾潜阳。

【临床应用】

1. 用于心神不安，症见心悸怔忡、失眠、惊痫等，常与朱砂配伍。

2. 用于肾虚气喘，可与熟地、五味子等同用。

3. 用于肝肾阴虚、肝阳上亢导致的头晕目眩等，可与龙骨、牡蛎等药同用。

4. 用于肾虚导致的头晕目眩、目视不明、耳鸣、耳聋等，可与熟地黄、山茱萸、五味子等同用。

【用量与用法】9~30g，先煎。

本类药还有龙骨、琥珀等。

（二）养心安神药

养心安神药多为植物种仁，药性甘润，具有养心安神作用，主要用于心肝血虚、心脾两虚等证，症见心悸怔忡、虚烦失眠、健忘多梦等。

酸枣仁

【药用】本品为鼠李科植物酸枣 [*Ziziphus jujuba Mill. var. spinosa（Bunge）Hu ex H. F. Chou*] 的干燥成熟种子。秋末冬初采收成熟果实，除去果肉及核壳，收集种子，晒干。

Tranquillizing Medicinals

All the medicinals that have functions of tranquillizing, and are applied for uneasiness of heart-spirit are called tranquilizing medicinals. The medicinals mainly include minerals and plant seeds, and are mainly attributive to heart and liver meridians. They are classified into settling tranquillizing medicinals and heart-nourishing tranquillizing medicinals. Since mineral medicinals are apt consume stomach qi, they should not be used for long period of time and must be combined with spleen-stomach tonifying medicinalsl; some of the medicinals are toxic, and should be used with caution.

Settling tranquillizing medicinals

Most of the settling tranquillizing medicinals are minerals, shells and fossils. They have functions of tranquillizing by heavy settling, and are indicated for hyperactive heart fire syndrome and phlegm-fire harassing the heart syndrome, manifested as palpitation, insomnia, epilepsy, and mania. Some of the medicinals also have the functions of pacifying liver and subduing yang, and are indicated for ascendant hyperactivity of liver yang syndrome.

Magnetitum (Ci Shi)

【Source】It is the magnetic iron ore magnetite, mainly contains Fe_3O_4. It is mined and got rid of the impurity of stone.

【Taste and Nature】Salty and cold.

【Meridian Entry】Liver, heart, and kidney meridians.

【Function】Tranquilize by heavy settling, promote qi absorption and calm panting, nourish kidney and subdue yang.

【Indications】

1. For uneasiness of heart spirit, manifested as palpitation, insomia and epilepsy, it is used in combination with *Cinnabaris*.

2. For panting due to kidney deficiency, it is used together with *Radix Rehmanniae Praeparata*, *Fructus Schisandrae*.

3. For liver-kidney yin deficiency and hyperactivity of liver yang, marked by dizziness, It is used together with *Os Draconis*, *Concha Ostreae*.

4. For dizziness, blurred vision, tinnitus and deafness due to kidney deficiency, it is used together with *Radix Rehmanniae Praeparata*, *Fructus Corni*, and *Fructus Schisandrae*.

【Preparation and dosage】9-30 g, dedoct first.

There are other settling tranquillizing medicinals such as *Os Draconis* and *Succinum*.

Heart-nourishing tranquillizing medicinals

Most of the heart-nourishing tranquillizing medicinals are plant seeds, are of sweet and nourishing in nature, have functions of nourishing the heart to tranquilize, and are mainly applied for heart-liver blood deficiency and dual deficiency of heart-spleen, manifested as palpitation, deficiency-restlessness, insomnia, amnesia, and dream-disturbed sleep.

Semen Ziziphi Spinosae (Suan Zao Ren)

【Source】It is the dried ripe seed of *Ziziphus jujuba Mill.var.spinosa(Bunge)Hu ex H.F.Chou* of *Rhamnaceae*. The seeds are collected from the ripe fruits in late autumn and early winter. After the shell and flesh are removed, they are dried.

【Taste and Nature】Sweet, sour, and neutral.

【Meridian Entry】Liver, gall bladder, and heart meridians.

【性味】甘、酸，平。

【归经】归肝、胆、心经。

【功效】养心安神，敛汗生津。

【临床应用】

1．用于心肝血虚导致的虚烦失眠、心悸怔忡等，可与茯苓、柏子仁、丹参、熟地等同用。

2．用于体虚自汗、盗汗，可与牡蛎、浮小麦等同用。

【用量与用法】3~9g，煎服。

本类药还有柏子仁、合欢皮、首乌藤、远志等。

十六、补益药

凡以补充人体气血阴阳为主要功效，治疗各种虚证为主的药物，称为补益药，也称为补虚药。补益药分为补气药、补阳药、补血药和补阴药四类。补气药和补阳药药性多甘温，而补血药和补阴药药性或甘温、或甘寒。使用补益药应注意：实邪未尽者慎用，以免病邪留滞；要适当配伍健脾养胃助消化的药物，以增强脾胃运化功能，更好发挥疗效。

（一）补气药

补气药性味多甘温，主要具有补气作用，适用于气虚证，症见神疲乏力、少气懒言、倦怠、自汗、脉虚等症。本类药物易壅滞气机，湿盛中满者忌用。

人 参

【药用】本品为五加科植物人参（*Panax ginseng C. A. Mey.*）的干燥根。多于秋季采挖，洗净，晒干。

【性味】甘，微苦，微温。

【归经】归脾、肺、心经。

【功效】大补元气，补脾益肺，生津安神。

【临床应用】

1．用于大失血、剧烈吐泻及久病大病导致的气虚欲脱等，可单用一味人参煎服，也可与附子等同用。

2．用于脾胃虚弱，症见倦怠乏力、食欲不振、胸腹胀满以及久泻脱肛等，常与黄芪、白术、茯苓、山药、莲肉、砂仁等配伍。

3．用于肺虚气喘，可与蛤蚧、胡桃肉等同用。

4．用于热病耗伤津液导致的口渴及消渴病，可与麦冬、五味子配伍。

【Function】Nourish the heart to tranquilize, engender fluid and constrain sweat.

【Indications】

1. For palpitation and vexation and insomnia due to heart-liver blood deficiency, it is used together with *Poria*, *Semen Platycladi*, *Radix Salviae Miltiorrhizae*, and *Radix Rehmanniae Praeparata*.

2. For spontaneous sweating and night sweating due to weak constitution, it is used together with *Concha Ostreae*, and *Fructus Tritici Levis*.

【Preparation and dosage】3-9 g, decoct.

There are other heart-nourishing tranquillizing medicinals, such as *Semen Biotae*, *Cortex Albiziae*, *Caulis Polygoni Multiflori*, *Radix Polygalae*.

Tonifying and Replenishing Medicinals

All the medicinals that have the main functions of replenishing qi, blood, yin and yang, and are mainly indicated to various deficiency syndromes, are called tonifying and replenishing medicinals. The medicinals are categorized into four groups: qi-tonifying medicinals, yang-tonifying medicinals, blood-tonifying medicinals, and yin-tonifying medicinals. Both qi-tonifying medicinals and yang-tonifying medicinals are mainly sweet in flavor and warm in nature; both blood-tonifying medicinals and yin-tonifying medicinals are mainly sweet in flavor and warm or cold in nature. The medicinals should not be used if the exterior pathogen is not relieved in order to avoid the retention of pathogen; the medicinals should be used in combination with spleen-stomach tonifying medicinals and digestant medicinals, so as to reinforce the spleen and stomach fucntions and achieve better therapeutic effects.

Qi-tonifying medicinals

Most of the qi-tonifying medicinals are sweet in flavor, and warm or neutral in nature, and have main functions of tonifying qi, and are applied for qi deficiency syndrome, manifested as listlessness and lack of strength, reluctance to speak and breathlessness, lassitude, spontaneous sweating, weak pulse. Since the medicinals are apt to obstruct the qi flow, they are contraindicated for dampness harassment marked by distention.

Radix Ginseng (Ren Shen)

【Source】It is the dried root of *Panas Ginseng C. A. Mey*. Mainly it is collected in autumn, washed clean, and dried.

【Taste and Nature】Sweet, slightly bitter, and slightly warm.

【Meridian Entry】Lung, spleen, and heart meridians.

【Function】Replenish the primordial qi, tonify the spleen and lung, promote fluid production, and induce tranquilization.

【Indications】

1. For severe bleeding, vomitting and diarrhea, prolonged disease causing qi collapse syndrome, it can be used alone or combined with *Radix Aconiti*.

2. For spleen-stomach qi deficiency syndrome, manifested as lassitude, lack of strength, poor appetite, epigastric and abdominal distention, and proctoptosis due to prolonged diarrhea, it is usually combined with *Radix Astragali*, *Rhizoma Atractylodis Macrocephalae*, *Poria*, *Rhizoma Dioscoreae*, *Semen Nelumbinis*, and *Semen Euryales*.

3. For dyspnea due to lung qi deficiency, it can be combined with *Gecko*, and *Semen Juglandis*.

4. For thirst and wasting-thirst due to consumption of body fluid, it can be used with *Radix Ophiopogonis*, and *Fructus Schisandrae*.

5. For syndrome of both qi and blood deficiency and agitation of heart spirit, manifesting as palpa-

5. 用于气血两亏、心神不安，症见心悸怔忡、失眠健忘等，常与酸枣仁、茯神、远志等同用。

【用量与用法】3~9g，另煎兑入汤剂服；野山参若研粉吞服，一次2g，一日2次。

【使用注意】实证、热证、肝阳上亢者均忌用。反藜芦，畏五灵脂。

黄 芪

【药用】本品为豆科植物蒙古黄芪［*Astragalus membranaceus（Fisch）Bge. var. mongholicus（Bge.）Hsiao*］或膜荚黄芪［*Astragalus membranaceus（Fisch.）Bge.*］的干燥根。春、秋二季采挖，除去须根及根头，晒干。

【性味】甘，温。

【归经】归脾、肺经。

【功效】补气升阳，固表止汗，利水消肿，托毒生肌。

【临床应用】

1. 用于脾胃虚弱导致的气虚衰弱、倦怠乏力，常与党参、白术等配伍。

2. 用于中气下陷导致的脱肛、子宫脱垂等，常与党参、升麻、柴胡等合用。

3. 用于表虚不固的自汗及体虚外感，自汗常与麻黄根、浮小麦、牡蛎等配伍；体虚易感风寒者可与防风、白术同用。

4. 用于气血不足、疮疡内陷、脓成不溃或久溃不敛者。疮疡内陷、或久溃不敛，可与党参、肉桂、当归等配伍；脓成不溃，可与当归、银花、白芷、穿山甲、皂角刺等同用。

5. 用于气虚水停，常配伍白术、茯苓等。

【用量与用法】9~30g，煎服。

【使用注意】表实邪盛、气滞湿阻、食积内停、阴虚阳亢、疮痈毒盛者，均不宜用。

本类药还有党参、白术、甘草、山药、大枣等。

（二）补阳药

补阳药药性多甘温，主要具有温补阳气作用，适用于阳虚证，症见畏寒、肢冷、完谷不化、小便清长、阳痿、宫寒不孕、冷汗淋漓、面色白、脉微等。本类药物阴虚火旺者忌用。

tions, fearful throbbing, insomnia and bad memory, it can be combined with *Semen Ziziphi Spinosae*, *Poria cum Radice Pino*, and *Radix Polygalae*.

【Preparation and dosage】3–9 g, It should be simmered separately and later mixed with decoction of other medicinal herbs for oral administration. As to wild ginseng, it is ground into powder for swallows, 2 g each time, twice per day.

【Caution】It is contraindicated in patients with excess syndrome, heat syndrome, and hyperactivity of liver yang syndrome. It should not be used in combination with *Rhizoma et Radix Veratri*, and *Faeces Trogopterorum*.

Radix Astragali (Huang Qi)

【Source】It is the dried root of *Astragalus membranaceus* (*Fisch*) *Bge var. mongholicus* (Bge). It is excavated and collected in spring and autumn. After removal of its rootlets and root-heads, it is dried by natural sunlight.

【Taste and Nature】Sweet and warm.

【Meridian Entry】Spleen and lung meridians.

【Function】Tonify qi and raise yang, strengthen the defensive and stop sweating, induce diuresis to alleviate edema, and expel toxin and promote tissue regeneration.

【Indications】

1. For lassitude, lack of strength due to spleen-stomach qi deficiency, it is usually combined with *Rhizoma Atractylodis Macrocephalae*, and *Radix Codonopsis*.

2. In cases of proctoptosis due to prolonged diarrhea, prolapse of uterus, it is usually combined with *Radix Codonopsis*, *Rhizoma Cimicifugae*, *Radix Bupleuri*.

3. For spontaneous sweating due to exterior deficiency, it is used in combination with *Mahuanggen*, *Fructus Tritici Levis*, and *Concha Ostreae*. For external contraction, it is combined with *Radix Saposhnikoviae* and *Rhizoma Atractylodis Macrocephalae*.

4. It is applied for unruptured ulcers or unhealed ulcers after rupture due to deficiency syndrome of qi and blood. For deep rooted ulcers which fail to heal for a long period, it is usually combined with *Radix Codonopsis*, *Cortex Cinnamomi*, and *Radix Angelicae Sinensis*. For unruptured ulcers, it is used in combination with *Radix Angelicae Sinensis*, *Flos Lonicerae*, *Radix Angelicae Dahuricae*, *Squama Manitis*, and *Spina Gleditsiae*.

5. For edema due to qi deficiency, it is used with *Rhizoma Atractylodis Macrocephalae*, and *Poria*.

【Preparation and dosage】9–30 g, decoct.

【Caution】It should not be used in patients with syndrome of exterior excess, qi stagnation and dampness obstruction, food accumulation, yin deficiency with yang hyperactivity, ulcer and abcess with excess toxin.

There are other qi-tonifying medicinals such as *Radix Codonopsis*, *Rhizoma Atractylodis Macrocephalae*, *Radix Glycyrrhizae*, *Rhizoma Dioscoreae*, and *Fructus Jujubae*.

Yang-tonifying medicinals

Most of the yang-tonifying medicinals are sweet in flavor and warm in nature, have main functions of tonifying yang qi, and are applied for yang deficiency syndrome manifested as inrolerance of cold, cold limbs, undigested food in stool, frequent urination, impotence, and infertility due to cold-uterus, pallor complexion, and weak pulse. These medicinals are contraindicated for patients of yin deficiency with fire effulgence.

鹿　茸

【药用】本品为鹿科动物梅花鹿（*Cervus nippon Temminck*）或马鹿（*Cervus elaphus Linnaeus*）的雄鹿未骨化密生茸毛的幼角。夏、秋二季锯取鹿茸，切片，阴干或烘干。

【性味】甘、咸，温。

【归经】归肾、肝经。

【功效】补肾壮阳，强筋健骨，固冲止带，托毒起陷。

【临床应用】

1. 用于肾阳不足，症见阳痿、肢冷、腰膝酸软、宫冷不孕、小便清长等，以及精血亏虚导致的筋骨无力、小儿发育不良、骨软行迟等。本品可单味服用，也可配合熟地、山萸肉、菟丝子、肉苁蓉等同用。

2. 用于冲任虚损导致的崩漏带下等，可与阿胶、当归、熟地、山萸肉、山药、白芍等配伍同用。

3. 用于疮疡久溃不敛、阴疽内陷不起等，可与黄芪等同用。

【用量与用法】1～2g，研末冲服。

【使用注意】本品宜从小量开始，缓缓加量，以免阳升风动，或伤阴动血。凡阴虚内热及外感实热忌用。

本类药还有淫羊藿、续断、海马、仙茅、巴戟天、补骨脂、益智仁、菟丝子、肉苁蓉、锁阳、蛤蚧、韭菜子。

（三）补血药

补血药味多甘，药性或温、或寒、或平，主要具有补血作用，适用于血虚证，症见面色萎黄、唇甲苍白、头晕、耳鸣、心悸、健忘、失眠、妇女月经不调等症。本类药物多滋腻，湿阻中焦及脘腹胀满者慎用。

熟地黄

【药用】本品为玄参科植物地黄（*Rhemannia glutinosa Libosch.*）的块根。秋季采挖，除去芦头、须根及泥沙，缓缓烘焙至约八成干，再经酒炖法或蒸发等炮制加工成。

【性味】甘，微温。

【归经】归肝、肾经。

【功效】补血养阴，填精益髓。

【临床应用】

1. 用于血虚阴亏、肝肾不足所致的眩晕、心悸、失眠及月经不调、崩漏等，常与当归、白芍、山茱萸等同用。

Cornu Cervi Pantotrichum (Lu Rong)

〖Source〗This medicinal is the hairy, non-ossified young horn of a stag of *Cervus Nippon Tmminck* or *Crvus elphhus Linnaeus*. The hair, non-ossified young horn of a stag is sawed-off in summer and autumn, sliced, and dried in shade or baked until dry.

〖Taste and Nature〗Sweet, salty and warm.

〖Meridian Entry〗Kidney and liver meridians.

〖Function〗Tonify kidney and strengthen yang, strengthen tensons and bones, regulate thoroughfare vessel and stop leucorrhea, stop invasion of toxin and expel sores.

〖Indications〗

1. It is indicated for kidney yang deficiency syndrome, manifested as impotence, cold limbs, soreness and weakness in the loins and knees, infertility due to cold-uterus, frequent urination, and essence-blood insufficiency syndrome manifested as bone and tendon weakness, infantile maldevelopment, and retardation in bone or walking. It can be used alone or combined with *Radix Rehmanniae Praeparata*, *Fructus Corni*, *Semen Cuscutae*, *Herba Cistanchis*.

2. In cases of deficiency-cold in thoroughfare and conception vessels, metrorrhagia and leukorrhagia, it is usually combined with *Colla Corii Asini*, *Radix Angelicae Sinensis*, *Radix Rehmanniae Praeparata*, *Fructus Corni*, *Rhizoma Dioscoreae*, *Radix Paeoniae Alba*.

3. In case of unhealed chronic ulcers, or deep-rooted yin abscess, it is often prescribed with *Radix Astragali*.

〖Preparation and dosage〗1-2 g, it is ground into powder for swallows.

〖Caution〗It should be taken in low dose at the beginning of treatment, and then the dosage could be increased gradually, in order to avoid upbearing yang-qi stirring wind, or consumption of yin and activating blood. It is contraindicated in patients with excess heat of external contraction syndrome and of internal heat of yin deficiency syndrome.

There are other yang-tonifying medicinals such as *Herba Epimedii*, *Radix Dipsaci*, *Hippocampus*, *Rhizoma Curculiginis*, *Radix Morindae Officinalis*, *Fructus Psoraleae*, *Fructus Alpiniae Oxyphyllae*, *Semen Cuscutae*, *Herba Cistanchis*, *Herba Cynomorii*, *Gecko*, and *Semen Allii Tuberosi*.

Blood-tonifying medicinals

Most of the blood tonifying medicinals are sweet in flavor, either warm, cold, or neutral in nature, mainly have the functions of replenishing blood, and are indicated for blood deficiency syndrome, manifested as sallow complexion, pallor lip and nails, dizziness, tinnitus, palpitations, amnesia, insomnia and irrgular menstruation. Lots of the blood tonifying medicinals are moisty and greasy, and they should be used with caution in patients with retention of dampness in the middle energizer and epigastric and abdominal distention.

Radix Rehmanniae Praeparata (Shu Di Huang)

〖Source〗This medicinal is the prepared root tuber of *Rehmannia ghutinosa libosch* (*Fam. Scrophulariaceae*). It is excavated and collected in autumn. After removel of top of roots, fibrous roots and sand, baking to 70%-80% dried, then mixtured with wine and processed with a series steaming for use.

〖Taste and Nature〗Sweet and slightly warm.

〖Meridian Entry〗Liver and kidney meridians.

〖Function〗Nourish yin, replenish blood, and replenish essence and marrow.

〖Indications〗

1. For blood and yin deficiency syndrome and liver-kidney yin deficiency syndrome, manifested as

2. 用于肾阴不足导致的骨蒸潮热、盗汗、遗精等，常与丹皮、龟板、知母、黄柏等同用。

【用量与用法】9~15g，煎服。

【使用注意】脾胃虚弱者慎用。

当 归

【药用】本品为伞形科植物当归 [Angelica sinensis (Oliv.) Diels] 的干燥根。秋末采挖，除去须根及泥沙，用烟火熏干。

【性味】甘、辛，温。

【归经】归肝、心、脾经。

【功效】补血调经，活血止痛，润肠通便。

【临床应用】

1. 用于血虚导致的月经不调、痛经、经闭等，常与熟地、白芍、川芎等配伍。

2. 用于产后瘀滞腹痛，可与益母草、川芎、桃仁等配伍。

3. 用于风湿痹痛，可与羌活、独活、防风、秦艽等配伍。

4. 用于经络不利、筋骨酸痛，可与桂枝、白芍等同用。

5. 用于外伤瘀痛，可与红花、桃仁、赤芍等品配伍。

6. 用于血虚肠燥便秘，常与肉苁蓉、生首乌等配伍。

【用量与用法】3~9g，煎服。

【使用注意】湿盛中满，大便泄泻者忌用。

本类药还有白芍、阿胶、龙眼肉等。

（四）补阴药

补阴药药性多甘寒，主要具有养阴生津作用，适用于阴虚证，症见咽干口燥、潮热、五心烦热、颧红、盗汗、舌红少苔、脉细数等。本类药物不宜应用于脾肾阳虚、痰湿内阻者。

沙 参

【药用】可分北沙参、南沙参。北沙参为伞形科植物珊瑚菜 (Glehnia littoralis Fr. Schmidt ex Miq.) 的干燥根。夏、秋二季采挖，洗净，去皮，干燥。或洗净直接干燥。南沙参为桔梗科植物轮叶沙参 [Adenophora tetraphylla (Thunb.) Fisch.] 或沙参 (Adenophora stricta Miq.) 的干燥根。春、秋二季采挖，洗净，去皮，干燥。

【性味】北沙参：甘、微苦，微寒。南沙参：甘，微寒。

【归经】归肺、胃经。

dizzness, palpitations, insomnia, irregular menstruation, metrorhagia and metrostaxis, it is used in combination with *Radix Angelicae Sinensis*, *Radix Paeoniae Alba*, and *Fructus Corni*.

2. For kidney yin deficiency syndrome, manifested as bone-steaming and tidal fever, night sweating, tinnitus, and seminal emission, it is used in combination with *Cortex Moutan*, *Plastron Testudinis*, *Rhizoma Anemarrhenae*, and *Cortex Phellodendri*.

【Preparation and dosage】9－15 g, decoct.

【Caution】It should be cautiously used in patients with spleen-stomach deficiency.

Radix Angelicae Sinensis (Dang Gui)

【Source】It is the dried root of *Angellica sinensis*(*Oliv.*) *Didls.* (*Fam. Umbelliferac*). It is excavated in late autumn. After removal of fibrous roots and sand, it is dried on smoke and fire.

【Taste and Nature】Sweet, pungent, and warm.

【Meridian Entry】Liver, heart, and spleen meridians.

【Function】Replenish blood and regulate menstruation, activate blood to relieve pain, and moisten the intestines to relax the bowels.

【Indications】

1. For irregular menstruation, amenorrhea and menorrhagia due to blood deficiency, it is often used together with *Radix Rehmanniae Praeparata*, *Radix Paeoniae Alba*, and *Rhizoma Chuanxiong*.

2. For post partum abdominal pain, it is used with *Herba Leonuri*, *Rhizoma Chuanxiong*, and *Semen Persicae*.

3. For wind-dampness arthralgia, it is used together with *Rhizoma seu Radix Notopterygii*, *Radix Angelicae Pubescentis*, *Radix Saposhnikoviae*, and *Radix Gentianae Macrophyllae*.

4. For malfunction of merdians and collaterals, soreness and pain in the tendons and bones, it is combined with *Ramulus Cinnamomi*, *Jixueteng*, and *Radix Paeoniae Alba*.

5. For traumatic injury pain, it is combined with *Flos Carthami*, *Semen Persicae*, and *Radix Paeoniae Rubra*.

6. For constipation due to blood deficiency with intestinal dryness, it is often used in combination with *Herba Cistanchis*, and *Radix Achyranthis Bidentatae*.

【Preparation and dosage】3－9 g, decoct.

【Caution】It is contraindicated in patients with excessive abdominal fullness and diarrhea.

There are other yang-tonifying medicinals such as *Radix Paeoniae Alba*, *Colla Corii Asini*, and *Longyanrou*.

Yin-tonifying medicinals

Yin-tonifying medicinals are mostly sweet in taste and cold in nature, mainly have functions of nourshing yin and promote fluid production, and are indicated for yin deficiency syndrome, manifested as dry throat and dry mouth, tidal fever, vexing heat in the chest, palms and soles, night sweating, red tongue with scanty tongue coating, and fine and rapid pulse. The medicinals should be used with caution in patients with spleen-kidney yang deficiency, internal obstruction of dampness and phlegm.

Radix Glehniae (Sha Shen)

【Source】It refers to two types of medicinals: *Radix Glehniae* and *Radix Adenophorae*. *Radix Glehniae* is the dried root of *Glehnia littoralis Fr. Schnidt ex Miq.* (*Fam. Umbelliferae*). It is excavated in summer and autumn. After being washed clean, it is peeled and dried by natural sunlight. *Radix Adenophorae* is the root of *Adenophora tetraphylia*(*Thunb.*) *Fisch.* or *Adenophora. strita Miq*(*Fam. Campanulaceae*). It is excavated in spring and summer. After being washed clean, it is peeled and dried by natural sunlight.

【功效】养阴清肺，益胃生津。

【临床应用】

1. 用于肺虚有热、干咳少痰，或久咳声哑等症，常与川贝、麦冬等配伍。

2. 用于胃阴耗伤、津少口渴等，常与麦冬、生地、石斛等品同用。

【用量与用法】北沙参：4.5~9g；南沙参：9~15g，煎服。

【使用注意】虚寒证忌服。反藜芦。

枸杞子

【药用】本品为茄科植物宁夏枸杞（*Lycium barbarum L.*）的干燥成熟果实。夏、秋二季果实呈红色时采收，干燥。

【性味】甘，平。

【归经】归肝、肾经。

【功效】补肾益精，养肝明目。

【临床应用】

1. 用于肝肾不足导致的遗精、腰膝酸痛，常与巴戟天、肉苁蓉、芡实等配伍。

2. 用于肝肾不足导致的头晕、目眩等，可与菊花、地黄、山萸肉等配伍。

【用量与用法】6~12g，煎服。

本类药还有麦冬、玉竹、黄精、石斛、天冬、桑椹、女贞子、龟甲等。

十七、固涩药

凡以收敛固涩为主要功效，治疗各种滑脱证候为主的药物，称为固涩药。滑脱诸症主要有自汗、盗汗、久泻、久痢、久咳、虚喘、遗精、遗尿、尿频及崩带不止等。本类药物药味多酸涩，主要归肺、脾、肾、大肠经。如外感表邪未解、或内有湿热以及郁热未清时，不宜使用固涩药，以免留邪。

五味子

【药用】本品为木兰科植物五味子［*Schisandra chinensis（Turcz.）Baill.*］的干燥成熟果实。秋季果实成熟时采摘，晒干。

【性味】酸、甘，温。

【归经】归肺、心、肾经。

【功效】敛肺滋肾，生津敛汗，涩精止泻，宁心安神。

【临床应用】

1. 用于久嗽虚喘，常与党参、麦冬、熟地、山茱萸等同用。

【Taste and Nature】 *Radix Glehniae*: sweet, slightly bitter, and sligthtly cold; *Radix Adenophorae*: sweet and slightly cold.

【Meridian Entry】Lung and stomach meridians.

【Function】Nourish yin and clear lung heat, reinforce the stomach and promote fluid production.

【Indications】

1. For yin deficiency and dryness-heat in the lung, manifested as dry cough with little sputum, dry throat with hoarse voice, it is used in combination with *Bulbus Fritillariae Cirrhosae*, and *Radix Ophiopogonis*.

2. For stomach yin deficiency and consumption of fluid, marked by thirst, it is used in combination with *Radix Ophiopogonis*, *Radix Rehmanniae*, and *Herba Dendrobii*.

【Preparation and dosage】*Radix Glehniae*: 4. 5-9 g; *Radix Adenophorae*: 9-15 g, decoct.

【Caution】It is contraindicated in patients with deficiency cold syndrome, and it is incompatible with *Rhizoma et Radix Veratri*.

Fruvtus Lycii Barbary (Gou Qi Zi)

【Source】It is the dried ripe fruits of the *Machaka Lycium Barbarum L.* (*Fam. Solanaceae*). It is collected in summer and autumn when the fruit appears salmon pink and dried.

【Taste and Nature】Sweet and neutral.

【Meridian Entry】Liver and kidney meridians.

【Function】Nourish liver and kidney, replenish essence, and improve vision.

【Indications】

1. For liver-kidney deficiency manifested as aching and weakness in the loins and knees, spermatorrhea, it is used in combination with *Radix Morindae Officinalis*, *Herba Cistanchis*, and *Semen Euryales*.

2. For liver-kidney deficiency manifested as dizzness, it is used in combination with *Flos Chrysanthemi*, *Radix Rehmanniae*, and *Fructus Corni*.

【Preparation and dosage】6-9 g, decoct.

There are other yin-tonifying medicinals such as *Radix Ophiopogonis*, *Rhizoma Polygonati Odorati*, *Rhizoma Polygonati*, *Herba Dendrobii*, *Radix Asparagi*, *Fructus Mori*, *Fructus Ligustri Lucidi*, and *Carapax et Plastrum Testudinis*.

Astrigent Medicinals

All the medicinals that have the main functions of arresting discharge, and are applicable to various syndrome marked by abnormal discharge of body substances, including spontaneous sweating, night sweating, chronic diarrhea and dysentery, chronic recurring cough, dyspnea, seminal emission, enuresis, frequent micturition, dyspnea, metrorrhagia and metrostaxis, leucorrhea. Most of the merdicinals are sour and astringent in flavor, enter the lung, spleen, kidney, and large intestine meridians. If the exterior pathogen is not released, or there is internal dampness-heat or uncleared internal heat, the medicinals should not be used, in order to avoid retention of pathogen.

Fructus Schisandrae (Wu Wei Zi)

【Source】It is the ripe fruit of *Schisandra chinensis* (*Tuecz*) *Baill.* of *Magnoliaceae*. It is collected in autumn when the fruit ripe and dried in the sunshine.

【Taste and Nature】Sour, sweet, and warm.

【Meridian Entry】Lung, heart, and kidney meridians

【Function】Astringe the lung and nourish kidney, engender body fluid and stop sweating, astringe es-

2．用于津少口渴，可与麦冬、生地、天花粉等同用。

3．用于体虚多汗，可配党参、麦冬、浮小麦、牡蛎等。

4．用于精滑不固、小便频数、久泻不止等，可与桑螵蛸、菟丝子、补骨脂、肉豆蔻等同用。

【用量与用法】1.5~6g，煎服。

本类药还有乌梅、金樱子、浮小麦、诃子、赤石脂、覆盆子、莲须、芡实。

（朴元林　董振华　张孟仁）

sence and stop diarrhea, and pacify the heart to tranquilize.

【Indications】

1. For chronic cough and dyspnea, it is used in combination with *Radix Codonopsis*, *Radix Ophiopogonis*, *Radix Rehmanniae Praeparata*, and *Fructus Corni*.

2. For thirst due to deficiency of body fluids, it is used in combination with *Radix Ophiopogonis*, *Radix Rehmanniae*, and *Radix Trichosanthis*.

3. For excessive sweating due to deficiency syndrome, it is used in combination with *Radix Codonopsis*, *Radix Ophiopogonis*, *Fructus Tritici Levis*, and *Concha Ostreae*.

4. For spermatorrhea, frequent micturition, chronic diarrhea, it is often used together with *Ootheca Mantidis*, *Semen Cuscutae*, *Fructus Psoraleae*, and *Semen Myristicae*.

【Preparation and dosage】1. 5-6 g, decoct.

There are other astrigent medicinals such as *Fructus Mume*, *Fructus Rosae Laevigatae*, *Fructus Tritici Levis*, *Fructus Chebulae*, *Halloysitum Rubrum*, *Fructus Rubi*, *Stamen Nelumbinis*, and *Semen Euryales*.

(*Piao Yuanlin   Zhang Wen*)

第九章　方　　剂

第一节　方剂学总论

方剂学是阐明和研究方剂配伍规律及临床应用的一门学科。方剂是在辨证审因确定治法的基础上，选择合适的药物，酌定用量，按照组方结构的要求，妥善配伍而成的。因此，辨证是治法的前提，治法是组方的依据，方剂是治法的体现；法随证立，方从法出，方以药成。

一、方剂的组成原则

方剂是以中医基本理论为指导，在辨证立法的基础上，按照一定的原则，选择适当的药物组合而成的。组方的原则称为"君、臣、佐、使"。其具体含义如下：

1. 君药　又称为方剂的主药，是针对主证或主病起主要治疗作用的药物。

2. 臣药　又称为方剂的辅药。作用有二：

（1）辅助君药加强治疗主病或主证。

（2）针对兼病及兼证起治疗作用。

3. 佐药　意义有三：

（1）佐使药：配合君臣药以加强其治疗作用，或直接治疗次要症状的药物。

（2）佐制药：减弱或消除君臣药毒性，以防机体产生不良反应的药物。

（3）反佐药：与主要药物性味相反，而在治疗中又起相成作用的药物，用于因病重拒药加以从治者。

4. 使药　分引经药和调和药。

（1）引经药：能引方中诸药至病所的药物。

（2）调和药：具有调和方中诸药作用的药物。

每个方剂，君药必不可少。在简单的方剂中，臣、佐、使药则不一定俱全，应根

CHAPTER NINE　FORMULAS

Section 1　Overview of Formulas

Formula study is an academic discipline of clarifying and studying on composition principles and clinical applications of formulas. Formulas are based on the determination of treatments, and they are composed via the procedure of selecting the right medicine, deciding the amount of discretion, and appropriately combining the medicine in accordance with the request of the combination structure. Therefore, syndrome differentiation is a prerequisite for treatment, treatment is a basis for composition of prescription, and formula is a manifestation of treatment; treatment follows the clarification of syndrome differentiation, prescription is based on the treatment, and prescription achieves success by means of medicines.

Composition Principle of Formula

Formulas, guided by the basic theory of TCM are based on the syndrome differentiation and certain principles, are combinations of appropriately chosen Chinese medicinals. Formula principle is named as "sovereign, minister, assistant and courier," with its special meaning as follows:

Sovereign medicinal: also known as chief, which plays major therapeutic role for the main syndrome or the primary disease.

Minister medicinal: also known as deputy, which has two functions:

(1) Accentuating and enhancing the effect of the chief ingredient to treat the main disease or the principle syndrome.

(2) Directly treating a coexisting disease or a coexisting syndrome.

Assistant medicinal: has three meanings:

(1) Helping assistant: accentuates and enhances the therapeutic effect of the sovereign medicinals and the minister medicinals, or directly treats secondary symptoms.

(2) Correcting assistant: moderates or eliminates the toxicity of the sovereign medicinal or the minister medicinals, so as to prevent their adverse reactions.

(3) Counteracting assistant: which nature and moving tendency are opposite to the chief ingredient but which is helpful in fulfilling the therapeutic effect, and which may be used in case of severve condition that rejects medicine and by means of following-treatment.

Courier medicinal: also known as envoy, which is classified as guide and harmonizing.

(1) Guide: guides the rest ingredients of the formula to the place where the main pathological changes exist.

(2) Harmonizing: harmonizes and integrates the actions of the other ingredients of the formula.

Each formula must have the sovereign(medicinal), but the minister, assistant, and courier(medicinals) are not necessary, which are based on the demand of the syndrome differentiation and clinical treatment.

据临床辨证立法的需要而定。

二、方剂的变化

方剂的组成，固然有一定的原则，但在临床应用时，还需根据病情的缓急以及患者的体质、年龄和生活环境等不同，予以灵活加减、化裁运用，使之更加切合病情。方剂组成的变化，一般有药味加减的变化、药量加减的变化和剂型更换的变化三种形式。

1. 药味加减的变化　方剂是由药物组成的，药物是决定方剂功用的主要因素，因此方剂中的药味增加或减少，必然使方剂功用发生变化。药味变化包括两种形式：

一是佐使药的加减。因为佐使药的药力较小，不发生主要配伍变化，所以一般不会引起功用的根本变化，只是主治的兼证不同而已。如主治少阳病的小柴胡汤，若口渴，主治证仍是少阳证，但口渴是津液不足，故去半夏加瓜蒌根。

二是臣药的加减。这种加减改变了君臣配伍关系，必然使方剂的功用发生根本变化。如麻黄汤功能主要为发汗解表、散风寒，兼有宣肺平喘之功，是主治外感风寒、无汗而喘的常用方剂。三拗汤君药虽然仍是麻黄，但因为缺少桂枝的配合，发汗力弱，且以杏仁为臣，与麻黄配伍，功专宣利肺气、发散风寒，故为治疗风寒犯肺咳喘的常用方剂。

2. 药量加减的变化　这种变化是指组成方剂的药物不变，但药量有了变化，因而改变了该方的功用和主治证候。例如，枳术汤和枳术丸都由枳实、白术两味药组成，但前方枳实倍于白术，故以消积导滞为主；后者白术用量则倍于枳实，故以健脾和中为主。因此，药味虽同，用量改变时，其方剂的作用也随着改变，适应证也随之变化。

三、方剂的剂型

方剂在组成以后（药物在使用前），根据病情与药物的特点制成一定的形态，称为剂型。常用剂型有：

1. 汤剂　汤剂是以药物配成方剂，加水煎煮去渣，制成汤液。汤剂疗法是中医临床治疗方法中最主要的疗法之一。既可以内服，也可以外用。汤剂具有吸收快、作用强的优点。汤剂可以根据临床具体病症灵活加减，故治疗疾病的针对性强，临床上应用最广。

2. 丸剂　丸剂是指药材细粉或药材提取物加适宜的粘合辅料制成的球形或类球形制剂。其吸收较慢，药效持久，节省药材，便于携带与服用。

3. 膏剂　是将药物用水或植物油煎熬浓缩而去渣而成。有内服和外用两种。

Variation of Formula

The composition of formula definitely has certain rules, but when used in clinical practice, the formula should be modified and verified freely, according to the condition which is either urgent or chronic, and the difference of the age, constitution and environment of the patients, so as to make it fit with the condition better. Generally, the variation of formula includes modification of ingredients, modification of dosage, and changing of the preparation form.

Variation of ingredients

Formula is composed of medicinals, and medicinals are main factors that decide the indication of a formula, thus, adding or reducing the ingredients results in the change of the indication of a formula. The variation of ingredients has two forms:

First is variation of assistant and courier. Generally it would not lead to fundermental change of functions, since the effects of assistant and courier are relatively weak, and there are no vital changes of composition but different co-exist symdromes to treat. For example, the indication of "Small Bupleurum Decoction" is lesser yang disease syndrome. In case of thirst, since the main syndrome is still lesser yang syndrome, and thirst refers to deficiency of fluid, so *Rhizoma Pinelliae* should be reduced and *Fructus Trichosanthis* should be added.

Second is variation of minister, which can change the relationships between the sovereign and the minister, and results in fundermental changes in the function of the formula. For example, "Ephedra Decoction" is a common used formula for asthma without sweating due to external contraction of wind-cold, and it has functions of promoting sweating to release the exterior, dissipating wind-cold and diffusing the lung to calm panting. The sovereign medicinal of "Three Crude Drugs Decoction" is the same as that of Ephedra Decoction, it is *Herba Ephedrae*. Since *Herba Ephedrae* has no minister of *Ramulus Cinnamomi*, the latter formula's function of sweating is weak, and its own minister is *Semen Armeniacae Amarum* which helps *Herba Ephedrae* focus on diffusing the lung to soothe the qi, and dissipating wind-cold, thus, the latter formula is a common formula for the treatment of cough and asthma results from wind-cold invading the lung.

Variation of the dosage

This change refers to no change of components but the change of the dosages, which results in the change of the formula's function and indication. For example, both "Aurantium-Atractylodes Decoction" and "Aurantium-Atractylodes Pill" are composed of *Fructus Aurantii Immaturus* and *Rhizoma Atractylodis Macrocephalae*, the dosage of *Fructus Aurantii Immaturus* is two times as that of *Rhizoma Atractylodis Macrocephalae* in the former, whereas, the dosage of *Rhizoma Atractylodis Macrocephalae* is two times as that of *Fructus Aurantii Immaturus* in the latter, thus, the former has main function of promoting digestion and removing food stagnation; the latter has main function of fortifying the spleen and harmonizing the spleen and stomach. Therefore, although the ingredients are the same, if the dosages are changed, the formulas's functions will be changed and the indications will be changed too.

Preparation Form of Formula

Preparation form refers to preparing the formula in a certain shape according to its ingredients' properties and the conditions, after the completion of the composition of a formula. Commonly used forms are described as below.

1. Decoction

Decoction is a liquid medicine prepared by boiling the ingredients in water, and taken after the dregs are removed. Decoction treatment is the most important treatment in clinical treatments of TCM. It is not

4．散剂　系一种或数种药物均匀混合而制成的干燥粉末状制剂。供内服或外用。

5．酒剂　古称"酒醴"。是用白酒或用黄酒浸制药物，或加温隔水炖煮，所得药液供内服或外用。酒剂多用于治疗风寒湿痹及跌打损伤等。

6．糖浆剂　系指含有药物、药材提取物或芳香物质的口服浓蔗糖水溶液。因含有糖，可以掩盖某些药物的不适气味，便于服用，适用于小儿及虚弱病人，尤多见于小儿用药，但不宜用于糖尿病患者。

7．片剂　是将药材细粉或药材提取物与辅料混合压制而成的小的片状的制剂。片剂用量准确，体积小，易于服用。

8．胶囊剂　系指将药物填装于空心硬质胶囊中或密封于弹性软质胶囊中而制成的固体制剂。

第二节　方剂各论

一、解表剂

解表剂是以解表药为主组成，具有宣散表邪、发汗解肌、透疹消疮等作用，主要治疗表证的方剂以及麻疹初期、疮疡初起，并兼有发热、恶寒、头痛、身痛、脉浮等表证者。属"八法"中的"汗法"。

临床使用解表剂，必须是外邪所伤而致的表证，无表证者不能使用。解表剂多为辛散轻扬之品，不宜久煎，以免功效减弱。解表剂取汗以微汗出为宜，若汗出不彻，则病邪不解；若汗出过多，易致耗气伤津。

解表剂可分为辛温解表、辛凉解表和扶正解表三类。

only for oral applicaton, but also for external use, and has merits of quick absportion and strong effects. Decoction can be freely modified according to the condition of clinical diseases or syndromes, so it is well-directed, and it is the most extensively used in clinical practice.

2. Pills

Pills are solid forms of preparation made into the spherical shapes by adding appropriate amount of excipient to the finely ground medicinals or extracts of medicinals. Pills are slower to be absorbed, persistent for the efficacy, economical to save the medicinal materials and convenient to be taken and carried compared with decoctions.

3. Plaster

Plaster is made by decocting the medicinals with water or vegetable oil, with the drugs removed. There are two types, one for oral administration, and another for external application.

4. Powder

Powder refers to the preparation of one or multiple medicinal materials ground and evenly mixed into dry powder. For internal administration or for external applications.

5. Medicated wine

Medicated wine is also called sweet wine(Jiu Li) in the ancient time. It is made by soaking the medicinals in liquor or yellow wine or stewing the medicinals in wine, and the liquid is used for oral and external application. Medicinal wine is mainly used to treat injury and impediment disease due to wind-cold-dampness.

6. Syrups

Syrups are concentrated solution of sugar containing the medicinal materials, the extract of meidicinals or aromatic substances. Containing sugar, it covers up some certain uncomfortable smells of some medicinals, and it is convenient to take. It is applicable to children and weak patients, especially for children, whereas, contraindicated for patients with diabetes.

7. Tablets

Tablets are small flattened pills of compressed powdered medicine or extract of medicine with formative agents. Tablets are accurate in dosage and small in volume, and convenient for oral application.

8. Capsules

Capsules are solid preparation forms in which a drug filled in a hollow hard capsule or sealed in a flexible soft capsule.

Section 2　Different Formula Forms

Exterior-releasing Formulas

The exterior-releasing formulas are the formulas which mainly consist of exterior-releasing medicinals, have the functions of diffusing and dispelling the exterior pathogens, promoting sweating to release the flesh, outbursting rashes, and releasing sores, and mainly treat exterior syndromes, and the early stage of measles or sores and ulcer, and concurrent with exterior symptoms such as fever, aversion to cold, headache, aching pain and floating pulse. The formulas belong to the "diaphoresis" of the "eight therapeutic methods."

The formulas must be indicated for the exterior syndromes due to invasion of exterior pathgens, and contraindicated for cases without the exterior syndromes. Most of the formulas are pungent-diffusing, light and upward-rising, and should not be decocted for long time to avoid the reduction of the effects. When promoting sweating with the exterior-releasing formulas, it should be mild sweating. If the sweating is not

（一）辛温解表剂

辛温解表剂适用于外感风寒表证。症见恶寒发热，头项强痛，肢体酸痛，口不渴，舌苔薄白，脉浮紧或浮缓等。代表方剂：麻黄汤、桂枝汤。

麻黄汤

【来源】《伤寒论》

【组成】麻黄（9克）桂枝（6克）杏仁（6克）甘草（3克）

【功用】发汗散寒，宣肺平喘。

【主治】外感风寒表实证。症见恶寒发热，头痛身疼，无汗而喘，舌苔薄白，脉浮紧。

【方解】方中麻黄辛苦温，善开泄腠理而发汗，祛在表之风寒；开郁闭之肺气，宣肺平喘，故为君药。桂枝透营达卫为臣药，解肌发表，温经散寒，既助麻黄解表，使发汗之力增加；又畅行营阴，使疼痛之症得解。二药相须为用，是辛温发汗的典型组合。佐药杏仁降气利肺，与麻黄相伍，宣降并用，以恢复肺气之宣肃，加强宣肺平喘之功，是为宣肃肺气的常用组合。炙甘草为使药，既能调和麻、杏之宣肃，又能缓和麻、桂相合之峻烈，使汗出不致过猛而耗伤正气。四药配伍，表寒得解，营卫得通，肺气得宣。

【注意事项】本方为辛温发汗之峻剂，药味虽少，但发汗力强，不可过服，否则，汗出过多必伤正气。

【加减】若喘急胸闷、咳嗽痰多、表证不甚者，去桂枝，加苏子、半夏以化痰止咳平喘。若鼻塞、流涕重者，加苍耳子、辛夷以宣通鼻窍。若夹湿邪而兼见骨节酸痛，加苍术、薏苡仁以祛风除湿。

completely, the pathogen will not be released; if the sweating is too excessive, then it results in the consumption of qi and fluid.

The exterior-releasing formulas are classified into three types: pungent-warm exterior-releasing formulas, pungent-cool exterior-releasing formulas, and renforcing healthy qi and exterior-releasing formulas.

Pungent-warm exterior-releasing formulas

Pungent-warm exterior-releasing formulas are indicated for exterior syndrome of wind-cold with external contraction, marked by aversion to cold, fever, headache and stiff neck, soreness and pain in the extremities, no thirst, a thin and white tongue coating, floating and tight or floating and tardy pulse. The representative formulas are "Ephedra Decoction" and "Ramulus Cinnamomi Decoction".

Ephedra Decoction(Ma Huang Tang)

【Source】*Treatise on Cold Damage Diseases*.

【Composition】*Herba Ephedrae* (9 g), *Ramulus Cinnamomi* (6 g), *Semen Armeniacae Amarum* (6 g), and *Radix Glycyrrhizae Praeparata* (3 g).

【Functions】Promote sweating and dissipate cold, diffuse the lung to calm panting.

【Indications】Exterior-excess syndrome due to exogenous wind-cold, marked by aversion to cold, fever, headache, general achiness, asthma, no sweating, thin and white tongue coating, and floating and tight pulse.

【Explanation】In the formula, *Herba Ephedrae* with bitter and acrid flavor and warm nature is good at effusing the interstices to induce sweating, and it dispels the exterior wind-cold, moreover, it opens and frees the depressed lung qi, and diffuses the lung to relieve asthma. Thus, *Herba Ephedrae* serves as the sovereign medicinal. *Ramulus Cinnamomi* as the minister medicinal drives pathogenic factors from the nutrient aspect to the defense aspect, it diffuses the flesh and promotes sweating, and warms the channels to dipel cold. It not only helps *Herba Ephedrae* to release the exterior and enhance the power of promoting sweating, but also goes freely in the nutrient aspect and relieves pain. The usage of *Herba Ephedrae* together with *Ramulus Cinnamomi* reinforces their efficacy mutually; it is a typical combination for promoting sweating with pungent-warm medicinals. *Semen Armeniacae Amarum* as the assistant medicinal descends and promotes lung qi. It is used together with *Herba Ephedrae*, effusing together with descending, so as to recover the fuctions of diffusing and descending of lung qi and reinforce its function of diffusing lung to relieve asthma; the combination is a typical combination of diffusing and descending lung qi. *Radix Glycyrrhizae Praeparata* as the courier medicinal not only mediates diffusing *Herba Ephedrae* and descending *Semen Armeniacae Amarum*, but also alleviates the drastic nature of *Herba Ephedrae* and *Ramulus Cinnamomi* combination, so as to avoid severe sweating which results in the consumption of healthy qi. The four ingredients jointly achieve the actions of relieving the exterior and dispelling cold, freeing the nutrient and defense aspects, and diffusing the lung qi.

【Note】It is a strong formula of the pungent-warm exterior-releasing formulas. Though its ingredients are small in the numbers, its action of sweating is strong. It should not be overtaken; otherwise, excessive sweating would result in consumption of healthy qi.

【Variation】In case of mild exterior syndrome concurrent with asthma and fullness in the chest, cough and productive phlegm, one should remove *Ramulus Cinnamomi* and add *Fructus Perillae* and *Rhizoma Pinelliae* to resolve phlegm and arrest cough and asthma. In case of nasal obstruction and severe running nose, add *Fructus Xanthii* and *Flos Magnoliae* to diffuse and open the orifices of the nose. In case of concurrence with dampness manifested as soreness and pain in the bones and joints, add *Rhizoma Atractylodis* and *Semen Coicis* to dispel wind and dampness.

桂枝汤

【来源】《伤寒论》

【组成】桂枝（9克）芍药（9克）生姜（9克）大枣（3枚）甘草（6克）

【功用】解肌发表，调和营卫。

【主治】外感风寒表虚证。症见发热头痛，汗出恶风，口不渴，舌苔薄白，脉浮缓。

【方解】本方以桂枝为君药，解肌发表，散外感风寒；以芍药为臣，益阴敛营。桂枝、白芍相合，一治卫强，一治营弱，合则调和营卫，是相须为用。生姜辛温，既助桂枝解肌，又能和胃止呕。大枣甘平，既能益气补中，又能滋脾生津。姜、枣相合，还可以生发脾胃之气而调和营卫，所以共为佐药。炙甘草之用有二：一为佐药，益气和中，合桂枝以解肌，合芍药以益阴；一为使药，调和诸药。本方虽只有五味药，但配伍严谨，发中有补，散中有收，滋阴和阳，调和营卫，是解肌发汗之总方。

【注意事项】表实无汗，或表寒里热，不汗出而烦躁，以及温病初起，见发热口渴，咽痛脉数时，皆不宜使用。

【加减】恶风寒较甚者，宜加防风、荆芥、淡豆豉疏散风寒；体质素虚者，可加黄芪益气，以扶正祛邪；兼见咳喘者，宜加杏仁、苏子、桔梗宣肺止咳平喘。

（二）辛凉解表剂

辛凉解表剂适用于外感风热表证或温病初起。症见发热、微恶风寒、头痛咽痛，或口微渴，咳嗽、咯黄痰或痰白而粘，苔薄白或微黄，脉浮数。代表方剂：银翘散、桑菊饮。

银翘散

【来源】《温病条辨》

【组成】连翘（30克）银花（30克）桔梗（18克）薄荷（18克）竹叶（12克）生甘草（15克）荆芥穗（12克）淡豆豉（15克）牛蒡子（18克）芦根（30克）

【功用】疏散风热，清热解毒。

【主治】温病初起。发热、微恶风寒，无汗或有汗不畅，头痛口渴，咳嗽咽痛，舌尖红，苔薄白或薄黄，脉浮数。

【方解】方中重用连翘、银花为君药，既有辛凉解表、清热解毒的作用，又具有

Ramulus Cinnamomi Decoction(Gui Zhi Tang)

【Source】*Treatise on Cold Damage Diseases.*

【Composition】*Ramulus Cinnamomi* (9 g), *Radix Paeoniae Lactiflorae* (9 g), *Rhizoma Zingiberis Recens* (9 g), *Fructus Jujubae* (3 pieces), and *Radix Glycyrrhizae Praeparata* (6 g).

【Functions】Release the flesh and the exterior, harmonize the nutrient and defense aspects.

【Indications】Exterior-deficiency dyndrome caused by exogenous wind-cold, marked by fever, headache, sweating, aversion to wind, no thirst, thin and white tongue coating, and floating and slow pulse.

【Explanation】In the formula, *Ramulus Cinnamomi* as sovereign medicinal, releases the flesh and diffuses the exterior, dispels the exterior pathogens of wind-cold; *Radix Paeoniae Alba* as minister medicinal, nourishes yin and restrains the nutrient aspect. *Ramulus Cinnamomi* and *Radix Paeoniae Alba*, the former treats the excess of the defense aspect, the latter treats the deficiency of the nutrient aspect, both of the two medicinals combined together, and modulate the defense and nutrient aspects, and the combination is mutual reinforcement. *Rhizoma Zingiberis Recens* is acrid and warm, it not only helps *Ramulus Cinnamomi* release the flesh, but also harmonizes the stomach to check vomiting. *Fructus Jujubae* is sweet and neutral, it not only tonifys the middle qi, but also nourishes the spleen and engenders fluid. Both *Rhizoma Zingiberis Recens* and *Fructus Jujubae* combined together to engender the spleen and stomach qi, and to modulate the defense and nutrient aspects, serve as the assistant medicinals. *Radix Glycyrrhizae Praeparata* has two effects: on one hand, it is the assistant medicinal to tonify the middle qi, combined with *Ramulus Cinnamomi* to release the flesh, combined with *Radix Paeoniae Alba* to nourishes yin; on the other hand, it is the courier medicinal to mediate all the ingredients. Though the formula merely consists of five ingredients; it is carefully and precisely composed of formation and structure. The formula is composed of tonification in releasing, with astringency inside dispelling, and have the functions of nourishing yin and modulating yang, and harmonizing the nutrient and defense aspects, and it is the principle formula of the releasing-flesh and promoting sweating formulas.

【Note】The formula should not be used in cases of exterior excess syndromes marked by no sweating, exterior cold with interior heat syndromes marked by restlessness with no sweating, and the early stage of warm diseases marked by fever, thirst, sore throat and rapid pulse.

【Variation】For severe aversion to wind and cold, add *Radix Saposhnikoviae*, *Spica Schizonepetae*, and *Semen Sojae Praeparatum* to dispel wind and coldness; for patients of weak constitution, add *Radix Astragali* to tonify qi, so as to reinforce the healthy qi and eliminate the pathogenic factors; and for concurrence with cough and asthma, add *Semen Armeniacae Amarum*, *Fructus Perillae*, and *Radix Platycodi* to diffuse the lung, suppress cough, and calm panting.

Pungent-cool exterior-releasing formulas

Pungent-cool exterior-releasing formulas are applicable to exterior syndromes of wind-heat or the early stage of febrile diseases, marked by fever, slight aversion to wind and cold, sore throat, or mild thirst, cough, yellow phlegm, or white and sticky phlegm, thin tongue coating with color of white or yellow, floating and rapid pulse. The representative formulas are: "Lonicera-Forsythia Powder" and "Morus-Chrysanthemum Decoction".

Lonicera-Forsythia Powder(Yin Qiao San)

【Source】*Systematized Identification of Warm-induced Diseases.*

【Composition】*Fructus Forsythiae* (30g), *Flos Lonicerae* (30g), *Radix Platycodi* (18g), *Herba Menthae* (18g), *Herba Lophatheri* (12g), *Radix Glycyrrhizae* (crude) (15g), *Schizonepetae* (12g), *Semen Sojae Preparatum* (15g), *Fructus Arctii* (18g), and *Rhizoma Phragmitis* (30g).

芳香避秽的功效。薄荷、牛蒡子疏散风热，清利头目，且解毒利咽；荆芥穗、淡豆豉辛而微温，加强辛解透表之力，助君药解表热，此四味共为臣药。竹叶清热除烦清上焦之热，且能生津，芦根清热生津，桔梗宣肺止咳，三者同为佐药。甘草合桔梗清利咽喉为佐，又调和诸药为使。

【注意事项】不宜久煎。

【加减】若口渴甚者，加知母、天花粉等清热生津；咳嗽甚者，加杏仁、前胡、紫菀、款冬花等止咳化痰；肺热咽痛明显，可加马勃、玄参等加强清肺热利咽喉；痰中带血者，去荆芥、淡豆豉等温热之品，加白茅根、丹皮、侧柏叶等凉血止血。

桑菊饮

【来源】《温病条辨》

【组成】桑叶（7.5克）菊花（3克）杏仁（6克）连翘（5克）薄荷（2.5克）桔梗（6克）甘草（2.5克）芦根（6克）

【功用】疏风清热，宣肺止咳。

【主治】风温初起。咳嗽，身热不甚，口微渴，苔薄白，脉浮数。

【方解】本方用桑叶清透肺热，菊花清散上焦风热，共为君药。臣以辛凉之薄荷，助桑叶、菊花散上焦风热，桔梗、杏仁，一升一降，宣肺止咳。连翘清热透表，芦根清热生津止渴，为佐药。甘草调和诸药，是使药之用。诸药配合，有疏风清热、宣肺止咳之功。

【注意事项】寒性咳嗽禁用本方。不宜久煎。

【加减】如肺热甚，咯黄痰者，可加黄芩、桑白皮和浙贝母以清热化痰；口渴者，加天花粉以清热生津止渴。

【Functions】Disperse wind-heat, clear heat, and detoxify.

【Indications】The onset stage of febrile diseases, marked by fever, slight aversion to wind and cold, no sweating, or unsmooth sweating, headache, thirst, cough, sore throat, red tip of the tongue, thin tongue coating with white or yellow color, and floating and rapid pulse.

【Explanation】In the formula, *Fructus Forsythiae* and *Flos Lonicerae* which serve as the sovereign medicinals in high dose, have the functions of pungent-cool releasing the exterior, clearing heat and detoxifying toxins, and dispelling filth with aroma. *Herba Menthae* and *Fructus Arctii* dispel wind-heat, clear the heat of the head and eyes, detoxify and soothe the throat; *Spica Schizonepetae* and *Semen Sojae Praeparatum* are acrid and slightly warm, enforce the functions of pungent-releasing the exterior, and help the sovereign medicinals dispel the exterior heat. The above-mentioned four ingredients are the minister medicinals. *Rhizoma Phragmitis* clears heat and relieves restlessness, clears the heat of upper energizer and engenders fluid; *Rhizoma Phragmitis* clears heat and engenders fluid; *Radix Platycodi diffuses* the lung to surpress cough, all of the above three ingredients are the assistant medicinals. *Radix Glycyrrhizae* combined with *Radix Platycodi* clears heat and soothes the throat as the assistant medicinal; it harmonizes all the ingredients as the courier medicinal as well.

【Note】The formula should not be decocted for long time.

【Variation】For severe thirst, add *Rhizoma Anemarrhenae* and *Radix Trichosanthis* to clear heat and engender fluid; for severe cough, add *Semen Armeniacae Amarum*, *Radix Peucedani*, *Radix Asteris*, and *Flos Fartarae* to surpress cough and resolve phlegm; for severe sore throat due to lung heat, add *Lasiosphaera seu Calvatia* and *Radix Scrophulariae* to promote the actions of clearing the lung to soothe the throat; for bloody sputum, add *Rhizoma Imperatae*, *Cortex Moutan*, and *Cacumen Platycladi* to cool the blood to stop bleeding.

Morus-Chrysanthemum Decoction(Sang Ju Yin)

【Source】*Systematized Identification of Warm-induced Diseases.*

【Composition】*Folium Mori* (7. 5 g), *Flos Chrysanthemi* (3 g), *Semen Armeniacae Amarum* (6 g), *Fructus Forsythiae* (5 g), *Herba Menthae* (2. 5 g), *Radix Platycodi* (6 g), *Radix Glycyrrhizae* (2. 5 g), and *Rhizoma Phragmitis* (6 g).

【Functions】Disperse wind-heat, diffuse the lung to surpress cough.

【Indications】The onset stage of febrile diseases, marked by cough, mild fever, slight thirst, thin and white tonge coating, and floating and rapid pulse.

【Explanation】In the formula, both *Folium Mori* and *Flos Chrysanthemi* serve as sovereign medicinals, the former clears heat and diffuses the lung, the latter dispels wind-heat of the upper energizer. The minister medicinals are: *Herba Menthae* which helps the sovereign medicinals clear wind-heat of the upper energizer; *Radix Platycodi* and *Semen Armeniacae Amarum* diffuse the lung and suppress cough, as the former is upward and the latter is downward. *Fructus Forsythiae* clears heat and outthrusts through the exterior, *Rhizoma Phragmitis* clears heat and engenders fluid to arrest thirst, and both are the assistant medicinals. *Radix Glycyrrhizae* harmonizes all the ingredients, and serves as courier medicinal. All the ingredients together achieve the success of dispelling wind and clearing heat, diffusing the lung to suppress cough.

【Note】The formula is contraindicated for cough due to cold. The formula should not be decocted for long time.

【Variation】In case of severe heat in the lung marked by cough and yellow sputum, add *Radix Scutellariae*, *Cortex Mori Radicis*, and *Bulbus Fritillariae Thunbergii* to clear heat and dispel the phlegm; in case of thirst, add *Radix Trichosanthis* to clear heat, and engender fluid to relieve thirst.

（三）扶正解表剂

扶正解表剂适用于体质素虚又感外邪而致表证。体虚外感此时既要解表，又要补虚，所以常用补益药与解表药配合组成方剂，使表证得解、正虚不伤。代表方剂：败毒散。

败毒散

【来源】《小儿药证直诀》

【组成】柴胡　前胡　川芎　枳壳　羌活　独活　茯苓　桔梗　人参（各10克）甘草（6克）生姜　薄荷（各少许）

【功用】散寒祛湿，益气解表。

【主治】气虚外感风寒湿邪。憎寒壮热，头项强痛，肢体酸痛，无汗，鼻塞，咳嗽有痰，胸膈痞满，舌淡苔白，脉浮而按之无力。

【方解】方中羌活、独活发散风寒，除湿止痛，羌活长于祛上部风寒湿邪，独活长于祛下部风寒湿邪，合而用之，为通治一身风寒湿邪的常用组合，共为君药。川芎行气活血，并能祛风；柴胡解肌透邪，且能行气，二药既可助君药解表逐邪，又可行气活血加强宣痹止痛之力，俱为臣药。桔梗上行宣肺，枳壳下气宽胸，前胡化痰止咳，茯苓渗湿消痰，皆为佐药。方中人参亦属佐药，益气扶正，一则助正气以鼓邪外出；二则令全方散中有补，不致耗伤真元且防邪再入。生姜、薄荷为引，以助解表之力；甘草调和药性，兼以益气和中，共为佐使之品。全方邪正兼顾，而以祛邪为主。

【注意事项】本方多辛温香燥之品，外感风热及阴虚外感者忌用；若是暑温、湿热致下痢不爽者以及无表证者，均非本方所宜。

【加减】若正气未虚而表寒较甚者，去人参，加荆芥、防风以祛风散寒；气虚明显者，可重用人参，或加黄芪以益气补虚；湿滞肌表经络、肢体酸楚疼痛甚者，可酌加威灵仙、桑枝、秦艽、汉防己等祛风除湿、通络止痛；咳嗽重者，加杏仁、白前止咳化痰。

Renforcing healthy qi and exterior-releasing formulas

Renforcing healthy qi and exterior-releasing formulas are applicable to exterior syndromes due to weak physique and invading exogenous pathogenic factors. For exterior syndromes concurrent with weak physique, one should not only release the exterior, but also tonify healthy qi to treat conditions of deficiency, thus, use the formula which usually consists of the tonifying and replenishing medicinals and the exterior-releasing medicinals, to release the exterior syndromes without consumption of healthy qi. The representative formula is "Antiphlogistic Powder".

Antiphlogistic Powder(Bai Du San)

【Source】*Key to Therapeutics of Children's Diseases.*

【Composition】*Radix Bupleuri* (10 g), *Radix Peucedani* (10 g), *Rhizoma Ligustici Chuanxiong* (10 g), *Fructus Aurantii* (10 g), *Rhizoma et Radix Notopterygii* (10 g), *Radix Angelicae Pubescentis* (10 g), *Poria* (10 g), *Radix Platycodi* (10 g), *Radix Ginseng* (10 g), *Radix Glycyrrhizae* (6 g); add *Rhizoma Zingiberis Recens* and *Herba Menthae* (each small amount).

【Functions】Dissipate cold and dispel dampness, tonify qi and release the exterior.

【Indications】Exterior syndromes due to invasion of wind-cold-dampness with qi deficiency, marked by aversion to cold, severe fever, headache and stiff neck, soreness and pain in limbs, no sweating, stuffy nose, productive cough, oppressed sensation in the chest, pale tongue with white tonge coating, and floating pulse that feels weak on heavy pressure.

【Explanation】In the formula, *Rhizoma Curcumae Longae* and *Radix Angelicae Pubescentis* dispel wind-cold, dispel dampness and relieve pain. The former is good at dispelling wind-cold-dampness of the upper body; the latter is good at dispelling wind-cold-dampness of the lower body, both of them are the sovereign medicinals, of which the combination is commonly used to treat wind-cold-dampness of the whole body. *Rhizoma Chuanxiong* moves qi and activates the blood, and dispels wind; *Radix Bupleuri* releases the flesh, dispels the pathogen and moves qi. Both of them are minister medicinals that help the sovereign medicinals not only release flesh and dispel pathogen, but also enforce the actions of activating the blood and diffusing impediment to relieve pain. *Radix Platycodi* guides qi upward to diffuse the lung, whereas *Fructus Aurantii* guides qi downward to soothe the chest; *Radix Peucedani* resolves phlegm and suppresses cough; *Poria* drains dampness and resolves phlegm, all of the four medicinals are the assistant medicinals. In the formulas, *Ginseng* can replenish the healthy qi and it belongs to the assistant medicinals. On one hand, *Ginseng* helps the healthy qi to dispel the pathogenic factors outward; on the other hand, it makes the formula dispelling with replenishing, and preventing the re-invasion of pathogenic factors without consumption of the genuine qi. *Rhizoma Zingiberis Recens* and *Herba Menthae* are the guides, and help release the exterior; *Radix Glycyrrhizae* mediates all the ingredients with the simultaneous actions of benefiting qi and harmonizing the middle. The whole formula concerns both the healthy qi and pathogenic factors together, and focuses on eliminating pathogenic factors.

【Note】Most of the ingredients in the formula are acrid, aromatic, warm, and dry. The formula is contraindicated for the external contraction syndrome of wind-heat and syndrome of yin deficiency with external contraction; and the formula is unadvisable for unsmooth diarrhea due to summerheat or dampness-heat, or cases without the exterior syndromes.

【Variation】In case of severe exterior cold syndromes without deficiency of healthy qi, remove *Ginseng*, and add *Herba Schizonepetae* and *Radix Saposhnikoviae* to dispel wind-cold; in case of severe qi deficiency, use *Ginseng* in high dose, or add *Radix Astragali* to tonify qi and replenish deficiency; in case of severe soreness and pain in the extremities due to the channels and collaterals blocked by the exterior dampness, consider to add *Radix Clematidis*, *Ramulus Mori*, *Radix Gentianae Macrophyllae*, and *Radix*

二、泻下剂

泻下剂是以泻下药为主组成，具有通导大便、泻下肠胃积滞、荡涤实热、攻逐水饮等作用，治疗里实证的方剂。属"八法"中的"下法"。主要治疗肠胃积滞、实热内结、大便不通或寒积、蓄水等。

泻下剂除润下外，性均峻烈，故孕妇、妇女经期禁用；泻下剂易耗损正气，故得效即止，不可用量过大。年老体弱、产妇以及失血脱水者慎用。

根据泻下剂的不同作用，可分为寒下剂、温下剂、润下剂、逐水剂和攻补兼施剂五类。

（一）寒下剂

寒下剂主要适用于里热积滞之证。症见大便秘结，或热结旁流，或下痢后重，壮热，口渴，腹痛拒按，恶食，苔黄糙者。代表方剂：大承气汤。

大承气汤

【来源】《伤寒论》

【组成】大黄（12克）厚朴（24克）枳实（12克）芒硝（9克）

【功用】峻下热结。

【主治】①阳明腑实证。大便不通，频转矢气，脘腹痞满，腹痛拒按，按之硬，甚或潮热谵语，手足漐然汗出。舌苔黄燥起刺，或焦黑燥裂，脉沉实；②热结旁流。下利清水，色纯青，脐腹疼痛，按之坚硬有块，口舌干燥，脉滑实；③里热实证之热厥、痉病或发狂等。

【方解】方中君药大黄泻热通便，荡涤肠胃。臣药芒硝助大黄泻热通便，并能软坚润燥，二药相须为用，峻下热结之力甚强；厚朴、枳实行气散结，消痞除满，并可助大黄、芒硝荡涤积滞以加速热结之排泄，共为佐使。

【注意事项】本方为泻下峻剂，如气虚阴亏，或胃肠无积滞，或年老体弱均不宜使用；孕妇禁用。

【加减】痞满重者，可重用厚朴；阴津不足者，宜加玄参、生地等以滋阴润燥。

Stephaniae to dispel wind-dampness, and to free collaterals and relieve pain; for severe cough, add *Semen Armeniacae Amarum* and *Rhizoma Cynanchi Stauntonii* to suppress cough and resolve phlegm.

Purgation Formulas

Purgation formulas are the formulas which consist of purgative medicinals, have functions of relaxing bowels, removing gastrointestinal retention, clearing excess heat, and expelling retention fluid. The formulas belong to the "purgation" of the "eight therapeutic methods," and are mainly indicated to gastrointestinal retention, internal excessive heat, constipation, cold accumulation, and water-retention.

Except for lubricant laxative formulas, the formulas are drastic and contraindicated for women during periods of pregnancy and menstruation. The formulas are apt to consume healthy qi, and should not be used with overdosage; one should stop the administration once the effect is achieved. The formulas should be used with caution for the elderly with weak physique, puerpera, and patients of blood depletion or fluid depletion.

According to the difference of functions, the purgation formulas are classified into five types: cold purgative formulas, warm purgative formulas, lubricant laxative formulas, expelling water by purgation formulas, and purgation with reinforcement formulas.

Cold purgative formulas

Cold purgative formulas are applicable to the excess syndromes of heat accumulation, marked by constipation, or unsmooth defecation, or diarrhea, high fever, thirst, abdominal pain with aversion to touch, aversion to foods, thick and yellow tongue coating. The presentative formula is "Potent Purgation Decoction".

Potent Purgation Decoction(Da Cheng Qi Tang)

【Source】*Treatise on Cold Damage Diseases.*

【Composition】*Radix Rhizoma Rhei* (12 g), *Cortex Magnoliae Officinalis* (24 g), *Fructus Aurantii Immaturus* (12 g), and *Natrii Sulfas* (9 g).

【Functions】Drastically purgate the heat accumulation.

【Indications】a) Yang brightness bowel pattern, exhibiting constipation, abdominal flatulence, pain and tenderness, hard if palpated, or even tidal fever, delirium, profuse sweating of limbs. Prickled tongue with dry and yellow coating, or fissured tongue with dry and black coating, and sunken and replete pulse. b) Watery diarrhea caused by heat, exhibiting watery diarrhea with blue color, abdominal pain, hard mass will be palpated, dry tongue and mouth, slippery and replete pulse. And c) Excess syndrome with internal heat, exhibiting heat syncope, convulsive disease, manic psychosis.

【Explanation】In the formula, *Radix et Rhizoma Rhei* serves as the sovereign medicinal, it purgates heat and relaxes the bowels, and eliminates the accumulation in the gastrointestine. As the minister medicinal, *Natrii Sulfas* helps *Radix et Rhizoma Rhei* purgate heat and relax the bowels, and it moistens the dryness and softens hardness. The sovereign and minister medicinals are used as mutual reinforcement to enforce the power of drastic purgation. *Cortex Magnoliae Officinalis* and *Fructus Aurantii Immaturus* promote qi flow and dispel stagnation, dispel accumulation and relieve fullness, and help *Radix et Rhizoma Rhei* and *Natrii Sulfas* relax the bowels, so as to promote purgation of accumulation of heat. Both *Cortex Magnoliae Officinalis* and *Fructus Aurantii Immaturus* are the assistant and courier medicinals.

【Note】The formula is drastic purgative formula, and it is not advisable to qi deficiency or yin depletion syndromes, or cases without gastrointestinal accumulation, or the elderly with weak physique; the formula is contraindicated for pregnant women.

【Variation】In case of severe distention, use *Cortex Magnoliae Officinalis* in high dose; in case of the

（二）温下剂

温下剂主要用于寒邪与积滞互阻肠道的寒积里实证。症见腹痛便秘，面色苍白，手足厥逆，苔白滑，脉弦紧者。代表方剂：大黄附子汤。

大黄附子汤

【来源】《金匮要略》

【组成】大黄（9克）制附子（12克）细辛（3克）

【功用】温里散寒，通便止痛。

【主治】寒积里实证。腹痛便秘，胁下偏痛，发热，手足厥冷，舌苔白腻，脉弦紧。

【方解】本方重用大辛大热之附子，温里散寒，止胁腹疼痛；以苦寒之大黄，泻下通便，荡涤积滞，共为君药。细辛辛温宣通，散寒止痛，助附子温里散寒，是为臣药。大黄虽性味苦寒，但配伍附子、细辛之辛散大热之品，则寒性被抑而泻下之功犹存，为去性取用之法。三味合力，而成温散寒凝、苦辛通降之剂，具有温下之功。

【注意事项】有实热或阳亢者不能使用。

【加减】腹痛甚、喜温，加肉桂加强温里祛寒止痛；腹胀满，可加厚朴、木香以行气导滞。

（三）润下剂

润下剂主要用于热邪伤津，或素体火盛，所致肠燥便秘者。代表方剂有：麻子仁丸。

麻子仁丸

【来源】《伤寒论》

【组成】麻子仁（500克）芍药（250克）枳实（250克）大黄（500克）厚朴（250克）杏仁（250克）【注：丸剂用量】

【功用】润肠通便。

【主治】肠胃燥热，津液不足。大便干结，小便频数，舌苔微黄，脉细涩。

【方解】方中火麻仁性味甘平，质润多脂，功能润肠通便，重用为君药。杏仁上肃肺气、下润大肠，白芍养血敛阴、缓急止痛，共为臣。大黄泻热通便，枳实下气破结，厚朴行气除满，三药共为佐药。蜂蜜润肠通便为使药。本方具有下不伤正、滋而不腻、攻润相合的特点，使燥热去、阴液复而大便调。

depletion of yin and fluid, add *Radix Scrophulariae* and *Radix Rehmanniae* to nourish yin and moisten dryness.

Warm purgative formulas

Warm purgative formulas are applicable to interior excess syndromes of cold accumulation in the intestines, marked by abnominal pain, constipation, pale complexion, cold hands and feet, white and slippery tongue coating, string-like and tight pulse. The representative formula is "Rhei and Aconiti Lateralis Praeparata Decoction".

Rhei and Aconiti Lateralis Praeparata Decoction(Da Huang Fu Zi Tang)

【Source】*Synopsis of Prescriptions of the Golden Chamber.*

【Composition】*Radix Rhizoma Rhei* (9 g), *Radix Aconiti Lateralis Praeparata* (12 g), and *Herba Asari* (3 g).

【Functions】Warm the interior to dispel cold, relax the bowl, and relieve pain.

【Indications】Excess syndrome due to accumulation of cold, marked by consitipation with abdominal pain, hypochondriac pain, fever, cold limbs, greasy white tongue, and string-like and tight pulse.

【Explanation】In the formula, *Radix Aconiti Lateralis Praeparata*, which is extremely acrid and hot is in high dose, warms the interior and dispels cold and relieves the pain in the abdomen and hypochondrium; *Radix Rhizoma Rhei*, which is bitter and cold, relaxes the bowels, and eliminates accumulation. Both of them are sovereign medicinals. The acrid and warm *Herba Asari* dispels cold and relieves pain, and helps *Radix Aconiti Lateralis Praeparata* warm the interior and dispel cold, it serves as the minister medicinal. Though *Radix Rhizoma Rhei* is bitter and cold, when it is used together with the extremely pungent and hot *Radix Aconiti Lateralis Praeparata* and *Herba Asari*, the cold nature is suppressed, and its function of purgation still remains. The combination is called remaining the function with elimination of nature. The three ingredients are used jointly as the formula of warm-pungent dispelling cold, and bitter-acrid moving and descending with warm purgation.

【Note】Contraindicated for syndromes of excess heat or syndromes of hyperactivity of yang.

【Variation】In case of abdominal pain concurrent with preference to warmth, add *Cortex Cinnamomi* to rienforce the actions of warming the interior and dispelling cold and relieving pain; for distention, add *Cortex Magnoliae Officinalis* and *Radix Aucklandiae* to promote qi flow and move stagnation.

Lubricant laxative formulas

Lubricant laxative formulas are applicable to fluid depletion due to heat, or constipation due to dryness in the intestines with constant excessive heat. The representative formula is "Cannabis Pills".

Cannabis Pills(Ma Zi Ren Wan)

【Source】*Treatise on Cold Damage Diseases.*

【Composition】*Fructus Cannabis* (500 g), *Radix Paeoniae Lactiflorae* (250 g), *Fructus Aurantii Immaturus* (250 g), *Radix Rhizoma Rhei* (500 g), *Cortex Magnoliae Officinalis* (100 g), and *Semen Armeniacae Amarum* (250g) [note: dosage for pills].

【Functions】Lubricate the intestine to induce bowel movement.

【Indications】Dryness-heat in the stomach and intestines and fluid deficiency, manifested as constipation, frequent micturition, mild yellow tongue fur, and fine and rough pulse.

【Explanation】In the formula, the sweet and neutral *Fructus Cannabis* with moist texture and profuse grease has functions of moistening the intestines and relaxing the bowels, used in high dose as the sovereign medicinal. *Semen Armeniacae Amarum* descends lung qi in the above and moistens the bowels in the below; *Radix Paeoniae* nourishes the blood and restrains body fluid, and relieves spasm and pain, both are

【注意事项】本方虽为润肠缓下之剂，但含有攻下破滞之品，故津亏血少者不宜常服，孕妇慎用。

【加减】痔疮便秘者，可加桃仁、当归以养血和血、润肠通便；痔疮出血属胃肠燥热者，可酌加槐花、地榆以凉血止血；燥热伤津较甚者，可加生地、玄参、麦冬以增液通便。

三、和解剂

凡具有调和机体机能，用来治疗少阳病、肝脾不调、寒热错杂以及疟疾等病证的方剂。属于"八法"中的"和法"。

和解剂通常性平和，尽管无明显寒热补泻之偏，仍勿滥用。凡邪在肌表、未入少阳，或已入里、阳明热盛者，均不宜使用；若劳倦内伤、饮食失调、气虚血弱而症见寒热者，也非本类方剂所宜。

和解剂分为和解少阳、调和肝脾、调和肠胃三类。

（一）和解少阳剂

和解少阳剂适用于伤寒邪在少阳证。症见寒热往来，胸胁苦满，心烦喜呕，默默不欲饮食，口苦咽干，目眩，脉弦等。代表方剂：小柴胡汤。

小柴胡汤

【来源】《伤寒论》

【组成】柴胡（24克）黄芩（9克）人参（9克）炙甘草（9克）半夏（9克）生姜（9克）大枣（4枚）

【功用】和解少阳。

【主治】

（1）伤寒少阳证。往来寒热，胸胁苦满，默默不欲饮食，心烦喜呕，口苦，咽干，目眩，舌苔薄白，脉弦。

（2）热入血室。妇人经水适断，寒热发作有时。

（3）疟疾、黄疸以及内伤杂病而见少阳证者。

【方解】方中柴胡苦辛微寒，轻清升散，并能疏泄气机之郁滞，使少阳半表之邪得以清解疏散，为君药。黄芩苦寒，能清泻少阳半里之热，为臣药。君臣相合，一散一清，相使为用，和解少阳。半夏、生姜和胃降逆止呕，人参、大枣益气健脾、扶正祛邪，共为佐药。炙甘草助参、枣扶正，并调和诸药，为使药。诸药合用，以和解少阳为主，兼补胃气，使半表半里之邪得解，少阳枢机得利，上焦通而胃气和，

the minister medicinals.*Radix et Rhizoma Rhei* clears heat and relaxes the bowels; *Fructus Aurantii Immaturus* descends qi and breaks mass; and *Cortex Magnoliae Officinalis* moves qi and eliminates stagnation.These three ingredients are the assistant medicinals.The formula has characteristics of purgation without consumption of healthy qi, nourishing without retention, and eliminating with moistening.It removes dryness-heat and restores yin and body fluid to relieve constipation.

【Note】Though the formula is one of lubricant laxative formulas, it contains purgative and stagnation-removing ingredients, thus, long-time administration of the formula is unadvisable for deficiency of the blood and body fluid.The formula should be cautiously used in pregnant women.

【Variation】In case of hemorrhoids and constipation, add *Semen Persicae* and *Radix Angenicae Sinensis* to nourish and regulate the blood, and moisten the intestines and promote defecation; in case of hemorrhoids with bleeding due to dryness-heat of the stomach and intestines, consider to add *Flos Sophorae* and *Radix Sanguisobae* to cool the blood and check bleeding; in case of severe depletion of body fluid due to dryness-heat, add *Radix Rehmanniae*, *Radix Scrophulariae* and *Radix Ophiopogonis* to increase body fluid and promote defecation.

Harmonizing and Releasing Formulas

Harmonizing and releasing formulas are formulas that adjust functions of the body, and are indicated for lesser yang disease, liver-spleen disharmony syndrome, and cold-heat complex syndrome.The formulas belong to harmonizing method of "the eight therapeutic methods."

The harmonizing and releasing formula should not be abused, though it is usually mild and has no specific bias of cold or heat and tonifying or purgating.It should not be indicated when the pathogen exists in the surface and not being invaded into lesser yang, or the pathogen invaded the interior with concurrent excessive heat in yang brightness.In case of internal injury due to labour, eating disorders, or qi-blood depletion with fever and cold, the formula should not be indicated either.

Harmonizing and releasing formulas are classified into three types: harmonizing and releasing lesser yang formulas, harmonizing the liver and spleen formulas, and harmonizing the stomach and intestine formulas.

Harmonizing and releasing lesser yang formulas

Harmonizing and releasing lesser yang formulas are applicable to lesser yang syndrome of febrile diseases, marked by alternate fever and chills, fullness and choking feeling in the chest and costal region, dysphoria, nausea and loss of appetite, bitter taste in the mouth, dry throat, dizziness and string-like pulse. The representative formula is "Small Bupleurum Decoction".

Small Bupleurum Decoction(Xiao Chai Hu Tang)

【Source】*Treatise on Cold Damage Diseases*.

【Composition】*Radix Bupleuri* (24 g), *Radix Scutellariae* (9 g), *Radix Ginseng* (9 g), *Radix Glycyrrhizae Praeparata* (9 g), *Rhizoma Pinelliae Praeparata* (9 g), *Rhizoma Zingiberis Recens* (9 g), and *Fructus Jujubae* (4 pieces).

【Functions】Homonize and release the lesser yang.

【Indications】

a) Lesser yang disease syndrome, marked by alternate chills and fever, fullness in the chest and hypochondrium, poor appetite, restlessness, vomiting, bitter taste, dry throat, dizziness, thin white tongue fur, and string-like pulse.b) Heat in the blood chamber, manisfesting as alternate chills and fever in women right after the menstruation.And c) Lesser yang syndromes of diseases of malaria, jaundice, and other complicated internal diseases.

则诸症自除。

【注意事项】肝火偏旺或阴血虚者不宜服用。

【加减】若胸中烦而不呕，去半夏、人参，加瓜蒌以清热理气宽胸；若渴者，去半夏，加天花粉以生津止渴；若腹中痛者，去黄芩，加白芍以柔肝缓急止痛；若瘀血互结，少腹满痛，可去人参、甘草、大枣之甘壅，加延胡索、当归尾、桃仁以活血止痛。

（二）调和肝脾剂

调和肝脾剂，适用于肝脾不和的病证。症见脘腹胸胁胀痛，神疲食少，月经不调，大便溏薄等。代表方剂：逍遥散。

逍遥散

【来源】《太平惠民和剂局方》

【组成】柴胡　当归　白芍　白术　茯苓（各30克）炙甘草（15克）生姜　薄荷（各少许）

【功用】疏肝解郁，养血健脾。

【主治】肝郁血虚。两胁作痛，头痛目眩，口燥咽干，神疲食少，或寒热往来，或月经不调，乳房作胀，舌淡红，苔薄白，脉弦而虚者。

【方解】本方既有柴胡疏肝解郁，为君药；又有当归、白芍养血柔肝，为臣药。特别是当归之芳香可以行气，味甘可以缓急，更是肝郁血虚之要药。白术、茯苓健脾去湿，使运化有权，气血有源。生姜温胃和中，薄荷少许，助柴胡疏肝解郁且清热，皆为佐药。炙甘草补中益气，缓肝之急，并调和诸药，为佐使药。如此配伍既补肝体，又助肝用，气血兼顾，肝脾并治，故为调和肝脾之名方，又是妇科调经的常用方。

【注意事项】阴虚火旺、肝阳上亢者不宜服用。

【加减】用于肝郁血虚发热，或潮热自汗盗汗等，加丹皮、栀子；用于肝郁血虚所致的经前腹痛，加地黄。

〖Explanation〗In the formula,*Radix Bupleuri* is bitter,acrid,and slightly cold,and it is light and upward rising and can clear heat and expel the exterior pathogen,can soothe the qi stagnation,thus clear and dispel the pathogen exits in half exterior of lesser yang,serves as the sovereign.*Radix Scutellariae* is bitter and cold,serving as the minister,it can clear the heat exits in half interior of lesser yang.The sovereign together with the minister,dispelling with clearing,assiting with each other,harmonize and release the lesser yang.*Rhizoma Pinelliae* and *Rhizoma Zingiberis Recens* harmonize the stomach,and direct qi downward to relieve vomiting.*Ginseng* and *Fructus Jujubae* tonify spleen qi,enforce vigor qi and dispel pathogens,both are assistant medicinals.*Radix Glycyrrhizae Praeparata* is courier medicinal,and it helps *Ginseng* and *Fructus Jujubae* to enforce heathy qi,and modulates all the ingredients.All the ingredients together,concentrate on harmonizing and releasing the lesser yang,and tonify the stomach as well,so as to release the pathogens in the half-interior and half-exterior,and free the transmission of the lesser yang,thus,the upper energizer is soothed and the stomach qi is harmonized,and the symptoms are relieved consequently.

〖Note〗Contraindicated in case of excessive heat of the liver and depletion of yin and the blood.

〖Variation〗In case of fullness in the chest,concurrent with restlessness without vomiting,remove *Rhizoma Pinelliae* and *Ginseng*,add *Fructus Trichosanthis* to clear heat,soothe qi and ease the chest;in case of thirst,remove *Rhizoma Pinelliae* and add *Radix Trichosanthis* to engender fluid and arrest thirst;in case of abdominal pain,remove *Radix Scutellariae* and add *Radix Paeoniae Alba* to emolliate the liver and alleviate pain;in case of fullness and pain in the lower abdomen due to blood stasis,remove *Ginseng*,*Radix Glycyrrhizae*,and *Fructus Jujubae*,which are sweet and might accumulate qi and the blood,and add *Rhizoma Corydalis*,*Radix Angelicae Sinensis*,and *Semen Persicae* to activiate the blood to alleviate pain.

Harmonizing the liver and spleen formulas

Harmonizing the liver and spleen formulas are applicable to disharmony syndrome of the liver and spleen,manifesting as chest stuffiness,hypochondriac pain,epigastric and abdominal pain,fatigue,anorexia,irregular menstruation,and loose stools.The representative formula is "Free and Easy Wanderer Powder".

Free and Easy Wanderer Powder(Xiao Yao San)

〖Source〗*Prescriptions from the Great Peace Imperial Grace Pharmacy.*

〖Composition〗*Radix Bupleuri* (30 g),*Radix Angenicae Sinensis* (30 g),*Radix Paeoniae* (30 g),*Rhizoma Atractylodis Macrocephalae* (30 g),*Poria* (30 g),*Radix Glycyrrhizae Praeparata* (15 g),*Rhizoma Zingiberis Recens* (small pieces),and *Herba Menthae* (a little).

〖Functions〗Soothe the liver to remove qi stagnation,nourish the blood,and strengthen the spleen.

〖Indications〗Liver qi stagnation with blood deficiency,marked by hypochondriac pain,headache,dizziness,dry mouth and throat,mental fatigue,poor appetite,or alternate fever and chills,or irregular menstruation,distention of breast,pale-red tongue,thin white tongue coating,string-like and vacuous pulse.

〖Explanation〗In this formula,*Radix Bupleuri*,as the sovereign medicinal,soothes the liver to remove qi stagnation,while *Radix Angelicae Sinensis* and *Radix Paeoniae* as the minister medicinals nourish the blood and soften the liver.Particularly,the aroma of *Radix Angelicae Sinensis* promotes blood circulation without hindering qi flow;the sweet taste of *Radix Angelicae Sinensis* relieves spasm. *Radix Angelicae Sinensis* is the prime medicinal to cure liver qi stagnation and blood deficiency.*Rhizoma Atractylodis Macrocephalae* and *Poria* strengthen the spleen and remove dampness to enhance the transporting function and the source of qi and blood.The *Rhizoma Zingiberis Recens* warms the stomach,mediates the middle energizer,while a bit of *Herba Menthae* assists *Radix Bupleuri* to disperse liver qi to remove qi stagnation,both the two ingredients are the assistant medicinals.*Radix Glycyrrhizae Praeparata* invigorates qi and tonifies

（三）调和肠胃剂

调和肠胃剂适用于邪犯肠胃，寒热错杂、升降失常，而致心下痞满，恶心呕吐，脘腹胀痛，肠鸣下利等证。代表方剂：半夏泻心汤。

半夏泻心汤

【来源】《伤寒论》

【组成】半夏（12克）黄芩　干姜　人参　炙甘草（各9克）黄连（3克）大枣（4枚）

【功用】和胃降逆，散结消痞。

【主治】寒热错杂、胃气不和之痞证。症见心下痞满，但满而不痛，或呕吐，肠鸣下利，舌苔薄黄腻，脉弦滑。

【方解】方中半夏辛开散结，苦降止呕，为君药。干姜温中散寒；黄芩、黄连苦寒泻热，为臣药。人参、大枣甘温，补益脾气以复升降之职，为佐药。炙甘草加强益气和中之功，并调和诸药，为佐使药。诸药配伍，分解寒热，开结除痞，标本兼顾。为体现调和寒热、辛开苦降治法的代表方。

【注意事项】不宜使用于气滞或食积所致的心下痞满。

【加减】湿热蕴积中焦，中气不虚，呕甚而痞，或舌苔厚腻者，可去人参、甘草、大枣、干姜，加枳实、生姜下气消痞止呕。

四、清热剂

清热剂是根据"热者寒之"的原则立法，以清热药物为主组成用以治疗里热证的方剂。属于"八法"中的"清法"。

清热剂适用于里热证。即表邪已解而热已入里、且里热已盛而尚未结实者。

清热剂易败胃气，损伤脾阳，病祛即止，不可久用，应注意保护胃气，用粳米、甘草、半夏、白术、茯苓等药以健脾和胃。清热剂根据功用不同，分为清气分热、清营凉血、清热解毒、清脏腑热、清热祛暑和清虚热六类。

the middle energizer, relieves emergency of the liver, and it is the assistant and courier medicinal. The so-formed formula not only tonifies the liver substance but also assists the liver functions, with consideration to both qi and blood, simultaneous treatment of the liver and spleen. It is the well-known formula of regulating the liver and spleen, also it is common used formula for regulating menstruation in gynecology.

【Note】Contraindicated for yin deficiency with effulgent fire syndrome and ascendant hyperactivity of liver yang syndrome.

【Variation】In case of liver qi stagnation and blood deficiency marked by fever or tidal fever, spontaneous sweating or nocturnal sweating, add *Cortex Moutan* and *Fructus Gardeniae*. For abdominal pain prior to menstruation due to liver qi stagnation and blood deficiency, add *Radix Rehmanniae*.

Harmonizing the stomach and intestine formulas

Harmonizing the stomach and intestine formulas are applicable to epigastric fullness, nausea, vomiting, epigastric and abdominal distension and pain, borborygmus and diarrhea caused by pathogenic factors invading the stomach and intestine, intermingled cold and heat, abnormal upbearing and downbearing functions. The representative formula is "Pinellia Decoction for Draining the Heart".

Pinellia Decoction for Draining the Heart(Ban Xia Xie Xin Tang)

【Source】*Treatise on Cold Damage Diseases.*

【Composition】*Rhizoma Pinelliae* (12 g), *Radix Scutellariae* (9 g), *Radix Zingiberis* (9 g), *Radix Ginseng* (9 g), *Radix Glycyrrhizae Praeparata* (9 g), *Rhizoma Coptidis* (3 g), and *Fructus Ziziphi Jujubae* (4 pieces).

【Functions】Hormonize the stomach and direct qi downward, relieve stagnation and dissipate binds.

【Indications】Stuffiness and fullness due to cold-heat complex or disorder of stomach qi, marked by epigastric fullness without pain, or vomiting, borborygmus, diarrhea, and thin, yellow and greasy tongue fur, and string-like and slippery pulse.

【Explanation】*Rhizoma Pinelliaeis* serves as the sovereign medicinal in this formula, its taste is acrid and it can dissipate stagnation; it has bitter nature which can descend qi and stop vomiting. *Rhizoma Zingiberis* (warms the interior and dispels cold), *Radix Scutellariae* and *Rhizoma Coptidis* (with bitter taste and cold nature clear heat) are the minister medicinals. *Radix Ginseng* and *Fructus Ziziphi Jujubae*, with sweet taste and warm nature benefit spleen qi to replenish its functions of upbearing and downbearing, serve as the assistant meidicinals; *Radix Glycyrrhizae Parepata* is the assistant and courier medicinal, has functions of enforcing the functions of tonifying qi and harmonying the middle, and harmonizing the other ingredients. All the ingredients in the formula combined together, possess the actions of separating the cold and heat, removing stagnation and dissipating binds, and treat both the root and the tip of diseases. It is the representative formula for modulating cold-heat complex syndrome by means of opening with acrid and descending with bitter.

【Note】The formula is contraindicated for stuffiness and fullness in the stomach due to retention and food accumulation or qi stagnation.

【Variation】In the case of invading dampness-heat in middle eneziger and without the middle qi deficiency, marked with serve vomiting and distetion, or thick greasy tongue fur, one should remove *Radix Genseng*, *Radix Glycyrrhizae*, *Fructus Jujubae* and *Rhizoma Zingiberis*, add *Fructus Aurantii Immaturus* and *Rhizoma Zingiberies Recens* to descend qi and soothe fullness and stop vomiting.

Heat-Clearing Formulas

Heat-clearing formulas are the formulas mainly composed of heat-clearing medicinals and are in accordance with the principle of "treating heat with cold," and are applicable for syndromes of interior heat.

（一）清气分热剂

清气分热的方剂，具有清热除烦、生津止渴的作用，适用于热在气分、热盛伤津之证。症见壮热烦渴，大汗，舌红苔黄，脉洪大或滑数。代表方剂：白虎汤。

白虎汤

【来源】《伤寒论》

【组成】石膏（50克）知母（18克）粳米（9克）甘草（6克）

【功用】清热生津。

【主治】伤寒阳明经证，或温病气分热证。壮热面赤，烦渴引饮，口舌干燥，大汗出，脉洪大有力。

【方解】方中辛甘大寒的石膏为君，清肺胃邪热，解肌透热，又可生津止渴。臣用知母苦寒质润，既助石膏清气分实热，又治已伤之阴。佐以粳米既可益胃护津，又可防止石膏大寒伤中。使以甘草调和诸药。

【注意事项】发热无汗、表证未解以及阴盛格阳、寒假热等情况不宜使用。

【加减】阳明气分热盛，兼见燥渴、汗多而脉浮大无力者，加人参（白虎加人参汤）；若兼有外热（里热重于外热），以身无寒但热，骨节疼烦为主证，加桂枝（白虎桂枝汤）；若兼有湿邪，如风湿热痹，可加苍术（白虎加苍术汤）。

（二）清营凉血剂

清营凉血方剂具有清营泻热、凉血散血的作用，适用于邪热入营，或热入血室的病证。症见身热烦扰，口渴或不渴，神昏谵语，吐血、衄血、斑疹，舌红绛，脉数等。代表方剂：清营汤、犀角地黄汤。

They belong to heat-clearing method of"the eight therapeutic methods."

Heat-clearing formulas are applicable to interior heat syndromes, which refer to the condition that the exterior pathogenic factors have been relieved, with heat entering the interior, or the interior excess heat without accumulation.

Heat-clearing formulas readily injure stomach qi and spleen yang, it should be stopped using as soon as the disease is relieved, and should not be indicated for a long period, and protection of stomach qi should be paid attention to, and *Fructus Oryzae Sativae*, *Radix Glycyrrhizae*, *Rhizoma Pinelliae*, *Rhizoma Atractylodis Macrocephalae*, and *Poria* should be added to tonify the spleen and harmonize the stomach. According to the difference of the functions, the heat-clearing formulas can be classified into six categories, formulas of clearing heat from qi aspect, formulas of clearing the nutrient aspect and cooling the blood aspect, formulas of clearing heat and removing toxins, formulas of clearing heat from viscera and bowels, formulas of expelling summer-heat, and formulas of clearing deficiency heat.

Formulas of clearing heat from qi aspect

Formulas of clearing heat from qi aspect have functions of clearing heat and relieving restlessness, generating fluid and relieving thirst, and are applicable to heat in the qi aspect, excess of heat and consumption of fluid syndromes, marked by high fever, thirst, profuse sweating, red tongue and yellow tongue coating, surging and large pulse, or rapid and slippery pulse. The representative formula is "White Tiger Decoction".

White Tiger Decoction (Bai Hu Tang)

【Source】*Treatise on Cold Damage Diseases.*

【Composition】*Gypsum Fibrosum* (50 g), *Rhizoma Anemarrhenae* (18 g), *Semen Oryzae Nonglutionosae* (9 g), *Radix Glycyrrhizae Praeparata* (6 g).

【Functions】Clear heat and generate fluid.

【Indications】Yang brightness syndrome of cold damage diseases, or heat in qi aspect of febrile diseases, marked by high fever, flushed face, thirst, dry mouth and tongue, profuse sweating, surging and large pulse with force.

【Explanation】In the formula, *Gypsum Fibrosum*, with acrid and sweet flavor and extremely cold nature, clears heat in the lung and stomach, expels pathogenic factors from the muscle to remove heat, and generates fluid and relieves thirst. *Rhizoma Anemarrhenae*, with bitter taste, which is cold and moist in nature, is minister medicinal, not only enforces *Gypsum Fibrosum* to clear excessive heat in qi aspect, but also replenishes consumed fluid. *Semen Oryzae Nonglutionosae*, as assistant medicinal, nourishes the stomach and protects fluid and prevents extremely cold *Gypsum Fibrosum* injurying the middle enerziger. *Radix Glycyrrhizae Praeparata* as courier medicinal modulates all the ingredients.

【Note】The formula is not applicable to fever without sweating due to unrelieved exterior pathogenic factors, excessive yin rejecting yang, and true-cold and false-heat syndrome.

【Variation】In case of excess heat of yang brightness syndomre, marked by dryness and thirst, profuse sweating, floating, surging and weak pulse, add *Radix Ginseng* ("White Tiger Plus Ginseng Decoction"); in case of external heat (interior heat is severer than exterior heat), mainly marked with fever without sweating, arthralgia and restlessness, add *Ramulus Cinnamomi* ("White Tiger Plus Cinnamon Twig Decoction"); in case of concurrence with dampness, such as impediment disease due to wind together with dampness-heat, add *Rhizoma Atractyloidis* ("White Tiger Plus Atractylodis Decoction").

Formulas for clearing the nutrient aspect and cooling the blood aspect

Formulas for clearing the nutrient aspect and cooling the blood aspect have functions of clearing the nutrient aspect, purging the heat, cooling the blood and dissipating blood stasis, and are applicable for ex-

清营汤

【来源】《温病条辨》

【组成】水牛角（30克）生地黄（15克）玄参（9克）竹叶心（3克）麦冬（9克）丹参（6克）黄连（5克）银花（9克）连翘（6克）

【功用】清营解毒，透热养阴。

【主治】热入营分证。身热夜甚，神烦少寐，时有谵语，口渴或不渴，斑疹隐隐，舌绛而干，脉细数。

【方解】本方用苦咸寒之水牛角清解营分之热毒为君。以生地黄滋阴凉血、麦冬清热养阴生津、玄参滋阴降火解毒，既可养阴保津，又可助君药清营凉血解毒，三药共为臣药。君臣相配，咸寒与甘寒并用，清营热而滋营阴，祛邪而扶正。温邪初入营分，故以银花、连翘、竹叶清热解毒，轻清透泄，使营分热邪透出气分而解，此即"入营犹可透热转气"之义；黄连苦寒，清心解毒；丹参清热凉血，活血散瘀，可防热与血结，共为佐药。以清营解毒为主，配以养阴生津和"透热转气"，使入营之邪透出气分而解，是本方的配伍特点。

【注意事项】使用本方应注意舌诊。如舌苔白滑，意味着湿重，不可单用本方，以防滋腻而助湿留邪。

【加减】热陷心包致窍闭神昏者，可合用安宫牛黄丸或至宝丹以清心开窍；若营热动风致痉厥抽搐者，可合用紫雪丹，或加水牛角、钩藤、地龙等以熄风止痉；若兼有热痰，可加天竺黄、川贝母等清热涤痰；如气分热邪犹盛，可重用银花、连翘、黄连，或加石膏、知母、大青叶、板蓝根等增强清热解毒之力。

cess heat in nutrient aspect, or heat entering the blood aspect, marked with fever and restlessness, thirst or without thirst, coma, delirium, hemoptysis, epistaxis, purple or black macula, deep red tongue, rapid pulse. The representative formulas are "Clearing Nutritive Qi Decoction" and "Cornus Rhinoceri Rehmannia Decoction".

Clearing Nutritive Qi Decoction(Qing Ying Tang)

【Source】*Systematized Identification of Warm(Pathogen)Diseases.*

【Composition】*Cornu Bufali* (30 g), *Radix Rehmanniae* (15 g), *Radix Scrophulariae* (9g), *Herba Lophatheri* (3 g), *Radix Ophiopogonis* (9 g), *Radix Salviae Miltiorrhizae* (6 g), *Rhizoma Coptidis* (5 g), *Flos Lonicerae* (9 g), and *Fructus Forsythiae* (6 g).

【Functions】Clear heat from the nutrient aspect and detoxify, outthrust and clear heat and nourish yin.

【Indications】Heat entering the nutrient aspect, marked by body fever worsened at night, dysphoria with insomnia, occasional delirium, thirst or without thirst, faint rashes, deep red dry tongue, and fine and rapid pulse.

【Explanation】In the formula, *Cornu Bubali* with bitter, salty taste and cold nature is the sovereign medicinal, it purges the heat and eliminates toxins in the nutrient aspect. *Radix Rehmanniae* nourishes yin and cools the blood, *Radix Ophiopogonis* clears heat, and nourishes yin and generates fluid, *Radix Scrophulariae* nourishes yin, clears heat and eliminates toxins. The above mentioned three medicinals not only nourish yin to protect fluid, but also help the sovereign medicinal clear heat in the nutrient aspect and detoxify in the nutrient aspect, all of them are the assistant medicinals; the sovereign medicinal combines with the assistant medicinals, the salty and cold combined with the sweet and cold, so as to clear heat in the nutrient aspect, nourish yin in the nutrient aspect, and dispel pathogenic factors and enforce the healthy qi. Since the pathogenic factors of febrile diseases just entered the nutrient aspect, add *Flos Lonicerae*, *Fructus Forsythiae*, and *Rhizoma Phragmitis* to clear heat and detoxify, which are light and outgoing, cool and heat-clearing, and can expel the heat from the nutrient aspect via the qi aspect and relieve the heat. This is the meaning of "when the pathogenic heat entered the nutrient aspect, it still can be outthrusted and cleared via the qi aspect". *Rhizoma Coptidis* with bitter and cold, clears heart and detoxify; *Radix Salviae Miltiorrhizae* clears heat and cools the blood, activates blood and removes stasis, and prevents the combination of the heat and stasis, those two medicinals are the assistant medicinals. The characteristic of combination the formula is, focusing on clearing heat and detoxifying in the nutrient aspect, accompanied with nourishing yin and generating fluid, and "outthrusting and clearing heat via qi aspect", so as to dispel the pathogenic heat which entered the nutrient aspect out to the qi aspect and disappear.

【Note】Pay attention to tongue diagnosis when using this formula. If the tongue coating is white and slippery, it means excessive dampness, the formula should not be used alone for fear that it might promote generation of greasiness and make dampness keep pathogenic factors.

【Variation】In case of coma due to the heat sunken in pericardium and orifices blocked, concurrently take "Bezoar Resurrection Pill or Precious Bolus" to clear the heart and open the orifices; in case of syncope and spasm due to wind and excessive heat in the nutrient aspect, add "Purple Snow Powder", or *Cornu Bubali*, *Ramulus Uncariae cum Uncis* and *Lumbricus* to extinguish wind to arrest convulsions; in case of intermingled heat-phlegm, add *Concretio Silicea Bambusae* and *Bulbus Fritillariae Cirrhosae* to clear heat and resolve phlegm; in case of excessive pathogenic heat in qi aspect, use *Flos Lonicerae*, *Fructus Forsythiae*, and *Rhizoma Coptidis* in high dose, or add *Gypsum Fibrosum*, *Rhizoma Anemarrhenae*, *Folium Isatidis*, and *Radix Isatidis* to enhance the potency of clearing heat and detoxifying.

犀角地黄汤

【来源】《备急千金要方》

【组成】水牛角［原为犀角］（30克）生地黄（24克）芍药（12克）牡丹皮（9克）

【功用】清热解毒，凉血散瘀。

【主治】热入血分证。

1. 热扰心神，身热谵语，舌绛起刺，脉细数。

2. 热伤血络，斑色紫黑、吐血、衄血、便血、尿血等，舌红绛，脉数。

3. 蓄血瘀热，喜忘如狂，漱水不欲咽，大便色黑易解。

【方解】方中水牛角为君，性味苦咸寒，凉血清心而解热毒。生地为臣，性味甘苦寒，凉血滋阴生津，一则助君清热凉血，又能止血；一则复已失之阴血。赤芍、丹皮为佐，性味苦微寒，清热凉血，活血散瘀。四药相合，共奏清热解毒、凉血散瘀之功。其特点是凉血与活血散瘀并用，使热清血宁而无耗血动血之弊，凉血止血又无冰伏留瘀之虑。

【注意事项】阳虚失血、脾胃虚弱者忌用。

【加减】若蓄血、喜忘如狂者，加大黄、黄芩，以清热逐瘀与凉血散瘀同用；若郁怒而夹肝火者，加柴胡、黄芩、栀子以清泻肝火；若热迫血溢之出血证，加白茅根、侧柏炭、小蓟等以增强凉血止血之功。

（三）清热解毒剂

以具有寒凉解毒作用的药物为主组成，治疗各种热毒病证的方剂。适用于一切急性火毒，如温疫、温毒及火毒或疮疡等证。代表方剂：黄连解毒汤。

黄连解毒汤

【来源】《外台秘要》

【组成】黄连（9克）黄芩（6克）黄柏（6克）栀子（9克）

【功用】泻火解毒。

【主治】一切实热火毒，三焦热盛之证。大热烦躁，谵语不眠，口燥咽干；或热病吐血、衄血；或热甚发斑，身热下痢，湿热黄疸；痈疽疔毒，小便黄赤，舌红苔黄，脉数有力。

【方解】方中黄连大苦大寒清泻心火为君，兼泻中焦之火。黄芩清上焦之火为臣。黄柏泻下焦之火；栀子清泻三焦之火，导热下行，引邪热从小便而出，共为佐

Cornus Rhinoceri Rehmannia Decoction (Xi Jiao Di Huang Tang)

【Source】*Essential Prescriptions Worth a Thousand Gold for Emergencies.*

【Composition】*Cornu Bubali* (30 g) (originally *Cornus Rhinocerotis*) , *Radix Rehmanniae* (15 g) , *Radix Paeoniae* (12 g) , and *Cortex Moutan Radicis* (9 g) .

【Functions】Clear heat and detoxify, cool blood, and dispel blood stasis.

【Indications】Heat entering the blood aspect.

(1) Heat harassing the heart spirit, marked by body fever, dilirum, deep red tongue with pricks, fine and rapid pulse.

(2) Heat injuried blood colleterals, marked by purple and dark rashes, hematemesis, nose bleeding, hematochezia, hematuria, deep red tongue, and rapid pulse.

(3) Blood amassment with heat, marked by forgetfulness like manic psychosis, gargling and aversion to swallow water, black stool, and easy to poop.

【Explanation】In the formula, the sovereign medicinal is *Cornu Bubali*, with bitter and salty taste, cold nature; it cools blood, purges heart heat and detoxicate heat-toxin. *Radix Rehmanniae* as minister medicinal, with sweet and acrid taste, cold nature, clears blood, nourishes yin and generates fluid; on one hand, it helps the sovereign medicinal clear heat, cool blood and stop bleeding, on another hand, it recovers consumted yin and blood. *Radix Paeoniae Rubra* and *Cortex Moutan* are the assistant medicinals, those are with acrid taste and cool nature, clear heat and cool blood, activate blood and remove stasis. The four ingredients forming the formula possess the actions of both clearing heat and detoxifying, and cooling blood and removing blood stasis. The characteristic of forming formula is the combination of cooling blood, activating blood to remove stasis, so as to cool heat and peacify blood without damaging and consuming blood, and cool blood to stop bleeding without retention of blood stasis due to ice-cold.

【Note】Contraindicated for bleeding due to yang deficiency syndrome and spleen-stomach deficiency syndrome.

【Variation】In case of blood amassment and manic and forgetting, add *Radix et Rhizoma Rhei* and *Radix Scutellariae*, to clear heat and remove stasis, together with cooling blood and dispelling stasis; in case of liver heat due to depression and anger, add *Radix Bupleuri*, *Radix Scutellariae*, and *Fructus Gardeniae* to clear liver heat; in case of bleeding due to excessive heat, add *Rhizoma Imperatae*, *Cacumen Platycladi Carbonisatus*, and *Herba Cephalanoploris* to rienforce the actions of cooling blood and stopping bleeding.

Formulas of clearing heat and removing toxins

Formulas of clearing heat and removing toxins are composed of medicinals with cool or cold nature and have functions of removing toxins, and to treat diseases and syndromes of heat-toxin, and are applicable to all acute fire toxin syndromes, such as pestilence, febrile toxin, fire toxin, sores and ulcer, etc. The representative formula is "Coptidis Detoxification Decoction."

Coptidis Detoxification Decoction (Huang Lian Jie Du Tang)

【Source】*Medical Secrets of an Official.*

【Composition】*Rhizoma Coptidis* (9 g) , *Radix Scutellariae* (6 g) , *Cortex Phellodendri* (6 g) , *Fructus Gardeniae* (9 g) .

【Functions】Purge fire and eliminate toxins.

【Indications】All syndromes of excess heat and heat toxin, and excessive heat in triple energizer, marked by high fever, dysphoria, delirium, insomnia, dry mouth and throat, or hemoptysis, bleeding due to febrile diseases, or macula due to sever heat, or body fever with diarrhea, or jaundice due to dampness and

药。四药合用，苦寒直折，热清毒解，去三焦之火邪。

【注意事项】本方大苦大寒，久服或过量易伤脾胃。

【加减】便秘者，加大黄以泻下焦实热；吐血、衄血、发斑者，加玄参、生地、丹皮以清热凉血；发黄者，加茵陈、大黄以清热祛湿退黄；疔疮肿毒者，加蒲公英、银花、连翘以增强清热解毒之力。

（四）清脏腑热剂

具有清解脏腑热邪的作用，用于热邪偏盛于某一脏腑的里热证。根据不同脏腑热盛之不同，清脏腑热常分为清心、清肺、清肝、清胃等治法。代表方剂：龙胆泻肝汤、泻白散、清胃散、白头翁汤。

龙胆泻肝汤

【来源】《医方集解》

【组成】龙胆草（6克）黄芩（9克）山栀子（9克）泽泻（12克）木通（6克）车前子（9克）当归（3克）生地黄（9克）柴胡（6克）生甘草（6克）

【功用】泻肝胆实火，清肝经湿热。

【主治】①肝胆实火上扰，症见头痛目赤，胁痛口苦，耳聋、耳肿；②肝经湿热下注，症见阴肿阴痒，筋痿阴汗，小便淋浊，妇女湿热带下等。

【方解】方中龙胆草大苦大寒，既泻肝胆实火，又清肝经湿热，是泻火除湿两擅其功的君药。黄芩、栀子苦寒泻火，助龙胆草加强清热祛湿之力，为臣药。泽泻、木通、车前子清热利湿，使湿热从小便排出。肝主藏血，肝经有热，易耗伤阴血，故用生地、当归滋阴养血，以防伤阴，为佐药。柴胡为引诸药入肝胆而设，甘草调和诸药，为使药。全方泻中有补、利中有滋，以使火降热清、湿浊分清。

【注意事项】本方药物多为苦寒之性，内服易伤脾胃，故对脾胃虚寒和阴虚阳亢之证慎用。

【加减】若肝胆实火较盛，可去木通、车前子，加黄连以增强泻火之力；若湿盛热轻者，可去黄芩、生地，加滑石、薏苡仁以加强利湿之功；若玉茎生疮，或便毒悬痈，或阴囊肿痛红热甚者，可去柴胡，加连翘、黄连、大黄以加大泻火解毒之用。

heat, or sore and carbuncle, skin rashes or skin infection, yellow and dark urine, red tongue with yellow tongue fur, and rapid and forceful pulse.

【Explanation】In the formula, *Rhizoma Coptidis* is the sovereign medicinal. It is severe bitter and severe cold, therefore, it can purge heart fire and clear fire in the middle energizer. *Radix Scutellariae*, as the minister medicinal, clears fire in the upper energizer. *Cortex Phellodendri* purges the fire in the lower energizer; *Fructus Gardeniae* purges fire in the triple energizers, leads the heat downwards, and guides the pathogenic heat going out via urine, those two medicinals are assistant medicinals. The four ingredients with bitter taste and cold nature are used together in one formula to eliminate pathogenic fire, heat and toxin of triple energizers.

【Note】The formula consists of extremely bitter and cold ingredients. It should not be used for long time or in high dose to avoid damaging the spleen and stomach.

【Variation】In case of constipation, add *Radix et Rhizoma Rhei* to purge excessive heat in the lower energizer; for hemoptysis, bleeding or macula, add *Radix Scrophulariae*, *Radix Rehmanniae*, and *Cortex Moutan* to clear heat and cool blood; for jaundice, add *Herba Artemisiae Scopariae* and *Radix et Rhizoma Rhei* to clear heat, dispel dampness, and remove jaundice; for sores and carbuncle, skin rashes or skin infection, add *Herba Taraxaci*, *Flos Lonicerae*, and *Fructus Forsythiae* to clear heat and remove toxins.

Formulas of clearing heat from viscera and bowels

Formulas of clearing heat from viscera and bowels have functions of clearing pathogenic heat from viscera and bowels, and are applicable to fire and heat syndrome due to excessive pathogenic heat in certain viscera and bowels. According to the different viscera and bowels with which the pathogenic heat is related, the methods of clearing heat from viscera and bowels are classified into clearing heart heat, clearing lung heat, clearing liver heat, clearing stomach heat, etc. The representative formulas are "Gentiana Draining the Liver Decoction", "Draining the White Powder", "Clearing the Stomach Powder" and "Pulsatilla Decoction".

Gentiana Draining the Liver Decoction(Long Dan Xie Gan Tang)

【Source】*Collection of Formulas with Notes.*

【Composition】*Radix Gentianae* (6 g), *Radix Scutellariae* (9 g), *Fructus Gardeniae* (9 g), *Rhizoma Alismatis* (12 g), *Caulis Akebiae* (6 g), *Semen Plantaginis* (9 g), *Radix Angenicae Sinensis* (3 g), *Radix Rehmanniae* (9 g), *Radix Bupleuri* (6 g), and *Radix Glycyrrhizae* (6 g).

【Functions】Purge excessive fire of the liver and gallbladder, clear dampness-heat from the liver meridian.

【Indications】a) Sthenic fire flaming up syndrome of the liver and gallbladder, marked by headache, red eyes, hypochondriac pain, bitter taste in the mouth, deafness, swelling of ear, red tongue with yellow coating, taut, rapid and forceful pulse; and b) Downward flow of dampness and heat syndrome of the liver meridian, marked by swelling of vulva, pruritus, polyhidrosis around external genitals, stranguria with turbid urine, leukorrhagia with foul odor and yellow color, red tongue with yellow and greasy tongue coating, string-like, rapid and forceful pulse.

【Explanation】In the formula, *Radix Gentianae* with severe bitter and severe cold, as the sovereign medicinal, not only purges excessive fire of the liver and gallbladder, but also removes dampness and heat from the liver and gallbladder meridians. *Radix Scutellariae* and *Fructus Gardeniae* clear heat and purge fire, concurrently dry dampness, those two meidicinals are minister medicinals. *Rhizoma Alismatis*, *Caulis Akebiae*, and *Semen Plantaginis* remove heat and dampness, and drain the dampness-heat via urine excretion. *Radix Rehmanniae* and *Radix Angenicae Sinensis* as the assistant medicinals nourish yin and blood, and prevent the consumption of yin. *Radix Bupleuri* guides the other medicinals to enter the liver and gall-

泻白散

【来源】《小儿药证直诀》

【组成】地骨皮　桑白皮（各30克）甘草（3克）粳米（10克）

【功用】清泻肺热，止咳平喘。

【主治】肺热喘咳证。气喘咳嗽，皮肤蒸热，日晡尤甚，舌红苔黄，脉细数。

【方解】方中桑白皮甘寒性降，专入肺经，清泻肺热，平喘止咳，为君药。地骨皮甘寒入肺，助君药清降肺中伏火，以为臣药。君臣相伍，清泻肺热，使金清气肃。炙甘草、粳米养胃和中以扶肺气，共为佐使。四药合用，共达泻肺清热、止咳平喘之功。本方特点是清中有润、泻中有补。

【注意事项】风寒咳嗽或肺虚喘咳者不宜使用。

【加减】肺经热重者，可黄芩、知母等以增强清泻肺热之力；燥热咳嗽者，加瓜蒌、川贝母等润肺止咳；阴虚潮热者，加鳖甲以滋阴退热；热伤阴津、烦热口渴者，加花粉、芦根以清热生津。

清胃散

【来源】《脾胃论》

【组成】生地黄（6克）当归身（6克）牡丹皮（9克）黄连（6克）升麻（9克）

【功用】清胃凉血。

【主治】胃火牙痛。症见牙痛牵引头痛，面颊发热，牙齿喜冷恶热，或牙宣出血，或牙龈红肿溃烂，或唇舌腮颊肿痛，口气热臭，口干舌燥，舌红苔黄，脉滑数。

【方解】方中黄连苦寒泻火为君，直折胃腑之热。升麻甘辛微寒，一则清热解毒，治胃火牙痛；一则轻清升散透发，宣达郁遏伏火，有"火郁发之"之意，黄连得升麻，泻火而无凉遏之弊；升麻得黄连，散火而无升焰之虞。胃热侵及血分，耗伤阴血，故用生地凉血滋阴；丹皮凉血清热，皆为臣药。佐以当归养血活血，以助消肿止痛。升麻兼以引经为使。诸药配伍，清胃凉血，使上炎之火得降，血分之热得除，循经外发，诸症皆可因热毒内撤而解。

【注意事项】牙痛属风寒及肾虚火炎者不宜使用。

【加减】若兼大肠有热而大便秘结者，加大黄以泻热荡实、导热下行；兼有口渴者，可加元参、天花粉以生津，或加石膏清热生津。

bladder meridians ; *Radix Glycyrrhizae* mediates all the ingredients , *Radix Bupleuri* and *Radix Glycyrrhizae* are the courier medicinals. All the ingredients used together possess the characteristics of tonification within purgation , nourishing within promoting , and ascension with descension. By these methods , the formula descends fire , clears heat and removes dampness.

【Note】The formula mainly consists of bitter and cold ingredients , and easily impairs the spleen and stomach , thus , it should be used cautiously in patients with spleen-stomach deficiency syndrome and yin deficiency with excessive yang.

【Variation】If the excess fire of liver and gallbladder is severe , then remove *Caulis Akebiae* and *Semen Plantaginis* , and add *Rhizoma Coptidis* to promote clearing fire ; in case of excessive dampness and mild heat , remove *Radix Scutellariae* and *Radix Rehmanniae* , add *Talcum* and *Semen Coicis* to strengthen the potency of eliminating dampness ; in case of sores in the penis , swollen scrotum with severe pain and feverish sensation , remove *Radix Bupleuri* , add *Fructus Forsythiae* , *Rhizoma Coptidis* , and *Radix Rhizoma Rhei* to promote perging fire and removing toxins.

Draining the White Powder (Xie Bai San)

【Source】*Key to Therapeutics of Children's Diseases.*

【Composition】*Cortex Lycii Radicis* (30 g) , *Cortex Mori Radicis* (30 g) , *Radix Glycyrrhizae* (3 g) , *Oryzae Sativae* (10 g).

【Functions】Purge lung heat , relieve cough and dyspnea.

【Indications】Cough and asthma due to the lung heat , marked by cough , asthma , feverish skin aggravated in the afternoon , red tongue with yellow tongue fur , and fine and rapid pulse.

【Explanation】In the formula , *Cortex Mori Radicis* which is sweet , cold and of descending actions , enters the lung meridian , clears lung heat , relieves cough and asthma , it serves as the sovereign medicinal. *Cortex Lycii Radicis* with sweet taste and cold nature enters the lung meridian , helps the sovereign medicinal clear the hiding fire in the lung , and serves as the minister medicinal. *Radix Glycyrrhizae Praeparata* and *Semen Oryzae Nonglutionosae* tonify lung qi , and serve as the assistant medicinals. The four ingredients used together possess moistening within heat-clearing , tonification within purgation.

【Note】It is not suitable for cough due to wind-cold , and cough and asthma due to lung deficiency.

【Variation】In case of severe lung heat , add *Radix Scutellariae* and *Rhizoma Anemarrhenae* to enhance the potency of purging lung heat ; in case of cough due to dry heat , add *Fructus Trichosanthis* and *Bulbus Fritillariae Cirrhosae* to moisten lung and relieve cough ; in case of tidal fever due to yin deficiency , add *Carapax Trionycis* to nourish yin and clear deficiency heat ; in case of fluid consumption caused by heat , marked by restlessness , fever and thirst , add *Radix Trichosanthis* and *Rhizoma Phragmitis* to clear heat and generate fluid.

Clearing the Stomach Powder (Qing Wei San)

【Source】*Treatise on the Spleen and Stomach.*

【Composition】*Radix Rehmanniae* (9 g) , *Radix Angenicae Sinensis* (6 g) , *Cortex Moutan Radicis* (9 g) , *Rhizoma Coptidis* (6 g) , and *Rhizoma Cimicifugae* (9 g).

【Functions】Purge stomach heat and cool the blood.

【Indications】Toothache due to stomach fire , marked by headache radiated by toothache , feverish cheeks , dental preference to cold and aversion to heat , or gingival atrophy with oozing of bloody fluid and pus , or ulceration of gum with swelling , or swelling and pain of lips , tongue and cheeks , hot and foul breath , dry mouth and tongue , red tongue with yellow tongue coating , slippery and rapid pulse.

【Explanation】In the formula , *Rhizoma Coptidis* , which is bitter and cold and has function of purging

白头翁汤

【来源】《伤寒论》

【组成】白头翁（15克）黄柏（12克）黄连（6克）秦皮（12克）

【功用】清热解毒，凉血止痢。

【主治】热毒痢疾。症见腹痛，里急后重，肛门灼热，下痢脓血，赤多白少，渴欲饮水，舌红苔黄，脉弦数。

【方解】方中君药白头翁苦寒而入血分，清热解毒，凉血止痢。臣以黄连，苦寒泻火解毒，燥湿厚肠，为治痢要药；黄柏清下焦湿热，共助白头翁清热解毒，尤能燥湿治痢。佐以秦皮苦涩而寒，清热解毒，兼以收涩止痢。四药配伍，共奏清热解毒、凉血止痢之功。

【注意事项】痢疾属寒湿及虚寒者禁用。

【加减】若外有表邪，恶寒发热者，加葛根、连翘、银花以透表解热；若里急后重较甚，加木香、槟榔、枳壳以调气；若脓血多者，加赤芍、丹皮、地榆以凉血和血。

（六）清虚热剂

清虚热剂具有养阴透热、清热除蒸的作用。宜用于热病后期，邪热未尽、阴液已伤，而见暮热早凉、舌红少苔者；或因肝肾阴虚，而致骨蒸潮热或久热不退的虚热证。代表方剂：青蒿鳖甲汤。

fire, is used as sovereign medicinal to directly purge stomach fire. *Rhizoma Cimicifugae*, with acrid and sweet flavor and slightly cold nature, serves as minister medicinal, follows the therapeutic principle of "clearing and dispersing when there is depressed fire." It not only purges fire and removes toxin to treat toothache due to stomach fire, but also ascends and disperses the internal fire. *Rhizoma Coptidis*, with the help of *Rhizoma Cimicifugae*, purges fire without inhibiting cold; while *Rhizoma Cimicifugae*, with the assistance of *Rhizoma Coptidis*, disperses fire without incurring the flaming up. Since the stomach heat invaded the blood aspect, and consumed nutrient blood, *Radix Rehmanniae* is added to cool the blood and nourish yin, and *Cortex Moutan Radicis* is added to cool the blood and clear heat, both are the minister medicinals. *Radix Angenicae Sinensis*, as the assistant medicinal, nourishes and activates the blood to relieve swelling and pain. *Rhizoma Cimicifugae* concurrently serves as the guiding courier. All the ingredients together clear the stomach and cool the blood, descend the upburning fire downward, and disperse the heat in the blood. All the symptoms along with the channel of the stomach will disappear when the heat dispersed internally.

【Note】Contraindicated for toothache due to wind-cold or due to kidney deficiency with upbearing deficiency fire.

【Variation】In case of concurrent constipation due to heat of large intestine, add *Radix Rhizoma Rhei* to purge heat and dispel mass, guide the heat downwards; in case of concurrent thirst, add *Radix Scrophulariae* and *Radix Trichosanthis* to ascend fluid, or add *Gypsum Fibrosum* to clear heat and generate fluid.

Pulsatilla Decoction (Bai Tou Weng Tang)

【Source】*Treatise on Cold Damage Diseases.*

【Composition】*Radix Pulsatillae* (15 g) , *Cortex Phellodendri* (12 g) , *Rhizoma Coptidis* (6 g) , and *Cortex Fraxini* (12 g).

【Functions】Purge heat and remove toxin, cool the blood, and relieve dysentery.

【Indications】Dysentery due to heat and toxin, marked by abdominalgia, tenesmus, feverish sensation of anus, dysentery due to pus and blood accompanied by more red than white, thirst with desire for drinking, red tongue with yellow tongue fur, and string-like and rapid pulse.

【Explanation】The bitter cold *Radix Pulsatillae* enters the blood aspect and serves as the sovereign medicinal; it clears heat and removes toxin, cools the blood and checks dysentery. *Rhizoma Coptidis* clears heat and removes toxin as an important medicinal of treating dysentery. *Cortex Phellodendri* clears heat and dries dampness, these two medicinals are minister medicinals. *Cortex Fraxini*, with bitter taste, cold and astringent nature, clears heat, removes toxin, and concurrently astringes to check dysentery; it serves as the assistant medicinal. The four ingredients are used together in the formula to clear heat, remove toxin, check dysentery, and cure tenesmus.

【Note】The formula is contraindicated for dysentery due to dampness-cold or deficiency cold.

【Variation】In case of exterior pathogenic factors, aversion to cold and fever, add *Radix Puerariae*, *Fructus Forsythiae*, and *Flos Lonicerae* to relieve the exterior syndrome and remove heat; in case of severe tenesmus, add *Radix Aucklandiae*, *Semen Arecae*, and *Fructus Aurantii* to regulate qi; in case of profuse pus and blood, add *Radix Paeoniae Rubra*, *Cortex Moutan Radicis*, and *Radix Sanguisobae* to cool and harmonize the blood.

Formulas of clearing deficiency heat

Formulas of clearing deficiency heat have functions of nourishing yin and dispelling heat outsidely, clearing heat and relieving steaming, and are applicable to the late stage of febrile diseases and syndromes of residual heat with yin consumption marked by fever at dusk and chill in the morning, red tongue with scanty tongue coating; or deficiency heat syndrome marked by steaming bone and tidal fever or retention of

青蒿鳖甲汤

【来源】《温病条辨》

【组成】青蒿（6克）鳖甲（15克）生地（12克）知母（6克）丹皮（9克）。

【功用】养阴透热。

【主治】邪热内伏证。症见夜热早凉，热退无汗，能食形瘦，舌红少苔，脉数。

【方解】方中鳖甲咸寒滋阴，直入阴分，以退虚热；青蒿芳香清热透毒，引邪外出。二药相合，透热而不伤阴，养阴而不恋邪，为君药。生地甘凉滋阴，知母苦寒滋润，共助君药以退虚热，为臣药。丹皮凉血透热，助青蒿以透泄阴分之伏热，为佐药。

【注意事项】方中青蒿不耐高温，煎煮时间不宜太长，或用沸水泡服；阴虚欲作动风者，不宜用本方。

【加减】用于肺痨骨蒸，阴虚火旺时，可加沙参、麦冬清肺养阴；用于小儿夏季热，属于阴虚有热时，可加石斛、地骨皮、白薇等以退虚热。

五、温里剂

温里剂是根据《素问·阴阳应象大论篇》"寒者热之"的原则，用温热药组成，具有温里助阳、散寒通脉等作用，治疗里寒证的方剂。属于"八法"中的"温法"。温里剂辛温燥热，应用须辨清寒热之真假。温里剂分为温中散寒、回阳救逆、温经散寒三类。

（一）温中散寒剂

温中散寒剂主治寒邪入里而致脾胃虚寒或中焦虚寒证，症见脘腹冷痛，食欲不振，呕吐、腹泻，手足不温，舌淡苔白滑，脉沉细或沉迟。代表方剂：理中丸。

理中丸

【来源】《伤寒论》

【组成】人参　干姜　白术　甘草（各90克）（丸剂用量）

【功用】温中祛寒，补气健脾。

【主治】

1. 脾胃虚寒证。症见脘腹绵绵作痛，喜温喜按，呕吐，大便稀溏，脘痞食少，畏寒肢冷，口不渴，舌淡，苔白润，脉沉细或沉迟无力。

2. 阳虚失血证。症见吐血、衄血、便血或崩漏等，血色暗淡，质清稀。

fever due to liver and kidney yin deficiency.The representative formula is "Artemisiae Annuae and Carapax Trionycis Decoction".

Artemisiae Annuae and Carapax Trionycis Decoction(Qing Hao Bie Jia Tang)

【Source】*Essentials of Seasonal Febrile Diseases.*

【Composition】*Herba Artemisiae* (6 g) ,*Carapax Trionycis* (15 g) ,*Radix Rehmanniae* (12 g) ,*Rhizoma Anemarrhenae* (6 g) ,and *Cortex Moutan Radicis* (9 g) .

【Functions】Nourish yin and release heat.

【Indications】Pathogenic factors of heat hidden in the interior aspects,marked by fever at night and chill in the morning,relieved fever without sweating,able to eat but with weight loss,red tongue with scanty tongue fur,fine and rapid pulse.

【Explanation】In the formula,*Carapax Trionycis*,with salty flavor and cold nature,directly nourishes yin and enters yin aspects to clear deficiency heat.*Herba Artemisiae*,with bitter and acrid flavors,cold nature and aromatic smell,clears heat and drives heat out.The two medicinals are used together as sovereign medicinals to clear heat without consumption of yin,and to nourish yin without retention of pathogenic factors.*Radix Rehmanniae*,with sweet taste and cool nature,nourishes yin;*Rhizoma Anemarrhenae*,with bitter taste and cold nature,nourishes yin.Both of them help the sovereign medicinals clear deficiency heat,as the minister medicinals.*Cortex Moutan* cools blood and clear heat,helpls *Herba Artemisiae* expel the hidden heat in yin aspects,and serves as the assistant medicinal.

【Note】*Herba Artemisiae* is not heat-resistant,thus it should not be decocted for a long time,or should wrapped in boiled water;the formula is contraindicated for yin deficiency engendering wind.

【Variation】In case of pulmonary tuberlosis and steaming bone,excessive heat due to yin deficiency, add *Radix Glehniae* and *Radix Ophiopogonis* to clear lung and nourish yin.In case of infantile fever in summer,add *Herba Dendrobii*,*Cortex Lycii*,and *Radix Cynanchi Atrati* to clear deficiency heat.

Interior-warming formulas

Interior-warming formulas are based on the principle of"heating the cold"in the chapter of *Dissusion on Reflection of Yin Yang* in *Plain Questions*,and are composed of warm and hot medicinals,they have functions of warming the interior and promoting yang,dispelling cold,and freeing the meridians,and they are indicated to interior cold syndromes.The formulas are acrid,warm,dry,and hot.Doctors should indentify whether the syndrome of heat or cold is real or false before application.The formulas are classified into three types:formulas of warming the middle and dispelling cold,formulas of restoring yang to save from collapse,and formulas of warming meridians and dispelling cold.

Formulas of warming the middle and dispelling cold

Formulas of warming the middle and dispelling cold are applicable to asthenic cold of the middle syndrome or asthenic cold of the spleen and stomach syndrome due to invasion of the cold pathogens,marked by cold pain in the abdomen,poor appetite,vomiting and diarrhea,cold limbs,pale tongue with white and slippery tongue coating,sunken and fine pulse or sunken and slow pulse.The representative formula is "Regulating the Centre Pills".

Regulating the Centre Pills(Li Zhong Wan)

【Source】*Treatise on Cold Damage Diseases.*

【Composition】*Radix Ginseng*, *Rhizoma Zingiberis*, *Rhizoma Atractylodis Macrocephalae*, and *Radix Glycyrrhizae Prepata* (each 90 g)〔dosage for pills〕.

【Functions】Warm the middle energizer to expel cold,invigorate qi,and strengthen the spleen.

3. 脾胃虚寒所致的胸痹；或病后多涎唾；或小儿慢惊等。

【方解】方中干姜大辛大热，温脾阳，祛寒邪，扶阳抑阴，为君药。人参性味甘温，补气健脾，为臣药。君臣相合，温中健脾。白术甘温苦燥、健脾燥湿，为佐药。甘草一则助参、术益气健脾；二则调和药性，为佐使药。全方温补并用，以温为主，温中阳、益脾气、助运化，故曰"理中"。

【注意事项】湿热内蕴中焦或脾胃阴虚者禁用。

【加减】寒甚者，加制附片；脾气虚者，重用人参，加黄芪；下痢甚者，加淮山药、煨诃子；呕吐甚者，加半夏、丁香；失血者，加阿胶、三七、地榆炭。

（二）回阳救逆剂

回阳救逆剂用于肾阳虚衰，阴寒内盛，或阳气衰微欲脱等症。症见四肢厥逆，精神萎靡，恶寒倦卧，呕吐腹痛，下利清谷，脉沉细或沉微，甚者出现冷汗淋漓、脉微欲绝。代表方剂：四逆汤。

四逆汤

【来源】《伤寒论》

【组成】附子（15克）干姜（6克）炙甘草（6克）

【功用】温中祛寒，回阳救逆。

【主治】阳虚欲脱，冷汗自出，四肢厥逆，下利清谷，脉微欲绝。

【方解】方中君药附子大辛大热，入心脾肾经，是回阳救逆第一要药，其上助心阳，中温脾土，下壮肾阳，可复一身之阳气而回阳救逆。臣药干姜亦为辛热之品，温中散寒，助阳通脉，两药相辅相成，使温阳破阴之力更强。佐药炙甘草性温，既补脾胃而调诸药，又缓干姜、附子之辛散燥烈，解附子之毒。

【注意事项】非阳虚厥逆者勿用；若属真寒假热，服药格拒者，可将本汤凉服。

【加减】气虚欲脱者，加人参以益气固脱；汗多脉微者，可加龙骨、牡蛎以镇摄固脱。

【Indications】a) Asthenic cold of the spleen and stomach syndrome, marked by vomiting, diarrhea, abdominal pain relieved by warming and pressing, anorexia, aversion to cold, cold limbs, pale tongue with white tongue coating, deep and thread pulse. b) Yang deficiency with bleeding, marked by hematemesis, nosebleed, hemafecia, metrorrhagia, dull blood color and cold limbs. And c) Obstruction of chest qi due to asthenic cold of the spleen and stomach, chronic infantile lonvulsion, or pedilection for spitting saliva after recovery from diseases.

【Explanation】In the formula, the extremely acrid and hot *Rhizoma Zingiberis* warms spleen yang, dispels cold, nourishes yang and depresses yin, serves as the sovereign medicinal. *Ginseng* is sweet and warm, tonifys qi and enforces the spleen, serving as the minister medicinal. The sovereign medicinal and the minister medicinal are combined together to warm the middle and tonify the spleen. *Rhizoma Atractylodis Macrocephalae* is sweet, warm, bitter and dry, tonifys the spleen and drys dampness, serving as assistant medicinal. *Radix Glycyrrhizae* as the assistant and courier medicinal helps *Ginseng* and *Rhizoma Atractylodis Macrocephalae* tonify the spleen qi, it modulates all the ingredients natures as well. The formula warms yang of the middle, tonifys spleen qi, and promotes digestion. Thus the formula is named "Regulating the Center Pills".

【Note】Contraindicated for dampness-heat in middle energizer or yin deficiency of spleen and stomach.

【Variation】In case of severe cold, add *Radix Aconiti Praeparata* ; in case of deficiency of spleen qi, use *Radix Ginseng* in high dose, and add *Radix Astragali* ; in case of severe diarrhea, add *Rhizoma Dioscoreae* and *Fructus Chebulae* ; for severe vomiting, add *Rhizoma Pinelliae* and *Flos Caryophylli* ; for loss of blood, add *Colla Corii Asini*, *Radix Notoginseng* and *Radix Sanguisorbae Carbonisatus*.

Restoring yang to save from collapse formulas

Formulas of restoring yang to save from collapse are applicable to syndromes of kidney yang deficiency, excessive internal yin or yang collapse. The syndromes are marked by cold extremeties, mental fatigue, aversion to cold, drowsiness and falling, vomiting and abdominal pain, diarreahea, sunken and fine or sunken and weak pulse, even profuse cold sweating, extremely feeble pulse. The representative formula is "Four Rebellions Decoction".

Four Rebellions Decoction(Si Ni Tang)

【Source】*Treatise on Cold Damage Diseases.*

【Composition】*Radix Aconiti Praeparata* (15 g), *Rhizoma Zingiberis* (6 g), and *Radix Glycyrrhizae Praeparata* (6 g).

【Functions】Warm the middle and dissipate cold, restore yang, and save from collapse.

【Indications】Yang deficiency even to collapse, marked by profuse cold sweating, cold extremities, diarreahea, and extremely feeble pulse.

【Explanation】In the formula, *Radix Aconiti Preaeparata* with the extremely acrid taste and extremely hot nature, as the sovereign medicinal, enters the heart, spleen and kidney meridians. It is the most primary medicinal for restoring yang and saving from collapse. It helps heart yang in the upper aspect, and warms the spleen-earth in the middle aspect, strengthens kidney yang in the lower aspect, thus, restores yang of the whole body and saves from collapse. The minister medicinal *Rhizoma Zingiberis* is also of acrid taste and hot nature, it warms the middle and dissipates cold, helps yang and frees the channels, together with the sovereign medicinal, these two drugs help each other and reinforce the function of dissipating cold. The assistant medicinal *Radix Glycyrrhizae Praeparata* is of warm nature, not only helps spleen and stomach and harmonizes the ingredients, also mediates the dry and acrid nature of *Rhizoma Zingiberis* and *Radix Aconiti Praeparata*, and detoxifies the *Radix Aconiti Praeparata*.

（三）温经散寒剂

温经散寒剂主治阳气不足或外寒内袭，寒邪凝于经络之证。因寒凝血脉，血脉不利，故见肢体冷痛或肢端青紫、小腹冷痛。代表方剂：当归四逆汤。

当归四逆汤

【来源】《伤寒论》

【组成】当归（12克）桂枝（9克）芍药（9克）细辛（3克）通草（6克）大枣（8枚）炙甘草（6克）

【功用】温经散寒，养血通脉。

【主治】血虚寒厥证。手足厥冷，或腰、股、腿、足、肩臂疼痛，口不渴，舌淡苔白，脉沉细。

【方解】本方以桂枝汤去生姜，倍大枣，加当归、通草、细辛组成。方中桂枝辛温，温经散寒、温通血脉；当归甘温，养血和血，共为君药。细辛温经散寒，助桂枝温通血脉；白芍养血和营，助当归补益营血，同为臣药。通草通经脉，以畅血行；大枣、甘草益气健脾养血，皆为佐药。重用大枣，既助归、芍补养营血，又防桂枝、细辛燥烈大过，伤及阴血，甘草兼有调和药性亦为使药。本方的配伍特点是温阳与散寒并用，养血与通脉兼施，温而不燥，补而不滞。

【注意事项】本方只适用于血虚寒凝之手足厥冷，其他原因引起的四肢厥冷病证不宜使用本方。

【加减】血瘀重者，可加牛膝、木瓜等活血祛瘀之品；用治妇女血虚寒凝之经期腹痛及男子寒疝、睾丸掣痛牵引少腹冷痛、肢冷、脉弦者，可加乌药、茴香、香附等理气止痛。

【Note】It is contraindicated for the symptoms of cold extremeties if it is not due to yang deficiency; in case of true cold and fake heat, and the patient vomits after taking the decoction, take decoction after it becomes cool.

【Variation】In case of qi deficiency with possible collapse, add *Radix Ginseng* to benefit qi and prevent collapse; in case of profuse sweating and indistinct pulse, add *Os Draconis* and *Concha Ostreae* to prevent collapse.

Meridian-warming and cold-dissipating formulas

The meridian-warming and cold-dissipating formulas are applicable to cold in the meridians due to yang deficiency or invading of external cold. Because of cold in meridians, the blood circulation is not free, marked by cold pain in extrimities or purpura in tips of extrimities, cold in lower abdomen. The representative formula is "Angelica Four Rebellions Decoction".

Angelica Four Rebellions Decoction(Dang Gui Si Ni Tang)

【Source】*Treatise on Cold Damage Diseases.*

【Composition】*Radix Angenicae Sinensis* (9 g), *Ramulus Cinnamomi* (9 g), *Radix Paeoniae* (9 g), *Herba Asari* (3 g), *Medulla Tetrapanacis* (6 g), *Fructus Ziziphi Jujubae* (8 pcs), and *Radix Glycyrrhizae Preparara* (6 g).

【Functions】Warm the meridian to dissipate cold, and nourish the blood to free the channel.

【Indications】Cold syncope with blood deficiency marked by cold hands and feet, or pain of waist, thighs, legs, feet, shoulders and arms, absence of thirst, pale tongue with white tongue coating, and sunken and fine pulse.

【Explanation】The formula is that "Ramulus Cinnamomi Decoction" deletes *Rhizoma Zingiberis Recens*, doubles *Fructus Jujubae*, and adds *Radix Angelicae Sinensis*, *Medulla Tetrapanacis*, and *Herba Asari*. In the formula, the acrid and warm *Ramulus* warms meridians to dispel cold and to free the blood vessels; *Radix Angenicae Sinensis* with sweet taste and warm nature, nourish blood and harmonize blood, both of the above mentioned two drugs are the sovereign medicinals. *Herba Asari* warms the meridians to dissipate cold, and helps *Ramulus Cinnamomi* warm the meridians to free the blood vessels; *Radix Paeoniae Alba* nourishes blood to harmonize the nutrient aspect, and helps *Radix Angelicae Sinensis* nourish blood and harmonize blood, both of *Radix Paeoniae Alba* and *Radix Angelicae Sinensis* are the ministers. *Medulla Tetrapanacis* frees the meridians to promote blood circulation; *Fructus Ziziphi Jujubae* and *Radix Glycyrrhizae Praeparata* benefit qi, tonify spleen, and nourish blood, all of the three drugs are the assistants. The formula uses *Fructus Ziziphi Jujubae* in high dose, which not only helps *Radix Angelicae Sinensis* and *Radix Paeoniae Alba* nourish blood and the nutrient aspect, but also prevents the dry and hot *Ramulus Cinnamomi* and *Herba Asari* consuming the blood and yin fluid. *Radix Glycyrrhizae Praeparata* is the courier medicinal as well, which can harmonize all the ingredients. The formula's characteristic is applying warming yang and dispelling cold together, nourishing blood and freeing meridians together, thus, the formula is warm but not dry, tonifying but not sluggish.

【Note】The formula is only applicable for cold of hands and feet due to blood deficiency and cold blocking channels, and it is contraindicated for other reasons.

【Variation】In case of severe blood stasis, add *Radix Achyranthis Bidentatae* and *Fructus Chaenomelis* to activate the blood and dispel stasis; in case of abdominal pain during menstration due to blood deficiency and cold in meridians, and men's hernia, marked by pulling pain of testicle together with traction of lower abdominal cold pain, cold extremities and taut pulse, add *Radix Linderae*, *Fructus Foeniculi*, and *Rhizoma Cyperi* to modulate qi and relieve pain.

六、补益剂

补益剂是以补益药为主组成，具有补养人体气、血、阴、阳的作用，治疗各种虚证的方剂。属于八法中的"补法"。使用补法时首先辨别虚实真假。"大实有羸状"，若误用补益，则助邪伤正；"至虚有盛候"，若不补反泻，则虚者更虚。对于虚不受补的病人，宜先调理脾胃，或配合健脾和胃、理气消导之品，以资运化，使之补而不滞。若外邪未尽而素体偏虚者，切勿过早纯用补益剂，以免留邪为患。补益剂煎煮时间宜长，且以空腹服为佳。根据其作用不同，补益剂可分为补气剂、补血剂、气血双补剂、补阴剂和补阳剂。

（一）补气剂

补气剂，主治脾肺气虚证。临床症见肢体倦怠乏力，少气懒言，语音低微，动则气促，食少便溏，面色萎白，舌淡苔白，脉虚弱，或自汗，或脱肛、子宫脱垂等。代表方剂：四君子汤、补中益气丸。

四君子汤

【来源】《太平惠民和剂局方》

【组成】人参　白术　茯苓（各9克）炙甘草（6克）

【功用】益气健脾。

【主治】脾胃气虚证。面色萎白，语声低微，气短乏力，食少便溏，舌淡苔白，脉虚弱。

【方解】方中人参甘温益气，健脾养胃，为君药。白术苦温，健脾燥湿，加强益气助运之力，为臣药；茯苓甘淡，与白术相配，健脾渗湿，为佐药。炙甘草甘平，益气和中，调和诸药，为使药。四药相合，共奏益气健脾之功。

【注意事项】阴虚血热者慎用。

【加减】呕吐者，加半夏降逆止呕；胸膈痞满者，加枳壳、陈皮行气宽胸；心悸失眠者，加酸枣仁宁心安神；畏寒肢冷、脘腹疼痛者，加干姜、附子温中祛寒。

Tonifying Formulas

Tonifying formulas are mainly composed of tonifying medicinals, and have functions of tonifying qi, blood, yin and yang, and indicated for various deficiency syndromes. They belong to "tonifying method" of "the eight therapeutic principles." Before applying tonifying method, one should distinguish whether the syndrome of excess or deficiency is true or false. "Severe excessive syndrome might have weak-like appearance," if applying tonifying method by mistake, it would help the pathogen and damage the vigor qi; "severe deficiency syndrome might have strong-like manifestation," if not tonifying but deleting, then the deficiency would be worse. If the patient is too weak to undertake tonifying treatment, one should modify the spleen and stomach first, or one should combine with tonifying the spleen and modifying the stomach medicinals, and modulating qi and promoting digestion medicinals, in order to help digestion and make the formula nourishing but not sluggish. If the external pathogen is not dispelled and the patient's body is weak, the tonifying formulas should not be applied alone too early, in order to avoid retention of pathogen in the body. The tonifying formulas should be decocted for a rather long period of time, and should be taken on an empty stomach. According to the difference of functions, the tonifying formulas are classified into tonifying qi formulas, tonifying blood formulas, tonifying both qi and blood formulas, tonifying yin formulas, and tonifying yang formulas.

Tonifying qi formulas

Tonifying qi formulas are indicated for qi deficiency syndrome of the spleen and lung, clinically manifested as fatigue, shortness of breath, low and weak voice, dyspnea in motion, poor appetite and loose stool, pale complexion, pale tongue with white coating, weak pulse, or spontaneous sweating, or anal prolapse, or uterine prolapse. The representative formulas are "Four Gentlemen Decoction" and "Tonifying the Centre and Benefiting Qi Decoction".

Four Gentlemen Decoction(Si Jun Zi Tang)

【Source】*Prescriptions from the Great Peace Imperial Grace Pharmacy.*

【Composition】*Radix Ginseng* (9 g), *Rhizoma Atractylodis Macroephapae* (9 g), *Poria* (9 g), and *Radix Glycyrrhizac Pracparata* (6 g).

【Functions】Replenish qi and strengthen the spleen.

【Indications】Qi deficiency of the spleen and stomach, marked by pale complexion, low and weak voice, shortness of breath and fatigue, poor appetite, loose stools, pale tongue with white coating, and weak pulse.

【Explanation】In the formula, sweet and warm *Ginseng* tonifies qi, tonifies the spleen and nourishes the stomach, and it is the sovereign medicinal. The bitter and warm *Rhizoma Atractylodis Macrocephalae* tonifies the spleen and dries dampness, and it helps the sovereign medicinal tonify qi and promote digestion as minister medicinal. Sweet and bland *Poria*, concurrent with *Rhizoma Atractylodis Macrocephalae*, tonifies the spleen and eliminates dampness, serving as the assistant medicinal; *Radix Glycyrrhizae Praeparata*, being sweet and neutral, strengthenes qi, harmonizes the middle, and harmonizes the ingredients, serving as the courier medicinal. All the four ingredients together achieve the function of tonifying qi and strengthening the spleen.

【Note】Contraindicated for yin deficiency and blood heat.

【Variation】For nausea and vomiting, add *Rhizoma Pinelliae* to descend the adverse flow of qi and stop vomiting; for chest and epigastric fullness, add *Fructus Aurantii* and *Pericarpium Citri Reticulatae* to replenish qi and soothe the chest; for palpitation and insomnia, add *Semen Ziziphi Spinosae* to peacify the heart and tranquilize; for aversion to cold, cold extremities and abdominal pain, add *Rhizoma Zingiberis*

补中益气丸

【来源】《脾胃论》

【组成】黄芪（18克）甘草（9克）人参（6克）当归（3克）橘皮（6克）升麻（6克）柴胡（6克）白术（9克）

【功用】补中益气，升阳举陷。

【主治】

1. 脾胃气虚证。饮食减少，体倦肢软，少气懒言，面色苍白，大便溏薄，舌淡，脉大而虚软。

2. 气虚下陷证。脱肛，子宫脱垂，久泻，久痢，崩漏等，见气短乏力、舌淡、脉虚者。

3. 气虚发热证。身热，自汗，渴喜热饮，气短乏力，舌淡，脉虚大无力。

【方解】方中重用黄芪为君药，味甘微温，入肺脾经，补中益气，升阳固表。人参、炙甘草、白术为臣药，补气健脾，增强黄芪补中益气之功。当归养血和营，助参、芪以补气养血；陈皮理气和胃，使补而不滞，为佐药。用少量升麻、柴胡升阳举陷，助君药以升提下陷之中气，同为佐使之用。炙甘草调和诸药亦为使药。本方的配伍特点是补气养血以治脾胃气虚，升提阳气以求浊降清升。

【注意事项】阴虚内热、肝阳上亢者忌用。

【加减】兼有腹痛者，加白芍柔肝止痛；头痛者，加蔓荆子、川芎疏风活血止痛；头顶痛者，加藁本、细辛以疏风止痛；咳嗽者，加五味子、麦冬敛肺止咳；气滞者，加木香、枳壳理气解郁；虚人感冒，加苏叶以增强辛散之力；气虚下陷者，可倍用黄芪，并加枳壳；气虚自汗者，加白芍、五味子敛阴止汗；脾虚湿困，胸满体倦者，去当归，加苍术、木香健脾燥湿理气；胁痛者，加郁金、香附行气止痛；兼有食滞、不思饮食者，加焦三仙消食导滞。

and *Radix Aconiti* to warm the middle and dissipate cold.

Tonifying the Centre and Benefiting Qi Decoction(Bu Zhong Yi Qi Tang)

【Source】*Treatise on the Spleen and Stomach.*

【Composition】*Radix Astragali* (18 g) , *Radix Glycyrrhizae* (9 g) , *Radix Ginseng* (6 g) , *Radix Angelicae Sinensis* (3 g) , *Tangerine peel* (6 g) , *Rhizome Cimicifugae* (6 g) , *Radix Bupleuri* (6g) , and *Rhizoma Atractylodis Macroephapae* (9 g) .

【Functions】Tonify the centre, benefit qi, elevate yang, and lift sunken qi.

【Indications】

(1) Qi deficiency of spleen and stomach, marked by less food intake, fatigue, powerless of body, short breath and disinclination to talk, pale complexion, loose stools, pale tongue, vacuous and soft pulse.

(2)Sunken qi pattern due to qi deficiency, marked by hysteroptosis, gastroptosis, prolapse of uterus, prolonged diarrhea and protracted dysentery, metrostaxis, short breath, fatigue, pale tongue, and vacuous pulse.

(3)Fever due to qi deficiency, marked by fever with spontaneous sweating, thirst with desire for hot drink, short breath, fatigue, pale tongue, and vacuous rootless large pulse.

【Explanation】In the formula, *Radix Astragali* is the sovereign medicinal, it tastes sweet and of warm nature, it enters the meridians of lung and spleen, and tonifies the centre and benefits qi, elevates yang and strengthens the surface. *Radix Ginseng* , *Radix Glycyrrhizae Praeparata* , and *Rhizoma Atractylodis Macrocephalae* , as the minister medicinals, tonify qi, strengthen spleen, and reinforce *Radix Astragali* to tonify the centre and benefit qi. *Radix Angelicae Sinensis* nourishes blood and harmonizes the nutrient aspect, helping *Radix Ginseng* and *Radix Astragali* tonify qi and nourish the blood. *Pericarpium Citri Reticulatae* modulates qi and harmonizes the stomach, tonifying without retention. Both *Radix Angelicae Sinensis* and *Pericarpium Citri Reticulatae* are the assistant medicinals. Small amounts of *Rhizoma Cimicifugae* and *Radix Bupleuri* are used to elevate yang and lift sunken qi, helping the sovereign medicinal elevate the sunken middle qi; both are courier medicinals and assistants medicinals. *Radix Glycyrrhizae Praeparata* modulates all the ingredients as the courier medicinal. The characteristic of the formula is tonifying qi and nourishing the blood to treat qi deficiency of the spleen and stomach, elevating yang to downbear the turbid and upbear the clear.

【Note】Contraindicated for internal fever due to yin deficiency and ascendant hyperactivity of liver yang.

【Variation】In case of abdominal pain, add *Radix Paeoniae Alba* to emolliate the liver to relieve pain; for headache, add *Fructus Viticis* and *Rhizoma Chuanxiong* to activate blood and relieve pain; in case of headache in the top of the head, add *Rhizoma et Radix Ligustici* and *Herba Asari* to disperse wind to relieve pain; for cough, add *Fructus Schisandrae* and *Radix Ophiopogonis* to constrain the lung to suppress cough; in case of stagnation of qi, add *Radix Aucklandiae* and *Fructus Aurantii* to modulate qi and disperse stagnation; for cold of weak patients, add *Folium Perillae* to reinforce the power of dispersing; for sunken qi pattern, double the dosage of *Radix Astragali* and add *Fructus Aurantii* ; for spontaneous sweating due to qi deficiency, add *Radix Paeoniae Alba* and *Fructus Schisandrae* to constrain yin to arrest sweating; in case of spleen deficiency with dampness encumbrance marked by fullness in the chest and fatigue, remove *Radix Angelicae Sinensis* , and add *Rhizoma Atractylodis* and *Radix Aucklandiae* to tonify spleen, modulate qi, and dry dampness; for hypochondriac pain, add *Radix Curcumae* and *Rhizoma Cyperi* to promote qi and relieve pain; for food retention and poor appetite, add *Charred Triplet* to promote digestion and remove food accumulation.

（二）补血剂

补血剂，主治血虚证。症见面色萎黄，头晕目眩，唇爪色淡，失眠，舌淡，脉细，或妇女月经不调，量少色淡，或经闭不行等。"气能生血"，故补血时多配伍补气之品，以助气化，或着重补气以生血。因大失血而致血虚阳脱者，尤应补气以固脱，使气旺则血生。血虚可导致血瘀，配伍活血药可防止血瘀。代表方剂：四物汤、归脾汤。

四物汤

【来源】《仙授理伤续断秘方》

【组成】当归（9克）川芎（6克）白芍（9克）熟地（12克）

【功用】补血调血。

【主治】营血虚滞证。症见心悸失眠，头晕目眩，面色无华，妇人月经不调，量少或经闭不行，脐腹作痛，口唇、爪甲色淡，舌淡，脉细弦或细涩。

【方解】方中熟地性味甘温，味厚质润，长于滋阴养血，填精补肾，为君药。当归补血养肝、和血调经，为臣药。白芍养血柔肝和营；川芎活血行气、调畅气血，同为佐药。诸药相配，动静结合，以血中之血药熟地、白芍，养营补血；血中之气药当归、川芎，活血和营。全方配伍具有补血而不滞血、和血而不伤血的特点，是血虚能补、血燥能润、血溢能止、血瘀能行的调血剂。

【注意事项】脾胃阳虚、食少便溏、阴虚发热以及血崩气脱者不可应用。

【加减】伴气虚者，加党参、黄芪补气生血；瘀血重者，加桃仁、红花，并用赤芍易白芍，加强活血祛瘀之力；血虚有寒者，加肉桂、炮姜、吴茱萸等温通血脉；血虚有热者，加黄芩、丹皮，并用生地易熟地，清热凉血；妊娠胎漏者，加阿胶、艾叶，止血安胎；血滞痛经者，加香附、元胡、鸡血藤等养血行血、理气止痛。

Tonifying blood formulas

These formulas are indicated for blood deficiency, manifested as sallow complexion, dizziness, vertigo, pale nails and lips, insomnia, pale tongue and weak pulse, or amenorrhea with less amount and pale color, or dismenstration. "Qi generates blood," when nourishing blood, one should combine tonifying qi drugs to help the qi transformation, or emphasize on tonifying qi to generate blood. In case of blood deficiency and yang relapse due to big blood loss, one should particularly tonify qi to stop relapse and let the qi rich, then the blood generates. Blood deficiency results in blood stasis, the blood stasis can be prevented by combining with blood-activating medicinals. The representative formulas are "Four Substances Decoction" and "Restoring the Spleen Decoction".

Four Substances Decoction (Si Wu Tang)

【Source】*Secret Formulary Bestowed by Immortals for Treating Injuries and Mending Fractures.*

【Composition】*Radix Angelicae Sinensis* (9 g), *Rhizoma Ligustici Chuangxiong* (6 g), *Radix Paeoniae Alba* (9 g), and *Radix Rehmanniae Praeparata* (12 g).

【Functions】Enrich and regulate the blood.

【Indications】Deficiency and stasis of the blood, marked by palpitation, insomnia, dizziness and vertigo, pale complexion, or female irregular menstruation, scanty menstruation, or amenia with vague pain of lower abdomen, pale tongue, fine and string-like pulse, or fine and rough pulse.

【Explanation】In the formula, sweet and warm *Radix Rehmanniae Praeparata*, which taste is thick and nature is moist, is good at nourishing yin and enriching blood, supplying the essense and tonifying the kidney, and it is the sovereign medicinal. *Radix Angelicae Sinensis* is the minister medicinal, it nourishes the blood and emolliates the liver, harmonizes the blood and regulates menstruation. *Radix Paeoniae Alba* nourishes the blood, emolliates the liver, and harmonizes the nutrient aspect; *Rhizoma Chuanxiong* activates blood and promotes qi, and modulates and frees qi and blood. Both of *Radix Paeoniae Alba* and *Rhizoma Chuanxiong* are the assistant medicinals. All the ingredients act together, the dynamic combined with the still, using "the blood medicinals among the blood medicinals" —*Radix Rehmanniae Praeparata* and *Radix Paeoniae Alba* to harmonize the nutrient aspect and nourish the blood; using "the qi medicinals among the blood medicinals" *Radix Angelicae Sinensis* and *Rhizoma Chuanxiong* to activate blood and harmonize the nutrient aspect. All the ingredients combines together, nourishing the blood without blocking the blood, harmonizing the blood without consumption of the blood. The formula is a modulating blood formula which can nourish in case of blood deficiency, moisten in case of blood dryness, stop in case of bleeding, and activate in case of blood stasis.

【Note】Contraindicated for spleen-stomach yang deficiency marked by poor appetite and diarrhea, fever due to yin deficiency, and qi relapse due to severe bleeding.

【Variation】For concurrency of qi deficiency, add *Radix Codonopsis* and *Radix Astragali* to tonify qi and enrich the blood; for severe blood stasis, add *Semen Persicae* and *Flos Carthami*, and replace the *Radix Paeoniae Alba* with *Radix Paeoniae Rubra* to enforce the function of activating blood and removing stasis; in case of cold concurrent with blood deficiency, add *Cortex Cinnamomi*, *Rhizoma Zingiberis* , and *Fructus Evodiae* to warm the meridians and free the channels; in case of heat concurrent with blood deficiency, add *Radix Scutellariae* and *Cortex Moutan*, replace *Radix Rehmanniae Praeparata* with *Radix Rehmanniae* to clear heat and cool the blood; for vaginal bleeding during pregnancy, add *Colla Corii Asini* and *Folium Artemisiae* to stop bleeding and prevent abortion; for dysmenorrhea due to blood stagnation, add *Rhizoma Cyperi*, and *Rhizoma Corydalis* to nourish and activate the blood, modulate qi, and relieve pain.

归脾汤

【来源】《正体类要》

【组成】黄芪 白术 当归 白茯苓 远志 龙眼肉 酸枣仁（各3克）人参（6克）木香（1.5克）炙甘草（1克）加生姜、大枣

【功用】益气补血，健脾养心。

【主治】

1. 心脾两虚证。症见心悸怔忡，健忘失眠，盗汗，体倦食少，面色萎黄，舌淡，苔薄白，脉细弱。

2. 脾不统血证。症见便血，皮下紫癜，妇女崩漏，月经超前，量多色淡，或淋漓不止，舌淡，脉细弱。

【方解】方中以黄芪、龙眼肉为君，配人参、白术、当归等甘温之臣药，补益脾气以生血，使气旺而血生；茯苓、远志、酸枣仁宁心安神；木香辛温香散，理气醒脾，共为佐药；姜、枣调和脾胃，为使药。全方共奏益气补血、健脾养心之功，是治疗思虑过度、劳伤心脾、气血两虚之良方。本方的配伍特点：一则心脾同治，重点在脾，使脾旺则气血生化有源，方名归脾，寓意在此；二则气血双补，重在补气，意在气为血之帅，气旺则血自生，血足则心有所养；三则补气养血药中佐以木香理气醒脾，补而不滞。

【注意事项】本方药性偏温，对邪热内伏及阴虚脉数者忌用。

【加减】崩漏下血偏寒者，加艾叶炭、炮姜炭以温经止血；偏热者，加生地炭、阿胶珠、棕榈炭以清热止血。

（三）气血双补剂

气血双补剂，主治气血两虚证。症见面色无华，头晕目眩，心悸怔忡，食少倦怠，气短懒言，舌淡，脉虚无力等。代表方剂：八珍汤。

八珍汤

【来源】《瑞竹堂经验方》

【组成】人参 白术 白茯苓 当归 川芎 白芍药 熟地黄 炙甘草（各10克）生姜 大枣

【功用】补益气血。

【主治】气血两虚证。症见面色苍白或萎黄，头晕眼花，四肢倦怠，气短懒言，心悸怔忡，食欲减退，舌质淡，苔薄白，脉细虚。

Restoring the Spleen Decoction(Gui Pi Tang)

【Source】*Classification and Essential of Modifying the Body.*

【Composition】*Radix Astragali* (3 g) , *Rhizoma Atractylodis Macroephapae* (3 g) , *Poria* (3 g) , *Radix Polygalae* (3 g) , *Arillus Longan* (3 g) , *Semen Zizihi Spinosae* (3 g) , *Radix Ginseng* (6 g) , *Radix Aucklandia* (1.5g) , and *Radix Glycyrrhizae Praeparata* (1 g) , add *Rhizoma Zingiberis Recens* and *Fructus Jujubae.*

【Functions】Tonify qi , nourish the blood , tonify the spleen , and nourish the heart.

【Indications】

(1) Dual deficiency of the heart and spleen , manifesting as palpitation , amnesia and insomnia , nocturnal sweating , fatigue and poor appetite , sallow complexion , pale tongue with white tongue coating , fine and weak pulse.

(2) Spleen failing to control the blood , manifesting as hemafecia , subcutaneous purpura , metrorrhagia , menstruation ahead of the time , profuse light colored menstruation , or dribbling menstruation , pale tongue , fine and weak pulse.

【Explanation】The formula takes *Radix Astragali* and *Arillus Longan* as sovereign medicinals , combined with the warm and sweet *Radix Ginseng* , *Rhizoma Atractylodis Macrocephalae* , and *Radix Angelicae Sinensis* as minister medicinals , to tonify spleen qi to generate the blood , so as to enrich qi and generate the blood. The assistant medicinals *Poria* , *Radix Polygalae* , and *Semen Ziziphi Spinosae* peacify the heart and tranquilize. *Radix Aucklandiae* is acrid and warm , it modulates qi and tonifies the spleen. *Rhizoma Zingiberis Recens* and *Fructus Jujubae* are courier medicinals that modulate the spleen and stomach. The formula possesses the functions of tonifying qi and nourishing the blood , tonifying the spleen and nourishing the heart ; and it is a good prescription for dual deficiency of qi and the blood due to excessive thinking and worrying , and injury of the heart and spleen due to mental labour. The characteristics of the composition of the formula are : a) treating both the heart and the spleen at the same time , emphasizing on the spleen , so as to invigorate the spleen and enrich the source of qi and blood , the name of the formula as "restoring the spleen" comes from this point ; b) tonifying both the qi and the blood , emphasizing on the qi , considering qi as the marshal of blood. If qi is vigorous , then the blood can generate automatically ; and If the blood is rich then the heart is enriched ; and c) combining with the *Radix Aucklandiae* as the assistant medicinal with tonifying qi and nourishing the blood medicinals , so as to modulate qi and invigorate the spleen , and supplement without stagnation.

【Note】The formula is warm , it is contraindicated for retention of pathogenic heat and yin deficiency marked by rapid pulse.

【Variation】In case of flooding and spotting , if it is with cold , add *Folium Artemisiae Carbonisatus* and *Rhizoma Zingiberis Carbonisatus* to warm the meridians and stop bleeding ; if it is with heat , add *Radix Rehmanniae Carbonisatus* , *Colla Corii Asini* , and *Vagina Trichycarpi Carbonisatus* to purge heat and stop bleeding.

Tonifying both qi and blood formulas

These formulas are indicated for dual deficiency of qi and the blood , manifested as pale complexion , dizziness , palpitation , poor appetite , fatigue , short breath and disinclination to talk , pale tongue , and vacuous pulse. The representative formula is "Eight Pearls Decoction".

Eight Pearls Decoction(Ba Zhen Tang)

【Source】*Empirical Prescriptions of Ruizhutang.*

【Composition】*Radix Ginseng* (9 g) , *Rhizoma Atractylodis Macroephapae* (9 g) , *Poria* (9 g) , *Radix*

【方解】方中人参与熟地相配，益气养血，同为君药。白术、茯苓健脾渗湿，助人参益气补脾；当归、白芍养血和营，助熟地补益阴血，共为臣药。川芎行气活血，使之补而不滞，为佐药。炙甘草益气和中、调和诸药，为使药。姜、枣调和脾胃，亦为使药。

【注意事项】有热象者忌用。

【加减】脘腹胀满者，加枳壳、厚朴、木香以理气消胀；纳呆食滞者，加砂仁、麦芽、神曲以开胃消食导滞；便溏、浮肿者，加山药、薏苡仁、车前子以增强健脾利湿之效。

（四）补阴剂

补阴剂，主治阴虚证。症见形体消瘦，头晕耳鸣，潮热颧红，五心烦热，盗汗失眠，腰酸遗精，咳嗽咯血，口燥咽干，舌红少苔，脉细数。由于阴虚易从热化，故多配伍清热之品。补阴药常常会影响脾胃的运化，产生气滞，故可配伍理气药。代表方剂：六味地黄丸。

六味地黄丸

【来源】《小儿药证直诀》

【组成】熟地黄（24克）山萸肉　山药（各12克）泽泻　茯苓　丹皮（各9克）。

【功用】滋阴补肾。

【主治】肾阴虚证。症见腰膝酸软，头晕目眩，耳鸣耳聋，盗汗，遗精，消渴，骨蒸潮热，手足心热，舌燥咽痛，牙齿动摇，足跟作痛，小便淋沥，以及小儿囟门不合，舌红少苔，脉沉细数。

【方解】方中重用熟地，滋阴补肾，填精益髓，为君药。山萸肉酸温补养肝肾，并能涩精；山药甘平补益脾阴，亦能固精，同为臣药。三药相配，可滋养肝脾肾三脏之阴，称为"三补"。泽泻利湿泄浊，防熟地之滋腻恋邪；牡丹皮清泻相火，制山萸肉之温涩；茯苓淡渗脾湿，助山药之健运，均为佐药。三药渗湿浊、清虚热，防君臣之偏，而称为"三泻"。全方体现了"壮水之主，以制阳光"之旨。本方的配伍特点是三补三泻，其中补药用量重于泻药，故以补为主；肝脾肾三阴并补，但以补肾阴为主。

【注意事项】本方药性偏于滋腻，脾虚泄泻者慎用。

【加减】阴虚而火旺盛者，加知母、玄参、黄柏等以加强清热降火之功；若兼有

Angelicae Sinensis (9 g), *Rhizoma Ligustici Chuanxiong* (9 g), *Radix Paeoniae Alba* (9 g), *Radix Rehmanniae Praeparata* (9 g), *Radix Glycyrrhizae Praeparata* (9 g), *Rhizoma Zingiberis Recens*, and Fructus Jujubae.

【Functions】Tonify both qi and blood.

【Indications】Dual deficiency of qi and the blood, manifested as pale or sallow complexion, dizziness, lassitude of the extremities, short breath and disinclination to talk, palpitation, poor appetite, pale tongue with thin white coating, and fine and weak pulse.

【Explanation】In the formula, both *Ginseng* and *Radix Rehmanniae Praeparata*, tonify qi and nourish blood, serving as the sovereign medicinals. *Rhizoma Atractylodis Macrocephalae* and *Poria* tonify the spleen and eliminate dampness, helping *Ginseng* tonify qi and strengthen the spleen; *Radix Angelicae Sinensis* and *Radix Paeoniae Alba* nourish the blood and harmonize the nutrient aspect, helping *Radix Rehmanniae Praeparata* to nourish the blood. The above mentioned four medicinals serve as minister medicinals. *Rhizoma Chuanxiong* promotes qi and activates blood, so as to tonify without stagnation, serving as assistant medicinal. *Radix Glycyrrhizae Praeparata* tonifits qi and harmonizes the middle, and modulates all the ingredients, it is the courier medicinal. *Rhizoma Zingiberis Recens* and *Fructus Jujubae* modulate the spleen and stomach, serving as the courier medicinals.

【Note】Contraindicated for cases with manifestation of heat.

【Variation】For abdominal fullness, add *Fructus Aurantii*, *Cortex Magnoliae Officinalis*, and *Radix Aucklandiae* to modulate qi and resolve distention; for poor appetite and food accumulation, add *Fructus Amomi*, *Fructus Hordei Germinatus*, and *Massa Fermentata Medicinalis* to improve appetite and promote digestion; for diarrhea and edema, add *Rhizoma Dioscoreae*, *Semen Coicis*, and *Semen Plantaginis* to promote the function of fortifying the spleen and draining dampness.

Tonifying yin formulas

These formulas are indicated for yin deficiency syndromes, manifested as emaciation, vertigo, tinnitus, hectic fever, flushed cheeks, feverish sensation in the palms and soles, night sweating, insomnia, soreness of waist, emission, cough and hemoptysis, dry mouth and throat, red tongue with little coating, fine and rapid pulse. Yin deficiency is prone to transform heat, so the formulas mainly consist of heat-clearing medicinals. Yin-tonifying medicinals usually affect the digestion of the spleen and stomach, and generate qi stagnation, and qi-regulating medicinals should be applied together. The representative formula is "Six-Ingredient Rehmannia Pills".

Six-Ingredient Rehmannia Pills (Liu Wei Di Huang Wan)

【Source】*Key to Therapeutics of Children's Diseases.*

【Composition】*Radix Rehmanniae Praeparata* (24 g), *Fructus Corni* (12 g), *Rhizoma Dioscoreae* (12 g), *Rhizoma Alismatis* (9 g), *Poria* (9 g), and *Cortex Moutan Radicis* (9 g).

【Functions】Nourish the kidney yin.

【Indications】Kidney yin deficiency, manifested as weakness and soreness of waist and knees, dizziness, tinnitus, deafness, nocturnal sweating, emission, diabetes, steaming sensation in the bones, hectic fever, feverish sensation in the palms and soles, dry tongue and sore throat, gomphiasis, heal pain dribbling urination, as well as persistent opening of fontanelle, red tongue with little coating, and deep fine and rapid pulse.

【Explanation】In this formula, *Radix Rehmanniae Praeparata* in high dose is capable of nourishing yin and invigorating the kidney, and enriching the essence and replenishing the marrow, it is the sovereign medicinal. *Fructus Corni* possesses the functions of nourishing the liver and kidney, and astringing the essence; *Rhizoma Dioscoreae* can tonify the spleen and strengthen the body, and astringe the kidney. Both

脾虚气滞，可加焦白术、砂仁、陈皮等以防碍气滞脾。

（五）补阳剂

补阳剂主治肾阳虚证。症见面色苍白，形寒肢冷，腰膝酸痛，下肢软弱无力，小便不利，或小便频数，尿后余沥，少腹拘急，男子阳痿早泄，女子宫寒不孕，舌淡苔白，脉沉细、尺脉尤甚。代表方剂：肾气丸。

肾气丸

【来源】《金匮要略》

【组成】干地黄（24克）山药　山茱萸（各12克）茯苓　泽泻　丹皮（各9克）桂枝　附子（各3克）

【功用】温补肾阳。

【主治】肾阳不足证。症见腰膝酸软，畏寒肢冷，少腹拘急，小便不利或频数，舌质淡胖，尺脉沉细；以及痰饮喘咳、水肿脚气、消渴、久泄等。

【方解】方用附子大辛大热，温补肾阳；桂枝辛甘而温，温通阳气，共为君药，补肾阳之虚、助气化之复；"善补阳者，必于阴中求阳，则阳得阴助而生化无穷"，故用干地黄滋阴补肾，山茱萸、山药补肝脾益精血，同为臣药；茯苓、泽泻利水渗湿，配桂枝以温化痰饮，丹皮清热凉血，合桂枝调血分之滞，为佐药。本方配伍特点有二：一为阴阳并补，而以补阳为主；二为滋阴之中加入少量桂、附以温阳，达到阴中求阳，少火生气。

【注意事项】肾阴不足、肾火上炎者不宜用。

【加减】小便数而多，色白，体质羸弱者，可加补骨脂、益智仁、覆盆子等以温肾缩泉；腰膝酸软重者，加杜仲、狗脊以补肾强腰膝；小腹冷者，加巴戟天、沉香以温肾祛寒；治疗阳痿时，可加淫羊藿、补骨脂、巴戟天等壮阳起痿。

Fructus Corni and *Rhizoma Dioscoreae* serve as the minister medicinals.The above three ingredients,known as "three tonics," reinforce yin of the liver,spleen and kidney.*Rhizoma Alismatis* can promote diuresis to eliminate dampness and prevent *Radix Rehmanniae Praeparata* from generating dampness;*Cortex Moutan* possesses the functions of clearing heat from the liver and restricting the warm and astringent property of *Fructus Corni*;*Poria* eliminates dampness from the spleen and helps *Rhizoma Dioscoreae* to promote the digestion of the spleen,these three ingredients are the assistant medicinals,and called"three purgatives" which can eliminate dampness, clear deficiency heat, and prevent the biased nature of the sovereign medicinal and the assistant medicinals.The whole formula reflects the idea of"enriching the water to restrict the sunshine."The characteristic of the formula is"three tonics and three purgatives,"of which the dosages of tonics are heavier than those of the purgatives,and focusing on the former;the formula tonifies yin of liver,spleen and kidney,especially focusing on the kidney yin.

【Note】The nature of the formula is biased towards moistening and nourishing,so the formula is contraindicated for spleen deficiency marked by diarrhea.

【Variation】In case of yin deficiency heat,add *Rhizoma Anemarrhenae*,*Radix Scrophulariae*,and *Cortex Phellodendri* to reinforce the function of clearing heat and purging fire;if concurrency with spleen deficiency and qi stagnation,add *Fructus Amomi* and *Pericarpium Citri Reticulatae* to avoid qi stagnation and dysfunction of the spleen.

Tonifying yang formulas

These formulas are indicated for deficiency of kidney yang,manifested as pale complexion,chillness and cold limbs,soreness and weakness of waist and knees,dysuria,sexual impotence,premature ejaculation,inability of pregnancy due to cold womb,pale tongue with white tongue coating,sunken and fine pulse,especially pulse of the chi section.The representative formula is "Kidney-Qi Pills".

Kidney-Qi Pills(Shen Qi Wan)

【Source】*Synopsis of Prescriptions of the Golden Chamber.*

【Composition】*Radix Rehmanniae Praeparata* (24 g),*Rhizoma Dioscoreae* (12 g),*Fructus Corni* (12 g),*Poria* (9 g),*Rhizoma Alismatis* (9 g), *Cortex Moutan Radicis* (9 g), *Ramulus Cinnamomi* (3 g),and *Radix Aconiti* (3 g).

【Functions】Warm and tonify kidney yang.

【Indications】Deficiency of kidney yang,marked by weakness and soreness of waist and knees,cold feeling in the lower part of the body,stiffness in the lower abdomen,dysuria or polyuria,pale and swollen tongue,sunken and fine pulse in the chi section;cough and asthma due to phlegm and water retention,edema,beriberi,diabetes,prolonged diarrhea,etc.

【Explanation】In the formula, *Radix Aconiti* is of severe acrid and very hot,and it warms kidney yang;*Ramulus Cinnamomi* is acrid and sweet and with warm nature,it warms and frees the yang qi.Both *Radix Aconiti* and *Ramulus Cinnamomi*,as the sovereign medicinals,tonify the deficiency of kidney yang and promote restoring the function of qi transformation.It is said"one who is good at tonifying yang,must get yang from yin,so that yang gets the help of yin and generates endlessly,"so using *Radix Rehmanniae* to nourish kidney yin,*Fructus Corni* and *Rhizoma Dioscoreae* tonify the liver and spleen,and enrich the essence and the blood,all of the above are the minister medicinals.*Poria* and *Rhizoma Alismatis*,which promote diuresis and eliminate dampness,combined with *Ramulus Cinnamomi* to warm the dampness to resolve phlegm;*Cortex Moutan*,which can clear heat and cool blood,combined with *Ramulus Cinnamomi*, modulates the stasis in the blood aspect,these three medicinals are the assistant medicinals.The formula has two characteristics:one is tonifying both yin and yang,focusing on yang;the other is that when nourishing kidney yin,adding *Ramulus Cinnamomi* and *Radix Aconiti* in low dose to warm yang,so as to"get

七、理气剂

理气剂是以理气药为主要组成，具有疏畅气机、调理脏腑功能、治疗气机失常的一类方剂。主要治疗肝胆、脾胃气滞，症见胸胁胀痛，脘腹胀满，嗳气吞酸，恶心呕吐，呃逆，或疝气疼痛，或月经不调、痛经；或肺气上逆，咳喘等证。理气剂多辛温香燥，容易伤津耗气，勿用过量，孕妇慎用。根据作用不同，理气剂可分为行气剂和降气剂。

（一）行气剂

行气剂用于治疗气机郁滞之证。气滞一般以脾胃气滞证和肝气郁滞证多见。脾胃气滞证主要表现为脘腹胀满，嗳气吞酸，呕恶食少，大便失常等；肝气郁滞证主要表现为胸胁胀痛，或疝气疼痛，或月经不调，或痛经等。代表方剂：越鞠丸。

越鞠丸

【来源】《丹溪心法》

【组成】苍术　香附　川芎　神曲　栀子（各10克）

【功用】行气解郁。

【主治】气、血、痰、火、湿、食六郁证，症见胸膈痞闷，脘腹胀痛，吞酸呕吐，饮食不化，舌淡红，苔薄白，脉弦。

【方解】方中香附行气解郁消滞，治疗气郁胸闷脘腹胀满疼痛，为君药；苍术燥湿健脾，治疗湿郁水谷不化；川芎活血行气，治疗血郁诸痛；神曲消食和胃，治疗食郁呕吐，饮食不消；栀子清热除烦，治疗火郁嘈杂吞酸，共为佐药。痰郁多因气、火、湿、食诸郁所致，气行通畅，湿去火清，则痰郁随之而解，故不另用化痰药物。

【注意事项】本方所治诸郁均为实证，因虚所致的郁证不宜使用。

【加减】本方以行气解郁为主，临床应用时可根据诸郁的轻重不同而变换君药，并适当加减使用。气郁为主，则以香附为君，佐以本方其他各味，还可再加木香；若湿郁偏重者，以苍术为主，再加茯苓、泽泻；若食郁偏重者，以神曲为主，再加麦芽；若血郁偏重者，以川芎为主，再加桃仁、红花；若火郁偏重者，以栀子为主，再加黄连、青黛；若痰郁偏重者，可加胆南星、法半夏、瓜蒌等。

yang from yin"and"vigorous fire generates qi."

【Note】Contraindicated for patients of kidney yin deficiency or upbearing of kidney fire.

【Variation】In case of polyuria and whitish urination, weak constitution, add *Fructus Psoraleae*, *Fructus Alpiniae Oxyphyllae*, and *Fructus Rubi* to warm the kidney and astringe the urine; in case of severe soreness and weakness of waist and knees, add *Cortex Eucommiae* and *Rhizoma Cibotii* to reinforce the function of tonifying kidney and strengthening waist and knees; for cold in lower abdomen, add *Radix Morindae Officinalis* and *Lignum Aquilariae Resinatum* to warm kidney and dispel cold; for sexual impotence, add *Herba Epimedii*, *Fructus Psoraleae*, and *Radix Morindae Officinalis* to tonify yang and resolve impotence.

Qi-regulating Formulas

Qi-regulating formulas are formulas that mainly composed of qi-regulating medicinals, and have functions of modulating qi flow and modulating functions of viscera and bowels, they are indicated for abnormal qi flow. Qi-regulating formulas are mainly indicated for qi stagnation of liver and gallbladder, and stagnation of spleen and stomach, marked by fullness sensation in the chest and diaphragm, abdominal distention and pain, fetid eructation and acid regurgitation, nausea and vomiting, hiccup or hernia pain, or irregular menstruation and menorrhalgia; or cough and asthma due to lung qi ascending counterflow. Most of the ingredients of the formulas are acrid, warm, aromatic and dry in properties, and tend to consume qi, injure the fluid; the formulas should not be used in over dosage, and be used with caution in pregnant women. Qi-regulating formulas are classified into promoting qi flow formulas and directing-qi-downward formulas.

Promoting qi flow formulas

Promoting qi flow formulas are indicated for qi stagnation patterns. Spleen and stomach qi stagnation and liver qi stagnation are common patterns of qi stagnation. Stagnation of the spleen and stomach are mainly marked by fullness in the chest and abdomen. The representative formula is "Gardenia-Ligusticum Pills".

Gardenia-Ligusticum Pills(Yue Ju Wan)

【Source】*Danxi's Experiential Therapy.*

【Composition】*Rhizoma Atractylodis* (10 g), *Rhizoma Cyperi Rotundi* (10 g), *Radix Ligustici Chuanxiong* (10 g), *Massa Fermentata* (10 g), and *Fructus Gardeniae Jasminoidis* (10 g).

【Functions】Promote the flow of qi to resolve stagnation.

【Indications】Syndromes of six types of stagnation, involving qi, blood, phlegm, fire, dampness and food, manifested as stifling sensation in the chest and diaphragm, abdominal distention and pain, fetid eructation and acid regurgitation, nausea and vomiting, indigestion, light red tongue with white coating, string-like pulse.

【Explanation】In the formula, *Rhizoma Cyperi* promotes qi flow and resolves stagnation. It can treat qi stagnation marked by fullness and pain in the chest and abdomen, serving as the sovereign medicinal. *Rhizoma Atractylodis* dries dampness and tonifies the spleen, treats indigestion due to dampness stagnation; *Rhizoma Chuanxiong* activates blood circulation and promotes qi flow, treating various kinds of pain patterns due to blood stasis. *Massa Fermentata Medicinalis* promotes digestion and harmonizes the stomach, and it is indicated for food stagnation marked by vomiting and indigestion. *Fructus Gardeniae* clears heat and resolves restlessness, and it is indicated for fire stagnation marked by vomiting acid and burning sensation in the stomach. All the above ingridients are the assistant medicinals. Phlegm stagnation mainly results from qi, fire, dampness, and food stagnations. If the qi flow is free, dampness is eliminated and fire is purged, then phlegm stagnation will be cured accordingly, thus it is not nessecery to add dispelling-phlegm

（二）降气剂

降气剂用于治疗气机上逆之证。临床多见肺气上逆证和胃气上逆证。肺气上逆证症见咳嗽短气、胸闷气喘等；胃气上逆证症见呕吐、呃逆等。代表方剂：旋覆代赭汤。

旋覆代赭汤

【来源】《伤寒论》

【组成】旋覆花（9克）代赭石　人参（各6克）甘草　半夏（各9克）生姜（15克）大枣（4枚）

【功用】降逆化痰，益气和胃。

【主治】胃气虚弱，痰浊内阻，胃气上逆，症见胃脘胀满、嗳气、呃逆或恶心呕吐，苔白滑，脉弦滑无力者。

【方解】方中旋覆花苦辛性温，有下气化痰，降逆止噫之功，为君药。代赭石甘寒质重，降逆下气，助君药降逆止呕，为臣药。君臣相合，善治胃失和降所致的嗳气、呃逆、呕吐诸证。半夏辛温，燥湿化痰，和胃降逆；生姜辛温，祛痰散结，降逆止呕，以协助君、臣药，增强其降逆止呕之功；人参、大枣、甘草益气补中以疗胃虚，又可防金石之品伤胃，同为佐药。甘草又能调和诸药，兼使药之用。诸药相配，标本兼顾，共奏降逆化痰、益气和胃之功。

【加减】如果胃气不虚，可去人参、大枣，并加重代赭石用量，增强重镇降逆之功；痰多者，加茯苓、陈皮等化痰和胃。

medicinals(when treating phlegm stagnation).

【Note】The formula is indicated for stagnation of excess syndromes, and contraindicated for stagnation of deficiency syndromes.

【Variation】The formula focuses on promoting qi flow and eliminating stagnation, the sovereign medicinal can be altered and its dosage can be appropriately modified in accordance with the different type and the severity of the stagnation. In case of qi stagnation, *Rhizoma Cyperi* is used as sovereign medicinal, and it assists other ingridients of the formula; moreover, *Radix Aucklandiae* is added. In case of stagnation due to slightly severe dampness, using *Rhizoma Atractylodis* as the sovereign medicinal, and add *poria* and *Rhizoma Alismatis*. In case of stagnation due to food accumulation, using *Massa Fermentata Medicinalis* as the sovereign medicinal, add *Fructus Hordei Germinatus*. In case of blood stagnation, using *Rhizoma Chuanxiong* as the sovereign medicinal, add *Semen Persicae* and *Flos Carthami*. In case of stagnation with heat, using *Fructus Gardeniae* as the sovereign medicinal, add *Rhizoma Coptidis* and *Indigo Naturalis*. In case of stagnation due to phlegm, add *Arisaema cum Bile*, *Rhizoma Pinelliae*, and *Fructus Trichosanthis*.

Directing-qi-downward formulas

Directing-qi-downward formulas are indicated for syndromes of adverse rising qi, which are usually adverse rising qi of lung qi or stomach. The syndrome of adverse rising of lung qi marked by cough, shortness of breath, fullness in the chest, asthma, etc.; the syndrome of adverse rising of stomach qi marked by vomiting, hiccup, and so on. The representative formula is "Inula-Haematite Decoction".

Inula-Haematite Decoction(Xuan Fu Dai Zhe Tang)

【Source】*Treatise on Cold Damage Diseases.*

【Composition】*Flos Inulae* (9 g), *Haematitum* (6 g), *Radix Ginseng* (6 g), *Radix Glycyrrhizae Praeparata* (9 g), *Rhizoma Zingiberis Recens* (15 g), and *Fructus Jujubae* (4 pieces).

【Functions】Direct rebellious qi downward and transform phlegm, tonify qi, and harmonize the stomach.

【Indications】Up-rising stomach qi due to stomach deficiency and phlegm stagnation, marked by epigastric stuffiness and hard, unremitting belching, hiccough, regurgitation, nausea and vomiting, white and slippery fur, and string-like, slippery and weak pulse.

【Explanation】In the formula, *Flos Inulae* is the sovereign medicinal, which is astringent, acrid and warm, directs the rebellious qi downward, dissolves phlegm, and stops belching. *Haematitum* is sweet, and cold, and heavy; it suppresses the rebellious qi downward, helps the sovereign medicinal to direct adverse rising qi downward and stop vomiting, serving as the minister medicinal. Both the sovereign medicinal and the minister medicinal are good at treating the symptoms of bleching, hiccup, and vomiting due to disharmony of the stamoch. *Rhizoma Pinelliae* is acrid and warm. It dries the dampness, eliminates phlegm, harmonizes the stomach, and directs the adverse rising qi. *Ginseng*, *Fructus Jujubae*, and *Radix Glycyrrhizae* tonify the middle to treat stomach deficiency, and prevent metal and stone medicinals damaging the stomach. All of these are the assistant medicinals. Among them, *Radix Glycyrrhizae* also modultes all the ingridients, and it is used as the courier medicinal as well. All the ingredients together, treat both the primary and the secondary aspects, concurrently achieve the success of directing rebellious qi downward, eliminating phlegm, tonifying qi, and harmonizing the stomach.

【Variation】If the stomach is not deficient, remove *Ginseng* and *Fructus Jujubae* add *Haematitum* in high dose to enforce the effect of heavy-suppressing and downward-directing; and for excessive phlegm, add *Poria* and *Pericarpium Citri Reticulatae* to harmonize the stomach and transform the phlegm.

八、理血剂

理血剂是以理血药为主组成，具有活血化瘀、止血的作用，治疗瘀血、出血病证的方剂。

根据作用不同，理血剂可分为活血祛瘀剂和止血剂。活血祛瘀方剂多属攻破之剂，易耗血伤正，不宜过量或久服，且孕妇宜慎用或禁用。止血之剂有滞血留瘀之虞，使用时需适当配伍活血祛瘀之品，使血止而不留瘀。

（一）活血祛瘀剂

活血祛瘀剂适用于各种瘀血病证。如瘀血内阻所致的胸、胁、腹部疼痛，肿块，痛经，经闭，络脉瘀阻之半身不遂，外伤瘀肿等。代表方剂：血府逐瘀汤、补阳还五汤。

血府逐瘀汤

【来源】《医林改错》

【组成】桃仁（12克）红花 当归 生地（各9克）枳壳 赤芍 甘草（各6克）柴胡（3克）桔梗 川芎（各4.5克）牛膝（9克）

【功用】活血祛瘀，行气止痛。

【主治】胸中血瘀证。症见胸痛，头痛日久，痛如针刺而有定处，或呃逆日久不止，或内热烦闷，或心悸失眠，急燥易怒，入暮潮热，唇暗或两目暗黑，舌黯红或有瘀斑，脉涩或弦紧。

【方解】方中桃仁破血行滞而润燥，红花活血化瘀以止痛，为君药；赤芍、川芎助君药活血化瘀，牛膝通利血脉，引血下行，为臣药；生地、当归养血益阴，清热活血，祛瘀而不伤阴血，桔梗、枳壳一升一降，行气宽中，柴胡疏肝解郁，升达清阳，共为佐药，使气行则血行；桔梗载药上行，兼使药之用；甘草调和诸药，为使药。全方配伍，既能行血分瘀滞，又能解气分郁结，活血而不耗血，祛瘀又能生新。

【注意事项】方中活血祛瘀药较多，故孕妇忌服。

【加减】血瘀经闭、痛经者，加香附、益母草等活血调经止痛；胁下有痞块，属血瘀者，加郁金、丹参以活血祛瘀、消癥化积。

Blood-regulating formulas

Blood-regulating formulas are mainly composed of blood-regulating medicinals, and have functions of activating blood and removing stasis or arresting bleeding, and are used to treat blood stasis or bleeding. According to their different functions, blood-regulating formulas are classified into two categories: blood-activating and stasis-resolving formulas and hemostatic formulas. Blood-activating and stasis-resolving formulas mainly belong to formulas of attacking and dispelling, and trend to consume the blood and injure healthy qi, so these should not be used overdosage or for a long period of time, and they are contraindicated for pregnant women. For fear of retention of blood stasis when using hemostatic formulas, one should approapritely add blood-activating and stasis-resolving medicinals, so as to arrest bleeding without retention of stasis.

Blood-activating and stasis-resolving formulas

Blood-activating and stasis-resolving formulas are used to treat various disorders due to blood stasis, such as, pain in the chest, hypochondrium or abdomen due to internal blood stasis, mass, dysmenorrhea, amenorrhea, hemiplegia due to stasis obstructing the collaterals, trauma and bruising. The representative formulas are "Blood Mansion Eliminating Stasis Decoction" and "Tonifying Yang and Restoring Five-Tenths Decoction".

Blood Mansion Eliminating Stasis Decoction (Xue Fu Zhu Yu Tang)

【Source】*Correction of Errors in Medical Classics.*

【Composition】*Semen Persicae* (12 g), *Flos Carthami* (9 g), *Radix Angelica Sinensis* (9 g), *Radix Remanniae* (9 g), *Fructus Aurantii* (6 g), *Radix Paeoniae* (6 g), *Radix Glycyrrhizae* (6 g), *Radix Bupleuri* (3 g), *Radix Platycodi* (4.5 g), *Rizoma Ligustici Chuanxiong* (4.5 g), and *Radix Achyranthis Bidentatae* (9 g).

【Functions】Activate blood, dispel stasis, promote qi, and relieve pain.

【Indications】Syndrome of blood stasis in the chest marked by protracted chest pain and headache at fixed location as if pricked by needles, or protracted hiccup, or palpitation and fearful throbbing, insomnia with frequent dreaming, irritability, tidal fever at dusk, dark-purple lips or blackish eyelids, dark-red tongue with maculations, and rough or string-like and tight pulse.

【Explanation】In this formula, *Semen Persicae* and *Flos Carthami* promote blood circulation to remove blood stasis and relieve pain, both serve as the sovereign medicinals; *Radix Paeoniae Rubra* and *Rhizoma Chuanxiong* assist the sovereign medicinal to promote blood circulation to remove blood stasis, *Radix Achyranthis Bidentatae* promotes blood circulation to lead stasis downwards, the above three medicinals serve as the minister medicinals; *Radix Rehmanniae* and *Radix Angelicae Sinensis* nourish the blood and yin to avoid yin and blood consumption when dispelling blood stasis; *Radix Platycodi* disperses lung qi and carries all the other medicinals upwards, while *Fructus Aurantii* downbears lung qi, so these two medicinals normalize qi dynamic; *Radix Bupleuri* regulates liver function to promote qi flow, the above five medicinals serve as the assistant medicinals. *Radix Glycyrrhizae* harmonizes all the ingredients, serving as the courier medicinal. With all the ingredients combined together, this formula not only can activate blood to dispel stasis, but also can disperge qi to resolve stagnation, thus it activates blood without consumption of the blood, dispels the stasis while generating the fresh blood.

【Note】Contraindicated for pregnant woman, because the formula consists of lots of ingridients of activating blood and removing stasis medicinals.

【Variation】In case of amenorrhea and menorrhalgia due to stasis, add *Rhizoma Cyperi* and *Herba Leonuri* to activate blood, modulate menstruation, and relieve pain; for swelling or mass underneath of the

补阳还五汤

【来源】《医林改错》

【组成】黄芪（120克）赤芍（5克）当归尾（6克） 地龙 川芎 红花 桃仁（各3克）

【功用】补气，活血，通络。

【主治】中风。半身不遂，口眼㖞斜，语言謇涩，口角流涎，小便频数或遗尿不禁，舌黯淡，苔白，脉缓。

【方解】方中重用生黄芪，大补脾胃元气，且黄芪性走，周行全身，"气能行血"，故令气旺以促血行，瘀去络通，为君药。当归尾长于活血，且化瘀而不伤血，为臣药。川芎、赤芍、桃仁、红花助当归尾活血祛瘀，地龙通经活络，均为佐药。本方的配伍特点是大量补气药与少量活血药相合，使气旺则血行，活血而不伤正，共奏补气、活血、通络之功。

【注意事项】本方需久服缓治，疗效方显。愈后还应继续服用一段时间，以巩固疗效，防止复发。

【加减】偏寒者，加熟附子温经散寒；脾胃虚弱者，加党参、白术补气健脾；痰多者，加制半夏、天竺黄化痰；语言不利者，加石菖蒲、郁金、远志等开窍化痰。

（二）止血剂

用于各种出血证。如吐血、咯血、便血、尿血、崩漏等。代表方剂：十灰散。

十灰散

【来源】《十药神书》

【组成】大蓟、小蓟、荷叶、侧柏叶、白茅根、茜草、栀子、大黄、牡丹皮、棕榈皮（各9克）。

【功用】凉血止血。

【主治】血热妄行之吐血、咯血、嗽血、衄血。

【方解】方中大蓟、小蓟性味甘凉，长于凉血止血，又能祛瘀，为君药；荷叶、侧柏叶、茅根、茜草凉血止血，加强君药的作用。并配以棕榈皮收涩止血，共为臣药。栀子清热泻火；大黄导热下行，能折其上逆之势，而缓解上部出血用丹皮凉血祛瘀，使血止而不留瘀，同为佐药。诸药烧炭存性，可加强收涩止血作用。另用藕汁或萝卜汁磨京墨调服，意在增强清热凉血止血、导热降气之功。

【注意事项】虚寒性出血者忌用。

hydrochondria due to blood stasis, add *Radix Curcumae* and *Radix Salviae Miltiorrhizae* to activate blood, remove stasis, and eliminate the mass.

Tonifying Yang and Restoring Five-Tenths Decoction(Bu Yang Huan Wu Tang)

【Source】*Correction of Errors in Medical Classics.*

【Composition】*Radix Astragali seu Hedysari* (120 g), *Radix Paeoniae Rubra* (5 g), *Exremitas Agelicae Sinensis Radicis* (6 g), *Lumbricus* (3 g), *Rizoma Ligustici Chuanxiong* (3 g), *Flos Carthami* (3 g), and *Semen Persicae* (3 g).

【Functions】Tonify qi, activate blood, and free meridians.

【Indications】Sequelae of apoplexy, marked by hemiplegia, deviation of the eyes and mouth, difficult sluggish speech, drooling from the corner of the mouth, frequent micturition or enuresis, pale and dull tongue with white tongue fur, and slow pulse.

【Explanation】In this formula, as sovereign medicinal, *Radix Astragali* is used in high dose to tonify the spleen and stomach and replenish source qi. Moreover, *Radix Astragali* has function of promote qi flow all over the body. "Qi is able to promote blood", thus, *Radix Astragali* makes qi strong so as to promote blood circulation, and remove stasis and free collaterals, and it serves as sovereign medicinal. *Radix Angelicae Sinensis* is good at activating blood, and it removes stasis without consuming the blood, serving as the minister medicinal. *Radix Paeoniae Rubra*, *Rhizoma Chuanxiong*, *Semen Persicae*, and *Flos Carthami* are used as assistant medicinals to promote the blood circulation and remove the blood stasis. *Lumbricus* is also used as assistant medicinal; it frees meridians and collaterals. The compatible characteristic of the formula is the combination of heavy dosage of tonifying qi medicinal with light dosages of activating blood medicinals, by which it tonifies qi to activate the blood circulation and activates the blood without damaging healthy qi. Thus, the formula achevieves the success of tonifying qi, activating blood, and freeing meridians.

【Note】The formula should be administered for a long period of time to achieve its effect, and a certain period of administration is needed to consolidate the therapeutic effect after recovery to prevent recurrence.

【Variation】If concurrent with cold syndrome, add *Radix Aconiti Lateralis Praeparata* to warm the meridians and dispel cold; in case of spleen-stomach deficiency, add *Radix Codonopsis* and *Rhizoma Atractylodis Macrocephalae* to tonify spleen qi; if concurrent with copious phlegm, add *Rhizoma Pinelliae* and *Concretio Silicea Bambusae* to dispel phlegm; for difficult sluggish speech, add *Rhizoma Acori Tatarinowii*, *Radix Curcumae*, and *Radix Polygalae* to open orifices and dispel phlegm.

Hemostatic Formulas

Hemostatic formulas are indicated for various patterns of bleeding, such as hemoptysis, hemafecia, hematuria, and metrorrhagia. The representative formula is "Ten Ash Power".

Ten Ash Power(Shi hui san)

【Source】*Ten Prescriptions Holy Book.*

【Composition】*Herba seu Radix Cirsii* (9 g), *Herba seu Radix Cephalanoploris* (9 g), *Folium Nelumlinis* (9 g), *Folium Biotae* (9 g), *Rhizoma Imperatae* (9 g), *Radix Rubiae* (9 g), *Fructus Gardeniae* (9 g), *Radix et Rhizoma Rhei* (9 g), *Cortex Moutan Radicis* (9 g), and *Stipulae Fibra Trachycarpi* (9 g).

【Functions】Cool the blood to stop bleeding.

【Indications】Hemoptysis, hemafecia, hematuria, and nose bleed due to frenetic movement of blood-heat.

【Explanation】In the formula, *Herba seu Radix Cirsii* and *Herba seu Radix Cephalanoploris*, which are sweet in favor and cool in nature, are used to cool the blood to arrest bleeding and remove blood stasis, as

【加减】气火上逆，血热较盛者，可以本方改作汤剂使用，并加牛膝、代赭石等镇降之品，引血热下行。

九、祛湿剂

祛湿剂是以祛湿药为主组成，具有化湿行水、通淋泄浊等作用，治疗水湿为病的方剂。祛湿药多辛燥或渗泄，易于伤阴，故阴亏体虚者及孕妇应慎用本类方剂。常配伍理气药，使"气化湿亦化"。根据作用不同，祛湿剂分为化湿和胃、清热祛湿、利水渗湿、温化水湿、祛风胜湿五类。

（一）化湿和胃

适用于湿浊阻滞，脾胃失和所致的脘腹胀满，嗳气吞酸，呕吐泄泻，食少体倦等。代表方剂：平胃散。

平胃散

【来源】《简要济众方》

【组成】苍术（120克）厚朴（90克）陈橘皮（60克）甘草（30克）（散剂用量）

【功用】燥湿运脾，行气和胃。

【主治】湿困脾胃。症见脘腹胀满，不思饮食，口淡无味，呕吐恶心，嗳气吞酸，泄泻，肢体沉重、怠惰嗜卧，舌苔白腻，脉缓。

【方解】方中苍术苦辛温燥，芳香猛烈，最善燥湿健脾，重用为君；厚朴，苦温行气，燥湿除满，助苍术健脾燥湿，为臣药；陈皮，理气化滞健脾和胃，协厚朴下气降逆，散满消胀，而且陈皮、厚朴气味芳香，可辅助苍术醒脾调中开胃。炙甘草、生姜、大枣调和脾胃，以助健运，同为佐药。且炙甘草能补能和，可制苍术、厚朴、陈皮之燥烈太过，使本方祛湿而不伤脾土。

【注意事项】素体肝肾阴虚者更应慎用；孕妇不宜用。

【加减】若舌苔黄腻，口苦咽干，但不甚渴饮，为湿热俱盛之证，可加黄芩、黄连，使湿热两清；若脾胃寒湿，脘腹冷痛，畏寒喜热，加干姜、肉桂以温化寒湿；若兼食滞见腹胀、大便秘结者，加槟榔、莱菔子、枳壳以消导积滞、消胀除满，下气通便；若呕吐者，加半夏以和胃止呕；若兼外感而见恶寒发热者，加藿香、苏叶、白芷等，以解表化浊。

the sovereign medicinals.*Folium Nelumlinis*, *Folium Biotae*, *Rhizoma Imperatae* and *Radix Rubiae* are used to cool the blood to arrest bleeding, so as to strengthen the function of the sovereign medicinals; *Stipulae Fibra Trachycarpi* is used to astringe bleeding, all of the above medicinals serve as the minister medicinals.*Fructus Gardeniae* clears heat and drains fire; *Rhizoma Rhei* guides heat downward, it can break the upward rising of the heat, and arrest bleeding in the upper body; *Cortex Moutan Radicis* cools blood and removes stasis, it is used to stop bleeding without retention of stasis, these three medicinals are the assistant medicinals.All of these ingredients are bunt to ash, so as to restore the nature and strengthen the function of astringing and stopping bleeding.The lotus root juice or radish juice ground on inkslab is used to enhance the action of cooling blood to stanch bleeding, and directing the heat downward and desecending qi.

〖Note〗The formula should not be administered to bleeding due to deficiency cold.

〖Variation〗For counter flowing of qi and heat due to severe blood heat, prepare the formula in form of decoction, add heavy and downward-directing medicinals, such as *Radix Achyranthis Bidentatae* and *Haematitum*, to direct blood-heat downward.

Dampness-eliminating formulas

Dampness-eliminating formulas are those formulas which mainly consist of dampness-eliminating medicinals, with actions of eliminating dampness, promoting diuresis, freeing strangury, and discharging turbidity.They are used to treat disease caused by dampness.Composed of dampness-eliminating medicinals which are of acrid taste and aromatic flavor, or inducing diuresis, and are prone to consume yin, these formulas should be cautiously administered to patients with yin deficiency and constitutional deficiency or pregnant women.Usually they are combined with qi-regulating medicinals, based on the theory of "dampness elimination follows qi transformation."According to different functions, dampness-eliminating formulas are categorized as dampness-eliminating and stomach-harmonizing formulas, heat-clearing and dampness-dispelling formulas, dampness-draining diuretic formulas, warming to transform dampness formulas, and wind-dampness-dispelling formulas.

Dampness-eliminating and stomach-harmonizing formulas

These formulas are indicated for syndrome of spleen-stomach disharmony due to dampness and turbidity obstruction, marked by glomus and fullness in the stomach and abdomen, belching and acid regurgitation, vomiting and diarrhea, reduced food intake and fatigue.The representative formula is "Balancing the Stomach Power".

Balancing the Stomach Power(Ping Wei San)

〖Source〗*Simple Prescriptons for Saving the People.*

〖Composition〗*Rhizoma Atractylodis* (120 g), *Cortex Magnoliae* (90 g), *Pericarpium Citri Reticulatae* (60 g), *Radix Glycyrrhizae Praeparata* (30 g). [dosage for powder]

〖Functions〗Dry dampness to invigorate the spleen, and promote qi flow to harmonize the stomach.

〖Indications〗Syndrome of dampness obstructing the spleen and stomach marked by distention and fullness in the stomach and abdomen, no desire for food and drink, tastelessness, vomiting and nausea, belching, acid regurgitation, diarrhea, heavy sensation of the body, lassitude and sleepiness, white greasy tongue coating, and slow pulse.

〖Explanation〗In the formula, Rhizoma Atractylodis is bitter and acrid, warm and dry, aromatic and strong, and effective in drying dampness and tonifying the spleen, and it is used in high dose as the sovereign medicinal; *Cortex Magnoliae Officinalis* is bitter and warm which promotes qi flow, and dries dampness and resolves distention, helps *Rhizoma Atractylodis* invigorate the spleen and dry dampness as the

（二）清热祛湿

清热祛湿剂用于湿遏热伏，或湿从热化，湿热内盛所致的病证。湿热伏在气分者，症见头痛身重，胸脘痞闷不饥，口淡不渴，或口中黏腻，发热，午后身热较著，舌苔白腻或微黄，脉缓等。代表方剂：茵陈蒿汤。

茵陈蒿汤

【来源】《伤寒论》

【组成】茵陈（18 克）　栀子（12 克）　大黄（6 克）

【功用】清热利湿退黄。

【主治】湿热黄疸。症见一身面目俱黄，色泽鲜明，腹满，口渴，小便短赤，舌苔黄腻，脉沉数。

【方解】方中重用茵陈蒿，以其最善清利湿热、退黄疸，为主药；栀子清泻三焦湿热，为臣药；大黄降泄瘀热，为佐药。茵陈蒿配栀子，以使湿热从小便而出；茵陈蒿配大黄，以使瘀热从大便而解。三药配合，引湿热由二便而出。

【注意事项】阴黄忌用。

【加减】本方所治为湿热俱盛，若热重于湿，症见身热，口苦，心烦者，加黄柏、龙胆草以清热祛湿；若湿多热少，症见小便不利，大便溏，舌苔厚腻者，可去大黄，加茯苓、泽泻、猪苓利水渗湿。

minister medicinal; *Pericarpium Citri Reticulatae* modulates qi and removes distention, invigorates the spleen and harmonizes the stamoch, it helps *Cortex Magnoliae Officinalis* guide qi downward and descend the reversing qi, and dispel distention. Both *Pericarpium Citri Reticulatae* and *Cortex Magnoliae Officinalis* are aromatic, they help *Rhizoma Atractylodis* awake the spleen to modulate the middle and increase the appitite. *Radix Glycyrrhizae Praeparata*, *Rhizoma Zingiberis Recens* and *Fructus Jujubae* modulate the spleen and stomach to promote digestion, all of them are the assistant medicinals. Moreover, *Radix Glycyrrhizae Praeparata* not only tonifies but also modulates; it restricts the drying actions of *Rhizoma Atractylodis*, *Cortex Magnoliae Officinalis*, and *Pericarpium Citri Reticulatae*, so as to make the formula dry dampness without damaging the spleen-earth.

【Note】The formula should be used cautiously in patients of liver-kidney yin deficiency; it is contraindicated for pregnant women.

【Variation】In case of yellowish greasy tongue coating, bitter taste in the mouth and dry throat, without severe thirst, which refers to excess of both dampness and heat, add *Radix Scutellariae* and *Rhizoma Coptidis* to clear dampness-heat; in case of cold-dampness of the spleen and stomach, marked by cold pain in the stomach and abdomen, aversion to cold, and preference to warmth, add *Rhizoma Zingiberis* and *Cortex Cinnamomi* to warm the middle and resolve the cold-dampness; in case of food accumulation marked by distention and constipation, add *Semen Arecae*, *Semen Raphani*, and *Fructus Aurantii* to promote digestion, remove distention, downward regulate qi, and relax the bowels; in case of vomiting, add *Rhizoma Pinelliae* to harmonize the stomach and stop vomiting; in case of concurrency with external cold marked by fever with aversion to cold, add *Herba Agastachis*, *Folium Perillae*, and *Radix Angelicae Dahuricae* to release the exterior and resolve turbidity.

Heat-clearing and dampness-dispelling formulas

These formulas are applicable to internal excess of dampness-heat patterns which are dampness covers the heat inside, or dampness follows the heat and becomes dampness-heat. Dampness-heat in the qi aspect, marked by headache and heavy body, pale taste in the mouth and without thirst, or sticky and greasy in the mouth, fever especially after the noon, white and greasy or mild yellowish tongue coating, slow pulse. The representative formula is "Capillaris Decoction".

Capillaris Decoction(Yin Chen Hao Tang)

【Source】*Treatise on Cold Damage Diseases.*

【Composition】*Herba Artemisiae Capillaris* (18 g), *Fructus Gardeniae* (9 g), and *Radix ex Rhizoma Rhei* (6 g).

【Functions】Clear heat, eliminate dampness, and abate jaundice.

【Indications】Jaundice due to dampness-heat, marked by bright yellow coloration of skin and eyes, abdominal fullness, thirst, inhibited urination, yellow and greasy tongue coating, sunken and rapid pulse.

【Explanation】In the formula, the sovereign medicinal *Herba Artemisiae Scopariae* is used in high dose, and it is good at clearing heat, removing dampness, and abating jaundice; *Fructus Gardeniae*, as the minister medicinal, clears dampness-heat of the three energizers; *Radix et Rhizoma Rhei*, as the assistant medicinal, clears and guides the stasis and the heat downward. *Herba Artemisiae Scopariae*, together with *Fructus Gardeniae*, drains the dampness-heat from urination; *Herba Artemisiae Scopariae*, together with *Radix et Rhizoma Rhei*, eliminates blood stasis and promotes defecation to expel heat from stools. These three medicinals are used in combination to guide and drain downward, and expel dampness-heat from defecation and urination.

【Note】Contraindicated for jaundice of yin syndrome.

【Variation】The indication of the formula is both severe dampness and severe heat, if heat is heavier

（三）利水渗湿

利水渗湿剂，适用于水湿壅盛所致的癃闭、淋浊、水肿、泄泻等证。以利尿为主要手段，使湿邪自小便而出。代表方剂：五苓散。

五苓散

【来源】《伤寒论》

【组成】茯苓（9克）泽泻（15克）猪苓（9克）桂枝（6克）白术（9克）。

【功用】利水渗湿、温阳化气。

【主治】

1. 外有表证，内停水湿。症见头痛发热、烦渴欲饮、或水入即吐、小便不利、舌苔白，脉浮。

2. 水湿内停。症见水肿、泄泻、小便不利以及霍乱吐泻等证。

3. 痰饮。症见脐下动悸、吐涎沫而头眩或短气而咳者。

【方解】方中重用泽泻直达膀胱，渗湿利水，为主药；臣以茯苓、猪苓淡利渗湿，加强利水蠲饮之力；佐以白术健脾以助运化水湿之力；并佐桂枝，一来外解太阳之表，二来温化膀胱之气。全方可使水行气化，表解脾健，则蓄水停饮之证可除。至于水肿、泄泻、霍乱、痰饮诸病，由于脾虚不运，水湿泛溢所致者，皆可用本方加减治疗。

【注意事项】本方为温阳化气利水之剂，病属湿热者忌用。

【加减】黄疸而湿盛小便短少者，加茵陈。若脾胃湿盛，脘腹胀满，泄泻者，可与苍术、厚朴、陈皮合用。若湿盛兼有热象者，去桂枝，方名"四苓散"。

（四）温化水湿

温化水湿剂，适用于阳虚气不化水，水湿内停或湿从寒化所致的病证，如阴水、痰饮、淋浊、寒湿脚气等。故除小便不利，或癃闭、淋浊、水肿、泄泻等外，常有手足不温，口不渴，舌淡苔白，脉沉弦或沉迟，沉细等证候。代表方剂：真武汤。

than dampness marked by body heat, bitter taste in mouth, restlessness, add *Cortex Phellodendri* and *Radix Gentianae* to clear heat and dispel dampness; for more dampness and less heat, marked by inhibated urination, loose stools, thick and greasy tongue coating, remove *Radix et Rhizoma Rhei* and add *Poria*, *Rhizoma Alismatis*, and *Polyporus* to promote diuresis and drain dampness.

Dampness-draining diuretic formula

Dampness-draining diuretic formulas are applicable for diseases which result from excess of water and dampness, such as dribbling unrinary block, edema, diarrhea, etc. Their main method is promoting diuresis to dispel the dampness from the urine. The representative formula is "Five-Ingredient Poria Powder".

Five-Ingredient Poria Powder(Wu Ling San)

【Source】*Treatise on Cold Damage Diseases.*

【Composition】*Polyporus* (9 g), *Rhizoma Alismatis* (15g), *Rhizoma Atractylodis* (9 g), *Poria* (9 g), and *Ramulus Cinnamomi* (6 g).

【Functions】Promote diuresis, percolate dampness, and warm yang to transform qi.

【Indications】

(1) Exterior pattern in the exterior, water and dampness retention in the interior, marked by headache, fever, thirst with a desire for drinking, even immediate vomiting after drinking, inhibited urination, white tongue fur, and float pulse.

(2) Water and dampness retention, marked by edema, diarrhea, inhibited urination or vomiting and diarrhea due to cholera, etc.

(3) Phlegm and fluid retention marked by palpitation below the umbilical region, vomiting of phlegm and foam, dizziness, or with shortness of breath, or cough.

【Explanation】In the formula, *Rhizoma Alismatis* as the sovereign medicinal is used in high dose to reach the bladder directly, and to promote diuresis and percolate dampness; *Poria* and *Polyporus*, which promote diuresis and percolate dampness, and reinforce the power of promoting diuresis and eliminating fluid; assisted with *Rhizoma Atractylodis Macrocephalae* which assists the effect of transforming water and dampness, and assisted with *Ramulus Cinnamomi* which on one hand relieves the exterior of yang brightness syndrome, on the other hand warms to transform the bladder qi. All the ingredients are used in combination to promote the water metabolism and qi transformation, and to relieve the exterior and tonify the spleen. Thus, the formula itself or with rariation is applicable for edema, diarrhea, chorela, phlegm and fluid retention, due to spleen deficiency and excess of water and dampness.

【Note】The formula is a warming yang, transforming qi and promoting diuresis formula, it is contraindicated for diseases result from dampness-heat.

【Variation】In case of jaundice and excessive dampness marked by short urination, add *Herba Artemisiae Scopariae*. In case of excessive dampness in spleen and stomach, marked by distention and diarrhea, apply with *Rhizoma Atractylodis*, *Cortex Magnoliae* and *Pericarpium Citri Reticulatae*. In case of excessive dampness with heat, remove *Ramulus Cinnamomi*, and named "Four-Ingredient Poria Powder".

Warming to transform dampness formulas

These formulas are applicable for syndromes result from qi failing in transforming water due to yang deficiency, water and dampness retention, or dampness transforms with cold, such as yin-water, phlegm and fluid retention, turbid and stragury, beriberi due to cold-dampness, etc. Therefore, besides inhibited urination, or dribbling urinary block, strangury and turbidity, edema, diarrhea, commonly there are coldness in hands and feet, without thirst, pale tongue with white tongue coating, sunken and string-like pulse or sunken and slow pulse, sunken and fine pulse. The representive formula is "Zhen Wu Decoction".

真武汤

【来源】《伤寒论》

【组成】熟附子　茯苓　白芍（各9克）白术（6克）生姜（9克）。

【功用】温阳利水。

【主治】

1. 脾肾阳虚，水气内停所致的水肿，症见小便不利，肢体浮肿，四肢沉重、疼痛，恶寒，舌淡而润，苔白，脉沉细者。

2. 发汗过多，阳气太虚，寒水内动，水气凌心，症见心悸、头晕，身体振动而欲地，舌淡润，脉沉细者。

【方解】方中以大辛大热之附子为君，温壮肾阳，化气行水，即"益火之原以消阴翳"之意。然主水在肾，制水在脾，脾喜燥恶湿，得阳则运，故以苦甘性温之白术健脾燥湿，扶土制水，合附子温阳健脾以助运化。寒水既停，则当渗利以去之，又用甘淡渗湿之茯苓，利水健脾，与白术相合，则健脾利水之力益著，共为臣药。生姜辛温，温中散水，走而不守，既可助附子温化寒水，又助苓、术健运行水。白芍苦酸微寒，益阴敛阴，且能利小便，与附子同用，使邪水去而真阴不伤，同为佐药。全方于温阳健脾利水药中少佐酸敛护阴之品，温阳利水不伤阴，益阴护阴不碍邪，合为温肾散寒，健脾利水之剂。

【注意事项】阴虚者忌用。

【加减】咳者，加干姜、细辛、五味子以温肺化饮；腹泻较重者，去白芍之寒，加干姜、益智仁以温中止泻；呕者，加吴茱萸、半夏以温胃止呕。

（五）祛风胜湿

祛风胜湿剂具有祛除风湿的作用，是用于治疗外感风湿所致的头痛、身痛、腰膝顽麻痹痛以及脚气足肿等证的方剂。代表方剂：独活寄生汤。

独活寄生汤

【来源】《备急千金要方》

【组成】独活（9克）　桑寄生　杜仲　牛膝　细辛　秦艽　茯苓　肉桂心　防风　川芎　人参　甘草　当归　芍药　干地黄（各6克）

【功用】祛风湿，止痹痛，益肝肾，补气血。

【主治】痹证日久，肝肾两虚，气血不足证。症见腰膝疼痛、痿软，肢节屈伸不利，或麻木不仁，畏寒喜温，心悸气短，舌淡，苔白，脉细弱。

Zhen Wu Decoction(Zhen Wu Tang)

【Source】*Treatise on Cold Damage Diseases.*

【Composition】*Laterale Tuber Aconiti* (9 g),*Poria* (9 g),*Radix Alba Paeoniae* (9 g),*Rhizoma Atractylodis Macrocephalae* (6 g),and *Rhizoma Zingiberis* (9 g).

【Functions】Warm yang to induce diuresis.

【Indications】

(1)Edema due to yang deficiency of the spleen and kidney and water retention,marked by inhibited urination,swelling in limbs,pain or heavy sensation of the limbs and body,aversion to cold,pale moisten tongue with white tongue coating,and sunken and fine pulse.

(2)Severe sweating,severe deficiency of yang,cold water moving in the interior,water invades heart,marked by palpitation,dizziness,trembling,pale and moisten tongue,and sunken and fine pulse.

【Explanation】In the formula,the sovereign medicinal *Radix Aconiti* is used to warm the kidney yang to promote qi flow to induce diuresis,that is"tonifying the source of the fire to eliminate the shadow." Since the kidney governs water,the spleen restricts water;the spleen likes dryness and dislikes dampness, and it works when gets yang,the formula takes *Rhizoma Atractylodis Macrocephalae* which is bitter,sweet and of warm nature,to supplement earth to restrict water,and combines with *Radix Aconiti* to warm yang and tonify the spleen to promote digestion.Since the cold water stops generating,it should be removed by draining and promoting urinating;thus,poria,which is sweet and bland,promote uriesis and tonify the spleen;when combined with *Rhizoma Atractylodis Macrocephalae*,its effectiveness in tonifying the spleen and promoting diuresis get more powerful,both are the minister medicinals.*Rhizoma Zingiberis Recens* is acrid and warm,it warms the middle and disperse the water,it runs without staying,it not only helps *Radix Aconiti* warm to transform cold water,but also helps *Poria* and *Rhizoma Atractylodis Macrocephalae* transport water.*Radix Paeoniae Alba* is bitter and slightly cold,it nourishes and restricts yin,and promotes diuresis;when used with *Radix Aconiti*,it removes the pathogenic water without comsuption of yin,both are the assistant medicinals.The formula uses less sour and restricting ingredients to nourish yin,among ingredients whose functions are of warming yang and tonifying the spleen and promoting diuresis,thus,it warms yang and promotes diuresis without consumption of yin,and nourishes yin and protects yin without retention of the pathogen.All the ingredients combined together to be a formula which warms the kidney to disperse cold,tonifies the spleen to promote diuresis.

【Note】Contraindicated for yin deficiency.

【Variation】For cough,add *Rhizoma Zingiberis*,*Herba Asari*,and *Fructus Schisandrae* to warm lung and remove fluid;for severe diarrhea,remove cold *Radix Paeoniae Alba* and add *Rhizoma Zingiberis* and *Fructus Alpiniae Oxyphyllae* to warm the middle and check diarrhea;and for vomiting,add *Fructus Evodiae* and *Rhizoma Pinelliae* to warm the stomach and stop vomiting.

Wind-dampness-dispelling formulas

These formulas have functions of dispelling wind-dampness,and are applicable for syndrome of exogenous wind and dampness,marked by headache,generalized aching pain,numbness and pain in waist or knees,impediment,and foot swelling due to beriberi.The representative formula is " Angelicae Pubescentis and Loranthi Decoction".

Angelicae Pubescentis and Loranthi Decoction(Du Huo Ji Sheng Tang)

【Source】*Essential Prescriptions Worth a Thousand Gold for Emergencies.*

【Composition】*Radix Angelicae Pubescentis* (9 g),*Ramululus Loranthi* (6 g),*Cortex Eucommiae* (6 g),*Radix Achyranthis Bidentatae* (6 g),*Herba Asari* (6 g),*Radix Gentianae Macrophyllae* (6 g),*Poria*

【方解】方中独活、桑寄生祛风除湿，养血和营，活络通痹，共为君药；牛膝、杜仲、熟地黄补肝肾、强筋骨，均为臣药；川芎、当归、芍药补血活血；人参、茯苓、甘草益气扶脾，使气血旺盛，有助于风湿祛除；细辛搜风通痹止痛，肉桂祛寒止痛，同为佐药；秦艽、防风祛周身风寒湿邪，为使药。全方标本兼顾，扶正祛邪。

【注意事项】痹证之属湿热实证者忌用。

【加减】痹证疼痛较剧者，可加制附子、白花蛇等以助搜风通络，活血止痛；寒邪偏盛者，加附子、干姜以温阳散寒；湿邪偏盛者，去地黄，加汉防己、薏苡仁、苍术以祛湿消肿；正虚不甚者，可减地黄、人参。

十、祛痰剂

祛痰剂是以祛痰药为主组成，具有消除痰饮作用，治疗各种痰病的方剂。属消法范畴。湿痰、热痰、燥痰、寒痰及风痰均可运用本类方剂加减治疗。根据痰病的性质及其相应治法的不同，分为燥湿化痰、清热化痰、润燥化痰、温化寒痰、化痰熄风五类。

（一）燥湿化痰

燥湿化痰剂主治痰湿证。痰湿证多因脾不健运，湿聚成痰所致。症见咳嗽痰多易咯，胸脘痞闷，恶心呕吐，头眩心悸，四肢困倦，舌苔白滑或腻，脉缓等。代表方剂：二陈汤。

二陈汤

【来源】《太平惠民和剂局方》

【组成】半夏　橘红（各15克）白茯苓（9克）甘草（4.5克）生姜（7片）乌梅（1个）

【功用】燥湿化痰，理气和中。

【主治】痰湿内阻，脾胃不和，症见胸脘痞闷，呕吐恶心，或头眩心悸，或咳嗽痰多，舌苔白润，脉滑。

【方解】方中半夏辛温性燥，善于燥湿化痰，又降逆和胃，为君药。橘红理气燥湿祛痰，燥湿以助半夏化痰之力，理气可使气顺则痰消，为臣药。因痰由湿生，湿自脾来，故用茯苓健脾渗湿，使湿去脾旺，痰无由生；生姜降逆化饮，既制半夏之毒，又助半夏、橘红行气消痰，和胃止呕；乌梅收敛肺气，与半夏相伍，散中有收，使祛痰而不伤正，并有欲劫之而先聚之之意，共为佐药。甘草调和药性兼润肺和中，为使药。全方标本兼顾，燥湿化痰，理气和中，为祛痰的基本方剂。因方中半夏、

(6 g) , *Cortex Cinnamomi* (6 g) , *Radix Ledebouriellae* (6 g) , *Rhizoma Lingustici Chuan Xiong* (6 g) , *Radix Ginseng* (6 g) , *Radix Glycyrrhizae* (6 g) , *Radix Angelicae Sinensis* (6 g) , *Radix Paeoniae* (6 g) , and *Radix Rehmanniae* (6 g) .

【Functions】Dispel wind-dampness, arrest pain, nourish the liver and kidney, tonify qi, and replenish the blood.

【Indications】Chronic impediment due to liver-kidney deficiency or vacuity of qi and blood, marked by pain and wilting of the lumbus and knees, inhibited movement or numbness of joints, aversion to cold and preference to warmth, palpitation, shortness of the breath, pale tongue with white tongue coating, fine and weak pulse.

【Explanation】In the formula, both *Radix Angelicae Pubescentis* and *Ramulus Taxilli* are the sovereign medicinals; they dispel wind-dampness, nourish the blood, harmonize the nutrient aspect, activate the collaterals, and free the impediments. *Radix Achyranthis Bidentatae* , *Cortex Eucommiae* , and *Radix Rehmanniae Praeparata* nourish the liver and kidney, strengthen the tendon and bone, all of them are the minister medicinals. *Rhizoma Chuanxiong* , *Radix Angelicae Sinensis* , and *Radix Paeoniae Alba* nourish the blood and activate the blood circulation; *Ginseng* , *Poria* , and *Radix Glycyrrhizae* tonify qi and supplement the spleen, and make qi and blood vigorous, they are helpful for dispelling wind-dampness; *Herba Asari* seeks wind and frees impediment and relieves pain, *Cortex Cinnamomi* dispels cold and relieves pain; all of them are the assistant medicinals. *Radix Gentianae Macrophyllae* and *Radix Saposhnikoviae* dispel pathogens of wind-cold-dampness of the whole body as the courier medicinals. The whole formula treats the root and the tip together, reinforces the healthy qi, and eliminates the pathogenic factors.

【Note】Contraindicated for impediment of excess pattern of dampness-heat.

【Variation】For severe pain of impediment, add *Radix Aconiti* and *Bungarus Parvus* to reinforce the actions of seeking wind and freeing the collaterals, activating blood and relieving pain; for excessive cold, add *Radix Aconiti* and *Rhizoma Zingiberis* to warm yang and dispel cold; for excessive dampness, remove *Radix Rehmanniae* and add *Radix Stephaniae* , *Semen Coicis* , and *Rhizoma Atractylodis* to dispel dampness and remove swelling; if the deficiency is not severe, remove *Radix Rehmanniae* and *Ginseng* .

Phlegm-dispelling Formulas

Phlegm-dispelling formulas are composed of dispelling phlegm medicinals, and have the actions of dispelling phlegm and eliminating fluid, are indicated for various phlegm syndromes. The formulas belong to "eliminating" among the "eight therapeutic methods." The formulas can be modified and applied for syndromes of dampness-phlegm, heat-phlegm, dry-phlegm, cold-phlegm or wind-phlegm. According to the different of the natures of phlegm and their corresponding treating methods, the formulas are classified into five categories, drying dampness to resolve phlegm formulas, clearing and resolving heat-phlegm formulas, moistening dryness to resolve phlegm formulas, warming and resolving cold-phlegm formulas, and extinguishing wind and resolving phlegm formulas.

Drying dampness to resolve phlegm formulas

Drying dampness to resolve phlegm formulas are applicable for phlegm-dampness syndrome, which mainly results from indigestion due to spleen deficiency, and phlegm generated from dampness accumulation, marked by cough, profuse phlegm being easy to be spitted out, fullness and oppression in the chest and stomach duct, nausea and vomiting, dizziness, palpatition, fatigued limbs, white greasy tongue coating or white glossy tongue coating, and slow pulse. The representative formula is "Two Old Decoction".

Two Old Decoction(Er Chen Tang)

【Source】*Prescriptions from the Great Peace Imperial Grace Pharmacy.*

橘红以陈久者良，故以"二陈"为名。

【注意事项】本方因其性燥，故对阴虚肺燥及咳血者忌用。

【加减】.风痰者，加南星、竹沥；热痰者，加黄芩、胆星；寒痰者，加干姜、细辛；食痰者，加莱菔子、神曲；气痰者，加枳实、厚朴；皮里膜外之痰者，加白芥子等。

（二）清热化痰

清热化痰剂，适用于火热内盛、炼津成痰、痰热互结之证。临床症见咳痰黄稠，胸闷烦热，舌红苔黄，脉滑数。代表方剂：清气化痰丸。

清气化痰丸

【来源】《医方考》

【组成】陈皮 杏仁 枳实 黄芩 瓜蒌仁 茯苓（各10克）胆南星 制半夏（各15克）

【功用】清热化痰，理气止咳。

【主治】痰热咳嗽。症见咳嗽痰黄，黏稠难咯，胸闷气急，舌苔黄腻，脉滑数。

【方解】方中胆南星味苦性凉，清热化痰，治痰热之壅闭，为君药。瓜蒌仁甘寒，长于清肺化痰；黄芩苦寒，善能清肺泻火，同为臣药，两药合用，泻肺火，化痰热，增强胆南星之效。枳实下气消痞，"除胸胁痰癖"；陈皮理气宽中，燥湿化痰。"脾为生痰之源，肺为贮痰之器"，故治痰先治脾，用茯苓健脾渗湿，防止痰液生成；杏仁宣利肺气，半夏燥湿化痰，共佐药。全方共奏清热化痰、理气止咳之功。

【注意事项】本方性偏苦燥，阴虚燥咳者忌用。

【加减】身热口渴，肺热较甚者，加石膏、知母以清泻肺热；痰多气急而喘者，加桑白皮、鱼腥草等以下气祛痰。

【Composition】*Rhizoma Pinelliae* (15 g) , *Exocarpium Citri Grandis* (15g) , *Poria* (9 g) , *Radix Glycyrrhizae* (4. 5 g) , *Rhizoma Zingiberis Recens* (7 pieces) , and *Fructus Plum* (1 piece).

【Functions】Dry dampness, disperse phlegm, modulate qi, and harmonize the middle.

【Indications】Phlegm-dampness and disharmony of the spleen and stomach, marked by fullness and oppression in the chest and stomach duct, nausea and vomiting, or vertigo and palpitation, or cough with productive phlegm, white and moisten tongue fur, and slippery pulse.

【Explanation】In the formula, *Rhizoma Pinelliae* is acrid, warm and dry. It is effective in drying dampness and dispelling phlegm, it desends the reversing qi and harmonizes the stomach, servingas the sovereign medicinal.*Exocarpium Citri Rubrum* modulates qi, dries dampness, and dispels phlegm, serveing as the minister medicinal.Because the phlegm results from dampness, and the dampness results from the spleen, using *Poria* to tonify the spleen and drain dampness, so that the dampness is removed and the spleen is fortified, and the phlegm will generate from nowhere;*Rhizoma Zingiberis Recens* desends the rebelling qi and transforms the fluid, not only restricts the toxin of *Rhizoma Pinelliae* but also helps *Rhizoma Pinelliae* and *Exocarpium Citri Rubrum* to activate qi flow, dispel phlegm, harmonize the stomach, and arrest vomiting;*Fructus Mume* restricts the lung qi, and it is combined with *Rhizoma Pinelliae*, dispelling with restricting, dispelling phlegm without consumption of vigor qi, and the combination has a meaning of dispelling after collecting;all the above medicinals are the assistant medicinals.*Radix Glycyrrhizae*, as the courier medicinal, modulates the natures of all the ingredients and moistens the lung and harmonizes the middle.All the ingredients together concern both the root and the tip, dry dampness and transform phlegm, modulte qi, and harmonize the middle, and the formula is the basic formula of phlegm-dispelling formulas. Since *Rhizoma Pinelliae* and *Exocarpium Citri Rubrum* are considered the older the better, the formula is named as "Two Old Decoction".

【Note】The nature of the formula is dry, so it is contraindicated for lung dryness due to yin deficiency or hemoptysis.

【Variation】For wind-phlegm, add *Rhizoma Arisaematis* and *Succus Bambusae* ;for heat-phlegm, add *Radix Scutellariae* and *Arisaema cum Bile* ;for cold-phlegm, add *Rhizoma Zingiberis* and *Herba Asari* ;for food-phlegm, add *Semen Raphani* and *Massa Fermentata Medicinalis* ;for qi-phlegm, add *Fructus Aurantii Immaturus* and *Cortex Magnoliae Officinalis*;for phlegm exists between inner skin and outer membrane, add *Semen Sinapis Albae*.

Clearing and resolving heat-phlegm formulas

Clearing and resolving heat-phlegm formulas are applicable for the syndrome of phlegm-heat due to internal excess of heat or fire boiling fluid into phlegm, clinically marked by cough with yellow thick phlegm, fullness and oppression in the chest, restlessness and fever, red tongue with yellow tongue coating, slippery and rapid pulse.The representative formula is "Clearing Qi and Resolving Phlegm Decoction".

Clearing Qi and Resolving Phlegm Decoction (Qing Qi Hua Tan Tang)

【Source】*Textual Criticism on Prescriptions.*

【Composition】*Pericarpium Citri Reticulatae* (10 g) , *Semen Armeniacae Amarum* (10 g) , *Fructus Aurantii Immaturus* (10 g) , *Radix Scutellariae* (10 g) , *Semen Trichosanthis* (10 g) , *Poria* (10 g) , *Arisaema cum Bile* (15 g) , and *Rhizoma Pinelliae Praeparata* (15 g).

【Functions】Clear heat, disperse phlegm, modulate qi, and suppress cough.

【Indications】Cough due to phlegm-heat, marked by cough with thick yellow phlegm, being difficult to be expectorated, glomus and oppression in the chest, rapid breathing, yellow greasy tongue fur, and slippery and rapid pulse.

（三） 润燥化痰

润燥化痰剂，适用于外感燥热，或肺阴亏虚所致的燥痰证。症见干咳少痰，或痰稠而粘，咯痰不爽，或咯痰带血，咽喉干燥，声音嘶哑。代表方剂：贝母瓜蒌散。

贝母瓜蒌散

【来源】《医学心悟》

【组成】贝母（4.5克）瓜蒌（3克）花粉　茯苓　橘红　桔梗（各2.5克）

【功用】润肺清热，理气化痰。

【主治】燥痰咳嗽。症见咳嗽呛急，咯痰不爽，涩而难出，咽喉干燥哽痛，苔白而干。

【方解】方中川贝清热润肺、化痰止咳为君。臣以全瓜蒌清热润燥，利气涤痰。天花粉清热化痰，生津润燥；茯苓健脾渗湿；橘红化痰止咳；桔梗宣肺利咽，均为佐药。全方共奏润肺清热、理气化痰之功。

【注意事项】对于肺肾阴虚、虚火上炎之咳嗽，并非所宜。

【加减】若兼感风邪、咽痒而咳，微恶风者，加桑叶、蝉蜕、杏仁、牛蒡子等宣肺散邪；燥热较甚、咽喉干涩哽痛明显者，加玄参、麦冬、生石膏等清燥润肺；声音嘶哑、痰中带血者，可去橘红，加南沙参、白芨等养阴清肺、化痰止血。

【Explanation】In the formula, *Arisaema cum Bile*, bitter and of cool nature, can clear heat, remove phlegm, and treat the blocking of heat-phlegm, and it is the sovereign medicinal. *Fructus Trichosanthis* is sweet and cold, it is effective in clearing the lung and resolving phlegm; *Radix Scutellariae* is bitter and cold, it is effective in clearing the lung and and purging heat. Both *Fructus Trichosanthis* and *Radix Scutellariae* are the minister medicinals, they are combined together to purge the lung heat and resolve phlegm-heat and reinforce the effect of *Arisaema cum Bile*. *Fructus Aurantii Immaturus* desends qi, resolves distention, and eliminates phlegm in the chest and abdomen; *Pericarpium Citri Reticulatae* modulates qi and soothes the middle, drys dampness, and resolves phlegm; "the spleen is the origin of the phlegm, and the lung is the container of the phlegm", thus, treating phlegm should start with the spleen, using *Poria* to tonify the spleen and drain dampness, and prevent the generation of the phlegm; *Semen Armeniacae Amarum* soothes the lung qi, *Rhizoma Pinelliae* dries dampness and resolves phlegm; all the above-mentioned medicinals are the assistant medicinals. All the ingredients together achieve the success of clearing heat, resolving phlegm, modulating qi, and arresting cough.

【Note】The formula's nature is bitter and dry, and contraindicated for dry-cough due to yin deficiency.

【Variation】For severe lung-heat, marked by fever and thist, add *Gypsum Fibrosum* and *Rhizoma Anemarrhenae* to clear and purge lung-heat; in case of productive phlegm and uneven rapid breath and asthma, add *Cortex Mori* and *Herba Houttuyniae* to direct qi downward and dispel phlegm.

Moistening dryness to resolve phlegm formulas

Moistening dryness to resolve phlegm formulas are applicable for syndromes of dry-phlegm due to external dryness-heat invading or lung yin deficiency, marked by cough with less phlegm, or sticky and thick phlegm difficult to expectorate, dry throat, or bleeding while expectorating phlegm, hoarse voice. The representative formula is "Fritillaria and Trichosanthis Powder".

Fritillaria and Trichosanthis Powder(Bei Mu Gua Lou San)

【Source】*Medical Insights*.

【Composition】*Bulbus Fritillariae Cirrhosae* (4. 5 g), *Fructus Trichosanthis* (3 g), *Radix Trichosanthis* (2. 5 g), *Poria* (2. 5 g), *Exocarpium Citri Grandis* (2. 5 g), and *Radix Platycodi* (2. 5 g).

【Functions】Moisten lung, clear heat, modulate qi, and resolve phlegm.

【Indications】Cough due to dryness-phlegm, marked by cough, irritable and uneven rapid breath, being difficult to be expectorated, dry throat, and pain in the throat, white dry tongue coating.

【Explanation】In the formula, *Bulbus Fritillariae Cirrhosae* is the sovereign medicinal, and it clears heat and moistens the lung, resolves phlegm and arrests cough. *Fructus Trichosanthis*, as the minister medicinal, clears heat and moistens dryness, frees qi flow and cleanses phlegm. *Radix Trichosanthis* clears heat, resolves phlegm, generates fluid, and moistens dryness; *Poria* tonifies the spleen and drains dampness; *Exocarpium Citri Rubrum* transforms phlegm and arrests cough; *Radix Platycodi* diffuses the lung and soothes the throat. All of the above are the assistant medicinals. All the ingredients together achieve the success of moistening the lung, clearing heat, modulating qi, and resolving phlegm.

【Note】Not suitable for cough due to yin deficiency of lung and kidney, and upburning of deficiency heat.

【Variation】In case of concurrency of invaded wind, marked by itching in the throat, cough, aversion to wind, add *Folium Mori*, *Periostracum Cicadae*, *Semen Armeniacae Amarum* and *Fructus Arctii* to expel lung and dispel pathogen; for severe dryness-heat, marked by dryness and pain in the throat, add *Radix Scrophulariae*, *Radix Ophiopogonis*, and *Gypsum Fibrosum* to resolve dryness and moisten the lung; in case of hoarse voice and bleeding in phlegm, remove *Exocarpium Citri Rubrum*, add Radix *Adenophorae* and

（四）温化寒痰

温化寒痰剂，适用于寒痰证。症见咳痰清稀色白，自觉口中有冷气，身寒，手足不温，大便溏泄，舌苔水滑，脉沉。代表方剂：苓甘五味姜辛汤。

苓甘五味姜辛汤

【来源】《金匮要略》

【组成】茯苓（12克）甘草（9克）干姜（9克）细辛（3克）五味子（5克）

【功用】温肺化饮。

【主治】寒饮内停，症见咳嗽，痰稀色白量多，喜唾，胸满喘逆，舌苔白滑，脉沉迟。

【方解】方中干姜性味辛热，既温肺散寒以化饮，又温运脾阳以化湿，为君药。细辛辛散，温肺散寒，助干姜散其凝聚之饮；茯苓甘淡，健脾渗湿，不仅化既聚之痰，又能杜生痰之源，为臣药。五味子酸温，敛肺气而止咳，与细辛、干姜相伍，散中有收，使散不伤正、收不留邪，又能调和肺之开合，为佐药。甘草和中，调协诸药，为使药。

【注意事项】本方药力较峻，中气不足、脾肾阳虚、孕妇等皆需慎用。

【加减】痰多欲呕者，加半夏以化痰降逆止呕；兼有冲气上逆者，加桂枝以温中降冲；咳甚而颜面虚浮者，加杏仁宣利肺气而止咳。

十一、消导剂

消导剂是以消导药为主组成，具有消食健脾，除痞化积等作用，治疗食积停滞的方剂。消导剂虽功力较缓和，但终属攻伐之方，故不宜长期服用，而纯虚无实者更当禁用。根据作用不同，消导剂可分为消食化滞与健脾消食两类。

（一）消食化滞

消食化滞剂用于因饮食不节导致的食积停滞，症见胸脘痞满、腹胀时痛、嗳腐吞酸、呕恶厌食，或大便泄泻，舌苔厚腻而黄，脉滑。代表方剂：保和丸。

Rhizoma Bletillae to nourish yin, clear the lung heat, resolve phlegm and arrest bleeding.

Warming and resolving cold-phlegm formulas

Warming and resolving cold-phlegm formulas are applicable for cold-phlegm syndrome, marked by cough with white watery phlegm, sensation of cold air in the mouth, cold body and limbs, loose stools, watery tongue coating, sunken pulse. The representative formula is "Poria Licorice Schisandra Ginger and Asrum Decoction".

Poria Licorice Schisandra Ginger and Asrum Decoction
(Ling Gan Wu Wei Jiang Xin Tang)

【Source】*Treatise on Cold Damage Diseases.*

【Composition】*Poria* (12 g), *Radix Glycyrrhizae* (9 g), *Rhizoma Zingiberis* (9 g), *Herba Asari* (3 g), and *Fructus Schisandrae* (5 g).

【Functions】Warm the lung and resolve retained fluid.

【Indications】Cold retained fluid, marked by cough with profuse phlegm, white and watery phlegm, preference to spitting, fullness in the chest, asthma, white and greasy tongue coating, and sunken and slow pulse.

【Explanation】In the formula, the sovereign medicinal *Rhizoma Zingiberis*, which is acrid and hot, not only can warm the lung and dispel coldness to transform fluid, but also can warm the spleen yang to drain dampness. *Herba Asari* is acrid and has function of dispersing; it warms the lung to disperse coldness and helps *Rhizoma Zingiberis* to disperse condensed fluid. *Poria* is sweet and mild; it tonifies the spleen and drains dampness, transforms the condensed phlegm, and stops the generation of phlegm. *Herba Asri* and *Poria* serve as the minister medicinals. *Fructus Schisandrae* is sour and warm, and it restricts lung qi and arrests cough; when combined with *Herba Asari* and *Rhizoma Zingiberis*, it disperes pathogenic factors without comsuption of healthy qi and modulates the opening and closing fuctions of the lung, serving as the assistant medicinal. *Radix Glycyrrhizae* harmonizes the middle and modulates all the ingredients, serving as the courier medicinal.

【Note】The actions of the formula are strong, and it should be cautiously used in yang deficieny or qi deficieny of the middle, or in pregnant women.

【Variation】For profuse phlegm with desire to vomit, add *Rhizoma Pinelliae* to direct counterflow of qi downward to check vomiting and disperse phlegm; for concurrency with qi couterflow, add *Ramulus Cinnamomi* to warm the middle and direct qi downward; for severe cough and edema in the face, add *Semen Armeniacae Amarum* to direct lung qi downward and reliere cough.

Digestant Formulas

Digestant formulas are mainly composed of promoting digestion medicinals, and have functions of promoting digestion, tonifying the spleen, and removing accumulation. They are indicated for all kinds of food accumulation. Though the actions of the formulas are relatively mild, they belong to the therapeutic method of attacking and quelling. Thus, one should not apply the formulas for a long period of time, and the formulas are contraindicated for pure deficiency syndrome. According to their different fuctions, digestant formulas are classified as digestion-promoting and stagnation-dispersing formulas and spleen-tonifying and digestion-promoting formulas.

Digestion-promoting and stagnation-dispersing formulas

These formulas are indicated for food accumulation due to irregular diet, marked by glomus and fullness in the stomach duct and chest, turbid belching, distention and occasional abdominal pain, acid regurgitation, nausea, poor appetite, or diarrhea, yellow, thick greasy coating, and slippery pulse. The representa-

保和丸

【来源】《丹溪心法》

【组成】山楂（18克）神曲（6克）半夏　茯苓（各9克）陈皮　连翘　萝卜子（各3克）

【功用】消食和胃。

【主治】食积停滞，症见胸脘痞满，腹胀时痛，嗳腐吞酸，恶食，或呕吐泄泻，舌苔厚腻或黄，脉滑。

【方解】方中重用山楂为君药，能消一切饮食积滞，尤善消肉食油腻之积。臣以神曲消食健脾，善化酒食陈腐之积；莱菔子下气消食，长于消谷面之积。半夏和胃降气止呕，陈皮行气消滞止呕；茯苓健脾渗湿止泻；连翘清热疏风，此三者为佐药。全方共奏消食和胃、清热祛湿之功，以使食积得消，热清湿去，胃气得和。

【注意事项】本方虽药性平和，但毕竟为消导之品，故纯虚无实不可使用。孕妇慎用。

【加减】食滞较重者，可加枳实、槟榔等，以增强消食导滞之力；腹胀较重者，加枳实、厚朴等以行气消胀；食积化热较甚见苔黄、脉数者，加黄芩、黄连，以加强清热泻火之力；腹胀而大便不通或不利者，加大黄、槟榔以通便导滞；兼有脾虚腹泻者，加白术以益气健脾。夏令小儿腹泻属消化不良而见大便溏泄而酸臭、食欲不振、小便少、口渴者，加鸡内金、天花粉、麦冬等。小儿疳积，症见面黄肌瘦、低热困倦、胸痞腹胀、头大颈细、厌食、大便不爽者，加鸡内金、炮山甲、鳖甲等。

（二）健脾消食

健脾消食剂，用于脾胃虚弱，食积内停之证。临床症见脘腹痞满，不思饮食，面黄体瘦，倦怠乏力，大便溏薄等。代表方剂：健脾丸。

健脾丸

【来源】《证治准绳》

【组成】白术（15克）木香　黄连　甘草（各6克）白茯苓（12克）人参（9克）神曲　陈皮　砂仁　麦芽　山楂　山药　肉豆蔻（各6克）

【功用】健脾和胃，消食止泻。

【主治】脾虚食积证。症见食少难消，脘腹痞闷，大便溏薄，苔腻微黄，脉象虚弱。

【方解】方中白术、茯苓用量偏重，意在健脾渗湿以止泻，为君药；人参、山药

tive formula is "Preserving and Harmonizing Pills".

Preserving and Harmonizing Pills(Bao He Wan)

【Source】*Danxi's Experiential Therapy.*

【Composition】*Fructus Crataegi* (18 g) , *Massa Fermentata Medicinalis* (6 g) , *Rhizoma Pinelliae* (9 g) ,*Poria* (9 g) ,*Pericarpium Citri Reticulatae* (3 g) ,*Fructus Forsythiae* (3 g) , and *Semen Raphani* (3 g).

【Functions】Promote digestion and harmonize the stomach.

【Indications】Food accumulation , manifested as glomus , and fullness in the stomach duct and chest , distention , occational abdominal pain , tutrid belching , acrid regurgitation , aversion to food , nausea , or vomiting and diarrhea , thick and greasy fur or yellow fur , and slippery pulse.

【Explanation】In the formula , the sovereign medicinal *Fructus Crataegi* in high dose removes all kinds of food accumulation , and it is good at eliminating accumulation of greasy food and meat food. *Massa Fermentata Medicinalis* promotes digestion and tonifies the spleen , and it is good at dispersing stagnation of food and wine ; *Semen Raphani* precipitates qi and promotes digestion , and it is good at eliminating accumulation of grain food ; the above two medicinals serve as the minister medicinals. *Rhizoma Pinelliae* harmonizes the stomach and directs conterflow downward to check vomiting ; *Pericarpium Citri Reticulatae* moves qi and disperses stagnation to chectvomiting ; *Poria* tonifies the spleen and drains dampness to check diarrhea ; *Fructus Forsythiae* clears heat and dissipates wind , the above mentioned three medicinals are the assistant medicinals. All the ingridients are used together to achieve the actions of promoting digestion , harmonizing the stomach , clearing heat , and removing dampness , so as to remove food accumulation , remove dampness , clear heat , and harmonize the stomach qi.

【Note】Altough the effect of the formula is moderate , it still belongs to digestant formulas. It should not be used in conditions of pure deficiency without excess. The formula should be cautiously used in pregnant women.

【Variation】For severe food stagnation , add *Fructus Aurantii Immaturus* and *Semen Arecae* to reinforce the power of promoting digestion ; for severe distention , add *Fructus Aurantii Immaturus* and *Cortex Magnoliae Officinalis* to promote qi and relieve distention ; for severe heat pattern due to food accumulation , marked by yellow tongue coating and rapid pulse , add *Radix Scutellariae* and *Rhizoma Coptidis* to promote clearing heat and purging fire ; for distention and constipation , add *Radix et Rhizoma Rhei* and *Semen Arecae* to free the bowel and remove stagnation ; for concurrency of spleen deficiency marked by diarrhea , add *Rhizoma Atractylodis Macrocephalae* to tonify spleen qi. For summer diarrhea in children due to indigestion , marked by loose stools with sour and odor smell , poor appitite , short urination , and thirst , add *Endothelium Corneum Gigeriae Galli* , *Radix Trichosanthis* , and *Radix Ophiopogonis.* For infantile malnutrition with accumulation , marked by yellow complexion and thin , low fever , drowsiness , sensation of fullness in the chest , distention , big head and thin neck , aversion to food , and unsatisfied stool , add *Endothelium Corneum Gigeriae Galli* , *Squama Manitis* , and *Carapax Trionycis.*

Spleen-tonifying and digestion-promoting formulas

These formulas are applicable for internal food accumulation due to spleen-stomach deficiency syndrome , clinically marked by fullness in abdomen , averstion to foods and drinks , yellow complexion and thin , fatigue , drowsiness , and loose stools. The representative formula is "Tonfiying the Spleen Pills".

Spleen-tonifying Pills(Jian Pi Wan)

【Source】*Standards of Syndrome Identification and Treatment.*

【Composition】*Rhizoma Atractylodis* (15 g) ,*Radix Aucklandiae* (6 g) ,*Rhizoma Coptidis* (6 g) ,*Ra-*

益气健脾，助茯苓、白术健脾。山楂、神曲、麦芽能消食化滞，可消一切食积，共为臣药。木香、砂仁、陈皮理气和胃，助运消痞；肉豆蔻温涩，合山药涩肠止泻；黄连清热燥湿，清食积所化之热，同为佐药。甘草补中和药，是为佐使之用。全方消补兼施，健脾消食，祛湿清热。

【注意事项】实热者不宜使用。

【加减】积滞中焦，胃失和降而见呕吐者，加半夏、丁香以降逆止呕；中虚寒凝致腹痛较剧者，加干姜、木香、白芍以散寒行气止痛；大便溏薄、小便少者，加薏苡仁、茯苓以健脾渗湿止泻。

（张孟仁）

dix Glycyrrhizae (6 g) , *Poria* (12 g) , *Radix Ginseng* (9 g) , *Massa Fermentata Medicinalis* (6 g) , *Pericarpium Citri Reticulatae* (6 g) , *Fructus Amoni* (6 g) , *Fructus Hordei Germinatus* (6 g) , *Frutus Crataegi* (6 g) , and *Semen Myristicae* (6 g) .

〖Functions〗Fortify the spleen and harmonize the stomach , promote digestion , and check diarrhea.

〖Indications〗Food accumulation due to spleen deficiency , marked by less food intake , indigestion , fullness and oppression in the stomach duct and abdomen , loose stools , slightly yellow and greasy tongue fur , and weak pulse.

〖Explanation〗In the formula , *Poria* and *Rhizoma Atractylodis Macrocephalae* are used in major dosage to fortify the spleen and drain dampness to check diarrhea , both are the sovereign medicinals. *Gingseng* and *Rhizoma Dioscoreae* tonify qi , and help *Poria* and *Rhizoma Atractylodis Macrocephalae* to tonify the spleen ; *Fructus Crataegi* , *Massa Fermentata Medicinalis* , and *Fructus Hordei Germinatus* promote digestion , remove accumulation , and treat all kinds of food accumulation ; all the above mentioned ingredients are the minister medicinals. *Radix Aucklandiae* , *Fructus Amomi* , and *Pericarpium Citri Reticulatae* modulate qi , harmonize the stomach , promote digestion , and remove accumulation ; *Semen Myristicae* is warm and astringe , together with *Rhizoma Dioscoreae* , it can astringe the intestines and check diarrhea ; *Rhizoma Coptidis* clears heat and drys dampness ; all the above mentioned medicinals are the assistant medicinals. *Radix Glycyrrhizae* tonifies the middle and harmonizes all ingredients , serving as the assistant and courier medicinal. All the ingredients are used together to eliminate food accumulation , remove dampness , and clear heat.

〖Note〗Contraindicated for patients of excess heat syndrome.

〖Variation〗For vomiting due to accumulation in the middle and disharmony of the stomach , add *Rhizoma Pinelliae* and *Flos Caryophylli* to descend qi and stop vomiting ; for severe abdominal pain due to deficiency cold of the spleen and stomach , add *Rhizoma Zingiberis* , *Radix Aucklandiae* , and *Radix Paeoniae Alba* to disperse cold , promote qi , and relieve pain ; for loose stools and short urination , add *Semen Coicis* and *Poria* to tonify the spleen , eliminate dampness , and check diarrhea.

(*Piao Yuanlin   Zhang Wen*)

第十章　针　　灸

针灸学是以中医理论为指导，运用针刺和艾灸防治疾病的一门临床学科。针灸学的内容包括经络、腧穴、刺灸法、临床治疗、针灸古籍和实验针灸等。针灸具有适应证广泛、经济安全、操作方便、疗效显著等特点。世界卫生组织向世界各国推荐针灸治疗43种疾病，目前全世界已有一百多个国家和地区开展了针灸医疗、科研和教育。

第一节　经络的概念及其临床应用

经络是经脉和络脉的总称。经络是运行气血的通路。经和络既有联系又有区别。经，"径也"，有路径的含义，是较粗大的干线，经脉贯通上下，沟通内外，是经络系统中的主干；络，"网也"，有网络的含义，络脉是经脉别出的分支，较经脉细小，纵横交错，遍布全身。《灵枢·脉度》载："经脉为里，支而横者为络，络之别者为孙。"经络内属于脏腑，外络于肢节，沟通于脏腑与体表之间，将人体各部的组织器官联系成为一个有机的整体，从而运行气血，营养全身，使人体各部的功能活动得以保护协调和相对平衡。

一、经络系统的组成

经络系统是由经脉和络脉组成的，其中经脉包括十二经脉和奇经八脉，以及附属于十二经脉的十二经别、十二经筋、十二皮部。络脉有十五络脉、浮络、孙络等（图 10-1）。

（一）十二经脉

1. 十二经脉的命名　十二经脉的命名是结合手足、阴阳、脏腑三个方面而定的。分布于上肢的经脉，在经脉名称之前冠以"手"字；分布于下肢的经脉，在经脉名

CHAPTER TEN   ACUPUNCTURE AND MOXIBUSTION

The science of acupuncture and moxibustion is a subject dealing with the prevention and treatment of diseases by needling and moxibustion, based on TCM theory. The science of acupuncture and moxibustion includes meridians and collaterals, acupoints, acupuncture techniques, clinical treatment, acupunctural ancient books, and experimental acupuncture. Acupuncture has characteristics of wide range of indications, economic security, simple application, and good curative effect. The World Health Organization has recommended acupuncture treatment to treat 43 diseases all over the world. Currently over one hundred countries and area around the world carry out the acupuncture health care, education and scientific research.

Section 1   Concept of Meridian and Its Clinical Application

The meridians and collaterals are comprehensively termed "Jingluo" in TCM, which is the pathway of qi and blood. There are relations and differences between meridians and collaterals. The meridians, meaning paths, are the main trunks which longitudinally and interiorly-exteriorly within the body; while the collaterals, meaning networks, thinner and smaller than meridians, are the branches which run crisscrossly over the body. The chapter, Discussion on the Measurement of Meridians (Chapter 17) in *Miraculous Pivot* says, "the meridians are internal trunks, their transversing branches are collaterals, the subdivisions of collaterals are minute collaterals." The meridians and collaterals pertain to the viscera and bowels interiorly and extend to the extremities and joints exteriorly, integrating the viscera and bowels, tissues, and organs into an organic whole, by which they transport qi and blood and regulate yin and yang, keeping the functions and activities of all parts of the body in harmony and balance relatively.

The Composition of the System of the Meridians and Collaterals

The system of meridians and collaterals is composed of meridians and collaterals. The meridians include the twelve main meridians, eight extra meridians and those subordinating to the twelve main meridians, including the twelve meridian divergences, twelve meridian sinews and twelve cutaneous regions; while the collaterals are made up of the fifteen collaterals, superficial collaterals and minute collaterals. (Figure 10-1)

The Twelve Main Meridians

1. The nomenclature of the twelve main meridians

The twelve regular meridians' nomenclature is based on the three factors: hand or foot, yin or yang, and a zang-organ (viscera) or fu-organ (bowel). Meridians located in the upper limbs are preceded the

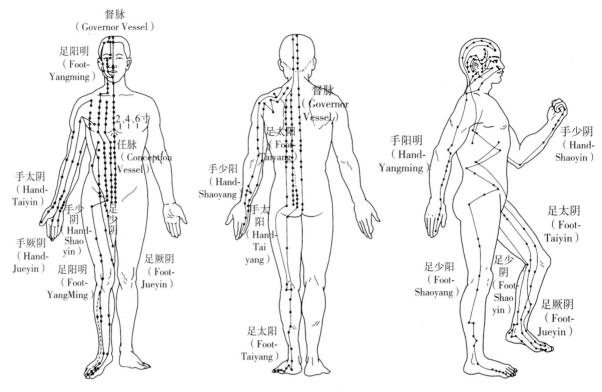

图 10-1 十四经脉循行分布示意图

(Distribution of the Fourteen Meridians)

称之前冠以"足"字。根据脏属阴、腑属阳、内侧为阴、外侧为阳的原则，肢体内侧面的前、中、后分别称为太阴、厥阴、少阴；肢体外侧面的前、中、后分别称为阳明、少阳、太阳。把各经所属脏腑结合循行于四肢的部位，定出各经的名称（表10-1）。

表 10-1　十二经脉名称及表里属络关系

手足	阴经（属脏）	阳经（属腑）	循行部位（阴经行于内侧，阳经行于外侧）	
手	太阴肺经	阳明大肠经	上肢	前线
	厥阴心包经	少阳三焦经		中线
	少阴心经	太阳小肠经		后线
足	太阴脾经	阳明胃经	下肢	前线
	厥阴肝经	少阳胆经		中线
	少阴肾经	太阳膀胱经		后线

word "hand" before their names; in turn, meridians located in the lower limbs, are dubbed the "foot" before their names. In accordance with the principles that viscera pertain to yin and bowels pertain to yang, interior is yin and exterior is yang; the anterior, medium and posterior of the inner sides of limbs are named "taiyin", "jueyin" and "shaoyin" respectively; and the anterior, medium and posterior sides of the outer sides of limbs are named "yangming", "shaoyang" and "taiyang." Each meridian's name is determinded by combining its related internal organ and its distribution of the limb (Table 10-1).

Table 10-1   The Names and Externally-Internally Pertaining Relationships of the Twelve Main Meridians

Hand or Foot	Yin Meridians (pertaining to zang-organs)	Yang Meridians (pertaining to *fu*-organs)	Circulation Region (the Yin Meridians run in the medial part, while the Yang Merians run in the lateral part)	
Hand	Lung Meridian of Hand-Taiyin	Large Intestine Meridian of Hand-Yangming	Upper Limbs	Anterior Line
	Pericardium of Hand-Jueyin	Triple Energizer Meridian of Hand-Shaoyang		Middle Line
	Heart Meridian of Hand-Shaoyin	Small Intestine Meridian of Hand-Taiyang		Posterior Line
Foot	Spleen Meridian of Foot-Taiyin	Stomach Meridian of Foot Yangming	Lower Limbs	Anterior Line
	Liver Meridian of Foot-Jueyin	Gallbladder Meridian of Foot-Shaoyang		Middle Line
	Kidney Meridian of Foot-Shaoyin	Bladder Meridian of Foot-Taiyang		Posterior Line

2. Distribution of the twelve main meridians

The meridians pertaining to six zang-organs (five zang and pericardium) are yin meridians; while the meridians pertaining to six fu-organs are yang meridians. The twelve main meridians are distributed symmetrically at the left and right sides of the head, face, trunk and four limbs, all over the body. The six yin meridians are distributed at the medial aspect of the limbs and ventrum, among which three of them at medial of upper limbs are three hand yin meridians, while three of them at medial of lower limbs are three foot yin meridians. The six yan meridians are mainly distributed at the lateral aspect of the limbs, head, face and trunk, among which three of them at lateral of upper limbs are three hand yang meridians, while three of them at lateral of lower limbs are three foot yang meridians.

Distribution of the twelve meridians in the head, truck, and four limbs: on the limbs, the anterior ones of three hand and foot yang meridians are Yangming, the medial ones of three hand and foot yang meridians are Shaoyang, the posterior ones of three hand and foot yang meridians are Taiyang; the anterior ones of three hand and foot yin meridians are Taiyin, the medial ones of three hand and foot yin meridians are Jueyin, the posterior ones of three hand and foot yin meridians are Shaoyin. The three foot yin meridians going in the lower half of leg and dorsal, the anterior one is Jueyin, the medial one is Taiyin, the posterior one is Shaoyin; while after the three foot yin meridians going to the eights *cun* beyond the medial malleolu and the foot Jueyin and the foot Taiyin crossing each other, the anterior one is Taiyin, the medial one is Jueyin, the posterior one is Shaoyin.

3. Externally-internally pertaining relationship of the twelve meridians

The twelve meridians pertain to viscus and fu-organs which have the externally-internally pertaining relationship of viscera and bowels, the yin meridians and yang meridians also have the externally-internally pertaining relationship. For example, the lung meridian of Hand-Taiyin pertains to the lung and connects the large intestine, while the large intestine meridian of Hand-Yangming pertains to the large intestine and connects the lung. The twelve meridians have six pairs of the externally-internally pertaining relationships (Table 10-1).

2. 十二经脉在体表的分布规律 凡属六脏（五脏加心包）的经脉称"阴经"，凡属六腑的经脉称为"阳经"。它们从左右对称地分布于头面、躯干和四肢，纵贯全身。六条阴经循行于四肢内侧及胸腹部，其中上肢内侧者为手三阴经，下肢内侧者为足三阴经；六条阳经多循行四肢外侧面及头面、躯干部，其中上肢外侧者为手三阳经，下肢外侧者为足三阳经。

十二经脉的头身四肢的分布规律是：手足三阳经为"阳明"在前，"少阳"在中，"太阳"在后；手足三阴经为"太阴"在前，"厥阴"在中，"少阴"在后。足三阴经在小腿下半部及足背，其排列是"厥阴"在前，"太阴"在中，"少阴"在后。至内踝上八寸处足厥阴经同足太阴经交叉后，循行在太阴与少阴之间，便成为"太阴"在前，"厥阴"在中，"少阴"在后。

3. 十二经脉的表里属络关系 十二经脉内属于脏腑，脏与腑有表里相合的关系，阴经与阳经有表里属络关系。阴经属脏络腑，阳经属腑络脏。如手太阴肺经属肺络大肠，手阳明大肠经属大肠络肺。十二经脉构成六对表里属络关系（表10-1）。

4. 十二经脉的循行走向规律 十二经脉的循行有一定的方向，其走向规律是：手三阴经从胸走手，手三阳经从手走头，足三阳经从头走足，足三阴经从足走腹（胸）。

5. 十二经脉的交接规律
（1）阴经与阳经在手足部交接。
（2）阳经与阳经在头面部交接。
（3）阴经与阴经在胸腹部交接。

走向与交接规律之间也有密切联系，两者结合起来，则是：手三阴经，从胸走手，交手三阳经；手三阳经，从手走头，交足三阳经；足三阳经，从头走足，交足三阴经；足三阴经，从足走腹（胸），交手三阴经。

6. 十二经脉的流注次序 经络是人体气血运行的通道，而十二经脉则为气血运行的主要通道，它们首尾相贯、依次衔接，因而脉中气血的运行也是循经脉依次传注的。由于全身气血皆由脾胃运化的水谷之精化生，故十二经脉气血的流注从起于手太阴肺经开始，依次流注各经，最后传至足厥阴肝经，复再回到手太阴肺经。

（二）奇经八脉

奇经八脉，包括督脉、任脉、冲脉、带脉、阳跷脉、阴跷脉、阳维脉、阴维脉的总称。它们与十二正经不同，既不直属脏腑，又无表里配合关系，故称"奇经八脉"。八脉中的任、督、冲脉皆起于胞中，同出会阴，称为"一源三岐"。其中督脉行于腰背正中线，上至头面；任脉行于胸腹正中，上抵颏部；冲、带、跷、维六脉的穴位均交汇于十二经与任、督脉中。

4. Distribution of the twelve meridians

The distribution of the twelve meridians has certain pattern: the three hand yin meridians go from the chest to hand, the three hand yang meridians go from hand to head, the three foot yang meridians go from head to foot, the three yin meridians go from foot to abdomen(chest).

5. Principle of connection of the twelve meridians

The yin meridians connect with the yang meridians in the hands and feet.

The yang meridians connect with the yin meridians in the head and face.

The yin meridians connect with the yin meridians in the chest and abdomen.

The principles of distribution and connection of the twelve meridians have close relationship. We make these two principles together and we get: the three hand yin meridians run from the chest to the hand, connecting with the three hand yang meridians; the three foot yang meridians run from the hand to the head, connecting with the three foot yang meridians; the three foot yang meridians run from the head to the foot, connecting with the three foot yin meridians; the three foot yin meridians run from the foot to the abdomen(chest), connecting with the three hand yin meridians.

6. Circle flow of qi in the twelve main meridians

The meridians and collaterals are pathways of qi and blood, while the twelve meridians are the main meridian of qi and blood running, they are intersecting, in sequence, thus the circulation of qi and blood of pulse is followed by injection of meridians. Since qi and blood is produced by the spleen and stomach, the flow of qi and blood of the twelve meridians starts from the lung meridian of Hand-Taiyin in the middle energizer, followed by each meridians in sequence, spreads to the liver meridian of Foot-Jueyin at last, then returns to the lung meridian of Hand-Taiyin.

Eight extra meridians

The eight extra meridians are the governor vessel, conception vessel, thoroughfare vessel, belt vessel, yang heel vessel, yin heel vessel, yang link vessel, and yin link vessel. They are different from the twelve main meridians because none of them pertains to the viscera or the bowels, and without exteriorly-interiorly relationships, and are called the eight extra meridians. The governor vessel, conception vessel, thoroughfare vessel all arise from the lower abdomen and emerge from the perineum. The governor vessel runs along the midline of the back and ascends to the head and face, while the conception vessel runs along the midline of the abdomen and the chest, and goes upward to the chin. All the acupuncture points of the thoroughfare vessel, belt vessel, heel vessels, and link vessels meet the twelwe main meridians, the governor vessel and conception vessel.

The eight extra meridians interact vertically and horizontally with the twelve meridians. All the points of the thoroughfare vessel, the belt vessel, the heel vessels, and the link vessels are affiliated to the twelve meridians, the conception vessel and the governor vessel. Since the conception vessel and the governor vessel have their own points, they are usually mentioned together with the twelve meridians, collectively known as the fourteen meridians(Figure 10-1).

The eight extra meridians mainly have two functions. One is strengthening the association among the meridians, and the other is the regulation functions of storing and irrigating of qi and blood flow of the twelve meridians.

The conception vessel: it meets all the yin meridians. It is described as "the sea of the yin meridians." Its function is to receive and bear the qi of the yin meridians.

The governor vessel: it meets all the yang meridians. It is described as "the sea of the yang meridians." Its function is to govern the qi of all the yang meridians.

奇经八脉的分布与十二经脉纵横交互，冲脉、带脉、跷脉、维脉六脉的腧穴都寄附于十二经与任、督脉之中。任、督二脉各有本经所属穴位，故与十二经脉相提并论，合称为"十四经"（图 10-1）。

奇经八脉作用主要体现于两个方面：其一，是沟通了十二经脉之间的联系；其二，是对十二经脉的气血运行起蓄积、渗灌调节作用。

1. 任脉　为诸条阴经交会之脉，称"阴脉之海"，具有调节全身阴经经气的作用。

2. 督脉　诸阳经均与其交会，称"阳脉之海"，具有调节全身阳经经气的作用。

3. 冲脉　十二经脉均与其交会，称"十二经之海"、"血海"，具有涵蓄十二经气血的作用。

4. 带脉　约束联系了纵行躯干部的诸经。

5. 阴维脉、阳维脉　分别调节六阴经和六阳经的经气，分别主管一身之表里，以维持阴阳协调和平衡。

6. 阴跷脉、阳跷脉　主持阳动阴静，共同调节下肢运动和眼睑的开合与睡眠。

由于十四经具有一定的循环路线和病候及其专属腧穴主治，它不但是经络系统的主干，而且在临床上还是辨证归经、诊断疾病和循经取穴施治的基础。

（三）十五络脉

十二经脉和任、督二脉各自别出一络，加上脾之大络，称为十五络脉。十二经脉的别络均从本经四肢肘膝关节以下的络穴分出，走向其相表里的经脉，即阴经别络于阳经，阳经别络于阴经。此外，从络脉分出的浮行于浅表部位的称为"浮络"，络脉中最细小的分支称为"孙络"。

四肢部的十二经别络，加强了十二经中表里两经的联系，沟通了表里两经的经气，补充了十二经脉循行的不足。躯干部的任脉别络、督脉别络和脾之大络，分别沟通了腹、背和全身经气，输布气血以濡养全身组织。

（四）十二经别

十二经别是十二正经离、入、出、合的别行部分，是正经别行深入体腔的支脉。十二经别多从四肢肘膝关节以上的正经别出（离），经过躯干深入体腔与相关的脏腑联系（入），再浅出于体表上行头项部（出），在头项部，阳经经别合于本经的经脉，阴经经别合于其相表里的阳经经脉（合）。十二经别按阴阳表里关系汇合成六组，在头项部合于六阳经脉，故有"六合"之称。

由于十二经别有离、入、出、合于表里之间的特点，不仅加强了十二经脉的内外联系，更加强了经脉所属络的脏腑在体腔深部的联系，补充了十二经脉在体内外循行的不足，扩大了手足三阴经穴位的主治范围。

The thoroughfare vessel: it meets all the twelve main meridians, and is termed as "the sea of the twelve main meridians" or "the sea of blood". Its function is to reserve qi and blood of the twelve main meridians.

The belt vessel: it goes around the waist as a girdle, controlling and associating all meridians running vertically around trunk.

The yin heel vessel and yang heel vessel: these two heel vessels regulate the qi of the six yin and six yang meridians respectively, manage the inferior and the external of the body, maintain the coordinate and balance of yin and yang.

The yin link vessel and yang link vessel: these two link vessels take charge of yin and yang, move and quiet, regulate the movement of the lower extremity and open and closing of the eyelids and sleep respectively.

Fifteen collaterals

The fifteen collaterals include the twelve collaterals which separate from the twelve regular channels, the collaterals of the conception vessel and the governor vessel and the major collaterals of the spleen. The collaterals of the twelve meridians all derive from the connecting points of their original meridians which are located in the lower regions of the elbow joints and the knee joints, and then they reach deeply to their externally-internally related meridians. Thus, the collaterals of yin meridians connect with the yang meridians, vice versa. In addition, superficial collaterals are those which are distributed on the superficial parts of the body. The smallest branches of the collaterals are called minute collaterals.

The twelve collaterals of the twelve meridians which are in the four limbs strengthen the association of the externally-internally related meridians of the body, they connect meridian qi of the externally-internally related meridians, and supplyment the insufficiency of the twelve meridians' circulation. The collaterals of the trunk, the collaterals of the conception vessel and governor vessel and the major collaterals of the spleen, respectively connect meridian qi of the whole body especially the abdomen and back, distributing qi and blood to nourish the whole body.

Twelve meridian divergences

The twelve meridian divergences are the branches which derive from, enter, emerge from, and join the twelve regular meridians which, in turn, reach the deeper parts of the body through these branches. Most of the twelve menidian divergences derive from the regular meridians at the upper and lower regions of the elbows and the knees and then enter the thoracic and abdominal cavities, where they connect their pertaining viscera or bowels to which they pertain. Then, they emerge from the body surface at the head and the neck. In the regions, the yang meridian divergenecs join the regulate channels, and the yin menidian divergences connect the internally-externally related yang meridian divergences. The twelve meridian divergences formed six groups based on their exterior-interior related relationships, they converge the six yang meridians in the head and neck, which are called six convergence.

Because the twelve meridian divergences have characteristics of departing, entering, exiting and emerging between the exterior and interior, they not only strengthen the association of the externally-internally related meridians of the body, but also promote the connection between the externally-internally related meridians and related viscera or bowels, supplyment the insufficiency of circulation of the twelve meridians, thus, they expand the scope of the treatment of three hand yin meridians and three foot yin meridians.

（五）十二经筋

十二经筋是十二经脉之气输布于筋肉骨节的体系，是十二经脉的外周联属部分。其循行分布均起始于四肢末端，走向躯干头面，行于体表，不入内脏，结聚于关节、骨骼部。经筋的作用主要是约束骨骼，利于关节屈伸活动，维持人体正常运动功能。经筋为病，多为转筋、筋痛、痹证等。

（六）十二皮部

十二皮部是十二经脉功能活动反映于体表的部位，也是络脉之气散布之所在。十二皮部的分布区域是以十二经脉在体表的分布范围。由于十二皮部居于人体最外层，又与经络气血相通，是体机的卫外屏障，起着保卫机体、抗御外邪和反映病证的作用。

上述十二经脉、奇经八脉、十五络脉、十二经别、十二经筋、十二皮部等共同组成经络系统，成为不可分割的整体。

二、经络的生理功能及经络学说在临床上的应用

（一）经络的生理功能

经络的功能活动，主要表现在沟通表里上下，联络脏腑器官，运行气血，感应传导及调节人体各部分机能平衡等方面。经络具有联系脏腑和肢体的作用。人体是由五脏六腑、四肢百骸、五官九窍、皮肉筋骨等组成。它们虽各有不同的生理功能，但又互相协作，使机体保持着协调和统一。十二经脉及其十二经别纵横交错，入里出表，通上达下，循行络属于脏腑和官窍之间；奇经八脉沟通于十二经之间；十二经筋、十二皮部联络筋脉皮肉。

1. 联络脏腑，沟通内外　经络具有联络脏腑和肢体的作用。经络能沟通表里、联络上下、将人体各部的组织器官联结成一个有机的整体。人体的五脏六腑、四肢百骸、五官九窍、皮肉筋骨等组织器官，之所以能保持相对的平衡与统一，完成正常的生理活动，是依靠经络系统的联络沟通而实现的。

2. 运行气血，协调阴阳　人体生命活动的物质基础是气血，其作用是濡润全身脏腑组织器官，使人体完成正常的生理功能。经络是人体气血运行的通道，通过经络系统将气血及营养物质输送到周身，从而完成和调于五脏、洒陈于六腑的生理功能。

3. 抗御外邪，保卫机体　由于经络能"行气血而营阴阳"，营气运行于脉中，卫气运行于脉外，使营卫之气密布于周身，加强了机体的防御能力。

4. 传导感应，调整虚实　针灸、按摩、气功等方法能防病治病，正是基于经络具有传导感应和调整虚实的作用。《灵枢·官能》说，"审于调气，明于经隧"，说明

Twelve meridian sinews

The twelve meridian sinews are the conduits which distribute the qi of the twelve regular meridians to the muscles, tendons, and joints, and they are the external connecting regions of the twelve regular meridians. All the distributions of the meridian sinews start from the tips of the limbs and turn on to the head and trunk. Instead of entering viscera and bowels, they travel along the body surface, and connect with the joints and bones. The main functions of the meridian sinews are controlling all the bones to ensure flexing and extending of the joints and maintain normal motion of the body. The diseases of the meridian sinews are mainly cramp, pain and impairment, etc.

Twelve cutaneous regions

The twelve cutaneous regions refer to the regions of the skin reflecting the functions of the twelve regular meridians respectively, also they are the regions where the qi of the collaterals spreads. The twelve cutaneous regions are in accordance with the domains of the twelve regular meridians. Since the cutaneous regions are the most superficial part of the body tissues, and they connect with the qi and blood of the twelve meridians, they are the protection to the organism, playing roles of protecting the body, resisting the external pathogenic factors, and manifesting the diseases.

The above-mentioned twelve regular meridians, eight extra meridians, fifteen collaterals, twelve meridian divergences, twelve meridian sinews and twelve cutaneous regions add up to the integrated system of the meridians and collaterals.

Physiological Functions of the Meridians and Collaterals and Clinical Application of the Theory of the Meridians and Collaterals

Physiological functions of the meridians and collaterals

The meridians and collaterals connect the upper and the lower, the interior and the exterior of the body, integrating all the five viscera and six bowels, transporting qi and blood, responsing, transmitting and regulating the balance of all parts of the human body. The meridians and collaterals have the function of connecting the viscera and bowels and the limbs. The human body is made upconsists of five viscera and six bowels, all limbs and bones, five sense organs, nine orifices, skins, muscles, tendons and bones, which have different physiological functions and, make the body maintain proper coordination and unification. The twelve regular meridians and the twelve meridian divergences run vertically and horizontally, communicate the upper and lower, the interior or exterior of the body, circulating and pertaining to all the viscera and bowels, sense organs, and orifices. The eight extra meridians communicate between the twelve meridians. The twelve meridian sinews, the twelve cutaneous regions connect tendons, vessels, skins, and muscles.

1. Connecting the viscera and bowels, communicating the interior and exterior

The meridians and collaterals have the function of connecting the viscera and bowels and the limbs. The meridians and collaterals run vertically and horizontally, communicate with all parts, upper and lower, interior or exterior of the body, integrating all the five viscera and six bowels, five sense organs, nine orifices, skins, muscles, tendons and bones of the human body into an organic whole, and ensuring a proper coordination and unification of the various functions of the body.

2. Transporting qi and blood and regulating yin and yang

The material basis of human life activity is qi and blood, whose role is moistening the viscera and bowels and tissues of the whole body to complete the normal physiological functions. The meridians and collaterals are channels transporting qi and blood, delivering qi, blood and nutrients to the whole body, thus completing the physiological function of nourishing the five viscera and six bowels.

运用针灸等治法要讲究"调气"，要明了经络的通路。针刺治疗必须"得气"，针刺中的"得气"现象是经络传导感应现象的表现。针灸就是通过相应的穴位和运用适量的刺激方法激发经络本身的功能，调节机体失常的机能使之趋向平衡。

（二）经络学说在临床上的应用

1. 说明病理变化　经络具有传注病邪、反映病候的功能。由于经络是人体通内达外的一个通道，在生理功能失调时，其又是病邪传注的途径，具有反映病候的特点，在临床某些病证的病理过程中，常常在经络循行通路上出现明显的压痛或结节、条索状等反应物，以及相应的部位皮肤色泽、形态、温度、电阻等的变化。通过望色、循经触摸反应物和按压等，可推断疾病的病理变化。当外邪侵犯人体时，病邪就沿着经络、自外而内，由表及里地传变。内脏病变也可以通过经络反映到体表的一定部位。有时内脏疾患还在头面五官等部位出现反应。如心火上炎可致口舌生疮；肝火上炎致耳目肿赤；肾气亏虚可使耳失聪。

2. 指导辨证归经　由于经络有一定的循行部位及所络属的脏腑及组织器官，根据体表相关部位发生的病理变化，可推断疾病的经脉和病位所在。临床上可根据所出现的证候，结合其所联系的脏腑，进行辨证归经。例如头痛可根据经脉在头部的循行分布规律加以辨别，如前额痛多与阳明经有关；巅顶痛则与足厥阴经、督脉有关。

3. 指导疾病的治疗及预防保健作用　针灸选穴，一般是在明确辨证的基础上，除选用局部腧穴外，常根据经脉循行和主治特点采用循经取穴进行治疗。例如，前额头痛与阳明经有关，可循经选取上肢的合谷穴、下肢的内庭穴治疗。还可用调理经络的方法，来预防保健。如灸大椎、风门可预防感冒；常灸足三里、关元、气海、三阴交可强壮身体、防病保健。

3. Resisting pathogens and protecting the body

The meridians and collaterals transport qi and blood and nourish yin and yang, and the nutrient qi runs within the interior vessels meridians, while the defensive qi runs outside the vessels, which making nutrient qi run along all the whole body to strengthen the resistance.

4. Transmitting needling sensation and regulating deficiency and excess conditions

The acupuncture, moxibustion and qigong prevent and treat diseases based on the meridians and collateral's functions of transmitting needling sensation and regulating deficiency and excess conditions. It is said in Miraculous Pivot that "one should consider carefully when regulating qi, and shoud fully understand the channels," which states that regulating qi is very important for above-mentioned therapies. Arrival of qi is critical for needling, which is the manifestation of meridians's transmitting needling sensation. The therapeutic actions of meridians acupuncture and moxibustion are realized mainly through the function of meridians and collaterals in regulating yin and yang. The treatment of acupuncture and moxibustion is to apply appropriate stimulation on certain points to promote the function of the meridians and collaterals, in order to regulate the disharmony towards a balance.

Clinical application of the theory of the meridians and collaterals

1. Explaining the pathogenic changes

The meridians and collaterals have the function of transmitting pathogenic factors and reflecting the disorders. Since the meridians and collaterals are channels from the interior to the exterior of the human body, and the channels transmitting pathogenic factors during the process of disorders, manifested as pressing pain, nodules, cords, and other reactants, or the change of skin color, shape, temperature, resistance in the corresponding parts. Through inspection of the complexion and by touching and pressing the reactants along the meridians, the disorders can be distinguished. The external pathogenic factors invade the human body from the exterior to the interior along the meridians. The disorders of internal organs can be manifested in the superficial skin through the meridians and collaterals. Sometimes the diseases of internal organs can be manifested in the head, face, and five sense organs. For example, heart fire flaming causes results in mouth and tongue sores, liver fire flaming upward causes red swollen eyes and ears, and kidney deficiency causes deafness.

2. Guiding the syndrome differentiation and channel entry

Meridians and collaterals have certain distribution location and pertaining viscera and bowels and tissues. According to the pathogenic changes of superficial skin, the location and meridian of disorder can be distinguished, guiding the syndrome differentiation and channel entry. For example, for the different kinds of headache, pain in the forehead concerns the yangming meridian; vertex pain concerns the liver meridian and the govorner vessel.

3. Guiding the treatment and prevention of diseases

The selection of points are based on the differentiation of syndromes, points are selected according to their indications and the course of meridians, in addition to the selection of local points. For example, Hegu (LI 4) in the upper limbs and Neiting (ST 44) in lower limbs are selected in case of pain in the forehead related to the stomach and large intestine meridians. In addition, regulating meridians and collaterals can prevent diseases. For example, moxibustion on Dazhui (GV 14) and Fengmen (BL 12) can prevent cold, moxibustion on Zusanli (ST 36), Guanyuan (KI 13), Qihai (KI 15) and Sanyinjiao (SP 6) can strengthen the body and prevent diseases.

第二节 腧穴学的概念及其临床应用

腧穴是人体脏腑经络气血输注于体表的部位。腧与"输"通，有传输的含义，"穴"即孔隙的意思。在历代文献中，腧穴有"砭灸处"、"节"、"会"、"气穴"、"骨空"等不同名称，俗称"穴位"。

人体的腧穴均分别归属于各经络，而经络又隶属于一定的脏腑，这就使腧穴、经络、脏腑间的相互联系成为不可分割的关系。腧穴是针灸施术的部位。

一、腧穴的分类

腧穴可分为十四经穴、奇穴、阿是穴三类。

（一）十四经穴

十四经穴为位于十二经脉和任督二脉的腧穴，简称"经穴"。它是腧穴的主体，现有 362 个经穴。经穴因其分布在十四经脉的循行线上，所以与经脉关系密切。它不仅可以反映本经经脉及其所属脏腑的病证，也可以反映本经脉所联系的其他经脉、脏腑的病证，同时又是针灸施治的部位。因此，腧穴不仅有治疗本经脏腑病证的作用，也可以治疗与本经相关经络、脏腑的病证。

（二）奇穴

奇穴是指未能归属于十四经脉的腧穴，它既有一定的穴名，又有明确的位置，又称"经外奇穴"。这些腧穴对某些病证具有特殊的治疗作用。奇穴因其所居人体部位的不同，其分布也不尽相同。有些位于经脉线外，如中泉、中魁；有些在经脉线内，如肘尖；有些是穴位组合之奇穴，如四神聪、四缝等穴。

（三）阿是穴

阿是穴又称压痛点、天应穴、不定穴等。这一类腧穴既无具体名称，又无固定位置，而是以压痛点或其他反应点作为针灸部位。阿是穴多位于病变的附近，也可在与其距离较远的部位。阿是穴是十四经穴与经外奇穴的补充，无一定数目。

二、腧穴的治疗作用

（一）近治作用

这是所有腧穴主治作用所具有的共同的特点。这些腧穴均能治疗该穴所在部位及邻近组织、器官的病症。如巅顶头痛取百会；胃痛取中脘；牙痛取下关；肩关节痛取肩髃等。

Section 2   Concept and Clinical Application of Acupuncture points

Acupuncture points are the sites through which the qi of the viscera and bowels and meridians is transported to the body surface. The Chinese characters "腧穴" respectively means "transportation" and "holes". In the medical literature of the past dynasties, acupuncture points have other terms such as "bianjiuchu(position for pressing or moxibustion)", "jie (cross)", "hui (joint)", "qixue (qi cell)", and "gukong(interspace between bones)", and are commonly known as acupoints.

Acupoints of the body are attributed to each meridian, while the meridians pertain to certain organs, which make the inter-linkages between the acupoints, meridians, organs into an inseparable organic whole. The acupuncture points are the sites of for acupuncture in the treatments.

Classification of acupuncture points

The acupuncture points fall into three categories: acupuncture points of the fourteen meridians, extra points, and Ashi points.

1. Acupuncture points of the fourteen meridians

Acupuncture points of the fourteen meridians are also known as "meridian points". They are distributed along the twelve main meridians, the governor vessels and the conception vessels. They form the main part of all acupuncture points, totally amounting to 362 at present. Since the acupuncture points of the fourteen meridians are distributed along the fourteen meridians, they have close relationships with the meridians and collaterals. They represent not only diseases of their pertaining meridians and organs but also diseases of the meridians and organs which have relationship with their pertaining meridians. At the same time, they are the locations for acupuncture and moxibution treatment. Therefore, acupuncture points play important roles in curing diseases not only of the organs pertaining the meridians, but also of the meridians, collaterals themselves.

2. Extra points

The extra points are points with specific names and definite locations, but are not attributed to the fourteen meridians. The extra points are also termed as "extraordinary points". They are effective in the treatment of certain diseases. The extra points are distributed on the different parts of the body, so they scattered over the body. Some extra points are distributed out of the courses of the fourteen meridians, such as Zhongquan(EX-UE 3) and Zhongkui(EX-UE 4), while some extra points are distributed along the course of the fourteen meridians, for example, Zhoujian(EX-UE 1); in addition, some extra points are a group of points, such as Sishencong(EX-HN 1) and Sifeng(EX-UE 10).

3. Ashi points

Ashi points are also called "tender spots", "reflexing points", or "unfixed points". Without specific names and definite locations, the tender spots and other sensitive spots are places for needling and moxibustion. Ashi points are generally located nearby the lesions, also located far from the lesions. Ashi points which have no certain number, are the supplement of the points of the fourteen meridians and the extra points.

The therapeutic properties of acupuncture points

1. Local and adjacent therapeutic properties

All the points in the body share the common feature in terms of their therapeutic properties. Each

（二）远治作用

这是十四经腧穴主治作用的基本规律。尤其是十二经脉在四肢肘、膝关节以下的腧穴，不仅能治疗局部病症，而且还能治疗本经循行所及的远隔部位的脏腑、组织、器官的病症，有的甚至具有影响全身的作用。例如外关穴，不仅能治疗手腕局部的病症，还能治疗偏头痛，同时还能治疗外感病的发热；合谷治疗面部疾患；足三里穴不仅能治疗下肢的病症，而且对于胃肠疾患有很好的治疗效果，并且对人体的防御免疫功能方面起很大的作用。

（三）特殊作用

某些腧穴有双相的良性调整作用。例如泄泻时，针刺天枢能止泻；便秘时，针刺天枢又能通便。针刺内关穴既治疗心动过速，也治疗心动过缓。此外，腧穴的治疗作用还具有相对的特异性，如大椎退热、承山通便、至阴矫正胎位等，均是其特殊的治疗作用。

三、特定穴

特定穴是指十四经上具有特殊治疗作用的腧穴。由于这类腧穴的分布和作用不同，因此各有特定的名称和含义。

（一）五输穴

手足三阴三阳经在肘膝关节以下各有五个重要腧穴，井、荥、输、经、合五穴，统称"五输穴"。五输穴按井、荥、输、经、合的顺序，从四肢末端向肘膝方向依次排列，是有具体含义的。古代医家把经气在经脉中运行的情况，比作自然界的水流，以说明经气的出入和经过部位的深浅及其不同作用。如经气所出，像水的源头，称为"井"；经气所溜，像刚出的泉水微流，称为"荥"；经气所注，像水流由浅入深，称为"输"；经气所行，像水在通畅的河中流过，称为"经"；最后经气充盛，进而汇合于脏腑，恰像百川汇合入海，称为"合"。

（二）俞、募穴

俞穴是脏腑经气输注于背腰部的腧穴，俞为阳；募穴是脏腑经气汇聚于胸腹部的腧穴，募为阴。它们均分布于躯干部，与脏腑有密切关系。多应用于各脏腑及相连属的组织器官的病症。

（三）原、络穴

原穴是脏腑原气之所过和留止的部位。十二经脉在腕、踝关节附近各有一个原穴，又名"十二原"。在六阳经上，原穴单独存在，排列在输穴之后，六阴经则以输代原。络脉在由经脉别出的部位各有一个腧穴，称为络穴。络脉由正经别出网络于周身。络穴具有联络表里两经的作用。

point is located on a particular site, and is able to treat disorders of this area and of nearby tissues and organs. For example, Baihui(GV 20) is used for vertex headache, Zhongwan(CV 12) is used for stomach ache, Xiaguan(ST 7) is used for toothache, and Jianyu(LI 15) is used for pain in the shoulder joint.

2. Remote therapeutic properties

This is the basic regularity of the therapeutic properties of the points of the fourteen meridians. The points of the fourteen meridians, especially those of the twelve main meridians located below the elbow and knee joints, are effective not only for local disorders but also for disorders of the tissues and viscera and bowels so far as the course of their pertaining meridians can reach. Some even have systemic therapeutic properties. For example, Waiguan(SJ 5) not only treats disorders of wrist, but also regulates treats migraine and external contraction heat syndrome; Hegu(LI 4) treats disorders of the face; Zusanli(ST 36) not only treats disorders of the lower limbs, but also has good effects on gastrointestinal diseases, even has certain effects on the defensive and immune reactions of the body.

3. Special therapeutic properties

Some acupuncture points have dual therapeutic effects when puncturing on different conditions. For example, in case of diarrhea, puncturing Tianshu (ST 25) can check diarrhea; in case of constipation, puncturing Tianshu (ST 25) can relax the bowels. Needling Neiguan(PC 6) not only can treat tachyrhythmia, but also can treat bradyarrhythmia. In addition, the therapeutic effects of the acupuncture points are relatively specific. Thus, the acupuncture points have their own specific therapeutic effects. For example, Dazhui(GV 14) can purge heat, Chengshan(BL 57) can relax the bowels, and Zhiyin(BL 67) can readjust the position of the fetus, etc.

Special points

Specific points refer to those of the fourteen meridians that have special therapeutic properties. Because of their locations and functions, they process specific names and meanings.

1. Five transport points

Each of the twelve main meridians has, below the elbow or knee, five specific and important points, namely well point, brook point, stream point, river point, and sea point, which are termed five transport points in general. They are situated in the above order from the distal end of extremities to the elbow or knee, and have specific significance. The situation of qi running along the meridians image the flow of meridians qi as the flow of water, which represents qi's locations of coming out, in, and through. The well point is situated in the place where the meridian qi starts to bubble. The brook point is where the meridian qi starts to gush. The stream point is where the meridian qi flourishes. The river point is where the meridian qi is pouring abundantly. Finally, the sea point signifies the confluence of the rivers enter the sea, where the meridian qi is the most flourishing.

2. Alarm points and transport points

Tansport points are specific points on the back where the qi of the respective viscera and bowels is infused, while alarm points are those points on the chest and abdomen where the qi of the repective viscera and bowels is infused and converged. Tansport points are yang, while alarm points are yin. They are all distributed at the trunk, and have close relationship with their respectively related viscera and bowels. They present abnormal reactions to the dysfunction of their corresponding viscera and bowels and tissues.

3. Source points and connecting points

Each of the twelve main meridians has a source point where the source qi is retained. These points are called twelve source points, which are distributed around the wrist joints and ankle joints. In the yang me-

十二经的络穴皆位于四肢肘膝关节以下，加之任脉络穴鸠尾位于腹，督脉络穴长强位于尾骶部，脾之大络大包位于胸胁部，共十五穴，又称"十五络穴"。多应用于脏腑病、表里两经病症。

（四）郄穴

"郄"有空隙之意，郄穴是各经经气深集的部位。十二经脉及阴阳跷、阴阳维脉各有一个郄穴，共十六个郄穴。多分布于四肢肘、膝关节以下。用于治疗各经的急性病症。

（五）下合穴

下合穴 是六腑经脉合于下肢三阳经的六个腧穴，主要分布于下肢膝关节附近。下合穴主治六腑疾患。

（六）八会穴

八会穴，是指人体全身脏、腑、气、血、筋、脉、骨、髓等精气所汇聚的八个腧穴，分布于躯干部和四肢部。

（七）八脉交会穴

奇经八脉与十二正经脉气相通的八个腧穴称为八脉交会穴，这八个穴位主要分布于肘膝关节以下。应用于奇经病症。两脉相合的腧穴互相配合应用。

四、腧穴的定位方法

在针灸治疗过程中，治疗效果的好坏与选穴是否准确有直接关系。

（一）自然标志取穴法

根据人体表面所具特征的部位作为标志，而定取穴位的方法称为自然标志定位法。人体自然标志有两种：

1. 固定标志　固定标志即是人体表面固定不移的部位。如人的五官、爪甲、乳头、肚脐等。

2. 活动标志　是依据人体某局部活动后出现的隆起、凹陷、孔隙、皱纹等作为取穴标志。如曲池屈肘取之。

ridians, the source points are located behind stream points, while in the yin meridians, the source points o-verlap with the stream points. Each of twelve main meridians has, on the limbs, a connecting point to link its exteriorly-interiorly related meridian. Each collateral has a point deriving from its exterior-interior related meridian, which is called the connecting point. The collaterals derive from meridians and run along the whole body. The connecting points have the function of connecting the exterior-interior related meridians.

The connecting points of twelve main meridians are distributed the areas inferior to the wrist joints and ankle joints, while the connecting point Jiuwei(CV 15) of the conception vessel is located at abdomen, the connecting point Changqiang(GV 1) of the governor vessel is located at sacrum, and the major collateral of the spleen is located at chest and rib-side. They are termed the "fifteen connecting points." A connecting point is used to treat disorders of organs and involving the two exteriorly-interiorly related meridians.

4.Cleft points

The cleft point is the site where the qi and blood of the meridian are deeply converged. Each of the twelve main meridians, yin heel vessel, yang heel vessel, yin link vessel, and yang link vessel has a cleft point on the limbs. There are sixteen cleft points in total. Most of them are distributed under the elbow or knee joints. The cleft point is used to treat acute disorders of its pertaining meridian.

5.Lower sea points of the bowels

The lower sea points of the bowels refer to the six points of the three yang meridians of hand and foot where the downward-flowing qi of the six bowels along the three yang meridians of foot. Most of them are distributed around the knee joints. The lower sea points of the bowels are mainly indicated in the disorders of the six bowels.

6.Eight meeting points

The eight meeting points are the eight points where the vital essence and the viscera, bowels, qi, blood, tendon, vessel, bone, and marrow join together. These points are distributed on the trunk and limbs.

7.Confluence points of the eight vessels

The confluence points of the eight vessels refer to the eight points where the eight extra meridians communicate with the twelve regular meridians. All of them are distributed in the regions inferior to the wrist joints and ankle joints. The confluence points of the eight vessels mainly cure the disorders of the eight extra meridians. The points of two related meridians should be used together.

Methods of locating acupuncture points

During the acupuncture and moxibustion treatment, the locations of acupuncture points, directly affect the therapeutic effects.

1.Location of points by natural landmarks

The location of points by natural landmarks refers to various anatomical landmarks of the body surface. The natural landmarks of the body fall into two categories.

(1) Fixed landmarks

The fixed landmarks are the landmarks of the body that would not change with body movement. For example, they include the five sense organs, nails, nipple and umbilicus.

(2) Moving landmarks

The moving landmarks will appear while the certain regions move volunatarily, such as apophysis, depressions, pores, and wrinkles. For example, when the arm is flexed and the cubital crease appears, Quchi (LI 11) can be located.

（二）手指同身寸取穴法

以患者手指为标准来定取穴位的方法。由于选取的手指不同，节段亦不同，可分为以下几种：

1. 中指同身寸法　是以患者的中指中节屈曲时内侧两端纹头之间作为 1 寸，可用于四肢部取穴的直寸和背部取穴的横寸（图 10-2）。

2. 拇指同身寸法　是以患者拇指指关节的横度作为 1 寸，适用于四肢部的直寸取穴（图 10-3）。

3. 横指同身寸法　又名"一夫法"，是令患者将示指、中指、无名指和小指并拢，以中指中节横纹处为标准，四指横量作为 3 寸（图 10-4）。

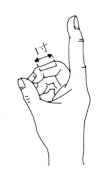
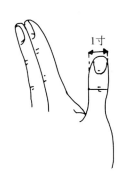
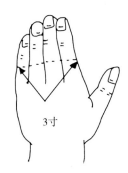

图 10-2　中指同身寸法　　　　　图 10-3　拇指同身寸法　　　　图 10-4　横指同身寸法

（Middle Finger *Cun* Measurement）　（Thumb *Cun* Measurement）　（Finger-Breadth *Cun* Measurement）

（三）简便取穴法

此法是临床上一种简便易行的方法。如垂手中指端取风市；两手虎口自然平直交叉，在示指端到达处取列缺穴等。

（四）骨度分寸定位法

骨度分寸法，是以患者骨节为主要标志测量周身各部的大小、长短，并依其比例折算尺寸作为定穴标准的方法（图 10-5，表 10-2）。

2.Location of point of figure *cun*

The length and width of the patient's finger(s) are taken as a standard for point locations. Due to different finger or segments, the following three methods are commonly used.

(1) Middle finger *cun* measurement

When the patient's middle finger is doubled into the palm, the distance between the two medial ends of the creases of the interphalangeal joints is taken as one *cun*. The methods is employed for measuring the vertical distance to locate the limb points, or for measuring the horizontal distance to locate the points on the back (Figure 10-2).

(2) Thumb *cun* measurement

The width of the interphalangeal joint of the patient's thumb is taken as one *cun*. The method is also employed for measuring the vertical distance to locate the point on the limbs (Figure 10-3).

(3) Finger-breadth *cun* measurement

The width of the four fingers (namely, the index finger, middle finger, ring finger, and little finger) brought close together side by side at the level of the dorsal skin crease of the proximal interphalangeal fold of the middle finger, which is taken as a unit of measurement of 3 *cun* (Figure 10-4).

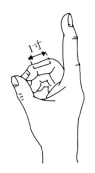

图 10-2   中指同身寸法
(Middle Finger *Cun* Measurement)

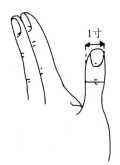

图 10-3   拇指同身寸法
(Thumb *Cun* Measurement)

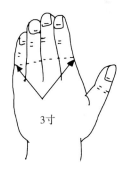

图 10-4   横指同身寸法
(Finger-Breadth *Cun* Measurement)

3.Simple location of points

These are simple methods of point location employed in clinical practice. For example, to locate Fengshi (GB 31) at the tip of the middle finger when at attention; when the index finger and thumbs of both hands are crossed with the index finger of one hand stretching, Lieque (LU 7) is in the place right under the tip of index finger.

4.Bone proportional *cun* measurement

Bone proportional *cun* measurement is a method of locating acupoints in which the patient's bone segments are taken as makers to measure the width or length of various portions of the body; and then, the measurements are converted proportionately into the acupoint-locating standards (Figure10-5, Table10-2).

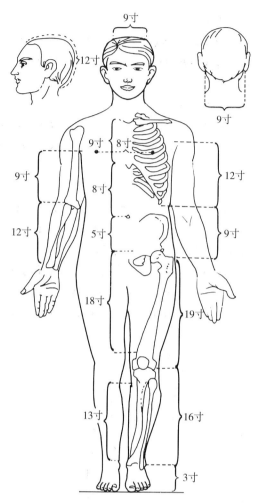

图 10-5　人体骨度分寸图

(Bone Proportional *Cun* Measurement)

表 10-2　常用骨度分寸表

分部	起止点	常用骨度	度量法	说　明
头部	前发际至后发际	12 寸	直寸	如前后发际不明，从眉心量至大椎穴作 18 寸，眉心至前发际 3 寸，大椎穴至后发际 3 寸
	耳后两完骨（乳突）之间	9 寸	横寸	用于量头部的横寸
胸腹部	天突至歧骨（胸剑联合）	9 寸		（1）胸部与肋部取穴直寸，一般根据肋骨计算，每一肋骨折作 1 寸 6 分
	歧骨至脐中	8 寸	直寸	
	脐中至横骨上廉（耻骨联合上缘）	5 寸		（2）"天突"指穴名的部位
	两乳头之间	8 寸	横寸	胸腹部取穴的横寸，可根据两乳头之间的距离折量。女性可用左右缺盆穴之间的宽度来代替两乳头之间的横寸

Table 10-2   Standards for Bone Proportional Cun Measurement

Body Part	Distance	Bone Proportional *cun* Measurement	Method	Explanation
Head	From anterior hairline to the posterior hairline	12 *cun*	Longitudinal measurement	If the anterior and posterior hairlines are indistinguishable, the distance from the glabella to Dazhui(GV 14) then is taken as 18 *cun*. The distance from the glabella to the anterior hairline is taken as 3 *cun*. The distance from Dazhui(GV 14) to the posterior hairline is taken as 3 *cun*
	Between the two mastoid processes(Rutu)	9 *cun*	Transverse measurement	This transverse measurement is also used to lacalize other points on the head
Chest and Abdomen	From the Tiantu (CV 22) to the sternocostal angle	9 *cun*	Longitudinal measurement	1.The longitudinal measurement of the chest and the hypochondriac region is generally based on the intercostals space.Every intercostals space equals 1 *cun* and 6 *fen*
	From the sternocostal angle to the center of the umbilicus	8 *cun*		2. "Tiantu(CV 22)"means the location of the point
	Between the centre of the umbilicus and the upper border of symphysis pubis	5 *cun*		
	Between the two nipples	8 *cun*	Transverse measurement	The longitudinal measurement of the chest and the hypochondriac region is generally based on the intercostals space. For women, the distance between the bilateral Quepen(ST12) can be used as the substitute of the transverse measurement of the two nipples
Back	From the area below Dazhui (GV 14) to the coccyx	21 *cun*	Transverse measurement	The longitudinal measurement on the back is based on the spinous processes of the vertebral column.In clinical practice, the lower angle of the scapula is about at the same level of the 7th thoracic vertebra, the iliac spine is about at the same level of the 4th lumbar vertebra
	Between the two spinal borders of scapula	6 *cun*	Transverse measurement	
Upper Extremities	Between the end of the axillary fold and the transverse cubital crease	9 *cun*	Longitudinal measurement	Used for the three Yin and the three Yang Meridians of the hand
	Between the transverse cubital crease and the transverse wrist crease	12 *cun*		
Lateral side of the chest	From the end of the axillary fold to the hypochondriac region	12 *cun*	Longitudinal measurement	"The hypochondriac region"means the tip of the 11th rib
Lateral part of the abdomen	From the area below the hypochondrium to the uppermost part of the lateral aspect of the thigh	9 *cun*	Longitudinal measurement	"The uppermost part of the lateral aspect of the thigh" means the prominence of the great trochanter

续表

分部	起止点	常用骨度	度量法	说　明
背腰部	大椎以下至尾骶	21寸	直寸	背部腧穴根据脊椎定穴。一般临床取穴，肩胛骨下角相当第七（胸）椎，髂嵴相当第16椎（第4腰椎棘突）
	两肩胛骨脊柱缘之间	6寸	横寸	
上肢部	腋前纹头（腋前皱襞）至肘横纹	9寸	直寸	用于手三阴、手三阳经的骨度分寸
	肘横纹至腕横纹	12寸		
侧胸部	腋以下至季胁	12寸	直寸	"季胁"指第11肋端
侧腹部	季胁以下至髀枢	9寸	直寸	"髀枢"指股骨大转子
下肢部	横骨上廉至内辅骨上廉（股骨内髁上缘）	18寸	直寸	用于足三阴经的骨度分寸
	内辅骨下廉（胫骨内髁下缘）至内踝高点	13寸		
	髀枢至膝中	19寸	直寸	(1) 用于足三阳经的骨度分寸
	臀横纹至膝中	14寸		(2) "膝中"的水平线：前面相当于犊鼻穴，后面相当于委中穴
	膝中至外踝高点	16寸		
	外踝高点至足底	3寸		

第三节　经络腧穴

十四经脉是十二经脉和任脉、督脉的总称。掌握每一条经脉的循行路线，了解腧穴的主治范围，是临床应用针灸治疗各种疾病的基础。

一、手太阴肺经

【主治概要】主治喉、胸、肺病，如咳嗽、气喘、胸部胀满、胸痛、喉痛、肩背痛等。

【本经腧穴】左右各11穴（图10-6）。

中府（LU 1）

【定位】胸前壁外上方，前正中线旁开6寸，平第一肋间隙处（图10-6）。

【解剖】当胸大肌、胸小肌处，内侧深层为第一肋间内、外肌；上外侧有腋动、静脉及胸肩峰动、静脉；布有锁骨上神经中间支、胸神经外侧支及第一肋间神经外侧皮支。

continued

Body Part	Distance	Bone Proportional *cun* Measurement	Method	Explanation
Lower Extremities	From the level of the border of symphsis pubis to the medial epicondyle of the femur	18 *cun*	Longitudinal measurement	Used for the three Yin Meridians of the Foot
	From the level of the border of the medial condyle of tibia to the tip of medial malleolus	13 *cun*		
	From the prominence of the great trochanter to the middle of patella	19 *cun*	Longitudinal measurement	1.Used for the three Yin Meridians of the Foot
	Between the crease of the buttock and the midpoint of the knee	14 *cun*		2. The anterior level of the centre of the paralla is about the same level of Dubi(ST 35) ,and the posterior level, about the same level of Weizhong(BL 40)
	Between the centre of patella and the tip of lateral malleolus	16 *cun*		
	From the tip of the lateral malleolus to the heel	3 *cun*		

Section 3   Meridians and Acupuncture Points

The twelve main meridians,together with the governor vessel and the conception vessel,are called the"fourteem meridians".Mastering distribution of each of the meridians and understanding the indications of acupoints are the basis for the clinical application of acupuncture and moxibustion treatment of various diseases.

The Lung Meridian of Hand-Taiyin

【Principal indications】Diseases of the throat,chest,and lung such as cough,asthma,chest fullness,chest pain,sore throat,and shoulder pain.

【Acupoints】11 points each side(Figure 10-6).

Zhongfu (LU 1)

【Location】The outer top of the anterior chest wall,6 *cun* lateral to the midline of the chest,and in the first intercostal space(Figure 10-6).

【Anatomy】Muscles:in m.pectoralis major and minor;deeper,m.intercostoles prima interni and externi.Blood vessels:superolaterally,the axillary artery and vein,the thoracoacromial artery and vein. Nerves:the intermediate supraclavicular nerve,the branches of the anterior thoracic nerve,and the lateral cutaneous branch of the first intercostal nerve.

【Indications】Cough,asthma,fullness of the lung,and pain in the chest and back.

【Manipulation】Puncture obliquely or subcutaneously 0. 5 - 0. 8 *cun* towards the lateral aspect of the chest.Do not deeply puncture inwards to avoid injuring the lung.

【Remarks】Alarm point of the lung,crossing point of the lung meridian of Hand-Taiyin and the

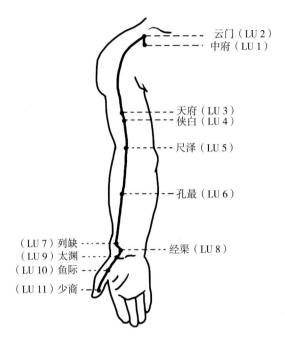

图 10-6　手太阴肺经腧穴总图

(The Lung Meridian of Hand-Taiyin)

【主治】咳嗽，气喘，肺胀满，胸痛，肩背痛。

【操作】向外斜刺或平刺 0.5~0.8 寸，不可向内深刺，以免伤及肺脏。

【附注】肺募穴；手、足太阴经交会穴。

尺泽（LU 5）

【定位】肘横纹中，肱二头肌肌腱桡侧缘（图 10-6）。

【解剖】在肘关节、肱二头肌肌腱的外方，肱桡肌起始部；有桡侧返动、静脉分支及头静脉；布有前臂外侧皮神经，直下为桡神经。

【主治】咳嗽，气喘，咳血，潮热，胸部胀满，咽喉肿痛，小儿惊风，吐泻，肘臂挛痛。

【操作】直刺 0.8~1.2 寸，或点刺出血。

【附注】手太阴经合穴。

列缺（LU 7）

【定位】桡骨茎突上方，腕横纹上 1.5 寸（图 10-7）。

【解剖】在肱桡肌腱与拇长展肌腱之间，桡侧腕长伸肌腱内侧；有头静脉，桡动、静脉分支；布有前臂外侧皮神经和桡神经浅支的混合支。

【主治】伤风，头痛，项强，咳嗽，气喘，咽喉肿痛，口眼㖞斜，齿痛。

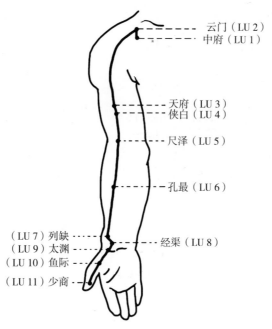

云门（LU 2）
中府（LU 1）

天府（LU 3）
侠白（LU 4）

尺泽（LU 5）

孔最（LU 6）

（LU 7）列缺
（LU 9）太渊
（LU 10）鱼际
（LU 11）少商

经渠（LU 8）

图 10-6   手太阴肺经腧穴总图
(The Lung Meridian of Hand-Taiyin)

spleen meridian of Foot-Taiyin.

Chize (LU 5)

【Location】On the cubital crease, and near the radial border of the tendon of m.biceps brachii(Figure 10-6).

【Anatomy】Muscles: the elbow joint, on the radial aspect of the tendon of m.biceps brachii and the origin of m.brachioradialis. Blood vessels: the cephalic vein and the branches of the radial recurrent artery and vein. Nerves: the lateral antebrachial cutaneous nerve and the radial nerve.

【Indications】Cough, asthma, hemoptysis, tidal fever, fullness in the chest, sore throat, infantile convulsion, vomiting and diarreah, and spasmodic pain of the elbow and arm.

【Manipulation】Puncture perpendicularly 0.8-1.2 *cun* , or prick the point to cause bleeding.

【Remarks】Sea point of the lung meridian of Hand-Taiyin.

Lieque (LU 7)

【Location】Superior to the styloid process of the radius and 1.5 *cun* above the transverse crease of the wrist(Figure 10-7).

【Anatomy】Muscles: between the tendons of m.brachioradialis and m.abductor pollicis longus; on the medical side of the tendon of m.extensor carpi radialis longus. Blood vessels: there are the cephalic vein and the branches of the radial artery and vein. Nerves: the lateral antebrachial cutaneous nerve and the superficial ramus of the radial nerve.

【Indications】Common cold, headache, stiffness of the neck, cough, asthma, sore throat, deviation of the mouth and eye, and toothache.

【Manipulation】Puncture 0.3-0.5 *cun* obliquely upwards.

【Remarks】Connecting point of the lung meridian of Hand-Taiyin, one of the confluence points of

【操作】 向上斜刺 0.3~0.5 寸。

【附注】 手太阴经络穴；八脉交会穴之一，通于任脉。

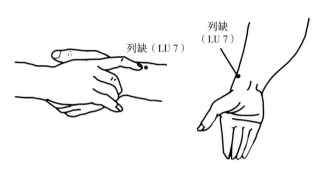

图 10-7 列缺

（Lieque）

太渊（LU 9）

【定位】 掌后腕横纹桡侧端，桡动脉的桡侧凹陷中（图 10-6）。

【解剖】 桡侧腕屈肌腱的外侧，拇展长肌腱内侧；有桡动、静脉；布有前臂外侧皮神经和桡神经浅支混合支。

【主治】 咳嗽，气喘，咳血，胸痛，咽喉肿痛，腕臂痛，无脉症。

【操作】 避开桡动脉，直刺 0.3~0.5 寸。

【附注】 手太阴经输穴；肺经原穴；八会穴之一，脉会太渊。

鱼际（LU 10）

【定位】 第一掌骨中点，赤白肉际处（图 10-6）。

【解剖】 有拇短展肌和拇指对掌肌；拇指静脉回流支；布有前臂外侧皮神经和桡神经浅支混合支。

【主治】 咳嗽，咳血，咽喉肿痛，失音，发热。

【操作】 直刺 0.5~0.8 寸。

【附注】 手太阴经荥穴。

二、手阳明大肠经

【主治概要】 主治头面、五官、咽喉病、胃肠病，如腹痛、肠鸣、泄泻、便秘、痢疾、咽喉痛、齿痛、鼻塞或鼻衄，以及本经循行部位的疼痛等。

【本经腧穴】 左右各 20 穴（图 10-8）。

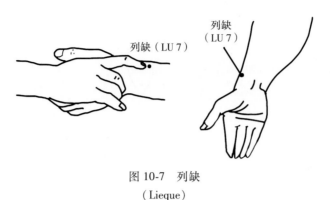

图 10-7　列缺
(Lieque)

the eight vessels, communicating with the conception vessel.

Taiyuan (LU 9)

【Location】At the radial end of the transverse crease of the wrist, in the depression on the radial side of the radial artery(Figure 10-6).

【Anatomy】Muscles: on the lateral side of the tendon of m.flexor carpi radialis and the medial side of the tendon of m.abductor pollicis longus.Blood vessels: the radial artery and vein.Nerves: the lateral antebrachial cutaneous nerve and the superficial ramus of the radial nerve.

【Indications】Cough, asthma, hemoptysis, chest pain, sore throat, pain in the wrist and arm, and pulseless disease.

【Manipulation】Away from the radial artery, puncture perpendicularly 0.3−0.5 *cun*.

【Remarks】Stream point and source point of the lung meridian of Hand-Taiyin.One of eight meeting points, with vessels meet in the point.

Yuji (LU 10)

【Location】At the midpoint of the palmar side of the first metacarpal bone, and on the junction of the red and white skin(Figure 10-6).

【Anatomy】Muscles: m.abductor pollicis brevis and m.opponens pollicis.Blood vessels: venules of the thumb draining to the cephalic vein.Nerves: the lateral cutaneous nerve of forearm and the superficial ramus of the radial nerve.

【Indications】Cough, hemoptysis, sore throat, aphonia, and fever.

【Manupilation】Puncture perpendicularly 0.5−0.8 *cun*.

【Remarks】Spring point of the lung meridian of Hand-Taiyin.

The Large Intestine Meridian of Hand-Yangming

【Principal indications】Diseases of the head, face, five sense organs, throat and gastrointestine.Such as, abdominal pain, borborygmus, diarrhea, constipation, dysentery, sore throat, toothache, nasal congestion, nosebleed, and other diseases in the regions along the course of this meridians.

【Acupoints】20 points each side(Figure 10-8).

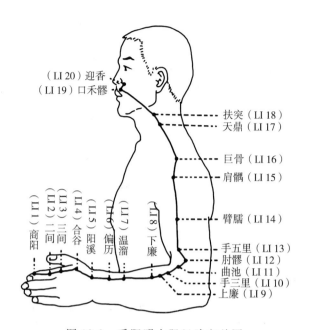

图 10-8 手阳明大肠经腧穴总图

(The Large Intestine Meridian of Hand-Yangming)

合谷 (LI 4)

【定位】手背，第一、二掌骨之间，约平第二掌骨桡侧中点处（图 10-9）。

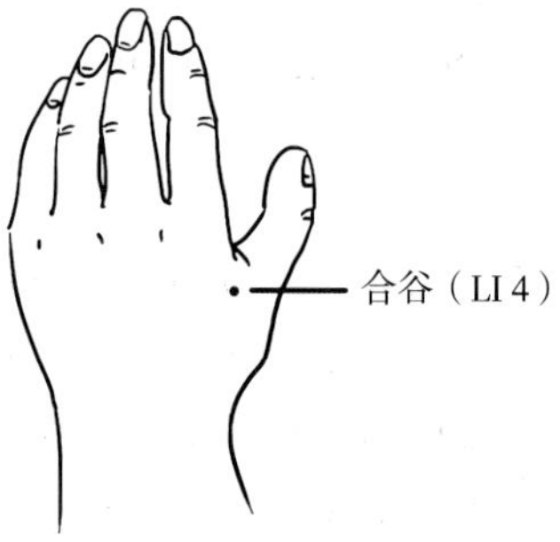

【解剖】在第一、二掌骨之间，第一骨间背侧肌中，深层有拇收肌横头；有手背静脉网，为头静脉的起始部，腧穴近侧正当桡动脉从手背穿向手掌之处；布有桡神经浅支的掌背侧神经，深部有正中神经的指掌侧固有神经。

图 10-9 合谷

(Hegu)

【主治】头痛，目赤肿痛，鼻衄，齿痛，牙关紧闭，口眼㖞斜，耳聋，痄腮，咽喉肿痛，热病无汗，多汗，腹痛，便秘，经闭，滞产。

【操作】直刺 0.5~1 寸，可灸。孕妇禁针灸。

【附注】手阳明经原穴。

手三里 (LI 10)

【定位】在阳溪与曲池连线上，曲池穴下 2 寸处（图 10-10）。

【解剖】有桡侧腕短伸肌、桡侧腕长伸肌，深层为旋后肌；有桡返动脉分支；布

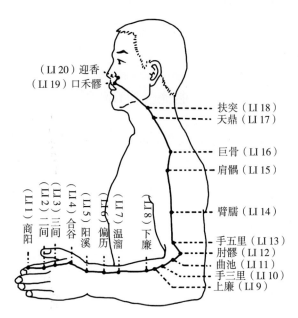

图 10-8   手阳明大肠经腧穴总图
(The Large Intestine Meridian of Hand-Yangming)

Hegu (LI 4)

【Location】On the dorsum of the hand, between the 1st and 2nd metacarpal bones and in the middle of the 2nd metacarpal bone on the radial side (Figure 10-9).

【Anatomy】Muscles: between the 1st and 2nd metacarpal bones, in the 1st m. interosseous dorsalis; deeper, the transverse part of m. adductor pollicis. Blood vessels: the origin of the cephalic vein, the venous network of the dorsum of the hand, proximal to the point where the radial artery passes through the dorsum to palm. Nerves: the dorsal nerve of hand derived from the superficial ramus of the radial nerve; deeper the palar proprial nerve coming from the median nerve.

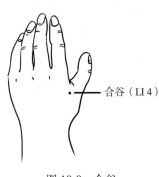

图 10-9   合谷
(Hegu)

【Indications】Headache, sore red swollen eyes, nosebleed, toothache, trismus, deviation of the mouth and eye, deafness, mumps, sore throat, anhidrosis in febrile diseases, hidrosis, abdominal pain, constipation, amenorahea and dystocia.

【Manipulation】Puncture perpendicularly 0.5 - 1 *cun*, moxibustion is applicable. Acupuncture and moxibustion are contraindicated for pregnant women.

【Remarks】Source point of the large intestine meridian of Hand-Yangming.

Shousanli (LI 10)

【Location】On the line joining Yangxi (LI 5) and Quchi (LI 11), 2 *cun* below Quchi (LI 11. Figure 10-10).

【Anatomy】Muscles: m. extensor carpi radialis brevis and longus; deeper m. supinator. Blood ves-

有前臂背侧皮神经及桡神经深支。

【主治】齿痛颊肿，上肢不遂，腹痛，腹泻。

【操作】直刺0.8~1.2寸。

曲池（LI 11）

【定位】屈肘，成直角，当肘横纹外端与肱骨外上髁连线的中点（图10-10）。

【解剖】桡侧腕长伸肌起始部，肱桡肌的桡侧；有桡返动脉的分支；布有前臂背侧皮神经，内侧深层为桡神经本干。

【主治】咽喉肿痛，齿痛，目赤痛，瘰疬，瘾疹，热病，上肢不遂，手臂肿痛，腹痛吐泻，高血压，癫狂。

【操作】直刺1~1.5寸。

【附注】手阳明经合穴。

肩髃（LI 15）

【定位】肩峰前下方，当肩峰与肱骨大结节之间。肩平举时，肩部出现两个凹陷，前面的凹陷中（图10-11）。

【解剖】三角肌上部中央；有旋肱后动、静脉；布有锁骨上神经、腋神经。

【主治】肩臂挛痛不遂，瘾疹，瘰疬。

【操作】直刺或向下斜刺0.8~1.5寸。

【附注】手阳明经与阳跷脉交会穴。

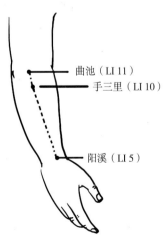

图 10-10　曲池、手三里、阳溪

（Quchi, Shousanli and Yangxi）

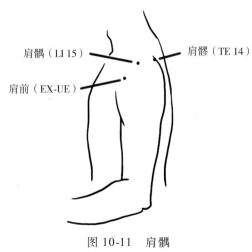

图 10-11　肩髃

（Jianyu）

sels: the branches of the radial recurrent artery. Nerves: the posterior antebrachial cutaneous nerve and deep ramus of the radial nerve.

【Indications】Toothache, swelling in the cheak, brachial palsy and pain, abdominal pain, and diarrhea.

【Manipulation】Puncture perpendicularly 0. 8-1. 2 *cun*.

Quchi (LI 11)

【Location】When the elbow is flexed to form a right angle, the point is at the midpoint of the line joining the lateral end of the transverse cubital crease and the lateral epicondyle of the humerus(Figure 10-10).

【Anatomy】Muscles: on the origin of m. extensor carpi radialis longus and on the radial side of m. brachio-radialis. Blood vessels: the branches of the radial recurrent artery. Nerves: the posterior antebrachial cutaneous nerve; deeper, on the medical side, the radial nerve.

【Indications】Sore throat, toothache, redness and pain of the eye, sceofula, urticarial, febrile diseases, brachial palsy and pain, swelling and pain of the hand and arm, abdominal pain, vomiting, diarrhea, hypertension, and manic-depressive psychosis.

【Manipulation】Puncture perpendicularly 1-1. 5 *cun*.

【Remarks】Sea point of the large intestine meridian of Hand-Yangming.

Jianyu (LI 15)

【Location】Antero-inferior to the acromion, between the acromion and the greater tuberosity of the humerus. When the arm is in abduction at 90°, there are two depressions on the shoulder. The point is in the anterior depression(Figure 10-11).

【Anatomy】Muscles: at the center of the upper portion of m. deltoideus. Blood vessels: the posterior circumflex humeral artery and vein. Nerves: the superaclavicular nerve and axillary nerve.

【Indications】Palsy and pain in the shoulder and arm, urticarial, and scrofula.

【Manipulation】Puncture perpendicularly or obliquely downwards 0. 8-1. 5 *cun*.

【Remarks】One of the confluence points of the eight vessels, where the large intestine meridian of Hand-Yangming meets the yang heel vessel.

迎香（LI 20）

【定位】鼻翼外缘中点，旁开 0.5 寸，当鼻唇沟中间（图 10-8）。

【解剖】在上唇方肌中，深部为梨状孔的边缘；有面动、静脉及眶下动、静脉分支；布有面神经与眶下神经的吻合丛。

【主治】鼻塞、鼻衄、口㖞、面痒、胆道蛔虫症。

【操作】斜刺或平刺 0.3~0.5 寸，不宜灸。

【附注】手、足阳明经交会穴。

三、足阳明胃经

【主治概要】主治胃肠病及头面部疾病，如肠鸣腹胀、水肿、胃痛、呕吐、口渴、消谷善饥、咽喉肿痛、口眼㖞斜，以及本经循行部位的疼痛、热病、发狂等。

【本经腧穴】左右各 45 穴（图 10-12）。

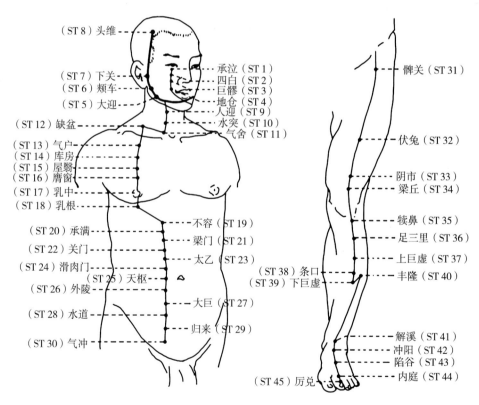

图 10-12　足阳明胃经腧穴总图

（The Stomach Meridian of Foot-Yangming）

Yingxiang（LI 20）

【Location】0. 5 *cun* lateral to the midpoint of the lateral border of ala nasi, in the nasolabial groove（Figure 10-8）.

【Anatomy】Muscles：in m.quadratus labii superioris, deeper the border of the aperture piriformis. Blood vessels：the facial artery and vein, the branches of the infraorbital artery and vein. Nerves：the anastomotic branch of the facial and infraorbital nerves.

【Indications】Nasal congestion, sniveling and nosebleed, wry mouth, itchy face, and biliary ascariasis.

【Manipulation】Puncture obliquely or subcutaneously 0. 3-0. 5 *cun*.Moxibustion is not advisable.

【Remarks】Crossing point for the large intestine meridian of Hand-Yangming and the stomach meridian of Foot-Yangming.

The Stomach Meridian of Foot-Yangming

【Principal indications】Gastrointestinal diseases and diseases of the head and face, such as borborygmus, abdominal distention, edema, stomach ache, vomiting, thirst, swift digestion with rapid hungering, sore swollen throat, deviated eyes, and mouth；and pain, febrile diseases and mania in the region along the course of this meridian.

【Acupoints】45 points each side（Figure 10-12）.

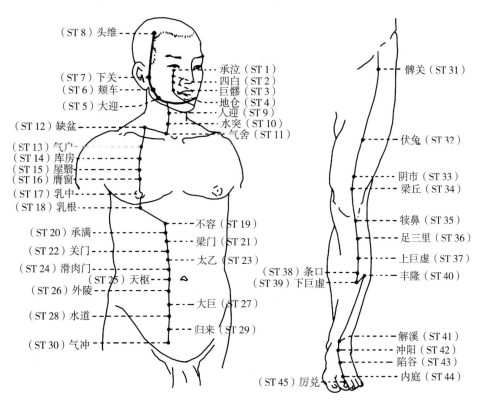

图 10-12　足阳明胃经腧穴总图
（The Stomach Meridian of Foot-Yangming）

地仓（ST 4）

【定位】口角旁0.4寸，巨髎穴直下取之（图10-12）。

【解剖】在口轮匝肌中，深层为颊肌；有面动、静脉；布有面神经和眶下神经分支，深层为颊肌神经的末支。

【主治】口㖞，流涎，眼睑瞤动。

【操作】斜刺或平刺0.5~0.8寸。

【附注】手、足阳明经与阳跷脉交会穴。

颊车（ST 6）

【定位】下颌角前上方一横指凹陷中，咀嚼时咬肌隆起最高点处（图10-12）。

【解剖】在下颌角前方，有咬肌；有咬肌动、静脉；布有耳大神经，面神经及咬肌神经。

【主治】口㖞，齿痛，颊肿，口噤不语。

【操作】直刺0.3~0.5寸，平刺0.5~1寸。

下关（ST 7）

【定位】颧弓下缘，下颌骨髁状突之前方，切迹之间凹陷中。合口有孔，张口即闭（图10-12）。

【解剖】当颧弓下缘，皮下有腮腺，为咬肌起始部；有面横动、静脉，最深层为上颌动、静脉；正当面神经颧眶支及耳颞神经分支，最深层为下颌神经。

【主治】耳聋，耳鸣，聤耳，齿痛，口噤，口眼㖞斜。

【操作】直刺0.5~1寸。

【附注】足阳明、足少阳经交会穴。

头维（ST 8）

【定位】额角发际直上0.5寸（图10-12）。

【解剖】在颞肌上缘帽状腱膜中；有颞浅动、静脉的额支；布有耳颞神经的分支及面神经额颞支。

【主治】头痛，目眩，眼痛，流泪，眼睑瞤动。

【操作】平刺0.5~1寸，不宜灸。

【附注】足阳明、足少阳经与阳维脉交会穴。

Dicang (ST 4)

【Location】0. 4 *cun* lateral to the angle of the mouth, directly below Juliao(ST 3)(Figure 10-12).

【Anatomy】Muscles: in m. orbicularis oris; deeper, m. buccinators. Blood vessels: the facial artery and vein. Nerves: superficially, the branches of the facial and infraorbital nerves; deeper, the terminal branch of the buccal nerve.

【Indications】Wry mouth, salivation, and twitching of eyelids.

【Manipulation】Puncture obliquely or subcutaneously 0. 5−0. 8 *cun*.

【Remarks】The crossing point of the stomach meridian of Foot-Yangming, the large instestine meridian of Hand-Yangming and the *yang* heel vessel.

Jiache (ST 6)

【Location】In the depression one finger-breadth anterior and superior to the angle of the mandible where m. masseter attaches at the prominence of the muscle when the teeth are clenched(Figure 10-12).

【Anatomy】Muscles: anterior to the lower angle of the mandible, there is m. masseter. Blood vessels: the masseteric artery and vein. Nerves: the great auricular nerve, facial nerve, and masseteric nerve.

【Indications】Wry mouth, toothache, swelling of the cheek, and trismus.

【Manipulation】Puncture perpendicularly 0. 3−0. 5 *cun*, or subcutaneously 0. 5−1 *cun*.

Xiaguan (ST 7)

【Location】At the lower border of the zygomatic arch and in the depression anterior to the condyloid process of the mandible. This point is located when the mouth is closed(Figure 10-12).

【Anatomy】Muscles: At the lower border of the zygomatic arch, parotid gland under the skin; at the origin of m. masseter. Blood vessels: superficially, the transverse facial artery and vein; in the deepest layer, the maxillary artery and vein. Nerves: the aygomatic branch of the facial nerve and the branches of the auriculotemporal nerve, and in the deepest layer, the mandibular nerve.

【Indications】Deafness, tinnitus, purulent ear, toothache, trismus, and deviation of the mouth and eyes.

【Manipulation】Puncture perpendicularly 0. 5−1 *cun*.

【Remarks】The crossing point of the stomach meridian of Foot-Yangming and the gallbladder meridian of Foot-Shaoyang.

Touwei (ST 8)

【Location】0. 5 *cun* directly above the hairline at the corner of the forehead(Figure 10-12).

【Anatomy】Muscles: in the galea aponeurotica of superior border of m. temporalis. Blood vessels: the frontal branches of the superficial temporal artery and vein. Nerves: the branch of the auriculotemporal nerve and the temporal branch of the facial nerve.

【Indications】Headache, blurred vision, ophthalmalgia, lacrimation, and twitching of eyelids.

【Manipulation】Puncture 0. 5−1 *cun* subcutaneously. Moxibustion is not applicable.

【Remarks】The crossing point of the stomach meridian of Foot-Yangming, the gallbladder meridian of Foot-Shaoyang and the yang link vessel.

天枢（ST 25）

【定位】脐旁 2 寸（图 10-12）。

【解剖】当腹直肌及其鞘处；有第九肋间动、静脉分支及腹壁下动、静脉分支；布有第十肋间神经分支。

【主治】腹胀肠鸣，绕脐痛，便秘，泄泻，痢疾，月经不调，癥瘕。

【操作】直刺 1~1.5 寸，可灸。

【附注】大肠募穴。

犊鼻（ST 35）

【定位】髌骨下缘，髌韧带外侧凹陷中（图 10-13）。

【解剖】在髌韧带外缘；有膝关节动、静脉网；布有腓肠外侧皮神经及腓总神经关节支。

【主治】膝痛，下肢麻痹，屈伸不利，脚气。

【操作】向髌韧带内后方斜刺 0.5~1 寸。

足三里（ST 36）

【定位】犊鼻穴下 3 寸，胫骨前缘一横指处（图 10-13）。

【解剖】在胫骨前肌，趾长伸肌之间；有胫前动、静脉；为腓肠外侧皮神经及隐

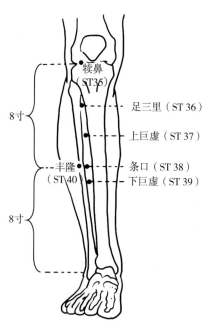

图 10-13 犊鼻、足三里、上巨虚、丰隆

（Dubi, Zusanli, Shangjuxu and Fenglong）

Tianshu (ST 25)

【 Location 】2 *cun* lateral to the umbilicus(Figure 10-12).

【 Anatomy 】Muscles：on m.rectus abdominis and its sheath.Blood vessels：the branches of the 9th intercostal and inferior epigastric arteries and veins.Nerves：the branch of the 10th intercostal nerve.

【 Indications 】Abdominal distension,borborygmus,pain around the umbilicus,constipation,diarrhea,dysentery,irregular menstruation,and abdominal mass.

【 Manipulation 】Puncture perpendicularly 0. 5-1 *cun*.Moxibustion is applicable.

【 Remarks 】Alarm point of the large intestine.

Dubi (ST 35)

【 Location 】At the lower border of the patella,in the depression lateral to the patellar ligament(Figure 10-13).

【 Anatomy 】Muscles：in the medial side,the patellar ligament.Blood vessels：the arterial and venous network around the knee joint.Nerves：the lateral sural cutaneous nerve and the articular branch of the common peroneal nerve.

【 Indications 】Pain,crural paralysis,numbness and motor impairment of the knee,and beriberi.

【 Manipulation 】Puncture 0. 5-1 *cun* obliquely backward towards the patellar ligament.

Zusanli (ST 36)

【 Location 】3 *cun* below Dubi(ST 35) ,one finger-breadth from the anterior crest of the tibia(Figure 10-13).

【 Anatomy 】Muscles：between m.anterior tibialis and m.extensor digitorum longus.Blood vessels：the anterior tibial artery and vein.Nerves：superficially,the lateral sural cutaneous nerve and the cutaneous branch of the saphenous nerve；deeper,the deep peroneal nerve.

【 Indications 】Gastric pain,vomiting,dysphagia-occlusion,abdominal distension,diarrhea,dysentery,constipation,acute mastitis,acute appendicitis,muscular atrophy,numbness pain and flaccidity of the lower extremities,edema,manic depressive psychosis,beriberi,and emaciation due to general deficiency.

【 Manipulation 】Puncture perpendicularly 1-2 *cun*.

【 Remarks 】Sea point of the stomach meridian of Foot-Yangming.

神经的皮支分布处，深层当腓深神经。

【主治】胃痛，呕吐，噎膈，腹胀，泄泻，痢疾，便秘，乳痈，肠痈，下肢痹痛，水肿，癫狂，脚气，虚劳羸瘦。

【操作】直刺 1~2 寸。

【附注】足阳明经合穴。

上巨虚（ST 37）

【定位】足三里穴下 3 寸（图 10-13）。

【解剖】在胫骨前肌中；有胫前动、静脉；布有腓肠外侧皮神经及隐神经的皮支，深层当腓深神经。

【主治】肠鸣，腹痛，泄泻，便秘，肠痈，下肢痿痹，脚气。

【操作】直刺 1~2 寸。

【附注】大肠经下合穴。

丰隆（ST 40）

【定位】外踝高点上 8 寸，条口穴外 1 寸（图 10-13）。

【解剖】在趾长伸肌外侧和腓骨短肌之间；有胫前动脉分支；当腓浅神经处。

【主治】头痛，眩晕，痰多咳嗽，呕吐，便秘，水肿，癫狂痫，下肢痿痹。

【操作】直刺 1~1.5 寸。

【附注】足阳明经络穴。

内庭（ST 44）

【定位】足背第二、三趾间缝纹端（图 10-12）。

【解剖】有足背静脉网；布有腓浅神经足背支。

【主治】齿痛，咽喉肿痛，口歪，鼻衄，胃病吐酸，腹胀，泄泻，痢疾，便秘，热病，足背肿痛。

【操作】直刺或斜刺 0.5~0.8 寸。

【附注】足阳明经荥穴。

四、足太阴脾经

【主治概要】主治脾胃病症，如腹胀、胃脘痛、呕吐、嗳气、便溏、黄疸、身重无力、舌根强痛、下肢肿胀、厥冷等病症。兼治妇科病及前阴病等。

【本经腧穴】左右各 21 穴（图 10-14）。

Shangjuxu (ST 37)

【 Location 】3 *cun* below Zusanli(ST 36) (Figure 10-13) .

【 Anatomy 】Muscles: in m.tibialis anterior.Blood vessels: the anterior tibial artery and vein.Nerves: superficially, the lateral sural cutaneous nerve and the cutaneous branch of the saphenous nerve; deeper, the deep peroneal nerve.

【 Indications 】Borborygmus, abdominal pain, diarrhea, constipation, acute appendicitis, muscular atrophy, numbness pain and flaccidity of the lower extremities, and beriberi.

【 Manipulation 】Puncture perpendicularly 1-2 *cun*.

【 Remarks 】The lower sea point of the large intestine.

Fenglong (ST 40)

【 Location 】8 *cun* superior to the external malleolus 1 *cun* lateral to Tiaokou(ST 38) (Figure 10-13) .

【 Anatomy 】Muscles: between the lateral side of m.extensor dogitorum longus and m.peroneus brevis.Blood vessels: the branch of the anterior tibial artery.Nerves: superificially, the superficial peroneal nerve.

【 Indications 】Headache, dizziness, copious phlegm and cough, vomiting, constipation, edema, manic-depressive psychosis, epilepsy, muscular atrophy, numbness pain, and flaccidity of the lower extremities.

【 Manipulation 】Puncture perpendicularly 1-1. 5 *cun*.

【 Remarks 】Connecting point of the stomach meridian of Foot-Yangming.

Neiting (ST 44)

【 Location 】Proximal to the vertical skin crease of the net work between the second and third toes (Figure 10-12) .

【 Anatomy 】Blood vessels: the dorsal venous network of foot.Nerves: the dorsal digital nerve derived from the superficial peroneal nerve.

【 Indications 】Toothache, sore throat, wry mouth, epistaxis, gastric pain, acid regurgitation, abdominal distension, diarrhea, dysentery, constipation, febrile diseases, and swelling and pain of the dorsum of the foot.

【 Manipulation 】Puncture perpendicularly or obliquely 0. 5-0. 8 *cun*.

【 Remarks 】Spring point of the stomach meridian of Foot-Yangming.

The Spleen Meridian of Foot-Taiyin

【 Principal indications 】Diseases of the spleen and stomach, such as abdominal distension, stomach duct pain, vomiting, belching eructation, loose stool, jaundice, heavy body and forceless, stiffness and pain of root of tongue, swelling and distention of the lower limbs, and reversal cold and diseases of the gynecopathies and genitals.

【 Acupoints 】21 points each side(Figure 10-14) .

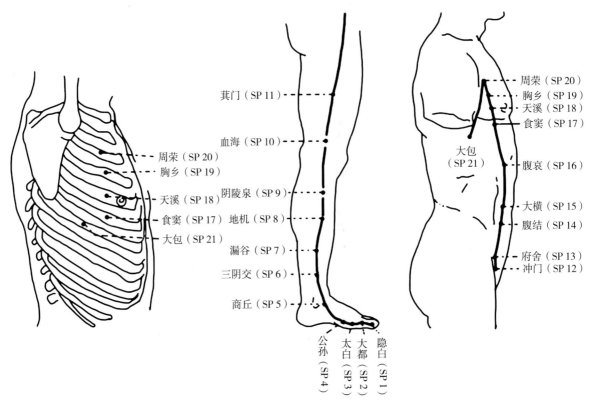

图 10-14 足太阴脾经腧穴总图

(The Spleen Meridian of Foot-Taiyin)

公孙 (SP 4)

【定位】第一跖骨基底前下缘，赤白肉际处（图 10-14）。

【解剖】在拇展肌中；有跗内侧动脉分支及足背静脉网；布有隐神经及腓浅神经分支。

【主治】胃痛，呕吐，腹痛，泄泻，痢疾。

【操作】直刺 0.6~1.2 寸。

【附注】足太阴经络穴；八脉交会穴之一，通于冲脉。

三阴交 (SP 6)

【定位】内踝高点上 3 寸，胫骨内侧缘后方（图 10-15）。

【解剖】在胫骨后缘和比目鱼肌之间，深层有屈趾长肌；有大隐静脉，胫后动、静脉；有小腿内侧皮神经，深层后方有胫神经。

【主治】肠鸣腹胀，泄泻，月经不调，带下，阴挺，不孕，滞产，遗精，阳痿，遗尿，疝气，失眠，下肢痿痹，脚气。

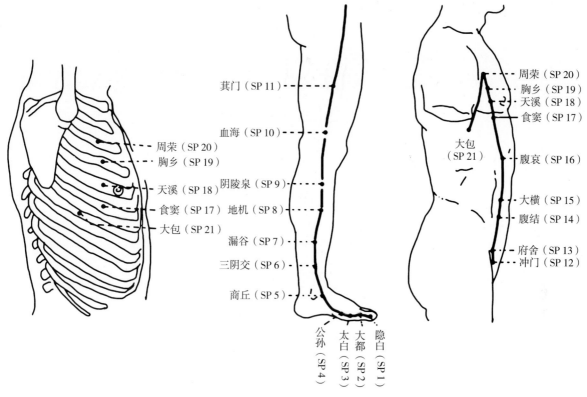

图 10-14   足太阴脾经腧穴总图
(The Spleen Meridian of Foot-Taiyin)

Gongsun (SP 4)

【Location】In the depression distal and inferior to the base of the first metatarsal bone, at the junction of the red and white skin(Figure 10-14).

【Anatomy】Muscles: in m. abductor halluces. Blood vessels: the branch of the medial tarsal artery and the dorsal venous network of the foot. Nerves: the saphenous nerve and the branch of the superficial peroneal nerve.

【Indications】Gastric pain, vomiting, abdominal pain, diarrhea, and dysentery.

【Manipulation】Puncture perpendicularly 0. 6-1. 2 *cun*.

【Remarks】Connecting point of the spleen meridian of Foot-Taiyin, one of the confluence points of eight vessels, linking to the thoroughfare vessel.

Sanyinjiao (SP 6)

【Location】3 *cun* directly above the tip pf the medial malleolus, on the posterior border of the medial aspect of the tibia(Figure 10-15).

【Anatomy】Muscles: between the posterior border of the tibia and m. flexer digitorum longus. Blood vessels: the great saphenous vein, the posterior tibial artery and vein. Nerves: superficially, the medical sural cutaneous nerve; deeper, in the posterior aspect, the tibial nerve.

【Indications】Borboryggnus, abdominal distension, diarrhea, irregular menstruation, leucorrhea, va-

【操作】直刺 1~1.5 寸，孕妇禁针。

【附注】足太阴、少阴、厥阴经交会穴。

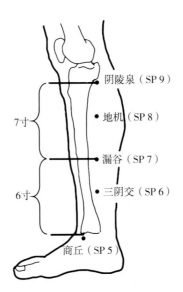

图 10-15 三阴交、阴陵泉

（Sanyinjiao and Yinlingquan）

阴陵泉（SP 9）

【定位】胫骨内侧髁后下缘凹陷中（图 10-15）。

【解剖】在胫骨后缘和腓肠肌之间，比目鱼肌起点上；前方有大隐静脉，膝最上动脉，最深层有胫后动、静脉；布有小腿内侧皮神经本干，最深层有胫神经。

【主治】腹胀，泄泻，水肿，黄疸，小便不利或失禁，膝痛。

【操作】直刺 1~2 寸。

【附注】足太阴经合穴。

血海（SP 10）

【定位】髌骨内上缘上 2 寸（图 10-14）。

【解剖】在股骨内上髁上缘，股内侧肌中间；有股动、静脉肌支；布有股前皮神经及股神经肌支。

【主治】月经不调，崩漏，经闭，瘾疹，湿疹，丹毒。

【操作】直刺 1~1.5 寸。

ginal protrusion, infertility, delivery stagnation, nocturnal emission, impotence, enuresis, hernia, insomnia, muscular atrophy, numbness pain and flaccidity of the lower extremities, and beriberi.

【Manipulation】Puncture perpendicularly 1−1. 5 *cun*. Acupuncture on this point is contraindicated in pregnant women.

【Remarks】The crossing point of the meridians of Foot-Tainyin, Foot-Shaoyin, and Foot-Jueyin.

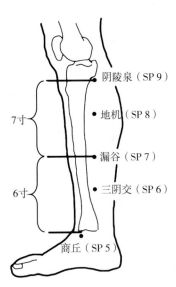

图 10-15　三阴交、阴陵泉
(Sanyinjiao and Yinlingquan)

Yinlingquan (SP 9)

【Location】In the depression of the lower border of the medial condyle of the tibia(Figure 10-15).

【Anatomy】Muscles: between the posterior border of the tibia and m.gastrocnemius, superior to the initial point of m. soleus. Blood vessels: anteriorly, the great saphenous vein, the genu suprema artery; deeper, the posterior tibial artery and vein. Nerves: superficially, the trunk of the medial sural cutaneous nerve; deeper, the tibial nerve.

【Indications】Abdominal distension, diarrhea, edema, jaundice, dysuria, incontinence of urine, and pain in the knee.

【Manipulation】Puncture perpendicularly 0. 5−1 *cun*.

【Remarks】Sea point of the spleen meridian of Foot-Taiyin.

Xuehai (SP 10)

【Location】2 *cun* directly above the medial border of the patella(Figure 10-14).

【Anatomy】Muscles: on the upper border of the epicondylus medialis femoris, in the middle of m. vastus medialis. Blood vessels: the muscular branches of the femoral artery and vein. Nerves: the anterior femoral cutaneous nerve and the muscular branch of the femoral nerve.

【Indications】Irregular menstruation, metrorrhagia and metrostaxia, amenorrhea, dormant papules, exzema, and erysilelas.

【Manipulation】Puncture perpendicularly 1−1. 5 *cun*.

五、手少阴心经

【主治概要】心、胸、神志病，如心动过速或过缓等，心律不齐、心绞痛、失眠、瘫痪、癫痫以及昏迷、上臂内侧痛等。

【本经腧穴】左右各9穴（图10-16）。

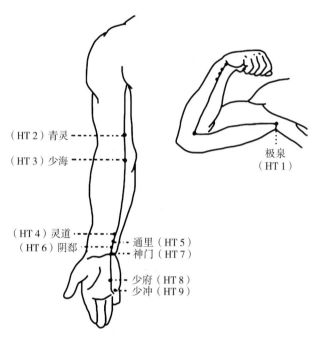

（HT 2）青灵
（HT 3）少海
（HT 4）灵道
（HT 6）阴郄
通里（HT 5）
神门（HT 7）
少府（HT 8）
少冲（HT 9）
极泉（HT 1）

图10-16　手少阴心经腧穴总图

(The Heart Meridian of Hand-Shaoyin)

极泉（HT 1）

【定位】在腋窝正中，腋动脉搏动处（图10-16）。

【解剖】在胸大肌的外下缘，深层为喙肱肌；外侧为腋动脉；布有尺神经、正中神经、前臂内侧皮神经及臂内侧皮神经。

【主治】心痛，咽干烦渴，胁肋疼痛，瘰疬，肩臂疼痛。

【操作】避开腋动脉，直刺或斜刺0.3~0.5寸。

通里（HT 5）

【定位】腕横纹上1寸，尺侧腕屈肌腱的桡侧（图10-16）。

【解剖】在尺侧腕屈肌与指浅屈肌之间，深层为指深屈肌；有尺动脉通过；布有前臂内侧皮神经，尺侧为尺神经。

The Heart Meridian of Hand-Shaoyin

【Principal indications】Diseases in the heart and chest and mental diseases, such as tachycardia, bradycardia, arrhythmia, angina, insomnia, paralysis, epilepsy, coma, and pain in the medial upper arm.

【Acupoints】9 points each side(Figure 10-16).

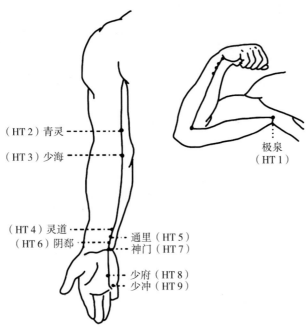

图 10-16   手少阴心经腧穴总图
(The Heart Meridian of Hand-Shaoyin)

Jiquan (HT 1)

【Location】In the center of the axilla, at the pulsating point of the axillary artery(Figure 10-16).

【Anatomy】Muscles: on the lateroinferior border of m.pectoralis majou; deeper, m.coracobrachialis. Blood vessel: laterally, the axillary. Nerves: the nlnar nerve, median nerve and medial brachial cutaneous nerve.

【Indications】Pain in the cardiac region, dryness of the throat and excessive thirst, pain in the castal region, scrofula, and pain of the shoulder and arm.

【Manipulation】Keeping away from the axillary artery; puncture perpendicularly 0.3−0.5 *cun*.

Tongli (HT 5)

【Location】1 *cun* above the transverse crease of the wrist, on the radial side of the tendon of m.flexor carpi ularis(Figure 10-16).

【Anatomy】Muscles: between the tendon of m, flexor carpi ulnaris and m.flexor digitorun superficialis; deeper, m.flexor digitorum profundus. Blood vessels: the ulnar artery. Nerves: the medial antebrachial cutaneous nerve; on the medial side, the ulnar nerve.

【Indications】Palpitation or severe palpitation, sudden loss of voice, aphasia with stiffness of the tongue, and pain in the wrist and forearm.

【主治】心悸，怔忡，暴喑，舌强不语，腕臂痛。

【操作】直刺0.3~0.5寸。

【附注】手少阴经络穴。

六、手太阳小肠经

【主治概要】头、项、耳、目、咽喉病、热病，如少腹痛、耳聋、耳鸣、颊肿、项背肩胛部疼痛以及肩臂外侧后缘痛等。

【本经腧穴】左右各19穴（图10-17）。

少泽（SI 1）

【定位】小指尺侧指甲角旁0.1寸（图10-17）。

【解剖】有指掌侧固有动、静脉，指背动脉形成的动、静脉网；布有尺神经手背支。

【主治】头痛，目翳，咽喉肿痛，乳痈，乳汁少，昏迷，热病。

【操作】浅刺0.1寸或点刺出血。

【附注】手太阳经井穴。

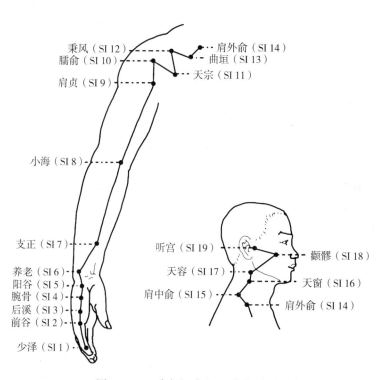

图10-17 手太阳小肠经腧穴总图

（The Small Instestine Meridian of Hand−Taiyang）

【Manipulation】Puncture perpendicularly 0. 3–0. 5 *cun*.

【Remarks】Connecting point of the heart meridian of Hand-Shaoyin.

The Small Instestine Meridian of Hand-Taiyang

【Principal indications】Diseases of the head, nape, ear, eye and throat, such as lesser abdominal pain, deafness, tinnitus, swelling in the cheek, pain in the back and scapular, and pain in the edge of the shoulder and lateral arm.

【Acupoints】19 points each side(Figure 10-17).

Shaoze (SI 1)

【Location】On the ulnar side of the little finger, about 0. 1 *cun* proximal to the corner of the nail (Figure 10-17)

【Anatomy】Blood vessels: the arterial and venous network formed by the palmar digital proprial artery and vein and the dorsal digital artery and vein. Nerves: the palmar digital proprial nerve.

【Indications】Headache, corneal opacity, sore throat, acute mastitis, scant breast milk, coma, and febrile diseases.

【Manipulation】Puncture subcutaneously 0. 1 *cun* or prick to cause bleeding.

【Remarks】Well point of the small intestine meridian of Hand-Taiyang.

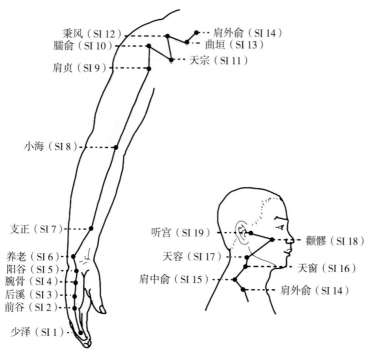

图 10-17   手太阳小肠经腧穴总图

(The Small Instestine Meridian of Hand-Taiyang)

后溪（SI 3）

【定位】握拳，第五指掌关节后尺侧，横纹头赤白肉际（图 10-18）。

【解剖】在小指尺侧，第五掌骨小头后方，当小指展肌起点外缘；有指背动、静脉，手背静脉网；布有尺神经手背支。

【主治】头项强痛，目赤，耳聋，咽喉肿痛，腰背痛，癫狂痫，疟疾，手指及肘臂挛痛。

【操作】直刺 0.5~1 寸。

【附注】手太阳经输穴；八脉交会穴之一，通于督脉。

颧髎（SI 18）

【定位】目外眦直下，颧骨下缘凹陷中（图 10-17）。

【解剖】在咬肌的起始部，颧肌中；有面横动、静脉分支；布有面神经及眶下神经。

【主治】口眼㖞斜，眼睑𥆧动，齿痛，颊肿。

【操作】直刺 0.3~0.5 寸，斜刺或平刺 0.5~1 寸。不宜灸。

【附注】手少阳、太阳经交会穴。

听宫（SI 19）

【定位】耳屏前，下颌骨髁状突的后缘，张口时呈凹陷处（图 10-19）。

【解剖】有颞浅动、静脉的耳前支；布有面神经及三叉神经第三支的耳颞神经。

【主治】耳鸣，耳聋，聤耳，齿痛，癫狂痫。

【操作】张口，直刺 1~1.5 寸。

【附注】手、足少阳与手太阳经交会穴。

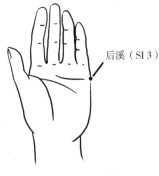

图 10-18　后溪

（Houxi）

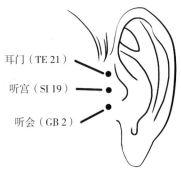

图 10-19　耳门、听宫、听会

（Ermen，Tinggong and Tinghui）

Houxi (SI 3)

【Location】When a fist is made, the point is on the ulnar side, proximaltothe 5th metacarphalangeal joint, at the end of the transverse creas and the junction of the red and white skin(Figure 10-18).

【Anatomy】Muscles: on the ulnar side of the little finger, posterior to the small end of the 5th metacarpal bome, lateral border of the origin of m.abductor digiti minimi manus. Blood vessels: the dorsal digital artery and vein, the dorsal venous network of the hand. Nerves: the dorasal metacarpal nerve.

【Indications】Pain and rigidity of the head and neck, redness of the eye, deafness, sore throat, lumbar pain, pain of the back, depressive psychosis, mania, epilepsy, maralia, and spasmodic pain of the finger, elbow and arm.

【Manipulation】Puncture perpendicularly 0. 5–1 *cun*.

【Remarks】Stream point of the small intestine meridian of Hand-Taiyang, one of the confluence points of the eight vessels, intersecting with the governor vessel.

Quanliao (SI 18)

【Location】Directly below the outer canthus, in the depression on the lower border of zygoma(Figure 10-17).

【Anatomy】Muscles: at the origin of the masseter and in m.zygomaticus major. Blood vessels: the branches of the transverse facial artery and vein. Nerves: the facial and infraorbital nerves.

【Indications】Facia paralysis, twitching of eyelids, toothache, and swelling of the cheek.

【Manipulation】Puncture perpendicularly 0. 3–0. 5 *cun*. Punctureobliquely or subcutaneously 0. 5–1 *cun*. Moxibustion is not advisable.

【Remarks】The crossing point of Hand-Shaoyang meridian and Hand-Taiyang meridian.

Tinggong (SI 19)

【Location】Anterior to the tragus and posterior to the condyloid process of the mandible, in the depression formed when the mouth is open(Figure 10-19).

【Anatomy】Blood vessels: the auricular branches of the superficial temporal artery and vein. Nerves: the facial nerve, the auriculotemporal nerve of the third branch of the trigeminal nerve.

【Indications】Tinnitus, deafness, otorrhea, toothache, depressive psychosis, mania, and epilepsy.

【Manipulation】Open mouth; puncture perpendicularly 1–1. 5 *cun*.

【Remarks】The crossing point of the Hand-Shaoyang, Foot-Shaoyang, and Hand-Taiyang meridians.

七、足太阳膀胱经

【主治概要】主治头、项、目、背、腰、下肢部病症，如小便不通、遗尿、癫狂、疟疾、头痛、目疾及项、背、腰、臀部以及下肢后侧本经循行部位疼痛等症。

【本经腧穴】左右各 67 穴（图 10-20）。

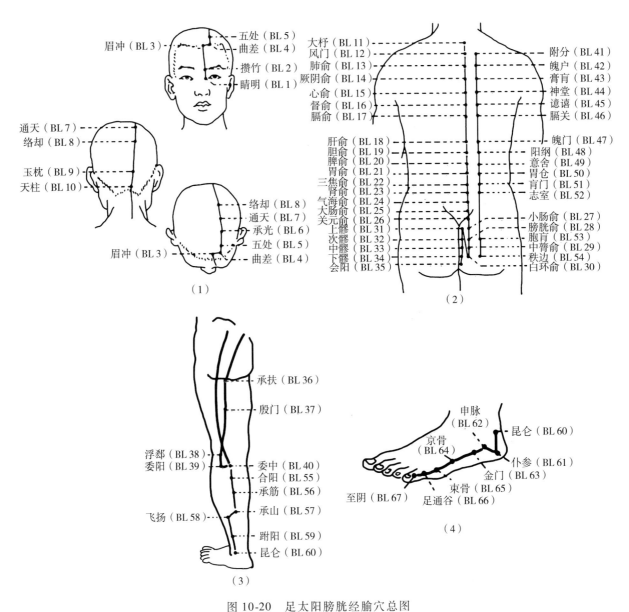

图 10-20　足太阳膀胱经腧穴总图

（The Bladder Meridian of Foot-Taiyang）

晴明（BL 1）

【定位】目内眦旁 0.1 寸（图 10-21）。

【解剖】在眶内缘睑内侧韧带中，深部为眼内直肌；有内眦动、静脉和滑车上下

The Bladder Meridian of Foot-Taiyang

【Principal indications】Diseases of the head, nape, eyes, back, lumbar region, and the lower extremities such as dysuria, enuresis, depressive psychosis, mania, maralia, headache, pain in the neck, back lumar, buttock and lower limbs, and other diseases in the regions along the course of this meridians.

【Acupoints】67 points each side (Figure 10-20).

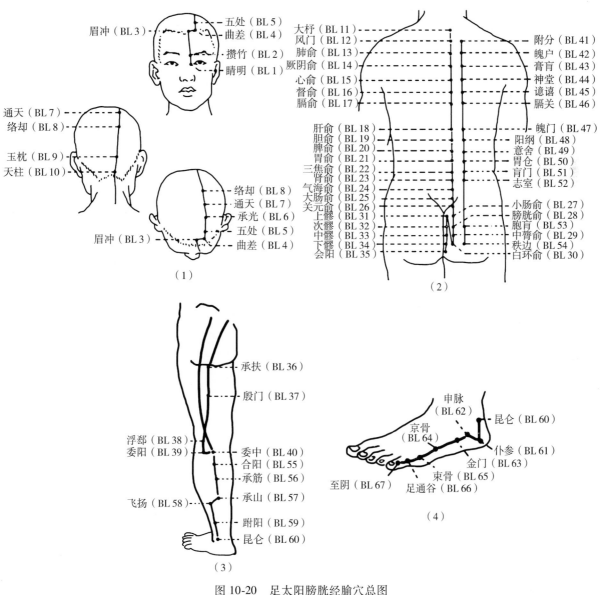

图 10-20　足太阳膀胱经腧穴总图
(The Bladder Meridian of Foot-Taiyang)

Jingming (BL 1)

【Location】0.1 *cun* superior to the inner canthus (Figure 10-21).

【Anatomy】Muscles: in the infraorbital medial palpebral ligament; deeper, m.rectus oculi medialis. Blood vessels: the angular artery and vein, the supratrochlear artery and vein and the infratrochlear arter-

动、静脉，深层上方有眼动、静脉本干；布有滑车上、下神经，深层为眼神经，上方为鼻睫神经。

【主治】目赤肿痛，流泪，视物不明，目眩，近视，夜盲，色盲。

【操作】嘱患者闭目，医者左手轻推眼球向外侧固定，左手缓慢进针，紧靠眶缘直刺0.5~1寸，不宜做大幅度提插和捻转，出针后按压针孔片刻，以防出血。禁灸。

【附注】手足太阳、足阳明、阴跷、阳跷五脉交会穴。

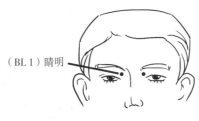

（BL 1）睛明

图 10-21　睛明

（Jingming）

攒竹（BL 2）

【定位】眉头凹陷中（图10-20）。

【解剖】有额肌及皱眉肌；当额动、静脉处；布有额神经内侧支。

【主治】头痛，口眼㖞斜，目视不明，流泪，目赤肿痛，眼睑瞤动，眉棱骨痛，眼睑下垂。

【操作】平刺0.5~0.8寸。禁灸。

风门（BL 12）

【定位】在背部，当第二胸椎棘突下，旁开1.5寸（图10-22）。

【解剖】有斜方肌、菱形肌、上后锯肌，深层为最长肌；有第二肋间动、静脉后支；布有第二、三胸神经后支内侧皮支，深层为第三胸神经后支外侧支。

【主治】伤风，咳嗽，发热头痛，项强，胸背痛。

【操作】斜刺0.5~0.8寸。

【附注】足太阳经与督脉交会穴。

肺俞（BL 13）

【定位】在背部，当第三胸椎棘突下，旁开1.5寸（图10-22）。

【解剖】有斜方肌、菱形肌，深层为最长肌；有第三肋间动、静脉后支；布有第

y and vein; deeper, superiorly, the ophthalmic artery and vein. Nerves: the supratrochlear and infratrochlear nerves; deeper, ophthalmic nerve; superiorly, the nasociliary nerve.

【Indications】Sore red swollen eyes, lacrimation, dim vision, bluerred vision, myopia, night blindness, and colour blindness.

【Manipulation】Ask the patient to close his eyes when pushing gently the eyeball to the lateral side and fixing it with the left hand. Puncture slowly perpendicularly 0.5−1 *cun* with the left hand. It is not advisable to twirl or lift and thrust the needle. To avoid bleeding, press the puncturing site for minutes after withdrawal of the needle. Moxibustion is not applicable.

【Remarks】The crossing point of the Hand-Taiyang, Foot-Taiyang, and Foot-Yangming meridians, and yin heel vessel, and yang heel vessel.

Cuanzhu (BL 2)

【Location】In the depression on the end of the eyebrow(Figure 10-20).

【Anatomy】Muscles: m. frontalis and m. corrugators supercilii. Blood vessels: the frontal artery and vein. Nerves: the medial branch of the frontal nerve.

【Indications】Headache, deviation of the mouth and eyes, blurred vision, lacrimation, sore red swollen eyes, twitching of eyelids, pain in the supraorbital region, and blepharoptosis.

【Manipulation】Puncture subcutaneously 0.5−0.8 *cun*. Moxibustion is not applicable.

Fengmen (BL 12)

【Location】On the back, 1.5 *cun* lateral to the lower border of the spinous process of the second thoracic vertebra(Figure 10-22).

【Anatomy】Muscles: m. trapezius, m. rhomboideus, m. serratus posterior superior; deeper, m. longissimus. Blood vessels: the posterior branches of the second intercostals artery and vein. Nerves: the medial cutaneous branches of the posterior rami of the second and third thoracic nerves; deeper, their lateral cutaneous branches of the third thoracic nerve.

【Indications】Common cold, cough, fever, headache, neck rigidity, and pain in the chest and back.

【Manipulation】Puncture obliquely 0.5−0.8 *cun*.

【Remarks】The crossing point of Foot-Taiyang meridian and governor vessel.

Feishu (BL 13)

【Location】On the back, 1.5 *cun* lateral to the lower border of the spinous process of the third thoracic vertebra(Figure 10-22).

【Anatomy】Muscles: m. trapezius, m. rhomboideus, m. serratus posterior superior; deeper, m. longissimus. Blood vessels: the posterior branches of the third intercostals artery and vein. Nerves: the medial cutaneous branches of the posterior rami of the third and fourth thoracic nerves; deeper, their lateral cutaneous branches of the third thoracic nerve.

【Indications】Cough, asthma, spitting of blood, fever due to yin-deficiency, tidal fever, night sweating, and nasal obstruction.

【Manipulation】Puncture obliquely 0.5−0.8 *cun*.

【Remarks】Tansport point of the lung meridian of Hand-Taiyin.

三或第四胸神经后支内侧皮支，深层为第三胸神经后支外侧支。

【主治】咳嗽，气喘，吐血，骨蒸，潮热，盗汗，鼻塞。

【操作】斜刺 0.5~0.8 寸

【附注】肺背俞穴。

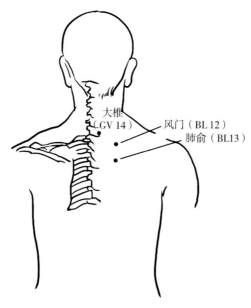

图 10-22　风门、肺俞

（Fengmen and Feishu）

心俞（BL 15）

【定位】在背部，当第五胸椎棘突下，旁开 1.5 寸（图 10-20）。

【解剖】有斜方肌、菱形肌，深层为最长肌；有第五肋间动、静脉后支；布有第五或第六胸神经后支内侧皮支，深层为第五胸神经后支外侧支。

【主治】心痛，惊悸，咳嗽，吐血，失眠，健忘，盗汗，梦遗，癫痫。

【操作】斜刺 0.5~0.8 寸。

【附注】心背俞穴。

膈俞（BL 17）

【定位】在背部，当第七胸椎棘突下，旁开 1.5 寸（图 10-20）。

【解剖】在斜方肌下缘，有背阔肌、最长肌；布有第七肋间动、静脉后支；布有第七或第八胸神经后支内侧皮支，深层为第七胸神经后支外侧支。

【主治】呕吐，呃逆，气喘，咳嗽，吐血，潮热，盗汗。

【操作】斜刺 0.5~0.8 寸。

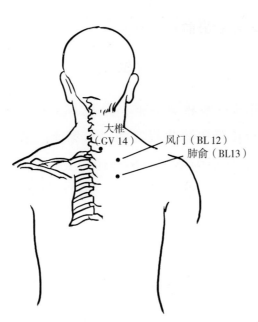

图 10-22   风门、肺俞
(Fengmen and Feishu)

Xinshu (BL15)

【Location】On the back , 1. 5 *cun* lateral to the lower border of the spinous process of the fifth thoracic vertebra (Figure 10-20).

【Anatomy】Muscles : m. trapezius , m. rhomboideus , m. serratus posterior superior ; deeper , m. longissimus. Blood vessels : the posterior branches of the fifth intercostals artery and vein. Nerves : the medial cutaneous branches of the posterior rami of the fifth and sixth thoracic nerves ; deeper , their lateral cutaneous branches of the fifth and sixth thoracic nerve.

【Indications】Cardiac pain , palpitation , cough , spitting of blood , insomnia , amnesia , night sweating , nocturnal emission , and epilepsy.

【Manipulation】Puncture obliquely 0. 5－1 *cun*.

【Remarks】Tansport point of the heart meridian of Hand-Shaoyin.

Geshu (BL 17)

【Location】On the back , 1. 5 *cun* lateral to the lower border of the spinous process of the seventh thoracic vertebra (Figure 10-21).

【Anatomy】Muscles : at the inferior border of m. trapezius ; m. latissimus dorsi , m. longissimus. Blood vessels : the medial branches of the posterior branches of the posterior branches of the seventh intercostals artery and vein. Nerves : the medial branches of the posterior rami of the seventh and eighth thoracic nerves ; deeper , their lateral branches of the the seventh thoracic nerve.

【Indications】Vomiting , hiccup , asthma , cough , spitting of blood , tidal fever , and night sweating.

【Manipulation】Puncture obliquely 0. 5－0. 8 *cun*.

【Remarks】One of the eight meeting points , point of the blood.

【附注】八会穴之一，血会膈俞。

脾俞（BL 20）

【定位】在背部，当第十一胸椎棘突下，旁开 1.5 寸（图 10-23）。

【解剖】在背阔肌、最长肌和髂肋肌之间；有第十一肋间动、静脉后支；布有第十一胸神经后支内侧皮支，深层为第十一胸神经后支外侧支。

【主治】腹胀，黄疸，呕吐，泄泻，痢疾，便血，水肿，背痛。

【操作】斜刺 0.5~0.8 寸。

【附注】脾背俞穴。

肾俞（BL 23）

【定位】在腰部，当第二腰椎棘突下，旁开 1.5 寸（图 10-24）。

【解剖】在腰背筋膜、最长肌和髂肋肌之间；有第二腰动、静脉后支；布有第一腰神经后支外侧支，深层为第一腰丛。

【主治】遗尿，遗精，阳痿，月经不调，白带，水肿，耳鸣，耳聋，腰痛。

【操作】直刺 0.5~1 寸。

【附注】肾背俞穴。

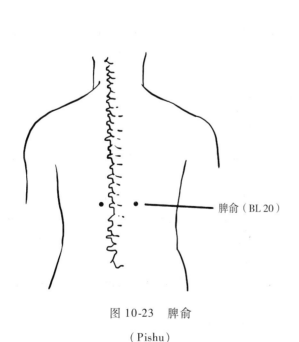

图 10-23　脾俞

（Pishu）

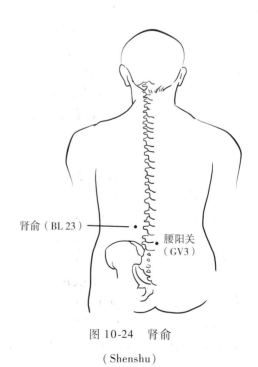

图 10-24　肾俞

（Shenshu）

Pishu (BL 20)

【Location】On the back, 1.5 *cun* lateral to the lower border of the spinous process of the eleventh thoracic vertebra(Figure 10-23).

【Anatomy】Muscles: m.latissimus dorsi, m.longissimus and m.iliocostalis. Blood vessels: the posterior branches of the eleventh intercostals artery and vein. Nerves: the medial cutaneous branches of the posterior rami of the eleventh and twelfth thoracic nerves; deeper, their posterior and lateral branches of the eleventh thoracic nerve.

【Indications】Abdominal distenstion, jaundice, vomiting, diarrhea, dysentery, blood stools, edema, and pain in the back.

【Manipulation】Puncture obliquely 0.5−0.8 *cun*.

【Remarks】Tansport point of the spleen meridian of Foot-Taiyin.

Shenshu (BL 23)

【Location】On the lumbar part, 1.5 *cun* lateral to the lower border of the spinous process of the second lumbar vertebra(Figure 10-24).

【Anatomy】Muscles: fascia lumbodorsalis, m.longissimus and m.iliocostalis. Blood vessels: the posterior branches of the second lumbar artery and vein. Nerves: the lateral cutaneous branch of the posterior ramus of the first lumbar nerve; the first lumber plexus.

【Indications】Enuresis, nocturnal emission, impotence, irregular menstruation, leukorrhagia, edema, tinnitus, deafness, and lower back pain.

【Manipulation】Puncture perpendicularly 0.5−0.8 *cun*.

【Remarks】Tansport point of the kidney meridian of Foot-Shaoyin.

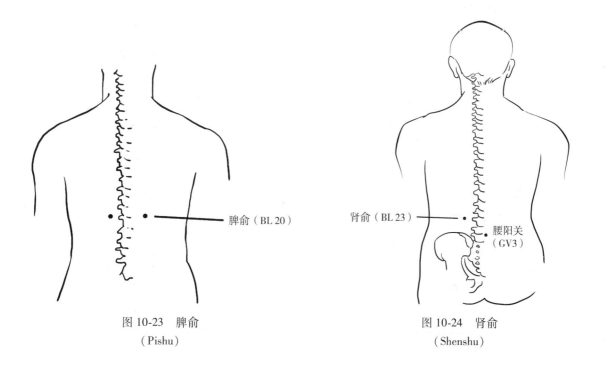

图 10-23   脾俞
(Pishu)

脾俞（BL 20）

肾俞（BL 23）

腰阳关
（GV3）

图 10-24   肾俞
(Shenshu)

大肠俞（BL 25）

【定位】在腰部，当第四腰椎棘突下，旁开1.5寸（图10-25）。

【解剖】在腰背筋膜、最长肌和髂肋肌之间；有第四腰动、静脉后支；布有第三腰神经皮支，深层为腰丛。

【主治】腹胀，泄泻，便秘，腰痛。

【操作】直刺0.8~1.2寸。

【附注】大肠背俞穴。

委中（BL 40）

【定位】在腘横纹中点，当股二头肌腱与半腱肌肌腱的中间（图10-26）。

【解剖】在腘窝正中，有腘筋膜；皮下有股腘静脉，深层内侧为腘静脉，最深层为腘动脉；有股后皮神经，正当胫神经处。

【主治】腰痛，下肢痿痹，腹痛，吐泻，小便不利，遗尿，丹毒。

【操作】直刺1~1.5寸，或用三棱针点刺腘静脉出血。

【附注】足太阳经合穴。

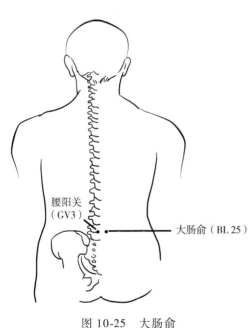

图 10-25　大肠俞

（Dachangshu）

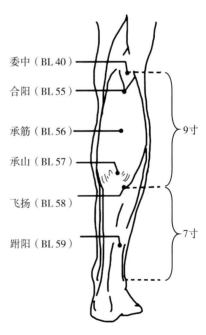

图 10-26　委中、承山

（Weizhong and Chengshan）

Dachangshu（BL 25）

【Location】On the lumbar part, 1. 5 *cun* lateral to the midpoint on the line joining the spinous processes of the fourth and fifth lumbar vertebrae(Figure 10-25).

【Anatomy】Muscles: fascia lumbodorsalis; m. sacrospinalis and m. longissimus. Blood vessels: the posterior branch of the fourth lumbar artery and vein. Nerves: the cutaneous branch of the third lumbar nerve; deeper, the lumbar plexus.

【Indications】Abdominal distension, diarrhea, constipation, and lower back pain.

【Manipulation】Puncture perpendicularly 0. 8 - 1. 5 *cun*.

【Remarks】Tansport point of the large intestine meridian of Hand-Yangming.

Weizhong（BL 40）

【Location】Midpoint of the transverse crease of the popliteal fossa, between the tendons of m. biceps femoris and m. semitendinosus(Figure 10-26).

【Anatomy】Muscles: in the popliteal fossa, there is the popliteal fascia. Blood vessels: superficially, femoropopliteal vein; deeper and medially, the popliteal vein; deepst, the popliteal artery. Nerves: the posterior femoral cutaneous nerve, the tibial nerve.

【Indications】Lumbar pain, muscular atrophy, pain, numbness pain and flaccidity of the lower extremities, abdominal pain, vomiting, diarrhea, dysuria, enuresis, and erysipelas.

【Manipulation】Puncture perpendicularly 1 - 1. 5 *cun*, or prick popliteal vein to cause bleeding with the three-edged needle.

【Remarks】Sea point of the bladder meridian of Foot-Taiyang.

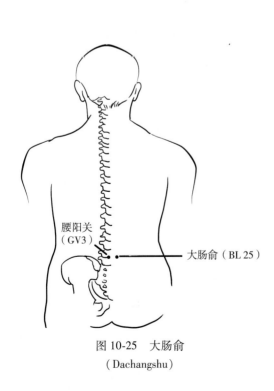

图 10-25 大肠俞
（Dachangshu）

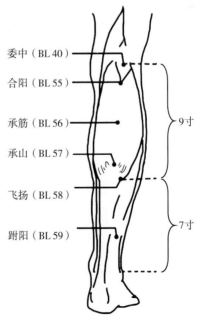

图 10-26 委中、承山
（Weizhong and Chengshan）

秩边（BL 54）

【定位】在臀部，平第四骶后孔，骶正中嵴旁开 3 寸。在骶管裂孔旁开 3 寸处（图 10-20）。

【解剖】有臀大肌，在梨状肌下缘；正当臀下动、静脉处；布有臀下神经及股后皮神经，外侧为坐骨神经。

【主治】小便不利，便秘，痔疾，腰骶痛，下肢痿痹。

【操作】直刺 1.5~2 寸。

承山（BL 57）

【定位】在小腿后面正中，当伸直小腿或足跟上提时，腓肠肌两肌腹之间凹陷的顶端（图 10-26）。

【解剖】在腓肠肌两肌腹交界下端；有小隐静脉，深层为胫后动、静脉；布有腓肠内侧皮神经，深层为胫神经。

【主治】痔疾，脚气，便秘，腰腿拘急疼痛。

【操作】直刺 1~2 寸。

昆仑（BL 60）

【定位】在足部外踝后方，当外踝高点与跟腱之间的凹陷处（图 10-20）。

【解剖】有腓骨短肌；有小隐静脉及外踝后动、静脉；布有腓肠神经。

【主治】头痛，项强，目眩，癫痫，难产，腰骶疼痛，足跟肿痛。

【操作】直刺 0.5~0.8 寸。

【附注】足太阳经经穴。

申脉（BL 62）

【定位】在足外侧部，外踝下缘凹陷中（图 10-20）。

【解剖】在腓骨长短肌腱上缘；有外踝动脉网及小隐静脉；布有腓肠神经的足背外侧皮神经分支。

【主治】头痛，眩晕，癫狂痫，腰腿酸痛，目赤痛，失眠。

【操作】直刺 0.3~0.5 寸。

【附注】八脉交会穴之一，通阳跷脉。

Zhibian (BL 54)

【Location】In the buttocks, parallel to the fourth posterior sacral foramina, 3 *cun* lateral to the median sacral crest, 3 *cun* lateral to the lsacral hiatus(Figure 10-20).

【Anatomy】Muscles: m. gluteus maximus, in the inferior border of m. piriformis. Blood vessels: the inferior gluteal nerve, the posterior femoral cutaneous nerve; laterally, the sciatic nerve.

【Indications】Dysuria, constipation, hemorrhoids, pain in the lumbosacral region, muscular atrophy, pain, and numbness and flaccidity of the lower extremities.

【Manipulation】Puncture perpendicularly 1. 5-2 *cun*.

Chengshan (BL 57)

【Location】on the posterior midline of the leg, in a pointed depression formed between the gastrocneminus muscle belly when the leg is stretched or the heel is lifted(Figure 10-26).

【Anatomy】Muscles: at the lower border of the junction of the two belies of m. gastrocnemius. Blood vessels: the small saphenous vein; deeper, the posterior tibial artery and vein. Nerves: the medial sural cutaneous nerve; deeper the tibial nerve.

【Indications】Hemorrhoids, beriberi, constipation, and contracture and pain of the lower back and leg.

【Manipulation】Puncture perpendicularly 1-2 *cun*.

Kunlun (BL 60)

【Location】In the posterior of the foot lateral malleolus, in the depression between the tip of the external malleolusandtendo calcaneus(Figure 10-20).

【Anatomy】Muscles: m. peroneus brevis. Blood vessels: the small saphenous vein, the posteroexternal malleolar artery and vein. Nerves: the sural nerve.

【Indications】Headache, neck rigidity, dizziness, epilepsy, dystocia, pain in the lumbosacral region, and heel pain and swelling.

【Manipulation】Puncture perpendicularly 0. 5-0. 8 *cun*.

【Remarks】River point of the bladder meridian of Foot-Taiyang.

Shenmai (BL 62)

【Location】In the lateral part of foot, in the depression on the inferior border of the external malleolus(Figure 10-20).

【Anatomy】Muscles: on the superior border of tendons of peroneus longus and peroneus brevis. Blood vessels: the external malleolar arterial network, the small saphenous vein. Nerves: the sural nerve.

【Indications】Headache, dizziness, depressive psychosis, mania, epilepsy, aching of the lower back and leg, redness and pain in the eyes, and insomnia.

【Manipulation】Puncture perpendicularly 0. 3-0. 5 *cun*.

【Remarks】One of the confluence points of the eight vessels, intersecting with the yang heel vessel.

至阴（BL 67）

【定位】在足小趾末节外侧，距趾甲角约0.1寸（图10-27）。

【解剖】有趾背动脉及趾跖侧固有动脉形成的动脉网；布有趾跖侧固有神经及足背外侧皮神经。

【主治】头痛，目痛，鼻塞，鼻衄，胎位不正，难产。

【操作】浅刺0.1寸。胎位不正用灸法。

【附注】足太阳经井穴。

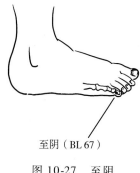

至阴（BL 67）

图 10-27 至阴

（Zhiyin）

八、足少阴肾经

【主治概要】主治妇科病、前阴病、肾、咽喉病及经脉循行部位其他病证，如遗精、阳痿、早泄、咳嗽、气喘、水肿、泄泻、便秘、耳鸣、失眠等。

【本经腧穴】左右各27穴（图10-28）。

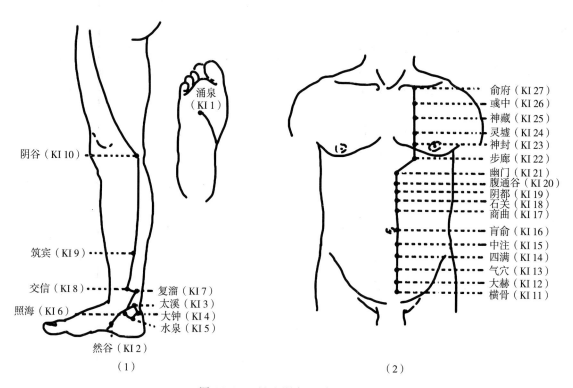

涌泉（KI 1）	
阴谷（KI 10）	俞府（KI 27）
	或中（KI 26）
	神藏（KI 25）
	灵墟（KI 24）
	神封（KI 23）
	步廊（KI 22）
	幽门（KI 21）
	腹通谷（KI 20）
	阴都（KI 19）
	石关（KI 18）
	商曲（KI 17）
筑宾（KI 9）	肓俞（KI 16）
	中注（KI 15）
	四满（KI 14）
交信（KI 8）　复溜（KI 7）	气穴（KI 13）
照海（KI 6）　太溪（KI 3）	大赫（KI 12）
大钟（KI 4）	横骨（KI 11）
水泉（KI 5）	
然谷（KI 2）	
（1）	（2）

图 10-28 足少阴肾经腧穴总图

（The Kidney Meridian of Foot-Shaoyin）

Zhiyin（BL 67）

【Location】One of the lateral side of the small toe, about 0. 1 *cun* lateral to the corner of the nail(Figure 10-27).

【Anatomy】Blood vessels: the network-formed by the dorsal digital artery and plantar digital proprial artery. Nerves: the plantar digital proprial nerve and the lateral dorsal cutaneous nerve of foot.

【Indications】Headache, pain in the eye, nasal obstruction, epistaxis, malposition of fetus, and dystocia.

【Manipulation】Puncture superficially 0. 1 *cun*. Malposition of fetus can be treated by moxibustion.

【Remarks】Well point of the bladder meridian of Foot-Taiyang.

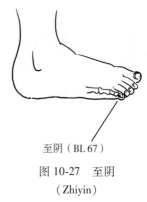

至阴（BL 67）

图 10-27   至阴
（Zhiyin）

The Kidney Meridian of Foot-*Shaoyin*

【Principal indications】Gynecological diseases, external genitalia diseases, and diseases of the kidney, throat and other diseases in the regions along the course of this meridian. For example, nocturnal emission, impotence, premature ejaculation, cough, asthma, edema, diarrhea, constipation, tinnitus, insomnia, etc.

【Acupoints】27 points each side(Figure 10-28).

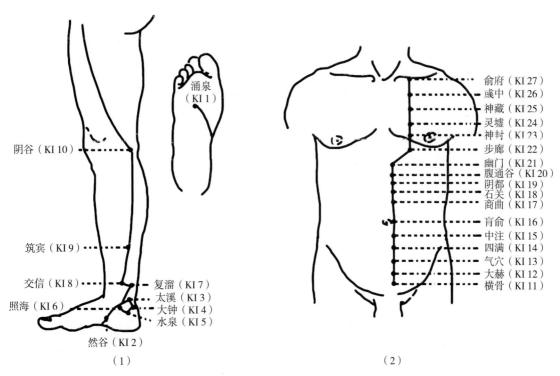

图 10-28   足少阴肾经腧穴总图
（The Kidney Meridian of Foot-Shaoyin）

涌泉（KI 1）

【定位】　在足底部，蹠足时足前部凹陷处（图 10-29）。

【解剖】　在足底第二、三跖骨之间，足底腱膜中，内有趾短屈肌腱、趾长屈肌腱，第二蚓状肌，深层为骨间肌；有来自胫前动脉的足底弓；布有足底内侧神经支。

【主治】　头痛，头昏，失眠，目眩，咽喉痛，舌干，失音，小便不利，大便难，小儿惊风，足心热，癫疾，霍乱转筋，昏厥。

【操作】　直刺 0.5~0.8 寸。

【附注】　足少阴经井穴。

太溪（KI 3）

【定位】　在足内侧，内踝后方，当内踝高点与跟腱之间的凹陷处（图 10-30）。

【解剖】　有胫后动、静脉；布有小腿内侧皮神经，当胫神经所过处。

【主治】　咽喉肿痛，齿痛，耳聋，耳鸣，咳嗽，气喘，胸痛咳血，消渴，月经不调，遗精，阳痿，小便频数。

【操作】　直刺 0.5~0.8 寸。可灸。

【附注】　足少阴经输穴、原穴。

照海（KI 6）

【定位】　在足内踝下缘凹陷处（图 10-28）。

【解剖】　后下方有胫后动、静脉；布有小腿内侧皮神经，当胫神经本干经过处。

【主治】　月经不调，带下，阴挺，阴痒，小便频数，癃闭，便秘，不寐，咽干，气喘。

【操作】　直刺 0.5~0.8 寸，可灸。

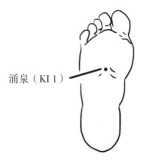

图 10-29　涌泉

（Yongquan）

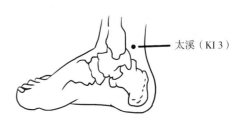

图 10-30　太溪

（Taixi）

Yongquan (KI 1)

【Location】In the bottom of the foot, in the depression when the foot is in plantar flexion(Figure10-29).

【Anatomy】Muscles: between the second and third plantar metatarsal bones, in the plantar aponeurosis; medially, the tendons of m. flexor digitorum brevis and longus, the second m. lumbricales; deeper m. interossei. Blood vessels: the plantar arterial arch derived from the anterior tibial artery. Nerves: the second common plantar digital nerve.

【Indications】Headache, dizziness, insomnia, blurred vision, sore throat, dry tongue, aphonia, dysuria, constipation, child fright wind, heat in the heart of the soles, madness, cholera cramps, and loss of consciousness.

【Manipulation】Puncture perpendicularly 0. 5-0. 8 *cun*.

【Remarks】Well point of the kidney meridian of Foot-Shaoyin.

Taixi (KI 3)

【Location】In the medial side of foot, posterior to the medial malleolus, in the depression between the tip of the medial malleolus and the tendo calcaneous(Figure10-30).

【Anatomy】Blood vessels: anteriorly, the posterior tibial artery and vein. Nerves: the medial crural cutaneous nerve, on the course of the tibial nerve.

【Indications】Sore throat, toothache, deafness, tinnitus, cough, shortness of breath, chest pain, hemoptysis, thirst, irregular menstruation, nocturnal emission, impotence, and frequent urination.

【Manipulation】Puncture perpendicularly 0. 5-0. 8 *cun*. Moxibustion is applicable.

【Remarks】Stream point and source point of the kidney meridian of Foot-Shaoyin.

Zhaohai (KI 6)

【Location】In the depression of the lower border of the tip of themedialmalleolus(Figure10-28).

【Anatomy】Blood vessels: posteroinferiorly, the posterior tibital artery and vein. Nerves: the medial crural cutaneous nerve; deeper, the tibial nerve.

【Indications】Irregular menstruation, leukorrhagia, prolapse of the uterus, pruritus vulvae, frequency of urination, retention of urine, constipation, insomnia, dry throat, and asthma.

【Manipulation】Puncture perpendicularly 0. 5-0. 8 *cun*. Moxibustion is applicable.

【Remarks】One of the confluence points of the eight vessels, connecting with the yin heel vessel.

【附注】八脉交会穴之一，通阴跷脉。

复溜（KI 7）

【定位】太溪穴上 2 寸，跟腱之前缘（图 10-28）。

【解剖】深层前方有胫后动、静脉；布有腓肠内侧皮神经和小腿内侧皮神经，深层为胫神经。

【主治】水肿，腹胀，泄泻，盗汗，热病汗不出，下肢萎痹。

【操作】直刺 0.5~1 寸，可灸。

【附注】足少阴经经穴。

九、手厥阴心包经

【主治概要】主治心、胸、胃、神志病，以及经脉循行部位的其他病证，如心痛、心悸、心烦、胸闷、癫狂、手臂挛急、掌心发热等。

【本经腧穴】左右各 9 穴（图 10-31）。

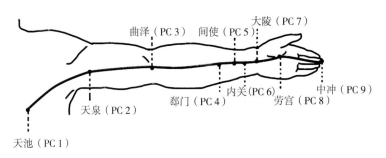

曲泽（PC 3）　间使（PC 5）　大陵（PC 7）
天泉（PC 2）　郄门（PC 4）　内关(PC 6)　劳宫（PC 8）　中冲（PC 9）
天池（PC 1）

图 10-31　手厥阴心包经腧穴总图

（The Pericardium Meridian of Hand-Jueyin）

内关（PC 6）

【定位】在前臂掌侧，当曲泽与大陵穴的连线上，腕横纹上 2 寸，掌长肌腱与桡侧腕屈肌腱之间（图 10-32）。

【解剖】有指浅屈肌，深层为指深屈肌；有前臂正中动、静脉，深层为前臂掌侧骨间动、静脉；布有前臂内侧皮神经，其下为正中神经掌皮支，深层为前臂掌侧骨间神经。

【主治】心痛，心悸，胸痛，胃痛，呕吐，呃逆，失眠，癫狂，痫证，郁证，眩晕，中风，偏瘫，哮喘，偏头痛，热病，肘臂挛痛。

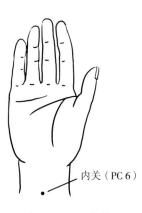

内关（PC 6）

图 10-32　内关

（Neiguan）

Fuliu (KI 7)

【Location】2 *cun* directly above Taixi(KI 3) , on the anterior border of tendo calcaneus(Figure10-28).

【Anatomy】Blood vessels: deeper, anteriorly, the posterior tibial artery and vein. Nerves: the medial sural and medial crural cutaneous nerves; deeper, the tibial nerve.

【Indications】Edema, abdominal distension, diarrhea, night sweating, febrile diseases without sweating, muscular atrophy, and numbness, pain, and flaccidity of the lower extremities.

【Manipulation】Puncture perpendicularly 0. 8-1 *cun*. Moxibustion is applicable.

【Remarks】River point of the kidney meridian of Foot-Shaoyin.

The Pericardium Meridian of Hand-*Jueyin*

【Principal indications】Diseases of the heart, chest and the stomach, mental diseases, and diseases in the regions along the meridian. For example, pain in the cardiac region, heart palpitations, irritability, oppression in the chest, manic depressive psychosis, heat in the heart of the hands, and spasmodic pain of the hand and arm, etc.

【Acupoints】9 points each side(Figure 10-31).

Neiguan (PC 6)

【Location】On the palmar side of the forearm, the line between Quze(PC 3) and Daling(PC 7) , 2 *cun* above the transverse crease of the wrist, between the tendons of m. palmarislongus and m. flexor radialis(Figure10-32).

【Anatomy】Muscles: There is m. flexor digitorum superficialis; deeper, m. flexor digitorum prefunds. Blood vessels: the median antebrachial artery and vein; deeper, the anterior interosseous artery and vein. Nerves: the rami cutaneus palmaris the medial of antebracnial cutaneous nerve; deeper, the median nerve; deepest, the anterior interosseous nerve.

【Indications】Pain in the cardiac region, heart palpitations, chest pain, gastric pain, vomiting, hiccup, insomnia, mania, epilepsy, depression, vertigo, stroke, paralysis, asthma, migraine, febrile diseases, and elbow and arm spasm pain.

【Manipulation】Puncture perpendicularly 0. 5-1 *cun*.

【Remarks】Connecting point of the pericardium meridian of Hand-Jueyin. One of the confluence points of the eight vessels, connecting the yin link vessel.

【操作】直刺 0.5~1 寸。

【附注】手厥阴经络穴；八脉交会穴之一，通阴维脉。

劳宫（PC 8）

【定位】在手掌心，当第二、三掌骨之间偏于第三掌骨，握拳屈指的中指尖处（图 10-33）。

【解剖】在第二、三掌骨间，下为掌腱膜；有指掌侧总动脉；布有正中神经的第二指掌侧总神经。

【主治】癫狂，痫证，口疮，口臭，鹅掌风。

【操作】直刺 0.3~0.5 寸。

【附注】手厥阴经荥穴。

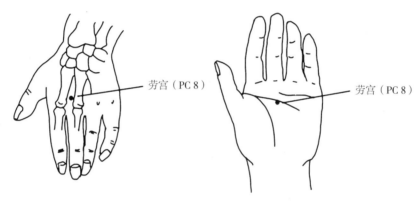

图 10-33 劳宫

（Laogong）

中冲（PC 9）

【定位】在手中指末节尖端中央（图 10-31）。

【解剖】有指掌侧固有动、静脉所形成的动、静脉网；为正中神经的指掌侧固有神经分布处。

【主治】中风昏迷，舌强不语，中暑，昏厥，小儿惊风，热病，舌下肿痛。

【操作】浅刺 0.1 寸，或用三棱针点刺出血。

【附注】手厥阴经井穴。

十、手少阳三焦经

【主治概要】主治侧头、耳、目、胸胁、咽喉部以及经脉循行部位的其他疾病，如水肿、遗尿、小便不利、耳鸣、耳聋、目赤、咽喉痛以及耳后、肩臂部外侧疼痛等。

Laogong (PC 8)

【Location】In the heart of palm, between the second and third metacarpal bones, close to the third metacarpal bone, when the fist is clenched, the point is just under the tip of the middle finger(Figure10-33).

【Anatomy】Muscles: between the 2nd and 3rd metacarpal bones of the palm; in the palmar aponeurosis. Blood vessels: the common palmar digital artery. Nerves: the second common palmar digital nerve of the median nerve.

【Indications】Manic depressive psychosis, epilepsy, aphtha, bad breath, and goose-foot wind.

【Manipulation】Puncture perpendicularly 0. 3−0. 5 *cun*.

【Remarks】Spring point of the pericardium meridian of Hand-Jueyin.

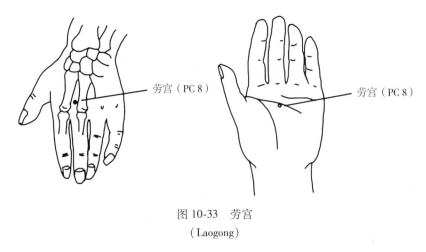

图 10-33   劳宫
(Laogong)

Zhongchong (PC 9)

【Location】In the center of the tip of the middle finger(Figure10-31).

【Anatomy】Blood vessels: the arterial and venous network formed by the palmar digital proprial artery and vein. Nerves: the palmar digital proprial nerve of the median nerve.

【Indications】Coma apoplectic, stiffness of the tongue impeding speech, summer heat stroke, fainting spell, child fright wind, febrile disease, and sublingual pain and swelling.

【Manipulation】Puncture subcutaneously 0. 1 *cun* or pick this point to cause bleeding with the three-edged needle.

【Remarks】Well point of the pericardium meridian of Hand-Jueyin.

The Triple Energizer Meridian of Hand-Shaoyang

【Principal indications】Diseases of the head, ear, eye, chest, hypochondrium and throat as well as diseases in the regions along this meridian. For example, edema, enuresis, difficult urination, tinnitus, deafness, red eyes, sore throat, pain in the ear and the lateral shoulder and arm, etc.

【Acupoints】23 points each side(Figure 10-34).

【本经腧穴】左右各 23 穴（图 10-34）。

中渚（TE 3）

【定位】在手背部，当指掌关节的后方，第四、五掌骨间凹陷处，液门穴后 1 寸（图 10-34）。

【解剖】有骨间肌；皮下有手背静脉网及掌背动脉；布有来自尺神经的手背支。

【主治】头痛，目眩，目赤，耳聋，耳鸣，喉痹，咽喉肿痛，手指不能屈伸，热病。

【操作】直刺 0.3~0.5 寸。

【附注】手少阳经输穴。

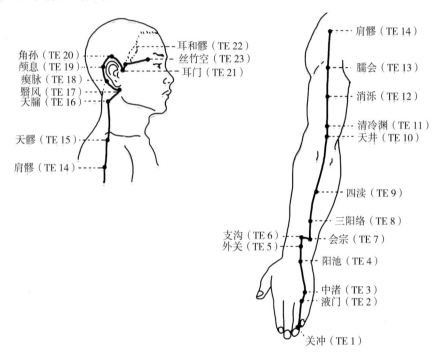

图 10-34　手少阳三焦经腧穴总图

(The Triple Energizer Meridian of Hand-Shaoyang)

外关（TE 5）

【定位】在前臂背侧，当阳池穴与肘尖连线上，腕背横纹上 2 寸，尺骨与桡骨之间（图 10-35）。

【解剖】在桡骨与尺骨之间，指总伸肌与拇长伸肌之间，深层有前臂骨间背侧动脉和前臂骨间掌侧动、静脉；布有前臂背侧皮神经和骨间背侧神经。

【主治】热病，头痛，耳聋，耳鸣，目赤肿痛，胁痛，瘰疬，上肢痹痛。

Zhongzhu（TE 3）

【Location】In the back of the hand, posterior of metacarpal joint, in the depression between the posterior borders of the small ends of the 4th and 5th metacarpal bones, 1 *cun* posterior of Yemen（TE 2）（Figure 10-34）.

【Anatomy】Muscles: the 4th m.interossei.Blood vessels: the dorsal venous network of hand and the dorsal metacarpal artery.Nerves: the dorsal metacarpal nerve derived from the ulnar nerve.

【Indications】Headache, dizziness, redness of the eye, deafness, tinius, throat impediment, sore throat, motor impairment of fingers, and febrile diseseas.

【Manipulation】Puncture perpendicularly 0. 3−0. 5 *cun*.

【Remarks】Stream point of the triple energizer meridian of Hand-Shaoyang.

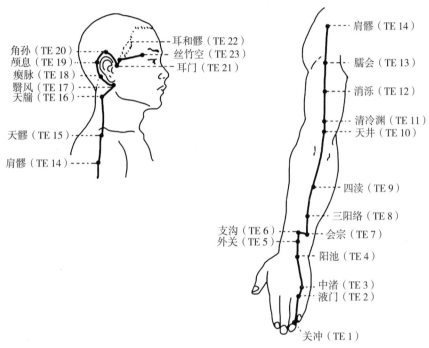

图 10-34　手少阳三焦经腧穴总图
（The Triple Energizer Meridian of Hand−Shaoyang）

Waiguan（TE 5）

【Location】On the line connecting Yangchi（TE 4）and the tip of olecranon, 2 *cun* above the transverse crease of the dorsum of wrist, between the radius and ulna（Figure 10-35）.

【Anatomy】Muscles: between the radius and ulna, between m.extensor digitorum communis and m. extensor pollicis longus.Blood vessels: deeper, the posterior antebrachial interosseous artery, the palmar antebrachial interosseous artery and vein.Nerves: the posterior antebrachial cutaneous nerve and posterior interosseous nerve.

【Indications】Febrile diseases, headache, deafness, tinnitus, sore red swollen eyes, pain in the hypochondriac region, scrofula, and pain and numbness of the upper extremities.

【Manipulation】Puncture perpendicularly 0. 5−1 *cun*.

【操作】直刺 0.5~1 寸。

【附注】手少阳经络穴；八脉交会穴之一，通阳维脉。

臑会（TE 13）

【定位】在臂外侧，当尺骨鹰嘴与肩髎穴的连线上，肩髎穴下 3 寸，当三角肌的后下缘（图 10-36）。

【解剖】在肱骨上端背面，肱三头肌中；有中侧副动、静脉；布有臂背侧皮神经，桡神经肌支，深层为桡神经。

【主治】瘿气，瘰疬，目疾，上肢痹痛。

【操作】直刺 0.5~1 寸。

肩髎（TE 14）

【定位】在肩部，肩髃后方，肩峰后下方，当臂外展时，于肩髃穴后下方呈现凹陷处（图 10-36）。

【解剖】在肩峰后下缘，三角肌中；有旋肱后动脉肌支；布有腋神经肌支。

【主治】臂痛，肩重不能举。

【操作】直刺 0.5~1.5 寸。

耳门（TE 21）

【定位】在面部，耳屏上切迹的前方，下颌骨髁状突后缘，张口有凹陷处（图 10-19）。

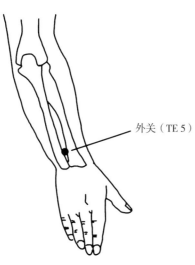

图 10-35 外关

（Waiguan）

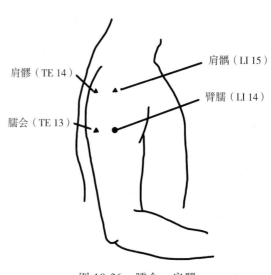

图 10-36 臑会、肩髎

（Naohui and Jianliao）

【Remarks】Connectiong point of the triple energizer meridian of Hand-Shaoyang. One of the confluence points of the eight vessels, connecting with the yang link vessel.

Naohui (TE 13)

【Location】On the line connecting Jianliao(TE 14) and the clecranon, 3 *cun* below Jianliao(TE 14), on the posterior border of m.deltoideus(Figure 10-36).

【Anatomy】Muscles: in the dorsum of superior humerus, m.triceps brachii. Blood vessels: The median collateral artery and vein. Nerves: The posterior branchial cutaneous nerve, the muscular branch of the radial nerve; deeper, the radial nerve.

【Indications】Goiter, scrofula, diseases of eyes, and pain and numbness of the upper extremities.

【Manipulation】Puncture perpendicularly 0. 5−1 *cun*.

Jianliao (TE 14)

【Location】On the shoulder, behind Jianyu(LI 15), posterior and inferior to the acromion, in the depression posterior to Jianyu (LI 15) when the arm is abducted(Figure 10-36).

【Anatomy】Muscles: on the posteroinferior border of the acromion, in m. deltoideus. Blood vessels: the muscular branch of the posterior circumflex humeral artery. Nerves: the muscular branch of the axillary nerve.

【Indications】Pain of the arm, inability to raise arm with a sensation of heaviness in the shoulder joint.

【Manipulation】Puncture perpendicularly 0. 5−1. 5 *cun*.

Ermen (TE 21)

【Location】On the face, in front of the superior notch of the anricula, in the depression on the posterior border of the mandibular condyloid process when open the mouth(Figure 10-19).

【Anatomy】Blood vessels: the superficial temporal artery and vein below the zygomatic arch. Nerves: the branches of the auriculotemporal nerve and facial nerve.

【Indications】Deafness, tinnitus, otitis media, and toothache.

【Manipulation】Open the mouth, puncture perpendicularly 0. 5−1 *cun*.

【解剖】有颞浅动、静脉；布有耳颞神经及面神经分支。

【主治】耳聋，耳鸣，聤耳，齿痛。

【操作】张口，直刺 0.5~1 寸。

丝竹空（TE 23）

【定位】在面部，当眉梢凹陷处（图 10-34）。

【解剖】有眼轮匝肌；颞浅动、静脉额支；布有面神经颧眶支及耳颞神经分支。

【主治】头痛，目眩，目赤痛，眼睑跳动，齿痛，癫痫。

【操作】平刺 0.5~1 寸，不宜灸。

十一、足少阳胆经

【主治概要】主治头、耳、目、咽喉病、神志病以及经脉循行部位的其他病证，如口苦、目眩、寒热交作、头痛，颔痛、目外眦痛，以及胸、胁、股、下肢外侧痛等。

【本经腧穴】左右各 44 穴（图 10-37）。

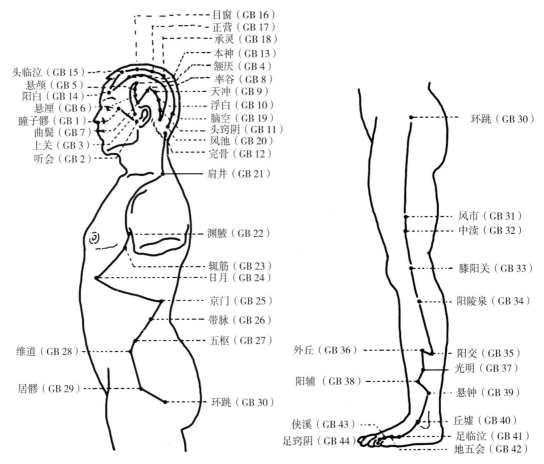

图 10-37 足少阳胆经腧穴总图

(The Gallbladder Meridian of Foot-Shaoyang)

Sizhukong（TE 23）

【Location】On the face, in the depression at the lateral end of the eyebrow(Figure 10-34).

【Anatomy】Muscles: subcutaneously, m.orbicularis oculi.Blood vessels: the frontal branches of the superficial temporal atery and vein.Nerves: the zygomatic temporal branch of the facial nerve and the branch of the auriculotemporal nerve.

【Indications】Headache, blurred vision, redness and pain of the eye, twitching of the eyelid, toochache, and epilepsy.

【Manipulation】Puncture subcutaneously 0. 5-1 *cun*.Moxibustion is not applicable

The Gallbladder Meridian of Foot-Shaoyang

【Principal indications】Diseases of the head, ear, eye, throat, mental diseases and the diseases in the regions along this meridian.For example, bitterness of mouth, dizziness, alternating cold and heat, headache, pain in the lower jaw, outer canthus of the eye, chest, rib-side, thigh, lateral lower extremity, etc.

【Acupoints】44 points each side(Figure 10-37).

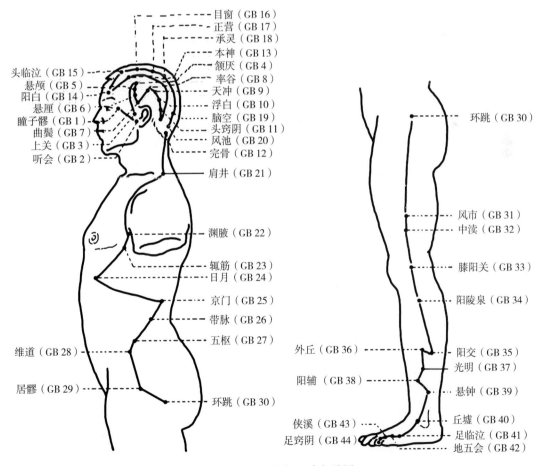

图 10-37　足少阳胆经腧穴总图

(The Gallbladder Meridian of Foot-ShaFoyang)

瞳子髎（GB 1）

【定位】在面部，目外眦旁约 0.5 寸，当眶骨外侧缘凹陷处（图 10-37）。

【解剖】有眼轮匝肌，深层为颞肌；当颧眶动、静脉分布处；布有颧面神经和颧颞神经，面神经的额颞支。

【主治】头痛，目赤，目痛，怕光羞明，迎风流泪，远视不明，内障，目翳，青盲。

【操作】向后刺或斜刺 0.3~0.5 寸；或用三棱针点刺出血。

【附注】手太阳、手少阳、足少阳经交会穴。

率谷（GB 8）

【定位】在头部，当耳尖直上入发际 1.5 寸处（图 10-38）。

【解剖】在颞肌中；有颞浅动、静脉顶支；布有耳颞神经和枕大神经会合支。

【主治】偏头痛，眩晕，呕吐，小儿惊风。

【操作】平刺 0.5~1 寸。

【附注】足太阳与足少阳经交会穴。

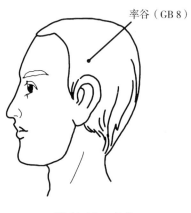

率谷（GB 8）

图 10-38　率谷

（Shuaigu）

肩井（GB 21）

【定位】在肩上，当大椎穴（督脉）与肩峰端连线的中点上（图 10-39）。

【解剖】有斜方肌，深层为肩胛提肌与冈上肌；有颈横动、静脉分支；布有腋神经分支，深层上方为桡神经。

【主治】肩背痹痛，手臂不举，颈项强痛，乳痈，瘰疬，难产。

Tongziliao（GB 1）

【Location】On the face, 0. 5 *cun* lateral to the outer canthus, in the depression on the lateral side of the orbit（Figure 10-37）

【Anatomy】Muscles: m.orbicularis oculi; deeper, m.temporalis. Blood vessels: the zygomaticoorbital artery and vein. Nerves: the zygomaticofacial and zygomaticotemporal nerves, the zemporal branch of the facial nerve.

【Indications】Headache, redness and pain of the eyes, photophoia, phengophobia, tearing on exposure to wind, farsightedness, internal obstruction, blurred vision, and optic atrophy.

【Manipulation】Puncture backwards obliquely 0. 3－0. 5 *cun*, or prick to cause bleeding with the three-edged needle.

【Remarks】The crossing point of the small intestine meridian of Hand-Taiyang, the triple energizer meridian of Hand-Shaoyang and the gallbaladder meridian of Foot-Shaoyang.

Shuaigu（GB 8）

【Location】On the head, superior to the apex of the auricle, 1. 5 *cun* within the hairline（Figure 10-38）.

【Anatomy】Muscles: within m. temporalis; Blood vessels: the parietal branches of the superficial temporal artery and vein. Nerves: the anastomotic branche of the auriculotemporal nerve and great occipital nerve.

【Indications】Migraine, vertigo, vomiting, and infantile convulsion.

【Manipulation】Puncture subcutaneously 0. 5－1 *cun*.

【Remarks】The crossing point of the gallbaladder meridian of Foot-Shaoyan and the bladder meridian of Foot-Taiyang.

Jianjin（GB 21）

【Location】On the shoulder, directly above the nipple, at the midpoint of the line connecting Dazhui（GV 14）and the acromion（Figure 10-39）.

【Anatomy】Muscles: m.trapezius; deeper, m.levator scapulae and m.supraspinatus. Blood vessels: the transverse artery and vein. Nerves: the posterior branche of the supraclavicular nerve; deeper, the accessory nerve.

【Indications】Numbness and pain of the arm and back, inability to raise arm with a sensation of heaviness in the shoulder joint, stiffness and pain of the neck, acute mastitis, scrofula, and dystocia.

【Manipulation】Puncture perpendicularly 0. 5－0. 8 *cun*. Due to the lung is below this point, deep insertion is contraindicated. Puncture is contraindicated in pregnant women.

【Remarks】The crossing point of the gallbaladder meridian of Foot-Shaoyan, of the triple energizer meridian of Hand-Shaoyang and the yang link vessel.

【操作】直刺 0.5~0.8 寸，深部正当肺尖，慎不可深刺。孕妇禁针。

【附注】手、足少阳经与阳维脉交会穴。

环跳（GB 30）

【定位】在股外侧部，侧卧屈股，当股骨大转子最凸点与骶管裂孔连线的外 1/3 与中 1/3 交点处（图 10-40）。

【解剖】在臀大肌、梨状肌下缘；内侧为臀下动、静脉；布有臀下皮神经，臀下神经，深部正当坐骨神经。

【主治】半身不遂，下肢痿痹，挫闪腰疼。

【操作】直刺 2~3 寸。

【附注】足少阳、太阳经交会穴。

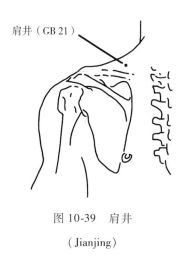

图 10-39　肩井

（Jianjing）

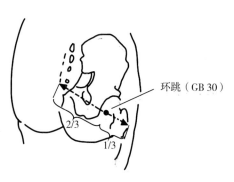

图 10-40　环跳

（Huantiao）

阳陵泉（GB 34）

【定位】在小腿外侧，当腓骨小头前下方凹陷处（图 10-41）。

【解剖】在腓骨长、短肌中；有膝下外侧动、静脉；当腓总神经分为腓浅神经及腓深神经处。

【主治】半身不遂，下肢痿痹、麻木，膝肿痛，脚气，胁肋痛，口苦，呕吐，黄疸，小儿惊风。

【操作】直刺或斜向下刺 1~1.5 寸。

【附注】足少阳经合穴；八会穴之一，筋会阳陵泉。

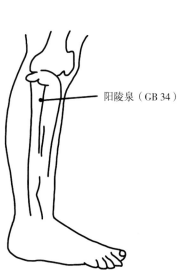

图 10-41　阳陵泉

（Yanglingquan）

Huantiao (GB 30)

【Location】On the lateral part of thigh, when take a lateral position and bend thigh, at the junction of the lateral 1/3 and medial 1/3 of the distance between the great trochanter of the femur and the hiatus of the sacrum(Figure 10-40).

【Anatomy】Muscles: on the inferior borders of m. gluteus maximus and m. piriformis. Blood vessels: medially, the inferior gluteal artery and vein. Nerves: the inferior gluteal cutaneous nerve, the inferior gluteal nerve; deeper, the sciatic nerve.

【Indications】Hemiplegia, muscular atrophy, numbness pain and flaccidity of the lower extremities, and lumbar pain due to contusion.

【Manipulation】Puncture perpendicularly 2–3 *cun*.

【Remarks】The crossing point of the gallbaladder meridian of Foot-Shaoyang and the bladder meridian of Foot-Taiyang.

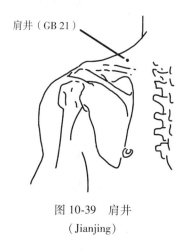

图 10-39 肩井
(Jianjing)

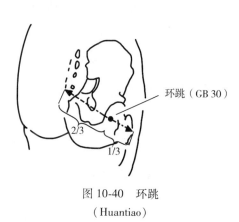

图 10-40 环跳
(Huantiao)

Yanglingquan (GB 34)

【Location】On the lateral part of crus, in the depression anterior and inferior to the small head of the fibula(Figure 10-41).

【Anatomy】Muscles: in m. peroneus longus and brevis. Blood vessels: the inferior lateral genicular artery and vein. Nerves: just where the common personal nerve bifurcates into the superficial and deep peroneal nerves.

【Indications】Hemiplegia, muscular atrophy, numbness pain and flaccidity of the lower extremities, numbness, swelling and pain of the knee, beriberi, hypochondriac pain, bitter taste in the mouth, vomiting, jaundice, and infantile convulsion.

【Manipulation】Puncture perpendicularly 1–1.5 *cun*.

【Remarks】Sea point of the gallbaladder meridian of Foot-Shaoyang; one of the eight meeting points, point of the tendon.

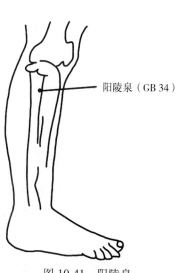

图 10-41 阳陵泉
(Yanglingquan)

光明（GB 37）

【定位】在小腿外侧，当外踝尖上 5 寸，腓骨前缘（图 10-37）。

【解剖】在趾长伸肌和腓骨短肌之间；有胫前动、静脉分支；布有腓浅神经。

【主治】目痛，夜盲，乳胀痛，膝痛，下肢痿痹，颊肿。

【操作】直刺 1~1.5 寸。

【附注】足少阳经络穴。

悬钟（GB 39）

【定位】在小腿外侧，当外踝尖上 3 寸，腓骨后缘（图 10-37）。

【解剖】在腓骨短肌与趾长伸肌分歧处；有胫前动、静脉分支；布有腓浅神经。

【主治】半身不遂，颈项强痛，胸腹胀满，胁肋疼痛，膝腿痛，腋下肿，咽喉肿痛，痔疾。

【操作】直刺 1~1.5 寸。

【附注】八会穴之一；髓会绝骨。

足临泣（GB 41）

【定位】在足背外侧，在第四、五跖骨结合部前方，小趾伸肌腱的外侧凹陷处（图 10-37）。

【解剖】有足背动、静脉网，第四趾背侧动、静脉；布有足背中间皮神经。

【主治】目赤肿痛，胁肋疼痛，月经不调，疟疾，中风偏瘫，肌痿痹痛，足跗肿痛，遗尿。

【操作】直刺 0.3~0.5 寸。

【附注】足少阳经输穴；八脉交会穴之一，通于带脉。

十二、足厥阴肝经

【主治概要】主治肝病、妇科病、前阴病，如头痛、胁痛、呃逆、小便不利、月经不调、疝气、少腹疼痛等。

【本经腧穴】左右各 14 穴（图 10-42）。

行间（LR 2）

【定位】在足背侧，当第一、二趾缝间，趾蹼缘的上方纹头处（图 10-42）。

【解剖】有足背静脉网，第一趾背侧动、静脉；腓神经的跖背侧神经分为趾背神经

Guangming (GB 37)

【Location】On the lateral part of crus, 5 *cun* above the tip of the external malleolus, on the anterior border of the fibula(Figure 10-37).

【Anatomy】Muscles: between m. extensor digitorum longus and m. peroneus brevis. Blood vessels: the branches of the anterior tibial atery and vein. Nerves: the superficial peroneal nerve.

【Indications】Pain of the eyes, night-blindness, distending pain of the breast, pain in the knee, muscular atrophy, numbness pain and flaccidity of the lower extremities, and swelling in the cheek.

【Manipulation】Puncture perpendicularly 1-1. 5 *cun*.

【Remarks】Connecting point of the gallbaladder meridian of Foot-Shaoyang.

Xuanzhong (GB 39)

【Location】On the lateral part of crus, 3 *cun* above the tip of the external malleolus, on the posterior border of the fibula(Figure 10-37).

【Anatomy】Muscles: on the bifurcate portion of m. peroneus brevis and m. extensor digitorum longus. Blood vessels: the branches of the anterior tibial artery and vein. Nerves: the superficial peroneal nerve.

【Indications】Hemiplegia, stiffness and pain of the neck, and chest distention, Abdominal distention, pain in the hypochondriac, pain in the knee, axillary swelling, sore throat, hemorrhoids.

【Manipulation】Puncture perpendicularly 1-1. 5 *cun*.

【Remarks】One of the eight meeting points, point of the marrow.

Zulinqi (GB 41)

【Location】On the outside dorsum of the foot, anterior to the junction of the 4th and 5th metatarsal bones, in the depression on the lateral side of the tendon of m. extensor digiti minimi of the foot(Figure 10-37).

【Anatomy】Blood vessels: the dorsal arterial and venous network of the foot, the 4th dorsal metatarsal artery and vein. Nerves: the intermediate dorsal cutaneous nerve of the foot.

【Indications】sore red swollen eyes, pain in the hypochondriac, irregular menstruation, maralia, paralysis due to stroke, muscular atrophy, numbness and pain, swelling and pain in the dorsum of foot, and enuresis.

【Manipulation】Puncture perpendicularly 0. 3-0. 5 *cun*.

【Remarks】Stream point of the gallbadder meridian of Foot-Shaoyang. One of the confluence points of the eight vessels, intersecting with the belt vessel.

The Liver Meridian of Foot-Jueyin

【Principal indications】Diseases of the liver, gynecopathies, diseases of the external genitalia and the diseases in the regions along this meridian. For example, headache, pain in the hypochondriac region, hiccup, dysuria, irregular menstruation, hernia, lesser abdominal pain, etc.

【Acupoints】14 points each side(Figure 10-42).

Xingjian (LR 2)

【Location】On the dorsum of the foot, between the first and second toes, proximal to the margin of

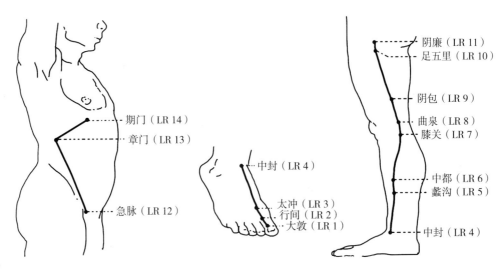

图 10-42　足厥阴肝经腧穴总图

(The Liver Meridian of Foot-Jueyin)

的分歧处。

【主治】月经过多，闭经，痛经，白带，遗尿，疝气，胸胁满痛，呃逆，咳嗽，泄泻，头痛，眩晕，目赤痛，青盲，中风，癫痫，口眼㖞斜。

【操作】斜刺 0.5~0.8 寸。

【附注】足厥阴经荥穴。

太冲（LR 3）

【定位】在足背侧第一、二跖骨结合部前下方凹陷处（图 10-43）。

【解剖】在拇长伸肌腱外缘；有足背静脉网，第一跖背侧动脉；布有跖背神经，深层为胫神经足底内侧神经。

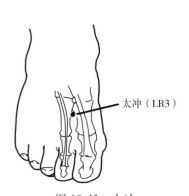

图 10-43　太冲

(Taichong)

【主治】头痛，眩晕，面瘫，疝气，月经不调，癃闭，遗尿，小儿惊风，癫狂，痫证，胁痛，腹胀，黄疸，呕逆，咽痛，目赤肿痛，下肢痿痹。

【操作】直刺 0.5~0.8 寸。

【附注】足厥阴经输穴、原穴。

章门（LR 13）

【定位】在侧腹部，当第十一肋游离端的下方（图 10-42）。

【解剖】有腹内、外斜肌及腹横肌；有第十肋间动脉末支；布有第十、十一肋间神经；右侧当肝脏下缘，左侧当脾脏下缘。

the web at the junction of the red and white skin(Figure 10-42).

【Anatomy】Blood vessels: the dorsal venous network of the foot and the first dorsal digital artery and vein. Nerves: the site where the dorsal digital nerves splite from the lateral dorsal metatarsal nerve of the deep peroneal nerve.

【Indications】Menometrorrhagia, amenorahea, dysmenorrhea, leucorrhea, enuresis, hernia, chest distention, abdominal distention, hiccup, cough, diarrhea, headache, dizziness, redness and pain of the eyes, clear-eye blindness, stroke, epilepsy, and deviation of the mouth and eyes.

【Manipulation】Puncture obliquely 0. 5−0. 8 *cun*.

【Remarks】Spring point of the liver meridian of Foot-Jueyin.

Taichong (LR 3)

【Location】On the dorsum of the foot, in the depression anterior to the junction of the first and second metatarsal bones(Figure 10-43).

【Anatomy】Muscles: on the lateral border of the tendon of m. extensor pollicis longus. Blood vessels: the dorsal venous network of the foot, the first dorsal metatarsal artery. Nerves: the branch of the deep personeal nerve.

【Indications】Headache, dizziness, facial paralysis, hernia, irregular menstruation, bling urinary block, enuresis, epilepsy, pain in the hypochondriac region, abdominal distention, jaundice, hiccup, sore throat, sore red swollen eyes, muscular atrophy, numbness pain and flaccidity of the lower extremities.

【Manipulation】Puncture perpendicularly 0. 5−0. 8 *cun*.

【Remarks】Stream point and source point of the liver meridian of Foot-Jueyin.

Zhangmen (LR 13)

【Location】On the lateral part of the abdomen, on the free end of the eleventh rib(Figure 10-42).

【Anatomy】Musles: in m. obliquus internus abdominis, m. obliquus externus abdominis and m. transversus abdomonis. Blood vessels: the terminal branch of the tenth intercostal artery. Nerves: the tenth and eleventh intercostal nerves. On the right of this point is the lower edge of the liver, while on the left of this point is the lower edge of the spleen.

【Indications】Abdominal distention, diarrhea, pain in the hypochondriac region, and mass in the abdomen.

【Manipulation】Puncture obliquely 0. 5−1 *cun*.

【Remarks】Alarm point of the spleen meridian of Foot-Taiyin. The crossing point of the liver meridian of Foot-Jueyin and the gallbladder meridian of Foot-Shaoyang. One of the eight meeting points, point of the viscera.

【主治】腹胀，泄泻，胁痛，痞块。

【操作】斜刺 0.5~1 寸。

【附注】脾募穴；足厥阴经与足少阳经交会穴；八会穴之一，脏会章门。

期门（LR 14）

【定位】在胸部，当乳头直下，第六肋间隙，前正中线旁开 4 寸（图 10-42）。

【解剖】在腹内、外斜肌腱膜中，有肋间肌；有第六肋间动、静脉；布有第六肋间神经。

【主治】胸胁胀满疼痛，呕吐，呃逆，吞酸，腹胀，泄泻，乳痈，胸中热，咳喘，奔豚，疟疾。

【操作】斜刺 0.5~0.8 寸。

【附注】肝募穴；足厥阴经、足太阴经与阴维脉交会穴。

十三、督脉（GV）

【主治概要】主治神志病，热病，腰骶、背、头项局部病证及相应的内脏疾病。

【本经腧穴】一名一穴，共 29 穴（图 10-44）。

腰阳关（GV 3）

【定位】在腰部，当后正中线上，第四腰椎棘突下凹陷中（图 10-45）。

【解剖】在腰背筋膜、棘上韧带及棘间韧带中；有腰动脉后支及棘突间静脉丛；布有腰神经后支的内侧支。

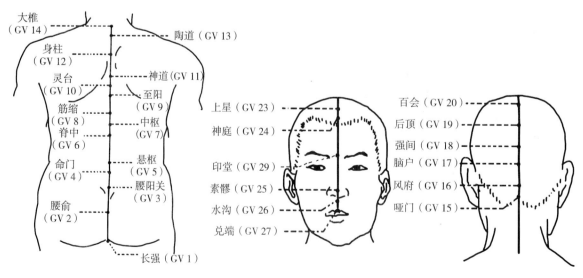

图 10-44　督脉腧穴总图

(The Governor Vessel)

Qimen (LR 14)

【Location】On the chest, directly below the nipple, in the sixth intercostal space, 4 *cun* lateral to the midline of the chest(Figure 10-42).

【Anatomy】Musles: in the aponeuroses of m.obliquus internus abdominis and m.obliquus externus abdominis, there are m.intercostales interni.Blood vessels: the sixth intercostal artery and vein.Nerves: the sixth intercostal nerve.

【Indications】Fullness and pain of the chest, vomiting, hiccup, acid regurgitation, abdominal distention, diarrhea, acute mastitis, heat vexation in the chest, running piglet, cough, asthma, and maralia.

【Manipulation】Puncture obliquely 0. 5−0. 8 *cun*.

【Remarks】Alarm point of the liver.The crossing point of the liver meridian of Foot-Jueyin, the bladder meridian of Foot-Taiyin and the yin link vessel.

The Governor Vessel

【Principal indications】Mental diseases, febrile diseases, local disesease of lumbosacral region, back, head and neck, and corresponding splanchnopathies.

【Acupoints】One name one point; totally 29 points(Figure 10-44).

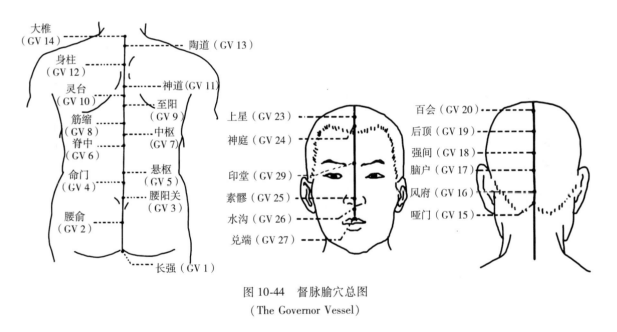

图 10-44   督脉腧穴总图
(The Governor Vessel)

Yaoyangguan (GV 3)

【Location】On the anterior midline of back, below the spinous process of the fourth lumbar vertebra (Figure 10-45).

【Anatomy】Muscles: fascia lumbodorsalis, aupraspinal and interspinal ligaments.Blood vessels: the posterior branch of the lumbar artery, the subcutaneous interspinal venous plexus.Nerves: the medial branch of the posterior ramus of the lumbar nerve.

【Indications】Pain in the lumbosacral, irregular menstruation, morbid leukorrhagia, nocturnal emission, impotence, muscular atrophy, and numbness, pain and flaccidity of the lower extremities.

【Manipulation】Puncture obliquely upwards 0. 5−1 *cun*.

【主治】腰骶疼痛，月经不调，赤白带下，遗精，阳痿，下肢痿痹。

【操作】向上斜刺 0.5~1 寸。

命门（GV 4）

【定位】在腰部，当后正中线上，第二腰椎棘突下凹陷中（图 10-45）。

【解剖】在腰背筋膜、棘上韧带及棘间韧带中；有腰动脉后支及棘突间静脉丛；布有腰神经后支内侧支。

【主治】虚损腰痛，脊强反折，遗尿，尿频，泄泻，遗精，阳痿，早泄，带下，手足逆冷。

【操作】向上斜刺 0.5~1 寸。

至阳（GV 9）

【定位】在背部，当后正中线上，第七胸椎棘突下凹陷中（图 10-44）。

【解剖】在腰背筋膜、棘上韧带及棘间韧带；有第七肋间动脉后支及棘突间静脉丛；布有第七肋间神经后支内侧支。

【主治】胸胁胀痛，黄疸，咳嗽气喘，脊强，背痛。

【操作】斜刺 0.5~1 寸。

大椎（GV 14）

【定位】在后正中线上，第七颈椎棘突下凹陷中（图 10-46）。

【解剖】在腰背筋膜、棘上韧带及棘间韧带中；有颈横动脉分支、棘突间静脉

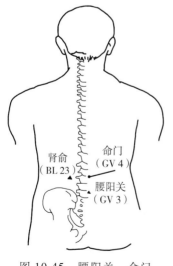

图 10-45　腰阳关、命门

（Yaoyangguan and Mingmen）

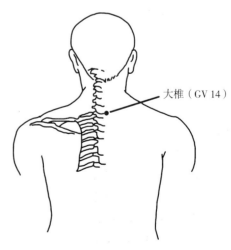

图 10-46　大椎

（Dazhui）

Mingmen (GV 4)

【Location】On the anterior midline of back, below the spinous process of the second lumbar vertebra(Figure 10-45).

【Anatomy】Muscles: fascia lumbodorsalis, aupraspinal and interspinal ligaments. Blood vessels: the posterior branch of the lumbar artery, the subcutaneous interspinal venous plexus. Nerves: the medial branch of the posterior ramus of the lumbar nerve.

【Indications】Lumbar pain due to vacuity detriment, arched-back rigidity, enuresis, frequent urination, diarrhea, nocturnal emission, impotence, premature ejaculation, leucorrhea, and counterflow cold of the extremities.

【Manipulation】Puncture perpendicularly upwards 0. 5–1 *cun*.

Zhiyang (GV 9)

【Location】On the anterior midline of back, below the spinous process of the seventh lumbar vertebra(Figure 10-44).

【Anatomy】Muscles: fascia lumbodorsalis, supraspinal and interspinal ligaments. Blood vessels: the posterior branch of the seventh intercostal artery, the subcutaneous interpinal venous plexus. Nerves: the medial branch of the posterior ramus of the seventh thoracic nerve.

【Indications】Fullness and pain of the chest and rib-side, jaundice, cough and asthma, stiffness of the back, and pain in the back.

【Manipulation】Puncture obliquely 0. 5–1 *cun*.

Dazhui (GV 14)

【Location】On the anterior midline of back, below the spinous process of the seventh cervical vertebra(Figure 10-46).

【Anatomy】Muscles: fascia lumbodorsalis superaspinal and interspinal ligaments. Blood vessels: the branch of the transverse cervical atery, the interspinal venous plexus. Nerves: the medial branch of the posterior ramus of the eighth cervical nerve.

【Indications】Febrile diseseas, malaria, cough and asthma, hectic, fever due to yin-deficiency, tidal fever, pain and rigidity of the head and neck, pain in the shoulder and back, summer heat stroke, and urticaria.

【Manipulation】Puncture obliquely 0. 5–1 *cun*. Moxibustion is applicable.

丛；布有第八颈神经后支内侧支。

【主治】热病，疟疾，咳嗽，喘逆，骨蒸潮热，头痛项强，肩背痛，中暑，风疹。

【操作】斜刺0.5~1寸，可灸。

百会（GV 20）

【定位】在头部，当后发际正中直上7寸，或两耳尖连线中点处（图10-47）。

【解剖】在帽状腱膜中；有左右颞浅动、静脉及左右枕动、静脉吻合网；布有枕大神经及额神经分支。

【主治】头痛，眩晕，惊悸，中风，失语，癫狂，痫证，痔疾，脱肛，阴挺，不寐。

【操作】平刺0.5~0.8寸。

【附注】督脉与足太阳经交会穴。

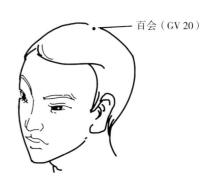

图10-47 百会

（Baihui）

神庭（GV 24）

【定位】在头部，当前发际正中直上0.5寸（图10-44）。

【解剖】在左右额肌之交界处；有额动、静脉分支；布有额神经分支。

【主治】头痛，眩晕，目赤肿痛，失眠，鼻渊，鼻衄，癫狂，热病。

【操作】平刺0.3~0.8寸。

【附注】督脉与足太阳、阳明经交会穴。

水沟（GV 26）

【定位】在面部，当人中沟的上1/3与中1/3交点处（图10-44）。

【解剖】在口轮匝肌中；有上唇动、静脉；布有眶下神经支及面神经颊支。

【主治】昏迷，晕厥，暑病，癫狂，痫证，小儿惊风，口眼㖞斜，腰脊强痛。

【操作】向上斜刺0.3~0.5寸。不灸。

【附注】督脉与手阳明、足阳明经交会穴。

印堂（GV 29）

【定位】在额部，当两眉头之中间（图10-48）。

【解剖】在掣眉间肌中；两侧有额内动、静脉分支；布有来自三叉神经的滑车上

Baihui (GV 20)

【Location】On the head, 7 *cun* directly above the midpoint of the posterior hairline, approximately on the midpoint of the line connecting the apexes of both ears(Figure 10-47).

【Anatomy】Muscles: in galea aponeurotica. Blood vessels: the anastomotic network formed by the superdicial temporal arteries and veins and the occipital arteries and veins on both sides. Nerves: the branches of the great occipital nerve and frontal nerve.

【Indications】Headache, dizziness, palpitation, stroke, aphasia, manic depressive psychosis, epilepsy, hemorrhoids, prolapse of the rectum, vaginal protrusion, and insomnia.

【Manipulation】Puncture horizontally 0. 5−0. 8 *cun*.

【Remarks】The crossing point of the governor vessel and the bladder meridian of Foot-Taiyang.

Shenting (GV 24)

【Location】On the head, 0. 5 *cun* directly above the midpoint of the anterior hairline(Figure 10-44).

【Anatomy】Muscles: at the junction of the left and right frontal muscles. Blood vessels: the branches of the frontal artery and vein. Nerves: the branch of the frontal nerve.

【Indications】Headache, dizziness, sore red swollen eyes, insomnia, rhinorrhea, nosebleed, epilepsy, and febrile diseases.

【Manipulation】Puncture subcutaneously 0. 3−0. 8 *cun*.

【Remarks】The crossing point of the governor vessel, the bladder meridian of Foot-Taiyang, and the stomach meridian of Foot-Yangming.

Shuigou (GV 26)

【Location】On the face, at the junction of the superior 1/3 and middle 1/3 of the philtrum(Figure 10-44).

【Anatomy】Muscles: in m.orbicularis oris. Blood vessels: the superior labial artery and vein. Nerves: the branch of the infraorbital nerve and the buccal branch of the facial nerve.

【Indications】Coma, apsychia, summer heat diseases, manic depressive psychosis, epilepsy, child fright wind, deviation of the mouth and eyes, and pain and stiffness of the lower back.

【Manipulation】Puncture obliquely upwards 0. 3−0. 5 *cun*. Moxibustion is not applicable.

【Remarks】The crossing point of the governor vessel and the large intestine meridian of Hand-Yangming and the stomach meridian of Foot-Yangming.

Yintang (GV 29)

【Location】In the frontal, the midpoint of the line between the medial ends of the two eyebrows (Figure 10-48).

【Anatomy】Muscles: m.corrugator supercilii. Blood vessels: on both sides, the branches of medial frontal artery and vein. Nerves: the supratrochlear nerve coming from the trigeminal nerve.

【Indications】Headache, faint, nasosinusitis, nosebleed, sore red swollen eyes, double tongue, vomiting, eclampsia, acute and chronic fright wind, insomnia, clove sore of face, and trigenminal neuralgia.

【Manipulation】Pinch the local skin, puncture subcutaneously downwards 0. 3−0. 5 *cun*, or prick to cause bleeding with the three-edged needle. Moxibustion is applicable.

神经。

【主治】头痛，头晕，鼻渊，鼻衄，目赤肿痛，重舌，呕吐，子痫，急、慢惊风，不寐，颜面疔疮以及三叉神经痛。

【操作】提捏局部皮肤，向下平刺 0.3～0.5寸，或用三棱针点刺出血，可灸。

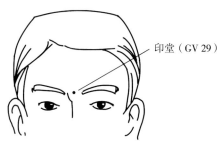

图 10-48　印堂

（Yintang）

十四、任脉

【主治概要】主治胸、腹、头面的局部病证，如疝气、带下、腹中结块等。

【本经腧穴】一名一穴，共 24 穴（图 10-49）。

中极（CV 3）

【定位】在下腹部，前正中线上，当脐下 4 寸（图 10-49）。

【解剖】在腹白线上，深部为乙状结肠；有腹壁浅动、静脉分支，腹壁下动、静脉分支；布有髂腹下神经的前皮支。

【主治】小便不利，遗尿，阳痿，遗精，疝气，月经不调，带下，崩漏，阴挺。

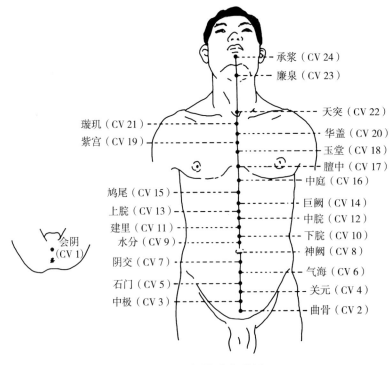

图 10-49　任脉腧穴总图

（The Conception Vessel）

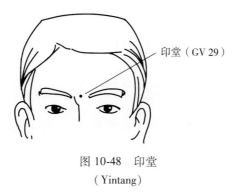

图 10-48 印堂

(Yintang)

The Conception Vessel

【Principal indications】Local diseseas of the abdomen, chest, head regions, such as hernia, leucorrhea, and glomus lumps in the abdomen.

【Acupoints】One name one point, totally 24 points(Figure 10-49).

Zhongji (CV 3)

【Location】On the hypogastrium, on the midline of the chest, 4 *cun* below the umbilicus(Figure 10-49).

【Anatomy】Muscles: on the linea alba; deeper, the sigmoid colon. Blood vessels: the branches of superficial epigastric artery and vein, and the branches of inferior epigastric artery and vein. Nerves: the branch of the iliohypogastric nerve.

【Indications】Dysuria, enuresis, impotence, nocturnal emission, hernia, irregular menstruation, leucorrhea, uterine bleeding, vaginal protrusion.

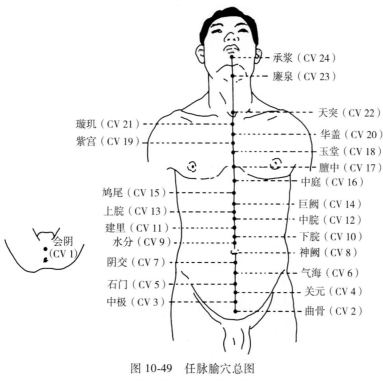

图 10-49 任脉腧穴总图

(The Conception Vessel)

【操作】直刺 1～1.5 寸。

【附注】任脉与足三阴经交会穴；膀胱募穴。

关元（CV 4）

【定位】在下腹部，前正中线上，当脐下 3 寸（图 10-50）。

【解剖】在腹白线上，深部为小肠；有腹壁浅动、静脉分支，腹壁下动、静脉分支；布有第十二肋间神经前皮支的内侧皮支。

【主治】遗尿，小便不利，疝气，遗精，阳痿，月经不调，崩漏带下，阴挺，不孕。本穴有强壮作用，为保健要穴。

【操作】直刺 1～2 寸，可灸。

【附注】任脉与足三阴经交会穴；小肠募穴。

气海（CV 6）

【定位】在下腹部，前正中线上，当脐下 1.5 寸（图 10-49）。

【解剖】在腹白线上，深部为小肠；有腹壁浅动脉、静脉分支，腹壁下动、静脉分支；布有第十一肋间神经前皮支的内侧皮支。

【主治】绕脐腹痛，水肿鼓胀，水谷不化，大便不通，泄痢，遗尿，遗精，疝气，月经不调，经闭，阴挺。本穴有强壮作用，为保健要穴。

【操作】直刺 1～2 寸。

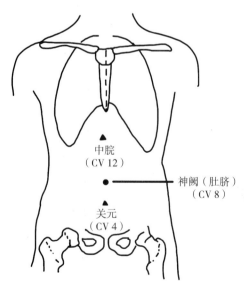

图 10-50　关元、神阙、中脘

（Guanyuan，Shenque and Zhongwan）

【Manipulation】Puncture perpendicularly 1−1. 5 *cun*.

【Remarks】The crossing point of the conception vessel, Foot-Taiyin, Foot-Shaoyin and Foot-Jueyin meridians; alarm point of the bladder.

Guanyuan（CV 4）

【Location】On the hypogastrium, on the midline of the chest, 3 *cun* below the umbilicus(Figure 10-50).

【Anatomy】Muscles: on the linea alba; deeper, the small intestine. Blood vessels: the branches of the superficial epigastric artery and vein and the branches of the inferior epigastric artery and vein. Nerves: the medial branche of the anterior cutaneous branch of the twelfth intercostal nerve.

【Indications】Enuresis, dysuria, hernia, nocturnal emission, impotence, irregular menstruation, uterine bleeding, leucorrhea, vaginal protrusion, sterility. One of the important points for tonification.

【Manipulation】Puncture perpendicularly 1−2 *cun*.

【Remarks】Alarm point of the small intestine. The crossing point of the conception vessel, Foot-Taiyin, Foot-Shaoyin and Foot-Jueyin meridians.

Qihai（CV 6）

【Location】On the hypogastrium, on the midline of the chest, 1. 5 *cun* below the umbilicus(Figure 10-49).

【Anatomy】Muscles: on the linea alba; deeper, the small intestine. Blood vessels: the branches of superficial epigastric atery and vein and the branches of inferior epigastric artery and vein. Nerves: the anterior cutaneous branch of the eleventh intercostal nerve.

【Indications】Periumbilical pain, water drum and swelling, non-transformation of grain and water, constipation, diarrhea, enuresis, nocturnal emission, hernia, irregular menstruation, amenorahea, and vaginal protrusion. One of the key points for tonification.

【Manipulation】Puncture perpendicularly 1−2 *cun*.

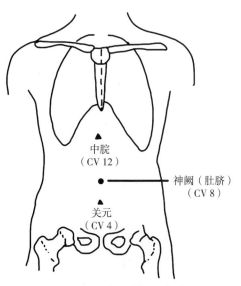

图 10-50　关元、神阙、中脘
(Guanyuan, Shenque and Zhongwan)

神阙 （CV 8）

【定位】 在腹中部，脐中央（图 10-50）。

【解剖】 在脐窝正中，深部为小肠；有腹壁下动、静脉；布有第十肋间神经前皮支的内侧皮支。

【主治】 中风脱证，腹痛，泄泻，脱肛，水肿，虚脱。

【操作】 多用艾条灸或艾炷隔盐灸。禁针刺。

中脘 （CV 12）

【定位】 在上腹部，前正中线上，当脐上 4 寸（图 10-50）。

【解剖】 在腹白线上，深部为胃幽门部；有腹壁上动、静脉；布有第七肋间神经前皮支的内侧支。

【主治】 胃痛，腹胀，泄泻，呕吐，翻胃，吞酸，黄疸，癫狂。

【操作】 直刺 1～1.5 寸。

【附注】 胃募穴；八会穴之一，腑会中脘；任脉与手太阳、少阳、足阳明经交会穴。

膻中 （CV 17）

【定位】 在胸部，当前正中线上，平第四肋间隙，两乳头连线的中点（图 10-49）。

【解剖】 在胸骨体上；有胸廓内动、静脉的前穿支；布有第四肋间神经前支的内侧皮支。

【主治】 咳嗽，气喘，胸痛，心悸，善太息，梅核气，产妇少乳，噎嗝，呕吐。

【操作】 平刺 0.3～0.5 寸。

【附注】 心包募穴；八会穴之一，气会膻中。

天突 （CV 22）

【定位】 在颈部前正中线上，胸骨上窝中央（图 10-49）。

【解剖】 在胸骨切迹中央，左右胸锁乳突肌之间，深层左右为胸骨舌骨肌和胸骨甲状肌；皮下有颈静脉弓、甲状腺下动脉分支；深部为气管，向下胸骨柄后方为无名静脉及主动脉弓；布有锁骨上神经前支。

【主治】 咳嗽，哮喘，胸痛，咽喉肿痛，暴喑，瘿气，噎嗝，梅核气。

【操作】 先直刺 0.2 寸，然后将针尖转向下方，沿胸骨柄后缘，气管前缘缓慢向下刺入 0.5～1 寸。本穴针刺不能过深，也不宜向左右刺，以防刺伤锁骨下动脉及肺尖。

【附注】 任脉与阴维脉交会穴。

Shenque (CV 8)

【Location】On the middle of abdomen, in the center of the umbilicus(Figure 10-50).

【Anatomy】In the center of the umbilicus; deeper, the small intestine. Blood vessels: the inferior epigastric artery and vein. Nerves: the anterior cutaneous branch of the tenth intercostal nerve.

【Indications】Collapse syndrome of apoplexy, abdominal pain, diarrhea, vaginal protrusion, edema, and collapse.

【Manipulation】More often, moxibustion with moxasticks is used, or moxibustion with ginger or salt is used. Puncture is prohibited.

Zhongwan (CV 12)

【Location】On the epigastrium, on the mideline of the chest, 4 *cun* above the umbilicus(Figure 10-50).

【Anatomy】Muscles: on the linea alba; deeper, the portio pylorica ventriculi. Blood vessels: the superior epigastric artery and vein. Nerves: the anterior cutaneous branch and the medial branch of the 7th intercostal nerve.

【Indications】Gastric pain, abdominal distension, diarrhea, vomiting, stomach reflux, acid regurgitation, jaundice, and manic depressive psychosis.

【Manipulation】Puncture perpendicularly 1-1. 5 *cun*.

【Remarks】Alarm point of the stomach. One of the eight meeting points, point of the bowels. The crossing point of the conception vessel, the small intestine meridian of Hand-Taiyang, the triple energizer meridian of Hand-Shaoyang, and the stomach meridian of Foot-Yangming.

Tanzhong (CV 17)

【Location】On the chest, on the midline of the chest, on the anterior midline, at the level with the fourth intercostal space, midway between nipples(Figure 10-49).

【Anatomy】Muscles: on the sternal body. Blood vessels: the anterior perforating branches of the internal mammary artery and vein. Nerves: the medial cutaneous branch of the anterior cutaneous branch of the fourth intercostal nerve.

【Indications】Cough, asthma, chest pain, palpitation, frequent sighing, globus hystericus, insufficient lactation, dysphagia, and vomiting.

【Manipulation】Puncture subcutaneously 0. 3-0. 5 *cun*.

【Remarks】Alarm point of the pericardium. One of the eight meeting points, point of qi.

Tiantu (CV 22)

【Location】On the anterior midline of the neck, in the center of the suprasternal fossa(Figure 10-49).

【Anatomy】Muscles: in the center of the sternal notch, between the left and right sternocleidomastoid muscles; deeper, m. sternohyoideus and m. sternothyroideus. Blood vessels: subcutaneously, the jugular venous arch and the branch of the inferior thyroid artery; deeper, the trachea; inferiorly, at the posterior aspect of the sternum, the innominate vein and aortic arch. Nerves: the anterior branch of the supraclavicular nerve.

【Indications】Cough, asthma, chest pain, sore throat, sudden loss of voice, goiter, dysphagia-occlu-

廉泉（CV 23）

【定位】在颈部，当前正中线上，结喉上方，舌骨体上缘中点处（图10-49）。

【解剖】在舌骨上方，有甲状舌骨肌、舌肌；有颈前浅静脉，甲状腺上动、静脉；布有颈皮神经，深层有舌下神经分支。

【主治】舌下肿痛，舌根急缩，舌纵涎出，舌强不语，暴喑，吞咽困难。

【操作】向舌根斜刺0.5~0.8寸。

【附注】任脉与阴维脉交会穴。

十五、经外奇穴

四神聪（EX-HN 1）

【定位】在头顶部，当百会前后左右各1寸处，共四穴（图10-51）。

【解剖】在帽状腱膜中；有枕动、静脉、颞浅动、静脉顶支和眶上动、静脉的吻合网；布有枕大神经、耳颞神经及眶上神经分支。

【主治】头痛，眩晕，失眠，健忘，癫狂，痫证，偏瘫，脑积水，大脑发育不全。

【操作】平刺0.5~0.8寸，可灸。

太阳（EX-HN 4）

【定位】在颞部，当眉梢与目外眦之间，向后约一横指的凹陷处（图10-52）。

【解剖】在颞筋膜及颞肌中；有颞浅动、静脉；布有三叉神经第二、三支分支及面神经颞支。

【主治】偏正头痛，目赤肿痛，目涩，牙痛，三叉神经痛。

【操作】直刺或斜刺0.3~0.5寸，或用三棱针点刺出血。禁灸。

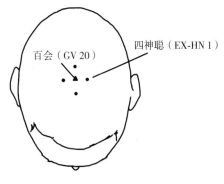

图10-51 四神聪

（Sishencong）

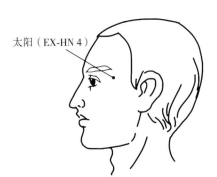

图10-52 太阳

（Taiyang）

sion, and globus hystericus.

【Manipulation】First puncture perpendicularly 0. 2 *cun* and then insert the needle tip downwards along the posterior aspect of the sternum 0. 5-1 *cun*.Do not puncture too deep and towards right or left to avoid demaging subclavian artery and the top of the lung.

【Remarks】The crossing point of the conception vessel and the yin link vessel.

Lianquan (CV 23)

【Location】On the anterior midline of the neck, above the laryngeal prominence, at the midpoint of the upper border of the hyoid bone(Figure 10-49).

【Anatomy】Muscles: above the hyoid bone, geniohyoid, muscles of tongue.Blood vessels: the anterior jugular vein, superiorthyroid artery and vein.Nerves: the cutaneous cervical nerve; deeper, the branche of hypoglossal nerve.

【Indications】Swelling and pain of the subglossal, stiffness of tongue root, salivation with flaccid tongue, aphasia with stiffness of the tongue, sudden loss of voice, and difficulty in swallowing.

【Manipulation】Puncture obliquely 0. 5-0. 8 *cun* towards the tongue root.

【Remarks】The crossing point of the conception vessel and the yin link vessel.

Extraordinary Points

Sishencong (EX-HN 1)

【Location】A group of 4 points, at the vertex, 1 *cun* respectively posterior, anterior, and lateral to Baihui(GV 20) (Figure 10-51).

【Anatomy】Muscles: in the galea aponeurotica. Blood vessels: the occipital arteries and veins, the temporal branches of the superficial temporal artery and vein and the anastomotic network formed by the supraorbital artery and veins and.Nerves: the branches of the great occipital nerve, the branch of the auriculotemporal nerve, and the supraprbital nerve.

【Indications】Headache, dizziness, rhinorrhea, insomnia, amnesia, manic depressive psychosis, epilepsy, paralysis, hydrencephalus, and cerebral agenesis.

【Manipulation】Puncture subcutaneously 0. 5-0. 8 *cun*.Moxibustion is applicable.

Taiyang (EX-HN 4)

【Location】In the tempora, in the depression about one finger breadth posterior to the midpoint between the lateral end of the eyebrow and the outer canthus(Figure 10-52).

【Anatomy】Muscles: in the fascia temporalis and m.temporalis.Blood vessels: the superficial temporal artery and vein.Nerves: the branches of the second and third branches of the trigeminal nerve and the temporal branch of the facial nerve.

【Indications】Headache, migraine, sore red swollen eyes, dry eyes, toothache, and trigenminal neuralgia.

【Manipulation】Puncture perpendicularly or obliquely 0. 3-0. 4 *cun*, or prick to cause bleeding with the three-edged needle.Moxibustion is forbidden.

四缝（EX-UE 10）

【定位】在第 2～5 指近端指关节掌侧面的中点，一侧四穴（图 10-53）。

【解剖】皮下有指纤维鞘、指滑液鞘、屈指深肌腱，深部为指关节腔；有指掌侧固有动、静脉分支；布有指掌侧固有神经。

【主治】疳积，百日咳，肠虫症，小儿腹泻，咳嗽气喘。

【操作】点刺 0.1～0.2 寸，挤出少量黄白色透明样黏液或出血。

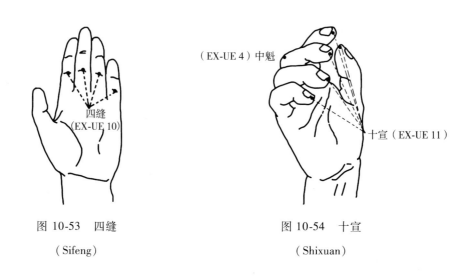

图 10-53 四缝
（Sifeng）

图 10-54 十宣
（Shixuan）

十宣（EX-UE 11）

【定位】在手十指指腹尖端，距指甲游离缘 0.1 寸，左右共十穴（图 10-54）。

【解剖】有指掌侧固有动、静脉形成的动、静脉网；布有指掌侧固有神经和丰富的痛觉感受器。

【主治】昏迷，晕厥，中暑，热病，小儿惊厥，咽喉肿痛，指端麻木。

【操作】直刺 0.1～0.2 寸，或用三棱针点刺出血。

内膝眼（EX-LE 4）

【定位】在膝部，在髌韧带内侧凹陷处（图 10-55）。

【解剖】在髌下韧带内侧，有膝关节动、静脉网；布有隐神经分支。

【主治】膝关节酸痛，鹤膝风，脚气，腿痛。

【操作】向膝中斜刺 0.5～1 寸，或透刺对侧犊鼻穴，可灸。

Sifeng (EX-UE 10)

【Location】On the palmer surface, in the midpoint of the transverse creases of the proximal interphalangeal joints of the second, third, fourth and fifth fingers, four points each side(Figure 10-53).

【Anatomy】Subcutaneously, fibrous sheaths of fingers, vaginae synoviales digitales manus, and tendon of the flexor digitorum profundus; deeper, finger joint cavity. Blood vessels: the branches of the proprial palmer digital artery and vein. Nerves: the proprial palmer digital nerve.

【Indications】Malnatrition, whooping cough, ascaridosis, diarrhea in children, cough, and asthma.

【Manipulation】Prick 0. 1−0. 2 *cun* and squeeze out a small amount of yellowish viscous fluid or blood.

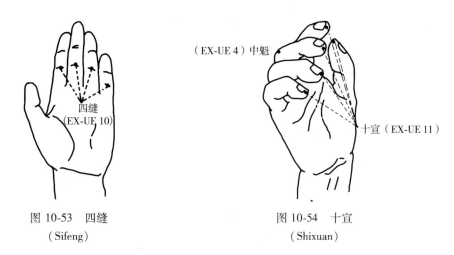

图 10-53　四缝
(Sifeng)

图 10-54　十宣
(Shixuan)

Shixuan (EX-UE 11)

【Location】On the tips of the ten fingers, about 0. 1 *cun* distal to the nails, a total of 10 points on both side(Figure 10-54).

【Anatomy】Blood vessels: the arterial and venous networks formed by the proprial palmer digital artery and vein. Nerves: the proprial palmar digital nerve, a large number of algesirecptors.

【Indications】Coma, apsychia, summer heat stroke, febrile diseases, child fright wind, sore throat, and numbness of extremities.

【Manipulation】Puncture perpendicularly 0. 1−0. 2 *cun*, or prick to cause bleeding with the three-edged needle.

Neixiyan (EX-LE 4)

【Location】A point in the olepressron, medial to the patellar ligament(Figure 10-55).

【Anatomy】Medial to the patellar ligament. Blood vessels: the arteral and venous networks of the knee. Nerves: the branches of the saphenous nerve.

【Indications】Aching and pain in the knee points, crane's-knee wind phlegm, beriberi, and leg pain.

【Manipulation】Puncture obliquely 0. 5−1 *cun*, or penetrate from the to. Moxibustion is applicable.

胆囊（EX-LE 6）

【定位】在小腿外侧上部，当腓骨小头前下方凹陷处（阳陵泉）直下 2 寸（图 10-55）。

【解剖】在腓骨长肌与趾长伸肌处；有胫前动、静脉分支；布有腓肠外侧皮神经、腓浅神经。

【主治】急、慢性胆囊炎，胆石症，胆道蛔虫症，胆绞痛，胁痛，下肢痿痹。

【操作】直刺 1~1.5 寸，可灸。

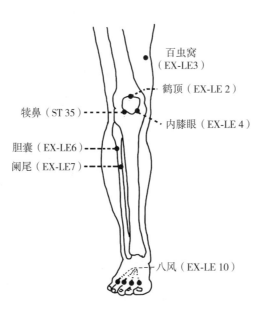

图 10-55　内膝眼、胆囊、阑尾

（Neixiyan，Dannang and Lanwei）

阑尾（EX-LE7）

【定位】当犊鼻下 5 寸，胫骨前缘旁开一横指（图 10-55）。

【解剖】穴下有胫骨前肌、小腿骨间膜和胫骨后肌；分布有腓肠外侧皮神经。

【主治】急、慢性阑尾炎，消化不良，胃炎，下肢瘫痪。

【操作】直刺 1.5~2 寸，可灸。

第四节　毫针刺法

一、进针法

在针刺时，一般用右手持针操作，称"刺手"，左手爪切按压所刺部位或辅助针

Dannang (EX-LE 6)

【Location】On the lateral part of crus, in the depression anterior and inferior to the small head of the fibula, 2 *cun* below Yanglingquan(GB 34)(Figure 10-55).

【Anatomy】Muscles: in m.peroneus logus and m.extensor digitorum logus. Blood vessels: the branches of the anterior tibial artery and vein. Nerves: the lateral cutaneous nerve of calf; deeper, the superfical peroneal nerve.

【Indications】Acute and chronic cholecystitis, cholelithiasis biliary ascariasis, biliary colic, pain in the hypochondriac region, muscular atrophy, and numbness, pain and flaccidity of the lower extremities.

【Manipulation】Puncture perpendicularly 1-1.5 *cun*. Moxibustion is applicable.

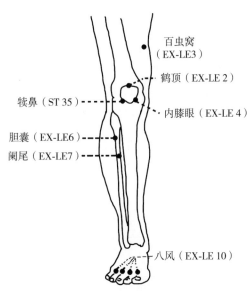

百虫窝（EX-LE3）

鹤顶（EX-LE 2）

犊鼻（ST 35）

内膝眼（EX-LE 4）

胆囊（EX-LE6）

阑尾（EX-LE7）

八风（EX-LE 10）

图 10-55　内膝眼、胆囊、阑尾
(Neixiyan, Dannang and Lanwei)

Lanwei (EX-LE 7)

【Location】5 *cun* below Dubi(ST 35), from the anterior crest of the tibia(Figure 10-55).

【Anatomy】Muscles: in m.tibialis anterior, crural interosseous membrane, and m.tibialis posterior. Nerves: the superficial peroneal nerves.

【Indications】Acute and chronic cholecystitis, indigestion, gastritis, and paralysis of lower limbs.

【Manipulation】Puncture perpendicularly 1.5-2 *cun*. Moxibustion is applicable.

Section 4　Needling Methods

Insertion

The needle should be inserted coordinately with the help of both hands. Generally the needle should be held with the right hand known as the puncturing hand. The left hand known as the pressing hand pushes firmly against the area close to the point or gives assistance to right hand. At the same time, the acu-

身，称"押手"。同时，医生持针应重视"治神"，全神贯注。《难经·七十八难》说："知为针者信其左，不知为针者信其右。"说明针刺操作时左右两手协同作用的重要性。右手持针的姿势，一般以拇、示、中三指夹持针柄，以无名指抵住针身，其状如持毛笔。

1. 单手进针法　术者以拇指、示指持针，中指端抵住腧穴，指腹紧靠针身下段。当拇、示指向下用力按压时，中指随之屈曲，将针刺入，直刺至所要求的深度。实际上，此法是以刺手的中指代替了押手的作用，具有简便、快捷、灵活的特点。该法多用于较短毫针的进针（图 10-56）。

2. 双手进针法　双手进针法是左右双手配合，协同进针。根据押手辅助动作的不同，又分为指切进针法、夹持进针法、提捏进针法、舒张进针法四种。

（1）指切进针法：又称爪切进针法，用押手拇指或示指端切按在腧穴位置旁，刺手持针，紧靠押手指甲面将针刺入。此法适宜于短针的进针（图 10-57）。

（2）夹持进针法：用押手拇、示二指持捏消毒干棉球，夹住针身下端，将针尖固定在腧穴表面，刺手捻动针柄，将针刺入腧穴，此法适用于长针的进针（图 10-58）。

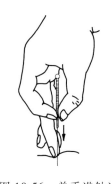

图 10-56　单手进针法

（Insertion with Single Hand）

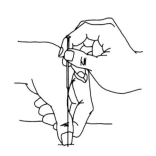

图 10-57　指切进针法

（Finger Press Insertion）

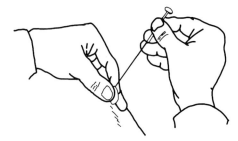

图 10-58　夹持进针法

（Pinch Needle Method）

（3）舒张进针法：用押手示、拇指将所刺腧穴部位的皮肤向两侧撑开，使皮肤绷紧，刺手持针，使针从左手拇、示二指的中间刺入。此法主要用于皮肤松弛部位的腧穴（图 10-59）。

（4）提捏进针法：用押手拇、示二指将针刺部位的皮肤捏起，刺手持针，从捏起的上端将针刺入。此法主要用于皮肉浅薄部位的进针，如印堂等（图 10-60）。

puncturist should pay attention to spirit, during the process of insertion. In the book *Classic on Medical problems*, it is discribed that "an experienced acupuncturist believes in the important function of the left hand, while an inexperienced believes in the important function of the right hand." It strengthens the importance of the coordination of the right and left hands on insertion. The position of the right hand holding the needle usually using the thumb, middle finger, and index finger to grip the needle handle, with the ring finger against the finger body, which likes hold a brush.

Insertion with single hand

The acupuncturist holds the needle with the thumb and the index finger with the middle finger against the acupuncture point, the finger pulp closing to the lower part of the needle body. When the thumb and index finger forcefully press downwards, the middle finger flex at the same time, and then insert the needle into the skin to the desired depth. In fact, the middle finger of the puncturing hand substitutes the function of the pressing hand, with the characteristics which is simple, fast and flexible. This method is suitable for puncturing with short needles(Figure 10-56).

Insertion with two hands

Insertion with two hands is the method of insertion by the combination of two hands' cooperation. According to the differently supporting action of the pressing hand, this method are divided into finger-press insertion, pinch-skin method, pinch-needle method, and tight-skin method.

1. Finger press insertion

Inserting the needle aided by the pressure of the finger of the pressing hand: press on the acupuncture point with the nail of the thumb, or the index finger or the middle finger of the left hand, hold the needle with the right hand and keep the needle tip closely against the border of the nail of the left hand, and then insert the needle into the skin. This method is suitable for puncturing with short needles(Figure 10-57).

2. Pinch needle method

Hold the dry sterilized cotton ball round the needle tip with the thumb and index finger of the left hand and fix the needle tip in directly over the selected point, and hold the needle handle with the right hand. Then, while the right hand presses the needle downward; the thumb and index finger of the left hand insert the needle tip swiftly into the skin. This method is suitable for puncturing with long needles (Figure 10-58).

3. Tight skin method

Put the thumb and the index finger, or the index and the middle finger on the skin where the point is located. Separate the two fingers and stretch the skin tightly, hold the needle with the right hand and insert it into the point. This method is suitable for puncturing the points on the areas where the skin is loose(Figure 10-59).

4. Pinch skin method

Pinch the skin up around the point with the thumb and the index finger of the left hand, hold the needle with the right hand, then insert the needle into the skin pinched up. This method is suitable for puncturing the points on the areas where the muscle and skin are thin(Figure 10-60).

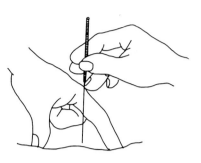 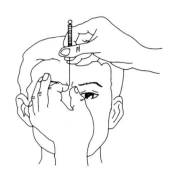

图 10-59　舒张进针法　　　　　图 10-60　提捏进针法

（Tight Skin Method）　　　　（Pinch Skin Method）

二、针刺的角度、深度和方向

在针刺过程中，角度、方向和深度非常重要。正确的针刺角度、方向和深度，是增强针感，提高疗效，防止意外事故发生的重要环节。取穴准确，不仅指其皮肤表面的位置，还必须与正确的针刺角度、方向和深度紧密地结合起来，才能充分发挥其治疗效果。同一腧穴，由于针刺角度、方向、深度的不同，所产生的针感强弱、方向和疗效常有明显差异。

1. 针刺的角度　针刺的角度，是指进针时的针身与皮肤表面所形所的夹角。其角度的大小，主要是根据腧穴所在部位的特点和医者针刺时所要达到的效果结合而定。一般分为直刺、斜刺和平刺三种（图 10-61）。

（1）直刺：针身与皮肤表面呈 90°角垂直刺入。此法适于大部分腧穴，尤以肌肉丰满处的腧穴常用。

（2）斜刺：针身与皮肤表面呈 45°角倾斜刺入。此法适用于肌肉较浅薄处或内有重要脏器或不宜于直刺、深刺的穴位。

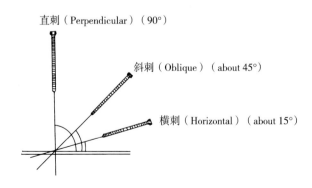

直刺（Perpendicular）（90°）

斜刺（Oblique）（about 45°）

横刺（Horizontal）（about 15°）

图 10-61　针刺角度

（Angle of Insertion）

Angle, Depth, and Direction of Insertion

In the process of insertion, the angle, depth, and direction are especially important in acupuncture. Correct angle, depth, and direction are very important parts of needling, which are helpful to promote the needling sensation, and enhance the desired therapeutic results and prevent side-effects. Appropiate selection of acupuncture points depends closely upon not only the locations of the points, but also the appropriate angle, depth and direction of insertion, which will help to guarantee its therapeutic purpose. Different angle, depth, and direction at the same point punctured might vary the needling sensation and therapeutic effect.

Angle of insertion

The angle of insertion refers to the angle formed by the needle and the skin surface as the needle is inserted. This angle depends upon the location's characteristic of the acupuncture points and the therapeutic purpose desired by the acupuncturists. Usually, there are three angles: perpendicular, oblique, and horizontal (Fig 10-61).

1. Perpendicular

The needle is inserted perpendicularly, forming a 90° angle with the skin surface. The angle of insertion is suitable for most points, especially for acupoints in the regions of thick musles of the body.

2. Oblique

The needle is inserted obliquely to form an angle of 45° with the skin surface. The method is used for the points on the thin skin or muscle, or the points under which there are important organs, or in which perpendicular insertion or deep insertion is not advisable.

3. Horizontal

Also known as suncutaneous or transverse insertion, the needle is inserted transversely to form an angle of 15°−20° with the skin. The method is suitable for the acupoints on the thin skin or muscle, such as acupoints of the head.

Depth of Insertion

The depth of needle insertion refers to the depth of the needle body within the skin. The depth of needle insertion of each acupuncture points has already been introduced in the former chapter. The introduction of the principle of the depth of insertion is as follows:

1. Constitution: for the thin and the weak, shallow insertion is advisable, while for the strong and the obese, deep insertion is advisable.

2. Age: for the elderly or the infants with delicate constitution, shallow insertion is advisable, while for the young and middle-aged with strong constitution, deep insertion is advisable.

3. Pathological condition: for yang diseases or new diseases, shallow insertion is advisable, while for yin diseases or long-lasting diseases, deep insertion is advisable.

4. Acupuncture location: for acupuncture points of head, face, chest, dorsum, and thin skin or muscle, shallow insertion is advisable; whereas, for limbs, breech, abdomen and thick skin or muscle, deep insertion is advisable.

There is a close relationship between the angle and the depth of insertion. Generally speaking, a deep insertion should be perpendicularly, whereas, a shallow insertion should be obliquely or horizontally.

Direction of insertion

In clinic, the direction of insertion is decided by the treatment needs. For example, in order to a-

（3）平刺：即横刺、沿皮刺。是针身与皮肤表面呈 15°～20°角沿皮刺入。此法适于皮薄肉少的部位，如头部的腧穴等。

2. 针刺的深度　指针身刺入人体内的深浅程度。每个腧穴的针刺深度，在腧穴各论中已有详述，在此仅根据下列情况作原则的介绍。

（1）体质：身体瘦弱浅刺，身强体肥者深刺。

（2）年龄：年老体弱及小儿娇嫩之体宜浅刺；中青年身强体壮者宜深刺。

（3）病情：阳证、新病宜浅刺；阴证、久病宜深刺。

（4）部位：头面和胸背及皮薄肉少处宜浅刺，四肢、臀、腹及肌肉丰满处宜深刺。

针刺的角度和深度关系极为密切，一般来说，深刺多用直刺；浅刺多用斜刺或平刺。

3. 针刺的方向　临床上针刺方向可根据治疗的需要而定。如为了达到"气至病所"，在针刺时针尖应朝向病痛部位；也可根据补泻的需要，如"迎随补泻"，根据辨证，有时要求针尖与所刺经脉循行方向一致，有时则要求针尖与所刺经脉循行方向相反。

三、治神

治神是指针灸医生通过对病人精神调摄和全神贯注，意念集中等，使针下得气甚而气至病所，提高临床疗效的方法。《素问·宝命全形论篇》说："凡刺之真，必先治神……。"《灵枢·官能篇》载"用针之要，无忘其神。"治神要贯穿于针刺操作的全过程，它直接影响到临床疗效，也是衡量针灸医生技术水平高低的标准。

四、行针与得气

行针也叫运针，是指医生将针刺入腧穴后，为了使之得气或进行补泻等目的而施行的各种针刺手法，这一过程称为行针。

得气也称针感，是毫针治病的关键之一，针刺必须在得气的情况下才可施行适当的补泻手法，才能获得满意的治疗效果。得气是指医生将针刺入腧穴后通过一定的手法操作，所产生的经气感应。当产生得气时，医生会感到针下有徐和或沉紧的感觉，同时病人也会在针下有相应的酸、麻、胀、重感，甚或沿着一定部位，向一定方向扩散传导的感觉。若没有得气，则医者感到针下空虚无物，患者亦无酸、胀、麻、重等感觉。得气与否及气至的迟速，直接关系到疗效，也可以借此窥测疾病的预后。临床上一般是得气迅速时，疗效较好；得气较慢时效果则差；若不得气，则可能无效。

chieve the result of "qi reaching the location of disorders," the tip of the needle should be towards the location of pain. According to the needs of reinforcing and reducing and the results of syndrome differentiation, sometimes the tip of the needle should be along the distribution of meridians, whereas sometimes opposite to it.

Mind Controlling

Mind controlling refers to the acupuncturist by means of regulating the patients' spirit and concentrating the spirit to help the arrival of qi, and even help the qi reach the region of diseases, which is a method to promote the therapeutic effects. *Plain Questions* said "one must control one's mind, this is the essence of needling." *Miraculous Pivot* states that "the principle of needling is not to forget the mind." Mind controlling should be conducted throughout the whole process of acupuncture operations, and it directly affects the clinical efficacy, also it is the measurement of the acupuncturist's level of needling technique.

Manipulations and Arrival of Qi

Needling manipulation, also known as needling transmission, refers to various manipulations of acupuncture to induce needling sensation and for the aim of reinforcing and reducing after the needle is inserted. This process also is termed as needling transmission.

The arrival of qi, also known as needling sensation, is a very important part of needling insertion. The appropriately reinforcing and reducing manipulations should be taken after the arrival of qi will make an effectively therapeutic result. The arrival of qi refers to induction of channel of qi after needle is inserted. During the needling sensation, the acupuncturist feels tempered and heavy, at the same time the patient has soreness, numbness, a distention feeling or heaviness around the point, even such feeling along certain direction diffuses and distributes to other place. If the qi fails to arrive, the acupuncturist feels empty, and the patient cannot feel the above feeling. Whether the qi arrives and whether the qi arrive timely directly decide the effectiveness and help to forecast prognosis. In the clinical practice, usually, the efficacy is better when the qi arrives quicker, whereas, the efficacy is poor when the qi arrives slow, if the qi does not arrive, it might be of no effect.

The reasons of failure of achievement of qi are diverse, including the acupuncturist's careless manipulation causing the inaccurate location, improper depth, angle and direction of insertion, imperfect syndrome differentiation, and patients' weak constitution and deficiency of qi influence the arrival of qi. During the insertion, the acupuncture should be based on appropriate location, angle, depth, and direction, proper syndrome differentiation, and perfect manipulation. Patients with diseases for a long time, in weak constitution, with deficiency of qi, or with partial insensitivity induced by other pathological factors will have a slow arrival of qi. Proper needling manipulations, such as pressing the skin along the course of the meridian, prolonged retaining, warming needle, and moxibustion, may promote the movement of meridian qi to reach the point. In addition, if the disease is improved, the meridian qi resumes, the qi will arrive. The failure of arrival of qi after the above manipulation means the collapse of organs and meridians, and other therapeutic methods should be considered.

针刺不得气的原因较多，可能由于医生用心失专，取穴不准确；或针刺角度、深浅及方向掌握的欠佳；或由于辨证失当；或由于病人的体质虚弱，经气不足等。针刺时要求医生用心要专一，全神贯注；合理调整针刺部位、角度、深度和方向；正确辨证，运用必要的手法，再次行针，一般即可得气。如患者病久体虚，以致经气不足，或因其他病理因素致局部感觉迟钝，而不易得气时，可采用行针推气或留针候气，或用温针，或加艾灸，以助经气的来复，或因治疗而随着疾病向愈，经气可逐步得到恢复，则可得气。若用上法仍不得气者，多为脏腑经络之气虚衰已极，当考虑配合或改用其他疗法。

1. 行针的基本手法

（1）提插法：是将针刺入腧穴的一定深度后，使针在穴内进行上、下进退的操作方法。把针从浅层向下刺入深层为插；由深层向上退到浅层为提。提插的幅度、频率可根据病情与腧穴部位而异。提插幅度大、频率快时，刺激量就大，若提插幅度小、频率慢时，刺激量就小（图 10-62）。

（2）捻转法：是将针刺入腧穴的一定深度后，以右手拇指和中、示二指持住针柄，进行一前一后的来回旋转捻动的操作方法。捻转的幅度、频率可根据病情与腧穴部位而异。捻转幅度大、频率快时，刺激量就大，若捻转幅度小、频率慢时，刺激量就小（图 10-63）。

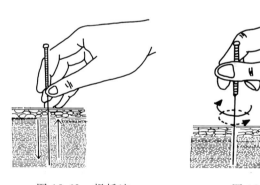

图 10-62　提插法　　　　　图 10-63　捻转法

（Lifting and Thrusting）　　　（Twirling or Rotating）

2. 辅助手法

（1）循法：是以左手或右手沿经脉的循行，进行徐和的循按的方法。此法可有行气，促经气达病所之功。

（2）刮柄法：是将针刺入一定深度后，用指甲由下而上刮动针柄的方法。此法可激发经气，促使得气。

The fundamental manipulation techniques

The fundamental manipulation techniques can be divided into two types:

Lifting and thrusting: this is a method by which the needle body is perpendicular lifted and thrusted in the point when the needle is inserted to a certain depth. Thrusting means to insert the needle from the superficial layer to the deep layer; lifting is to withdraw the needle from the deep layer to the superficial layer. The extent and frequency are decided by the condition and location of acupuncture points. A large extent and fast frequency of lifting and thrusting results in large stimulation, while a small extent and slow frequency lifting and thrusting results in small stimulation(Figure 10-62).

Twirling or rotating: this refers to the manipulation by which the needle body is twirled or rotated forward and backward continuously after the needle has reached its desired depth. The manipulation is done by the thumb, the middle finger and the index finger of right hand which hold the needle body. The extent and frequency are decided by the condition and location of acupuncture points. A large extent and fast frequency of twirling and rotating results in large stimulation, while a small extent and slow frequency of twirling and rotating results in small stimulation(Figure 10-63).

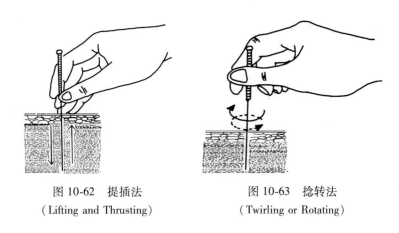

图 10-62　提插法　　　　　　　图 10-63　捻转法
(Lifting and Thrusting)　　　　(Twirling or Rotating)

The auxiliary manipulation techniques

The auxiliary manipulation techniques can be divided into three types:

Pressing: slightly press the skin up and down, slowly and softly along the course of the meridians with the fingers. It is a method of promoting qi by which the circulation of qi and blood is pushed and the meridian qi is promoted to reach the diseases part of the body.

Scraping: after the needle is inserted to a certain depth, scrape the handle with a finger nail upward from downward. It is used to promote meridian qi.

Plucking: after the needle is inserted to a certain point, pluck the needle handle slightly with the finger, make the needle tremble slightly, so as to promote moving of the meridian qi.

（3）弹针法：是将针刺入腧穴后，以手指轻轻弹针柄，使针身产生轻微的震动，而使经气速行。

五、针刺补泻

凡是能鼓舞人体正气，使低下的功能恢复旺盛的手法，即是补法。凡是能疏泄病邪、使亢进的功能恢复正常的手法，即是泻法。临床常用针刺补泻手法如下（表10-3）：

表10-3 常用单式补泻手法

手法	补法	泻法
提插补泻	先浅后深，重插轻提，提插幅度小，频率慢	先深后浅，轻插重提，提插幅度大，频率快
捻转补泻	左转时角度小，用力轻为补	右转时角度大，用力重为泻
疾徐补泻	进针慢、退针快，少捻转	进针快、退针慢，多捻转
迎随补泻	针尖随着经脉循行的方向，顺经斜刺为补	针尖迎着经脉循行的方向，迎经斜刺为泻
呼吸补泻	呼气时进针，吸气时退针为补	吸气时进针，呼气时退针为泻
开阖补泻	出针后迅速按压针孔为补	出针时摇大针孔为泻
平补平泻	进针后均匀地提插、捻转、得气后出针	

六、留针法与出针法

1. 留针法　一般病证，只要针下得气，施术完毕后即可出针，或酌留15～30分钟。但对一些慢性、顽固性、疼痛性、痉挛性病证，可适当增加留针时间，并加以行针，以增强疗效。对针感较差者，留针还可起到候气的作用。

2. 出针法　出针时，是以左手拇、示指持消毒干棉球，最好持止血钳夹消毒干棉球或消毒棉棍，按住针孔周围皮肤，右手持针轻微捻转并慢慢提至皮下，然后迅速拔出并用消毒干棉棍按压针孔片刻，防止出血；若施行针刺泻法则不按压针孔，最后检查针数，防止遗漏。

七、针刺异常情况的处理及预防

1. 晕针

【现象】针刺过程中出现心慌、精神疲倦、头晕目眩，或面色苍白、恶心欲呕、出冷汗、脉象沉细；严重者出现肢体厥冷、血压下降、二便失禁、不省人事等。

【原因】精神紧张、体质虚弱、饥饿疲劳、大汗、大泻、大出血后，或体位不当，或医者手法过重而致脑部暂时缺血。

Reinforcing and Reducing Methods of Acupuncture

The manipulation which is able to invigorate the body resistance and to strengthen the weakened physiological function is called reinforcing method, whereas, the manipulation which is able to eliminated the pathogenic factors and to harmonize the hyperactive physiological functions is called reducing method. Common reinforcing and reducing methods used in clinic are shown as follows(Table 10-3) :

Table10-3   Common reinforcing and reducing methods

Method	Reinforcing method	Reducing method
Reinforcing and reducing by lifting and thrusting the needle	From shallow to deep, thrust heavily and lift gently, lift and thrust with a small extent and slow frequency	From deep to shallow, lift heavily and thrust gently, lift and thrust with a large extent and fast frequency
Reinforcing and reducing by twirling and rotating the needle	Rotate towards left with a small angle and a small force	Rotate towards right with large angle and a large force
Reinforcing and reducing achieved by rapid and slow insertion and withdrawal of the needle	Slow insertion and rapid withdrawal of the needle with less twirling and rotating	Rapid insertion and slow withdrawal of the needle with more twirling and rotating
Reinforcing and reducing achieved by the direction the needle tip points to	Puncture a point following its meridian course	Puncture a point against its meridian course
Reinforcing and reducing achieved by means of respiration	Insert the needle when the patient breaches out and withdrawal the needle when the patient breathes in	Insert the needle when the patient breaches in and withdrawal the needle when the patient breathes out
Reinforcing and reducing by keeping the hole open or close	Withdraw needle slowly and press the needling hole quickly to close it	Withdraw the needle quickly and shake and enlarge the hole
Even reinforcing and reducing	After the needle is inserted, thrust and rotate the needle evenly, and then withdraw the needle after the arrival of qi	

Retaining and Withdrawing the Needle

Retaining

In general, the needle is retained for fifteen to thirty minutes after the arrival of qi. For some chronic, intractable, painful and spastic cases, the time for retaining of the needle may be appropriately prolonged, in addition, manipulations may be given to strengthen the therapeutic effects. For patients with a dull needling sensation, retaining the needle serves as a method of awaiting qi.

Withdrawing

When withdrawing the needle, take a sterilized dry cotton with the thumb and the index finger of left hand, then press the skin around the point, rotate the needle slightly, and lift it slowly to the subcutaneous level with the right hand, and then withdraw it quickly and press the punctured point with sterilized dry cotton for a while to prevent bleeding. For reducing methods, the punctured point should not be pressed. Checking the number of needles is necessary to avoid omission.

Management and Prevention of Possible Accidents

Fainting

【Manifestation】In the process of acupuncture treatment, adverse symptoms are shown as palpitation,

【处理】首先将针全部取出，使患者平卧，头部稍低，注意保暖，轻者在饮温开水或糖水后即可恢复正常；重者在上述处理的基础上，可指掐人中、素髎、内关穴，必要时应配合其他急救措施。

【预防】对于初次接受针刺治疗和精神紧张者，应先让他们放松；选择舒适的体位，取穴不宜太多，手法不宜过重；对于过度饥饿、疲劳者，不予针刺。留针过程中，医者应随时注意观察病人的神色，询问病人的感觉。

2. 滞针

【现象】进针后，出现提插捻转及出针困难，患者疼痛明显。

【原因】患者精神紧张。针刺入后，局部肌肉强烈收缩，或因毫针刺入肌腱，行针时捻转角度过大或连续进行单向捻转。

【处理】嘱患者消除紧张状态，使局部肌肉放松。因单向捻转而致者，需反向捻转。如属肌肉一时性紧张，可以按揉局部，或在附近部位加刺一针，随之将针取出。

【预防】对精神紧张者，先消除紧张顾虑，进针时避开肌腱，行针时捻转角度不宜过大，更不可单向连续捻转。

3. 弯针

【现象】针身弯曲，针柄改变了进针时刺入的方向和角度，提插捻转及出针均感困难，患者感觉疼痛。

【原因】医者进针手法不熟练，用力过猛，或碰到坚硬组织；留针中患者改变体位；针柄受到外物的压迫和碰撞以及滞针未得到及时正确地处理。

【处理】如系轻微弯曲，不能再行提插捻转，应慢慢将针退出；弯曲角度过大时，应顺着弯曲方向将针退出；如因患者改变体位而致，应嘱患者恢复原体位，使局部肌肉放松，再行退针，切忌强行拔针。

【预防】医生进针手法要熟练，指力要轻巧，患者体位要舒适，留针时不得随意改动体位，针刺部位和针柄不能受外物碰撞和压迫，如有滞针及时正确处理。

4. 断针

【现象】针身折断，残端留在患者体内。

【原因】针具质量欠佳，针身或针根有剥蚀损坏；针刺时，针身全部刺入；行针时，强力捻转提插，肌肉强烈收缩或患者改变体位；滞针和弯针现象未及时正确处理。

【处理】嘱患者不要紧张，不要乱动，以防断端向肌肉深层陷入。如断端还在体外，可用手指或镊子取出；如断端与皮肤相平，可挤压针孔两旁，使断端暴露体外，用镊子取出；如针身完全陷入肌肉，应在 X 线下定位，外科手术取出。

【预防】认真检查针具，对不符合质量要求的应剔出不用。选针时，针身的长度

fatigue, dizziness, vertigo, paleness, nausea, vomit, cold sweating, and thin and weak pulse. In severe cases, there may be symptoms such as cold extremities, drop of blood pressure, fecal and urinary incontinence, and loss of consciousness.

【Cause】Nervous tension, delicate constitution, hunger, fatigue; severe sweating, diarrhea or bleeding; improper position, or transient ischemic attack due to heavy manipulation of the practitioner.

【Management】Stop needling immediately and withdraw all the needles, then help the patient to lie down and lower the head, and keep the patient body warm. In mild case, the patient recovers immediately after drinking some warm or sweet water. In severe cases, in addition to the above management, press hard with the fingernail or needle the auncpuncture points of Renzhong(GV 26), Suliao(GV 25), and Neiguan (PC 6), together with other emergency methods if necessary.

【Prevention】For the patients who first receive acupuncture therapy and are nervous, let them relax. Keep a comfortable posture. Do not select too many points, and don't manipulate too forceful. For the patients who are too hungry and tired, insertion is prohibited. During the process of retaining the needle, pay attention to the patient's facial expression, and ask the patients' feeling.

Stuck needle

【Manifestation】After insertion, the needle is difficult to rotate, lift, thrust, and withdraw, while the patient feels apparently pain.

【Cause】This may arise from nervousness of the patient, strong spasm of the local muscle after the insertion, improper insertion into tendons, twirling the needle with too large amplitude or in one direction only.

【Management】Ask the patient to relax, and relax the local muscle. If the needle is stuck due to excessive rotation in one direction, the condition will release when the needle is twirled in the opposite direction. If the stuck needle is caused by the tension of the muscle temporarily, withdraw it by massaging the skin near the point or by inserting another needle nearby and then withdraw the needle.

【Prevention】Nervous patients should be encouraged to relax. Avoid the muscle tendons during insertion. Twirling with too large amplitude or in one direction should be prohibited.

Bent needle

【Manifestation】After the needle is inserted, it is found at times difficult or impossible to rotate, lift, and thrust the needle, with the patient feeling apparently pain.

【Cause】This may result from unskillful manipulation or too forceful manipulation, or the needle striking the hard tissue, or a sudden change of the patient's posture for different reasons, or form an improper management of the struck needle.

【Management】When the needle is bent, lifting, thrusting, and rotating shall in no case be applied. The needle may be removed slowly and withdraw by following the course of bend. In case the bent needle is caused by the change of the patient's posture, move him to his original position, relax the local muscle and then remove the needle. Never try to withdraw the needle with force.

【Prevention】Perfect insertion and gentle manipulation are required. The patient should have a proper and comfortable position. During the retaining period, change of the position is not allowed. The needling area in no case be impacted or pressed by an external force. A proper management should be taken after stuck needle.

Broken needle

【Manifestation】The needle body is broken during manipulation and the broken part is below the skin surface.

【Cause】This may arise from the poor quality of the needle or eroded base of the needle, from too strong manipulation of the needle, from too strong muscle spasm, or a sudden movement of the patient

要比准备刺入的深度长 0.5 寸。针刺时，不要将针身全部刺入，应留一部分在体外。进针时，如发生弯针，应立即出针，不可强行刺入。对于滞针和弯针，应及时正确处理，不可强行拔出。

5. 血肿

【现象】出针后，局部呈青紫色或肿胀疼痛。

【原因】针尖弯曲带钩，使皮肉受损或针刺时误伤小血管。

【处理】微量出血或针孔局部小块青紫，是毛细血管受损引起，一般不必处理，可自行消退。如局部青紫较重或活动不便者，在先行冷敷止血后，过 24 小时再行热敷，或按揉局部，以促使局部瘀血消散。

【预防】仔细检查针具，熟悉解剖部位，避开血管针刺。

6. 创伤性气胸

【现象】轻者感胸痛、胸闷、心慌、呼吸不畅；重者则出现呼吸困难、心跳加快、紫绀、出冷汗、烦躁，严重时发生血压下降、休克等危急现象等。体检时可见患侧胸部肋间隙增宽，触诊可见气管向健侧移位，患侧胸部叩诊呈鼓音，心浊音界缩小，肺部听诊呼吸音明显减弱或消失。X 线胸透可进一步确诊。

【原因】凡刺胸骨上窝，胸骨切迹上缘及第十一胸椎两侧，侧胸（胸中线）第八肋间，前胸（锁骨中线）第六肋间以上的腧穴，如针刺方向、角度和深度不当，都可能刺伤肺脏，使空气进入胸腔，导致创伤性气胸。

【处理】一旦有气胸发生，可作对症处理，采用半卧位休息，防止感染，镇咳，胸腔穿刺排气等。

【预防】为了有效地防止发生气胸，针刺以上部位时，医者思想必须高度集中，正确为患者选择体位，熟悉解剖部位，掌握好针刺方向、角度和深度。

when the needle is in place, or from an improper and timely management after stuck needle and bent needle.

【Management】When it happens, the patient should be asked to keep calm to from maing.If the broken part protrudes from the skin, remove it with forceps or fingers.If the broken part is at the same level of the skin, press the tissue around the site until the broken end is exposed, and then remove it with forceps. If it is completely under the skin, surgery should be resorted to.

【Prevention】To prevent accidents, careful inspection of the quality of the needle should be made prior to the treatment to reject the needles which are not in conformity with the requirements specified.The length of needle body should be 0. 5 *cun* longer than the depth of needle inserted into the body.The needle body should not be inserted into the body completely, and a little part should be exposed outside the skin. On needle insertion, if it is bent, the needle should be withdrawn immediately.Never try to insert a needle with too much force.For stuck needle and bent needle, make a proper manipulation, and forceful pulling out is not advisable.

Hematoma

【Manifestation】Local swelling, distension and pain after withdrawal of the needle.

【Cause】This may result from the bend needle tip with hook or from injury of the skin, muscle, and blood vessels during insertion.

【Management】Generally, a mild hematoma, due to the injuries of capillary vessel, will disappear by itself.If the local swelling and pain are serious, apply local pressing, or cold pressing or warming maxibustion to help disperse the hematoma.

【Prevention】A careful inspection of acupuncture tools should be taken before insertion.Grasp the anatomy location.Avoid injuring the blood vessels.

Traumatic pneumothorax

【Manifestation】In the mild cases, the patient feels chest pain, chest tightness, palpitation, shortness of breath;in the severe cases, the patient suffers from a serious of emergency, such as difficulty in breathing, rapid heartbeat, cyanosis, cold sweating, irritability, severe drop in blood pressure, and shock.On examination, it may be found that the intercostal space of the diseased side becomes wider.The trachea even is displaced to the healthy side.A hyperresonance may be got on thoracic percussion.The vesicular respiratory sound becomes weak or disappears.Further diagnosis of the condition is confirmed by chest X-ray examination.

【Cause】When acupuncture is applied to the points above the supraclavicular fossa, or the suprasternal notch, or both sides of the 11th thoracic vertebra, the points above the 8th intercostal space on the middle auxiliary line and above the 6th intercostal space on the midclavicular line, because of improper direction, angle or depth of the needle, the pleura and lung are sometimes injured and the air enters the thoracic cavity to cause pneumothorax.

【Management】Once pneumothorax takes place, ask the patient to rest in a half recumbent posture. Mild cases can be managed according to their symptoms and signs to prevent infections, antitussive and sacking out air by thoracentesis.

【Prevention】In order to effectively prevent the occurrence of pneumothorax, when inserting the above points, the acupuncturist must be highly concentrated, and select the correct posture for patients, and should be familiar with the anatomic site, and grasp the direction, angle, and depth of insertion.

第 五 节　灸　　法

一、灸法的概述

灸法是用艾绒为主要材料制成的艾炷或艾条点燃以后，在体表的一定部位熏灼，给人体以温热性刺激，通过经络的传导起到疏通经络，温通气血，回阳救逆，扶正祛邪，达到治疗疾病和预防保健目的的一种外治方法。

二、常用灸法

（一）艾炷灸

将纯净的艾绒放在平板上，用手指搓捏成圆锥形状，称为艾炷（图 10-64）。每燃烧一个艾炷称为一壮。艾炷灸分为直接灸和间接灸两类。

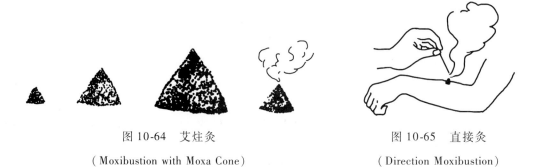

图 10-64　艾炷灸
（Moxibustion with Moxa Cone）

图 10-65　直接灸
（Direction Moxibustion）

1. 直接灸　将艾炷直接放在皮肤上施灸称直接灸（图 10-65）。分为瘢痕灸和无瘢痕灸。

（1）瘢痕灸：又称"化脓灸"，施灸前用大蒜捣汁涂敷施灸部位后，放置艾炷施灸。灸后一周左右，施术部位化脓（称"灸疮"），5~6 周后，灸疮自行痊愈，结痂脱落，留下瘢痕。

（2）无瘢痕灸：将艾炷置于穴位上点燃，当艾炷燃到 2/5 左右，病人感到灼痛时，即更换艾炷再灸。一般灸 3~5 壮，使局部皮肤充血为度。

2. 间接灸　艾炷不直接放在皮肤上，而用药物隔开放在皮肤上施灸。常用的有如下几种：

（1）隔姜灸：将新鲜生姜切成约 0.5cm 厚的薄片，中心处用针穿刺数孔，上置艾炷，放在穴位施灸，当患者感到灼痛时，可将姜片稍许上提，使之离开皮肤片刻，

Section 5   Moxibustion

Introduction of Moxibustion

Moxibustion treats and prevents diseases by applying heat stimulation to points or certain locations of the human body, with the help of meridians' transportation to induce the smooth of meridians and collaterals, warm and soothe qi and blood, restore yang and rescue patient from collapse of yang, strengthening body resistance to eliminate pathogenic factors, by ignition of moxa cones or moxa stricks produced by moxa.

Common Moxibustions

Moxibustion with Moxa Cones

Place a small amount of moxa wool on a board, knead and shape it into a cone with fingers, which called moxa cone(Figure 10-64). During treatment with moxibustion, one moxa cone used at one point is called one unit or one *zhuang*. Moxibustion with moxa cones may be direct moxibustion or indirect moxibustion.

1. Direct moxibustion

A moxa cone placed directly on the skin and ignited is called direct moxibustion(Figure 10-65). This type of moxibustion is subdivided into nonscarring moxibustuion and scarring moxibustion.

(1)Scarring moxibustion   Scarring moxibustion is also known as "festering moxibustion." Prior to moxibustion, apply some garlic juice into the point, then put the moxa cone on the point and ignite it until it completely burns out and extinguishes. After five or six weeks, the post-moxibustion sore may heal by itself and scab falls off, leaving scar on the skin.

(2)Nonscarring mosibustion   A moxa cone of proper size is placed directly on a point, when 2/5 of it is burnt or the patient feels pain, remove the cone and place another one. Generally, three to five *zhuang* are used each time, until the patient's local skin hyperemia.

2. Indirect moxibustion

The ignited moxa cone does not set on the skin directly but is insulated from the skin by materials. Commonly used types are as follows.

(1)Moxibustion with ginger

Cut a slice of ginger about 0.5 cm thick, punch numerous holes on it and place it on the point selected. On top of this piece of ginger, a large moxa cone is placed and ignited. When the patient feels it scorching, remove it from the skin and then put it on the skin, and repeat for several times, or put some pieces of paper and then put it on the skin until the local skin becomes ruddy(Figure 10-66). This method is indicated in symptoms caused by external contraction, and deficiency cold syndromes, such as cold, cough, wind-dampness impediment pain, vomiting, abdominal pain, diarrhea.

(2)Moxibustion with garlic

Cut a slice of a large single clove of garlic about 0.5 cm thick, punch numerous holes on it and place it on the point selected or a swelling lump. On top of this piece of garlic, a large moxa cone is placed and ignited. Generally five to seven *zhuang* is applied. When the patient feels it scorching, remove it and light another. This method is indicated in phthisis, lump in abdomen, the early stage of skin ulcer with boils, poisonous insect or snake bite, etc.

旋即放下，再行灸治，反复进行。或在姜片下衬一些纸片，放下再灸，直到局部皮肤潮红为止（图 10-66）。此法多用于治疗外感表证和虚寒性疾病，如感冒、咳嗽、风湿痹痛、呕吐、腹痛、泄泻等。

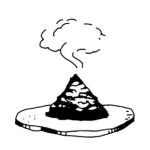

图 10-66　隔姜灸

（ Moxibustion with Ginger ）

（2）隔蒜灸：用独头大蒜切成约 0.5cm 厚的薄片，中间用针穿刺数孔，放在穴位或肿块上（如未溃破化脓的脓头处），用艾炷灸，可灸 5 ~ 7 壮。本法多用于治疗肺痨、腹中积块及未溃疮疖、虫蛇咬伤等。

（3）隔盐灸：本法只适于脐部。以纯白干燥的食盐，填平脐孔，再放上姜片和艾炷施灸。此方法对急性腹痛、吐泻、痢疾、四肢厥冷和虚脱等证，具有回阳救逆的作用。

（二）艾条灸

将点燃的一端艾条悬于施灸部位之上，一般艾火距皮肤有一定距离，灸 10 ~ 20 分钟，以灸至皮肤温热红晕，而又不致烧伤皮肤为度。操作方法又分为温和灸、雀啄灸和回旋灸。

1. 温和灸　将艾条的一端点燃，对准施灸处，距 0.5 ~ 1 寸进行熏烤，使患者局部有温热感而无灼痛。一般每处灸 5 ~ 10 分钟，至皮肤稍起红晕为度（图 10-67）。

2. 雀啄灸　艾条燃着的一端，与施灸处不固定距离，而是像鸟雀啄食一样，上下移动或均匀地向左右方向移动或反复旋转施灸（图 10-68）。

3. 回旋灸　施灸时，艾条点燃的一端与施灸皮肤虽保持一定的距离，但位置不固定，而是均匀地向左右方向移动或反复旋转地进行灸治。

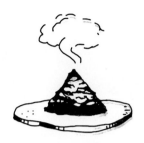

图 10-66   隔姜灸
(Moxibustion with Ginger)

(3) Moxibustion with salt

This method is only for umbilicus. Fill the umbilicus with dry salt to the level of the skin, place a piece of ginger and a large moxa cone and then ignite it. This method is effective in cases of acute abdominal pain, vomiting and diarrhea, dysentery, cold limbs, and collapse. In addition, moxibustion with salt has the function to restore to yang from collapse of yang.

Moxibustion with Moxa Sticks

Ignite one end of moxa sticks and put it over the selected point. Generally, the fire of moxa stick has certain distance away from the selected skin. Keep moxibustion for 10 to 20 minutes, until the skin warm and ruddy, without burning the skin. This method is divided into gentle moxibustion, pecking sparrow moxibustion and circling moxibustion.

1. Gentle moxibustion

Put the lighted end of a moxa stick over the selected point to warm it, and 0.5−1 *cun* away the point is recommended. It is good for the patient to feel warm, comfortable and painless. Gentle moxibustion for each point may last 5−10 minutes until the skin around the point becomes flushed (Figure 10-67).

2. Pecking sparrow moxibustion

Ignite one end of a moxa stick, the distance between the ignited end and the point is not stable Evenly peck the moxa stick over the point up and down, left and right or rotate repeatedly, just like a bird's pecking (Figure 10-68).

3. Circling moxibustion

Ignite one end of a moxa stick, and keep it at a fixed distance away from the patient's skin, and evenly move the ignited moxa stick left and right or repeatedly in a circular direction.

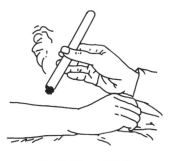

图 10-67　温和灸

（Gentle Moxibustion）

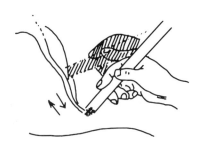

图 10-68　雀啄灸

（Pecking Sparrow Moxibustion）

（三）温针灸

温针灸是针刺与艾灸结合应用的一种方法，适用于既需要留针而又适宜用艾灸的病证。操作方法是，将针刺入腧穴得气后并给予适当补泻手法而留针时，将纯净细软的艾绒捏在针尾上，或用艾条一段长约 2 厘米，插在针柄上，点燃施灸。待艾绒或艾条烧完后除去灰烬，将针取出。此法是一种简而易行的针灸并用方法（图 10-69）。

三、灸法的适应证和禁忌证

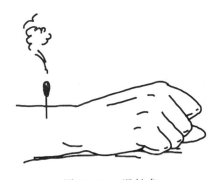

图 10-69　温针灸

（Warm Needling Moxibustion）

（一）适应证

1．慢性病及阳气不足的疾病。

2．一切虚寒病证。

（二）禁忌证

1．对实热证、阴虚发热者，一般不适宜灸疗。

2．对颜面、五官和有大血管的部位，不宜采用瘢痕灸。

3．孕妇的腹部、腰骶部也不宜施灸。

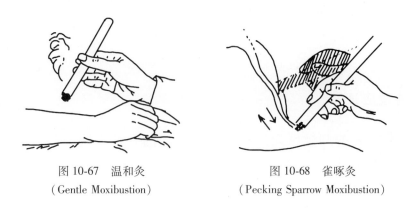

图 10-67　温和灸
（Gentle Moxibustion）　　　

图 10-68　雀啄灸
（Pecking Sparrow Moxibustion）

Warm needling moxibustion

Warm needling moxibustion is a method of acupuncture combined with moxibustion, and it is used for conditions in which both the retaining of the needle and moxibustion are needed. The manipulation is as follows:

After the needle is inserted and the qi is arrived and appropriated supplementation and draining manipulations are performed, and the needle is retained in the point in proper depth, wrap the handle of the needle with the moxa wool; or put the needle handle into a 2 cm long moxa stick, ignite the moxa wool or the moxa stick to perform moxibustion. After the moxa wool or moxa stick is burned completely, clean the ashes and remove the needle. It is a simple method to apply moxibustion combined with acupuncture (Figure 10-69).

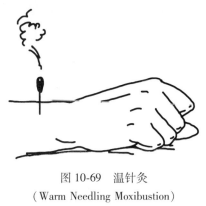

图 10-69　温针灸
（Warm Needling Moxibustion）

Indications and Contraindications of Moxibustion

Indications of Moxibustion

1. Chronic diseases and diseases due to yang-deficiency.

2. All the deficiency cold syndromes.

Contraindications of Moxibustion

1. Excess heat syndrome, and heat due to yin deficiency are not allowed to be treated by moxibustion.

2. Scarring moxibustion should not be applied to the face and head, or the area in the vicinity of the large blood vessels.

3. It is prohibited to use moxibustion on the abdominal or the lumbosacral region of a pregnant woman.

第六节 头针疗法

一、头针的适应证

头针是在头部特定的刺激区运用针刺防治疾病的一种方法，临床常用于脑源性疾患，如神经、精神系统疾病、脑血管疾病、假性球麻痹、失语、共济失调、震颤麻痹、舞蹈病等。此外，也可以治疗坐骨神经痛、三叉神经痛、头痛、运动神经元疾病、急性腰痛、肩周炎、消化系统疾病、胃下垂、膈肌痉挛等。

二、头部刺激区的定位和主治

（一）定位依据

常用的定位方法有两种：一是根据脏腑经络理论，在头部选取相关经穴进行治疗。二是根据大脑皮质的功能定位，在头皮上划分出相应的刺激区进行针刺。下面主要介绍第二种。

（二）定位线

划分刺激区的两条标准定位线：前后正中线：是从两眉间中点（正中线前点）至枕外粗隆尖端下缘（正中线后点）经过头顶的连线。眉枕线：是从眉中点上缘和枕外粗隆尖端的头侧面连线（图10-70）。

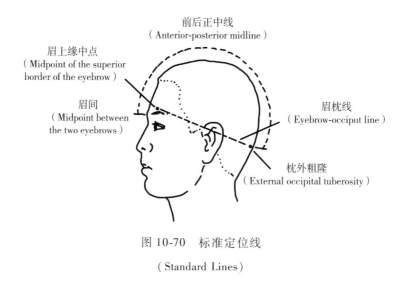

图 10-70　标准定位线

（Standard Lines）

（三）刺激区定位和主治作用

1. 运动区　运动区上点在前后正中线中点往后0.5cm处；下点在眉枕线和鬓角

Section 6   Scalp Acupuncture

Indications of the Scalp Acupuncture

The scalp acupuncture is a therapy to prevent and treat diseases by needling specific stimulation areas of the scalp. It is usually used to treat cerebral diseases including nervous system disease, psychiatric disorders, cerebrovascular diseases, pseudobulbar palsy, aphasia, ataxia, tremor, paralysis, chorea, etc. In addition, scalp acupuncture is also used to treat sciatica, trigeminal neuralgia, headache, motor neuron disease, acute low back pain, frozen shoulder, digestive diseases, prolapse of the stomach, diaphragm spasm, etc.

Division of Stimulation Areas and Main Indications

The principle of locating points

Two methods are commonly used for locating points. First, according to the theories of the viscera and bowels and meridians and collaterals, select meridian points in the head to treat diseases; the second method is based on the functional orientation of the cerebral cortex, and needling is performed in the stimulation areas on the scalp. The second method is mainly introduced as follows.

The standard lines

There are two standard lines which are used to divide the stimulation areas. One is called antero-posterior midline: the middle connecting the midpoint between the two eyebrows (the anterior point of antero-posterior midline) with the lower border of the tip of the external occipital tuberosity across the vertex (the posterior point of antero-posterior midline). The other is the eyebrow-occiput line: the line connecting the midpoint of the superior border of the eyebrow with the tip of the external occipital tuberosity horizontally along the lateral side of the head (Figure 10-70).

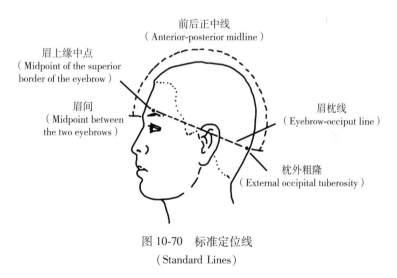

图 10-70   标准定位线

(Standard Lines)

Division of stimulation areas and their main indications

1. The motor area

Take the point 0.5 cm posterior to the midpoint of antero-posterior midline as the upper point, and

发际前缘相交处。如果鬓角不明显，可以从颧弓中点向上引垂直线，此线与眉枕线交叉处向前移 0.5cm 为运动区下点。上下两点连线即为运行区。运动区又可分为上、中、下三部（图 10-71）。

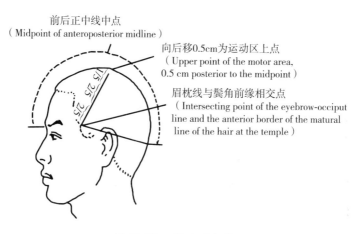

图 10-71　运动区定位

（Location of the Motor Area）

（1）上部：是运动区的上 1/5，为下肢、躯干运动区。主治对侧下肢、躯干部瘫痪。

（2）中部：是运动区的中 2/5，为上肢运动区。主治对侧上肢瘫痪。

（3）下部：是运动区的下 2/5，为面运动区，亦称言语一区。主治对侧中枢性面神经瘫痪，运动性失语（部分或完全丧失语言能力，但基本上保留理解语言的能力），流涎，发音障碍，假性球麻痹等。

2. 感觉区　感觉区在运动区向后移 1.5cm 的平行线即是本区。感觉区可分为上、中、下三部（图 10-72）。

（1）上部：是感觉区的上 1/5，为下肢、头、躯干感觉区。主治对侧腰腿痛、麻木、感觉异常、头后、颈项部疼痛、头晕、耳鸣。

（2）中部：是感觉区的中 2/5，为上肢感觉区。主治对侧上肢疼痛、麻木、感觉异常。

（3）下部：是感觉区的下 2/5，为面感觉区。主治对侧面部麻木，偏头痛，颞颌关节炎等。

3. 舞蹈震颤控制区　舞蹈震颤控制区在运动区向前移 1.5cm 的平行线（图 10-72）。主治舞蹈病，震颤麻痹，震颤麻痹综合征。

4. 晕听区　晕听区从耳尖直上 1.5cm 处，向前及向后各引 2cm 的水平线（图 10-72）。主治眩晕、耳鸣、听力降低。

the intersecting point of the eyebrow-occiput line and the anterior border of the matural line of the hair at the temple as the lower point. If the temple is not obvious, draw a vertical line from the midpoint of zygomatic arch, and 0. 5 cm forwards from the intersecting point of this line and eyebrow pillow line is the lower point. The connecting line between these two points is the motor area . The area is subdivided into 3 parts: the upper part, the middle part, and the lower part(Figure 10-71).

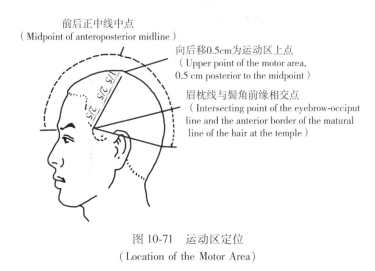

前后正中线中点
(Midpoint of anteroposterior midline)

向后移0.5cm为运动区上点
(Upper point of the motor area,
0.5 cm posterior to the midpoint)

眉枕线与鬓角前缘相交点
(Intersecting point of the eyebrow-occiput
line and the anterior border of the matural
line of the hair at the temple)

图 10-71   运动区定位
(Location of the Motor Area)

The upper part: the upper 1/5 of this area is the lower limb and trunk motor area. This motor area is used for contralateral paralysis of the lower limb and the trunk.

The middle part: the middle 2/5 of this area is the upper limb motor area area. This area is applied for contralateral paralysis of the upper limb.

The lower part: the lower 2/5 of this area is the face area, also called the 1st speech area. This area is for contallateral central facial paralysis, motor aphasia(partially lose the ability of speech, but basically retaining the ability of understanding) , salivation, and dysphonia.

2. The sensory area

The parallel line, 1. 5 *cun* behind the motor area, is the sensory area. The area is subdivided into 3 parts: the upper part, the middle part, and the lower part(Figure 10-72).

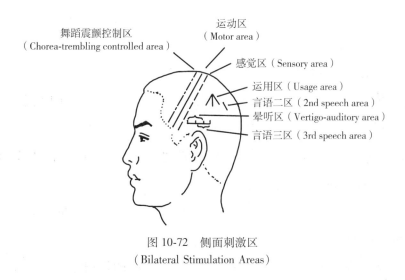

舞蹈震颤控制区
(Chorea-trembling controlled area)

运动区
(Motor area)

感觉区 (Sensory area)

运用区 (Usage area)

言语二区 (2nd speech area)

晕听区 (Vertigo-auditory area)

言语三区 (3rd speech area)

图 10-72   侧面刺激区
(Bilateral Stimulation Areas)

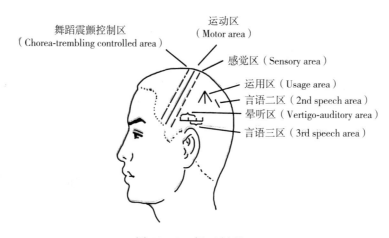

图 10-72 侧面刺激区

（Bilateral Stimulation Areas）

5. 言语二区　言语二区从顶骨结节后下方 2cm 处引一平行于前后正中线的直线，向下取 3cm 长直线（图 10-72）。主治命名性失语。

6. 言语三区　言语三区从晕听区中点向后引 4cm 长的水平线（图 10-72）。主治感觉性失语。

7. 运用区　运用区从顶骨结节起分别引一垂直线和与该线夹角为 40°的前后两线，长度为 3cm（图 10-72）。主治失用症。

8. 足运感区　足运感区在前后正中线的中点旁开左右各 1cm，向后引 3cm 长平行于正中线的直线（图 10-73）。主治对侧下肢瘫痪，疼痛，麻木，急性腰扭伤，夜尿多，皮质性多尿，子宫下垂等。

9. 视区　视区在前后正中线的后点旁开 1cm 处的枕外粗隆水平线上，向上引平行于前后正中线的 4cm 长直线（图 10-73）。主治皮层性视力障碍。

10. 平衡区　平衡区在前后正中线的后点旁开 3.5cm 处的枕外粗隆水平线上，向下引平行于前后正中线的 4cm 长直线（图 10-73）。主治小脑疾病引起的共济失调，平衡障碍，头晕，脑干功能障碍引起的肢体麻木瘫痪。

11. 胃区　胃区从瞳孔直上发际处为起点，向上行平行于前后正中线 2cm 长直线（图 10-74）。主治胃炎、胃溃疡等引起的胃痛、上腹部不适。

12. 胸腔区　胸腔区在胃区与前后正中线之间，发际上下各引 2cm 长直线（图 10-74）。主治支气管哮喘，胸部不适等症。

13. 生殖区　生殖区从额角处向上引平行于前后正中线的 2cm 长直线（图 10-74）。主治功能性子宫出血，盆腔炎，子宫脱垂等。

选穴方法，单侧肢体疾病，选用对侧刺激区；双侧肢体疾病，选用双侧刺激区；

(1)The upper part   The upper 1/5 of this area is the lower limb, head and trunk sensory area. This sensory area is used for contralateral lumber pain, pain of the leg, numbness, paresthesia, occipital headache, pain in the nape region, dizziness and tinnitus.

(2)The middle part   The middle 2/5 of this area is the upper limb sensory area. This sensory area is applied for contralateral upper limb pain, numbness and paresthesia.

(3)The lower part   The lower 2/5 is the face sensory area. This sensory area is indicated for contralateral facial numbness, migraine, trigeminal neuralgia, toothache and temporomandibular arthritis(Figure 10-72).

3. The chorea-trembling controlled area

The parallel line, 1. 5 cm in front of the motor area(Figure 10-72). This area is indicated for chorea, Parkinson's disease, and paralysis agitans syndrome.

4. The vertigo-auditory area

This area is a 4 cm horizontal straight line located on the site 1. 5 cm right above the auricular apex (Figure 10-72). This area is indicated for dizziness, tinnitus and hypoacusis.

5. The 2nd speech area

This area is a 3 cm straight line, starting from a point 2 cm posterior and inferior to the parietal tubercle, parallel to the anterposterior midline(Figure 10-72). This area is used for nominal aphasia.

6. The 3rd speech area

This area is 4 cm backward horizontal line from the midpoint of the vertigo-auditory area(Figure 10-72). This area is indicated for sensory aphasia.

7. The usage area

Take the parietal tubercle as a starting point, draw a vertical line from the point, at the same time draw the other two lines from the point separately forwards and backwards, at 40°with the vertical line, each of the three lines is 3 cm long(Figure 10-72). This area is indicated for apraxia.

8. The foot motor sensory area

Draw two 3 cm straight lines backwards parallel to the antero-posterior midline. Their starting points arc 1 cm bilateral to the midpoint of the midline(Figure 10-75). This area is indicated for contralateral lower limb paralysis, pain, numbnesss, acute lumber sprain, cerebrocortical polyuria, nocturia, uterine prolapse, etc.

9. The optic area

Draw a 4 cm straight line upwards, parallel to the antero-posterior midline, 1-cm evenly beside the external occipital protuberance(Figure 10-73). This area is indicated for cerebro-cortical visual disturbance.

10. The balance area

Draw a 4 cm straight line downwards, parallel to the antero-posterior midline, 3. 5 cm evenly beside the external occipital protuberance(Figure 10-73). This area is indicated for equilibrium disturbance, balance disorder, dizziness caused by cerebellum disease, and limb paralysis and numbness caused by functional disorder of brainstem.

11. The gastric area

Take the hair margin directly above the pupil as a starting point, draw a 2 cm straight line upwards, parallel to the antero-posterior midline(Figure 10-74). This area is indicated for gastric pain and epigastric discomfort due to gastritis or gastrohelcoma.

12. The thoracic area

Midway between the gastric area and the anteroposterior midline, take the hair margin as the midpoint, draw a 4 cm straight line, parallel to the antero-posterior midline(Figure 10-74). This area is used

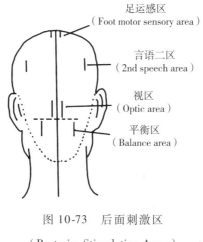

图 10-73　后面刺激区

(Posterior Stimulation Areas)

内脏全身疾病或不易区别左右的疾病，可双侧取穴，一般根据疾病选用相应的刺激区，并可选用有关刺激区配合治疗。如下肢瘫痪，可选下肢运动区配足运感区等。

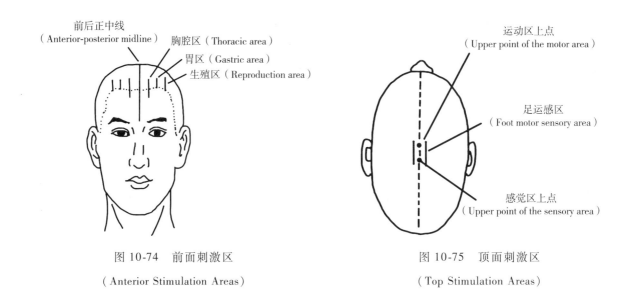

图 10-74　前面刺激区

(Anterior Stimulation Areas)

图 10-75　顶面刺激区

(Top Stimulation Areas)

三、头针的操作方法

病员采取坐位或卧位，分开头发，常规消毒，选用 28～30 号 1.5～2.5 寸长的不锈钢毫针，针与头皮呈 30°左右夹角快速将针刺入头皮下，快速捻转。当针达到帽状腱膜下层时，指下感到阻力减小，然后使针与头皮平行继续快速推进针体，根据不同穴区可刺入不同的长度。或用捻转法进针，一般以拇指掌侧面和示指桡侧面夹持针柄，以示指的掌指关节快速连续屈伸，使针身左右旋转，捻转速度每分钟可达 200

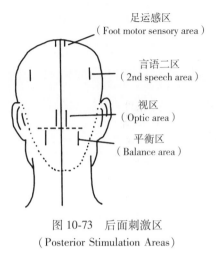

图 10-73　后面刺激区
(Posterior Stimulation Areas)

for bronchial asthma and chest pain.

13. The reproduction area

Draw a 2 cm straight line from the frontal angle upward, parallel to the antero-posterior midline (Figure 10-74). This area is indicated for functional uterine bleeding, pelvic inflammation, and uterine prolapse.

The method for selecting points: for diseases of one side, select the points of stimulation areas in opposite side; for diseases of both sides, select the points of stimulation areas in both sides; for the diseases of internal organs, the whole body or unable to distinguish right or left side, select he points of stimulation areas in both sides. Generally according the diseases, select the pertaining and the related stimulation areas. For example, for the paralysis of the lower extremities, select the motor area for the lower limbs and the foot motor sensory area.

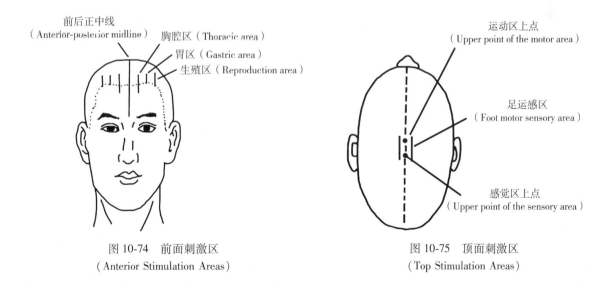

图 10-74　前面刺激区　　　　　　　　图 10-75　顶面刺激区
(Anterior Stimulation Areas)　　　　(Top Stimulation Areas)

Manipulation of the Scalp Acupuncture

The patient takes a sitting or lying position, separate the patient's hair and sterilize the stimulation area routinely, use a No. 28−30, 1. 5−2. 5 *cun* filiform needle along the subcutis at an angle of 30°with the scalp, insert the needle quickly into the skin or the subcutaneous muscle in a swiftly twirling manner.

次左右。进针后持续捻转 0.5~1 分钟，留针 5~10 分钟，反复操作 2~3 次即可起针。出针方法：如针下无沉紧感，可快速抽拔出针，也可缓缓出针，起针后必须用消毒干棉棍按压针孔片刻，以防止出血。一般每日或隔日针治一次，5 次为一个疗程。休息 2~3 天后，再继续下一疗程。

四、头针注意事项

1. 头部因长有头发，因此尤其须做到严密消毒，以防感染。

2. 毫针推进时术者手下如有抵抗感，或患者觉疼痛时，应停止进针，将针往后退，然后改变角度再进针。

3. 由于头针的刺激较强，刺激时间较长，术者须注意观察患者表情，以防晕针。

4. 对于脑血管病患者，只要患者生命指征平稳，早期就可配合头针治疗。缺血性脑梗死患者可在发病 48 小时后进行头针治疗；脑出血患者可在发病 1 周后进行头针治疗。

5. 凡并发有高热、心力衰竭等症时，不宜采用头针疗法。

第七节　耳针疗法

一、概述

耳针是在耳郭穴位用针刺等刺激防治疾病的一种方法。治病范围较广，操作方便。

二、常用耳穴

（一）耳郭表面解剖（图 10-76）

为了便于掌握耳针穴位的部位，必须熟悉耳郭解剖名称。

1. 耳轮　耳郭最外缘的卷曲部分；其深入至耳腔内的横行突起部分叫"耳轮脚"；耳轮后上方稍突起处叫"耳轮结节"；耳轮与耳垂的交界处叫"耳轮尾"。

2. 对耳轮　在耳轮的内侧，与耳轮相对的隆起部，又叫对耳轮体；其上方有两分叉，向上分叉的一支叫"对耳轮上脚"，向下分叉的一支叫"对耳轮下脚"。

3. 三角窝　对耳轮上脚和下脚之间的三角形凹窝。

4. 耳舟　耳轮与对耳轮之间凹沟，又称"舟状窝"。

5. 耳屏　指耳郭前面瓣状突起部，又叫"耳珠"。

6. 屏上切迹　耳屏上缘与耳轮脚之间的凹陷。

When the needle reaches the lower layer of epicranial aponeurosis, the finger feels the decreased resistance, and then rapidly insert the needle parallel with the scalp, according to the different points insert different lengths; or insert the needle by twisting needle method, usually hold the needle handle with the palmar surface of the thumb and the radial surface of the index finger, twist the needle with the help of the bending and stretching movement of the metacarpophalangeal joint of the index finger rapidly and continuously, the twisting speed may reach 200 times/min or so. Twist the needle continuously for 0. 5－1 minutes after the needle is inserted, retain the needle for 5－10 minutes, repeat the manipulation 2－3 times, and then withdraw the needle. For patients with hemiparalysis, let them move the limbs (passive movement for patients with severe hemiparalysis), according to the fact that twisting fast increase the stimulation electric needles also can be used by connecting an impulse electronic therapeutic meter in the main points after insertion to substitute the twisting by fingers. The intensity of stimulation is decided by the resistance of patients. Needle withdrawal method: if there is a feeling of heaviness, the needle can be quickly or slowly pulled out. The needle holes must be pressed by sterilized dry cotton stick for a moment to prevent bleeding. In general, the scalp needling therapy should be applied once a day or every other day, 5 times for one therapeutic course, start the next course after a rest of 2－3 days.

Precaution of the Scalp Acupuncture

Because of the hair in the head, a strict sterilization should be carried out to prevent infection.

If the acupuncturist feels resistance during the process of insertion, or the patient feels pain, the acupuncturist should stop needling, retreat the needle and change the angle of insertion, and re-insert the needle.

Because of the scalp acupuncture's strong and lasting stimulation, the acupuncturist should pay attention to observe the patients' facial expression to avoid fainting.

For patients with cerebrovascular diseases, if only the patients' vital signs are stable, the scalp acupuncture can be performed. Scalp acupuncture can be taken within 48 hours after the onset of ischemic cerebral infarction and a week after the onset of cerebral hemorrhage.

For the patients with high fever or heart failure, the scalp acupuncture is not advisable.

Section 7   Ear Acupuncture Therapy

Introduction

Ear acupuncture is a therapy that treats and prevents diseases by stimulating certain points on the auricle with needles. The therapy is characterized by wide indications and easy manipulation.

Commonly Used Ear Points

Anatomy of the Auricle Surface(Figure 10-76)

In order to facilitate the grasp of the parts of the ear acupuncture points, the acupuncturist must be familiar with the anatomy of the auricle surface.

(1) Helix   the curling rim of the most lateral border of the auricle; Helix crus: atransverse ridge of the helix continuing backward into the ear cavity; Helix tubercle: a small tubercle at the posterior-superior aspect of the helix; Helix cauda: the inferior part of the helix, at the junction of the helix and the lobule.

(2) Antihelix   at the medial aspect of the helix, an elevated ridge parallel to the helix is called "the principle part of antihelix." Its upper part branches out into "the superior antihelix crus" and "the inferior antihelix crus."

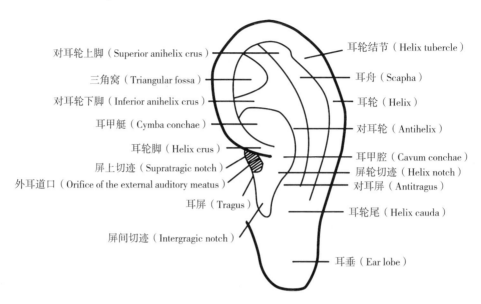

对耳轮上脚（Superior anihelix crus）
三角窝（Triangular fossa）
对耳轮下脚（Inferior anihelix crus）
耳甲艇（Cymba conchae）
耳轮脚（Helix crus）
屏上切迹（Supratragic notch）
外耳道口（Orifice of the external auditory meatus）
耳屏（Tragus）
屏间切迹（Intergragic notch）

耳轮结节（Helix tubercle）
耳舟（Scapha）
耳轮（Helix）
对耳轮（Antihelix）
耳甲腔（Cavum conchae）
屏轮切迹（Helix notch）
对耳屏（Antitragus）
耳轮尾（Helix cauda）
耳垂（Ear lobe）

图 10-76　耳郭表面解剖

(Anatomy of the Auricle Surface)

7. 屏轮切迹　对耳屏与对耳轮之间的稍凹陷处。

8. 对耳屏　对耳轮下方与耳屏相对的隆起部。

9. 屏间切迹　耳屏与对耳屏之间的凹陷。

10. 耳垂　耳郭最下部，无软骨的皮垂。

11. 耳甲艇　耳轮脚以上的耳腔部分。

12. 耳甲腔　耳轮脚以下的耳腔部分。

13. 外耳道开口　在耳甲腔内的孔窍。

（二）耳穴在耳郭上的分布规律

人体发生疾病时，常会在耳郭的相应部位出现"阳性反应"点，如压痛、变形、变色、水疱、结节、丘疹、凹陷、脱屑、电阻降低等，这些反应点就是耳针疗法的刺激点。

耳穴在耳郭的分布有一定规律，一般来说耳郭好像一个倒置的胎儿，头部朝下，臀部朝上。其分布规律是：与头面部相应的穴位在耳垂邻近；与上肢相应的穴位在耳舟；与躯干和下肢相应的穴位在对耳轮和对耳轮上、下脚；与内脏相应的穴位多集中在耳甲艇和耳甲腔；消化道在耳轮脚周围环形排列（图 10-77，图 10-78）。

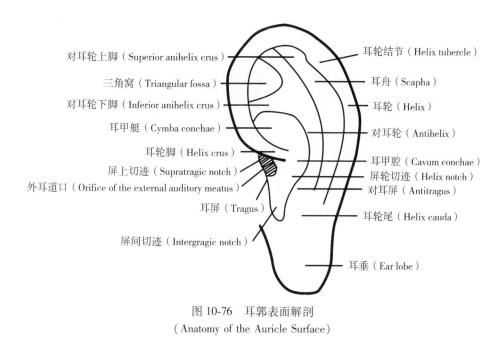

对耳轮上脚（Superior anihelix crus）   耳轮结节（Helix tubercle）
三角窝（Triangular fossa）   耳舟（Scapha）
对耳轮下脚（Inferior anihelix crus）   耳轮（Helix）
耳甲艇（Cymba conchae）   对耳轮（Antihelix）
耳轮脚（Helix crus）   耳甲腔（Cavum conchae）
屏上切迹（Supratragic notch）   屏轮切迹（Helix notch）
外耳道口（Orifice of the external auditory meatus）   对耳屏（Antitragus）
耳屏（Tragus）   耳轮尾（Helix cauda）
屏间切迹（Intergragic notch）
耳垂（Ear lobe）

图 10-76　耳郭表面解剖
（Anatomy of the Auricle Surface）

（3）Triangular fossa　the triangular depression between the two crura of the antihelix.

（4）Scapha　the narrow curved depression between the helix and the antihelix. It is also known as "the scaphoid fossa."

（5）Tragus　a curved flap in front of the auricle.

（6）Supratragic notch　the depression between the upper border of the tragus and the helix crus.

（7）Helix notch　the shallow depression between the antitragus and antihelix.

（8）Antitragus　a small tubercle opposite to the tragus and superior to the ear lobe.

（9）Intergragic notch　the depression between the tragus and antitragus.

（10）Ear lobe　the lowest part of the auricle where there is no cartilage.

（11）Cymba conchae　the cavum superior to the helix crus.

（12）Cavum conchae　the cavum inferior to the helix crus.

（13）Orifice of the external auditory meatus　the opening in the cavum concha.

Distribution of Auricular Point on the Auricle Surface

When the human body has disorders, some positively sensitive spots usually emerge in the related auricular area, such as pressing pain, heteromorphosis, skin color changes, tunercles, vesicle, tubercles, papule, depression, desquamation, and reduction of the electrical resistance. These reaction spots are the stimulation points for needling of ear acupuncture therapy.

There are some principles of the distribution of auricular points. The auricle is just like a fetus with the head downwards and the buttocks upwards. The distribution of auticular point is as follows: points located on the lobule are related to the head and facial region, those on the scapha to the upper limbs, those on the antihelix and its two crura to the trunk and lower imbs, those in the cavum and cymba conchae to the internal organs, and those around as a ring around helic crus to the digestive tract（Figure 10-77, Figure 10-78）.

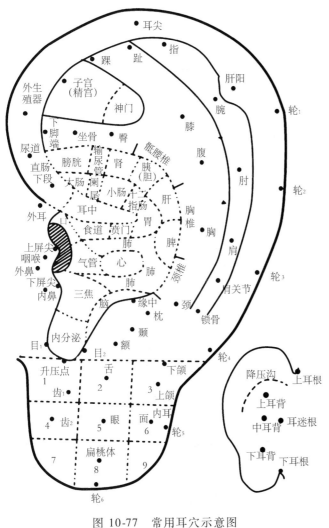

图 10-77　常用耳穴示意图

Figure 10-77　Distribution of Auricular Point on the Auricle Surface

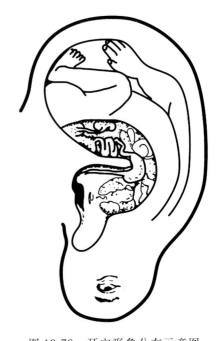

图 10-78　耳穴形象分布示意图

（Distribution Diagram of Auricular Point）

（三）常用耳穴的定位及主治（表 10-4）

表 10-4　常用耳穴解剖部位及主治表

分部	穴名	解剖部位	主治
耳轮	轮 1~6	自耳轮结节下缘至耳垂正中下缘分成五等分，共 6 点，自上而下依次为轮 1、轮 2、轮 3、轮 4、轮 5、轮 6	发热、扁桃体炎、高血压
耳轮脚	膈（耳中）	在耳轮脚	呃逆，黄疸，消化不良，皮肤瘙痒
耳舟	肘	在腕穴与肩穴之间	相应部位的疼痛、麻木
	肩关节	在肩与屏轮切迹平线之间	

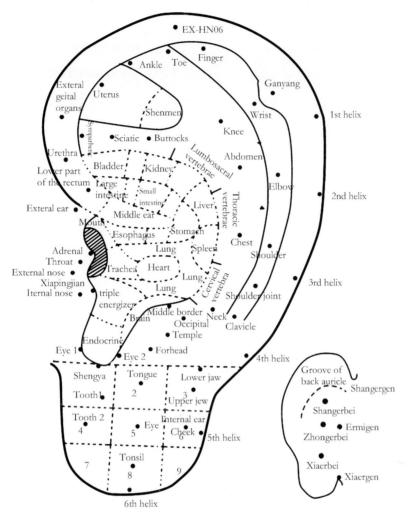

Figure 10-77 Distribution of Auricular Point on the Auricle Surface

Location and Indications of Auricular Points Commonly Used (Table 10-4)

Table10-4　Location and indications of auricular points commonly used

Body part	Name of auricular points	Anatomy location	Indications
The helix	1st - 6th helix	Divide the region from the lower edge of the helix nodules to middle of the lower edge of the ear lobe into five equal parts, totally six points, from top to bottom, 1st helix to 6th helix	Fever, tonsillitis, and hypertension
The helix crus	Pt. diaphragm (Pt. point middle ear)	On the helix crus	Hiccup, jaundice, indigestion, and itchy skin
The scapha	Pt. elbow	Between Pt. wrist and Pt. shoulder	Pain and numbness in the corresponding location
	Pt. shoulder joint	From the shoulder to the parallel line of the helix notch	

分部	穴名	解剖部位	主治
对耳轮上脚	趾	对耳轮上脚的外上角	相应部位的疼痛、麻木
	踝	对耳轮上脚的内上角	相应部位的疼痛、麻木
	膝	对耳轮上脚的起始部与对耳轮下脚上缘同水平	相应部位的疼痛、麻木
对耳轮下脚	臀	在对耳轮下脚的外侧1/2处	腰痛，坐骨神经痛
	坐骨神经	在对耳轮下脚的内侧1/2处	腰痛，坐骨神经痛
	交感（下脚端）	在耳轮下脚与耳轮内侧交界处	消化、循环系统功能失调、哮喘、急惊风、痛经等
对耳轮	腹	对耳轮上，与对耳轮下脚相平	腹腔疾病、消化妇科病
	胸	对耳轮上，与屏上切迹同水平	胸胁痛、乳腺炎
	颈	在轮屏切迹偏耳舟侧处	落枕、颈部扭伤、单纯性甲状腺肿
三角窝	子宫（精宫）	三角窝耳轮内侧缘的中点	月经不调、带下、痛经、盆腔炎；遗精、阳痿
	神门	在三角窝内靠耳轮上脚的下、中1/3交界处	失眠、多梦、烦躁、眩晕、咳嗽、哮喘、荨麻疹、炎症
耳屏	外鼻	耳屏外侧面的中央	鼻炎、鼻疖等
	咽喉	耳屏内侧面的上1/2处	咽喉肿痛
	肾上腺	在耳屏下部外侧缘	低血压，昏厥，无脉症、咳嗽、哮喘，感冒，中暑
对耳屏	脑点（缘中）	在对耳屏尖与轮屏切迹间的中点	遗尿症，功能性子宫出血
	颞（太阳）	额穴与枕穴连线的中点	偏头痛
屏间切迹	目1	屏间切迹前下	青光眼、近视、麦粒肿
	目2	屏间切迹后下	青光眼、近视、麦粒肿
	内分泌	在屏间切迹底部	更年期综合征、甲亢、皮肤病、肥胖等
	胃	在耳轮脚消失处	消化不良、腹胀、胃痛、呃逆
	大肠	在耳轮脚上方内1/3处	痢疾、肠炎、腹泻、便秘
耳甲艇	膀胱	在对耳轮下脚的下缘、大肠穴直上方	膀胱炎、尿潴留、遗尿
	肾	在对耳轮下脚的下缘、小肠穴直上方	生殖、泌尿、妇科疾病，腰痛，耳鸣，失眠，眩晕
	肝	在胃、十二指肠穴的后方	胁痛、眼病、月经不调、消化不良、胃胀、崩漏等
	脾	在肝穴下方，耳甲腔的外上方	消化不良、腹胀、胃痛、口腔炎、崩漏、血液病等
耳甲腔	心	耳甲腔正中	心血管系统疾病、中暑、急惊风
	肺	心穴的上、下、外三面	呼吸系统疾病、皮肤病
	三焦	在口、内分泌、皮质下和肺穴之间	便秘、浮肿、肥胖、糖尿病

continued

Body part	Name of auricular points	Anatomy location	Indications
The superior antihelix crus	Pt.toe	Lateral and superior angle of the superior antihelix crus	Pain and numbness in the corresponding location
	Pt.ankle	Medial and superior angle of the superior antihelix crus	Pain and numbness in the corresponding location
	Pt.knee	Middle portion of the superior antihelix crus	Pain and numbness in the corresponding location
The inferior antihelix crus	Pt.butlocks	At lateral 1/2 of the inferior antihelix crus	Pain in the lower back and sciatica
	Pt.sciatic	At the medial 1/2 of the inferior antihelix crus	Pain in the lower back and sciatica
	Pt.sympathetic (Pt.end of inferior antihelix crus)	The terminal of the inferior antihelix crus	Digestive, circulatory system dysfunction, asthma, acute convulsion, and dysmenorrhea
The antihelix	Pt.abdomen	On the border of the cavum conchae level to inferior antihelix crus	Celiac diseases, digestive system diseases, and gynecological diseases
	Pt.chest	On the border of the cavum conchae level to supratragic notch	Pain in the chest and rib-side, mastitis
	neck	near the scapha of the helix notch	Stiff neck, neck sprains, and simple goiter
The triangular fossa	Pt.uterus (Pt.seminal)	The midpoint of the bottom of the triangular fossa.	Irregular menstruation, leukorrhagia, dysmenorrheal, pelvic inflammatory disease, and impotence
	Pt.shenmen	At the bifurcating point between superior and inferior antihelix crus, and the lateral 1/3 of the triangular fossa	Insomnia, dream-disturbed, irritation, vertigo, cough, asthma, urticaria, and inflammation
The tragus	Pt.external nose	In the center of the lateral part of tragus	Rhinitis and nasal furuncle
	Pt.throat	Upper half of the medial aspect of the tragus	Sore throat
	Pt.adrenal	The lateral border of the lower protubercle	Hypotension, syncope, pulseless disease, cough, asthma, cold, and heat stroke
The antitragus	Pt.brain (Pt.middle border)	Midpoint between the antitragic apex and helixtragic notch	Enuresis and dysfunctional uterine bleeding
	Pt.temple (Pt.taiyang)	The midpoint of Pt.occiput and Pt.forehead	Migraine
The intertragic notch	Pt.eye 1	On the anterior and inferior side of the intertragic notch	Glaucoma, myopia, and hordeolum
	Pt.eye 2	On the posterior and inferior aspect of the intertragic notch	Glaucoma, myopia, and hordeolum
	Pt.endocrine	At the base of the cavum conchae in the intertragic notch	Climacteric syndrome, hyperthyroidism, skin diseases, and obesity
	Pt.stomach	Around the area where the helix crus terminates	Indigestion, abdomen distention, stomach pain, and hiccup
	Pt.large intestine	At medial 1/3 of the superior aspect of the helix crus	Dysentery, enteritis, diarrhea, and constipation

续　表

分部	穴名	解剖部位	主治
耳垂	眼	在耳垂 5 区的中央	青光眼、近视、麦粒肿等
	面颊	在耳垂 5、6 区交界线周围	三叉神经痛、面神经麻痹、痤疮
	内耳	在耳垂 6 区中央稍上方	耳鸣、听力减退、中耳炎、耳源性眩晕
	扁桃体	在耳垂 8 区中央	扁桃体炎
耳郭背面部	降压沟	在耳郭背面，由内上方斜向外下方行走的凹沟处	降血压
	耳迷根	在耳郭背与乳突交界处（相当于耳轮脚同水平）的耳根部	胃痛、胆道蛔虫症、腹泻、气喘、鼻塞

注：为使定位方便，把耳垂划分成"井"字的九等份，由内向外，由上到下，分别为 1、2、3 区，4、5、6 区，7、8、9 区。

三、耳针的临床应用及注意事项

（一）耳针适用范围

耳针在临床治疗的疾病很广，不仅用于治疗许多功能性疾病，而且对一部分器质性疾病，也有一定疗效。主要治疗以下几类病证：

1. 多种疼痛性病证，如软组织损伤、手术后疼痛、头痛、面痛、胁痛、腰腿痛、关节痛等。

2. 多种内脏病证，如眩晕、失眠、阳痿、遗精、月经不调、哮喘、泄泻、便秘、瘿、消渴、肥胖、小儿遗尿等。

3. 多种热病，如感冒、百日咳、丹痧、疟疾、痢疾等。

4. 皮肤病和五官病，如风疹、湿疹、目赤肿痛、牙痛、口疮、耳内流脓、过敏性鼻炎等。

此外，还可用于戒烟、戒酒、戒毒和催乳等方面。

（二）注意事项

1. 严密消毒，预防感染。针具、耳穴局部皮肤常规消毒。

2. 耳郭部针刺比较疼痛，注意预防晕针。

3. 有习惯性流产史的孕妇禁用耳针。年老体弱、严重贫血、过度疲劳等情况慎用耳针。

continued

Body part	Name of auricular points	Anatomy location	Indications
The cymba conchae	Pt.bladder	On the antero-inferior border of the inferior antihelix crus.Directly above Pt.large intestine	Cystitis,retention of urine,and enuresis
	Pt.kidney	On the lower border of the inferior antihelix crus, directly above Pt.small intestine	Diseases of the urinary and genital systems, gynecopathy,lumar pain,tinnitus,insomnia, and dizziness
	Pt.liver	Behind the Pt.stomach and Pt.duodenum	Hypochondriac pain,diseases of the eyes,irregular menstruation,indigestion,fullness of the stomach,and flooding and spotting
	Pt.spleen	At the lateral and superior aspect of the cavum conchae	Indigestion,distention of abdomen,stomach pain,stomatitis,flooding and spotting,blood diseases,etc.
The cavum conchae	Pt.heart	In the central depression of the cavum conchae	Cardiovascular diseases,heat stroke,and acute convulsion
	Pt.lung	Around the central depression of the cavum conchae	Respiratory diseases,and skin diseases
	Pt.triple energizer	Between Pt.mouth,Pt.endocrine,Pt.subcortex and Pt.lung	Constipation,edema,obesity,and diabetes
The ear lobe	Pt.eye	The middle of the 5th section	Glaucoma,myopia,and hordeolum
	Pt.cheek	Around the borderline of the 5th and 6th sections	Trigeminal neuralgia,facial paralysis,and acne
	Pt.internal ear	The upper part of the 6th section	Tinnitus,impaired hearing,tympanitis,and aural vertigo
	Pt.tonsil	The middle part of the 8th section	Tonsillitis
The back auricle	Pt.groove of back auricle	Through the backside of the superior antihelix crus and inferior antihelix crus,in the depression	Lower blood pressure
	Pt.ermigen	At the junction of back auricle and mastoid in root of ear vagus(equivalent level to crus of helix)	Stomach pain,ascariasis,diarrhea,asthma, and nasal congestion

Note:In order to easy location,the earlobe is divided into equal sections like Chinese character "井",these sections are numbered from the medial section laterally and from the upper section downward,respectively one to nine.

Clinical Applications of Ear Acupuncture and Precaution

Clinical Indications and Contraindications for Ear Acupuncture Therapy

Ear acupuncture is widely used in clinical treatment,not only for many functional diseases,but also for many organic diseases.The main diseases are as following:

(1)Various diseases marked with pain,such as soft tissue injury,pain after surgery,headache,facial pain,pain in the rib-side,pain in the waist and legs,and pain in the joints.

(2)Various diseases of viscera,such as dizziness,insomnia,impotence,seminal emission,irregular menstruation,asthma,diarrhea,constipation,goiter,diabetes,obesity,and enuresis in children.

(3)Various febrile diseases,such as influenza,whooping cough,cinnabar sand,malaria,and dysentery.

(4)Skin diseases and facial diseases,such as rubella,eczema,sore red swollen eyes,toothache,oral ulcer,purulent ear discharge,and allergic rhinitis.

In addition,ear acunpuncture therapy is indicated for quitting smoking,alcohol and drug,and promoting lactation.

第八节 拔罐疗法

一、拔罐的适应证

拔罐后，引起局部组织充血或皮下轻度的瘀血，使机体气血活动旺盛、经络通畅。因而本法具有行气止痛、消肿散结、祛风散寒、清热拔毒等作用，广泛地用于内、外、妇、儿、皮肤、五官、神经等多科病证。拔罐法无痛无创，使用安全，经常和针刺配合使用。

二、拔罐法的操作

（一）火罐法

火罐法是利用燃烧时消耗罐中部分氧气，并借火焰的热力使罐内的气体膨胀而排除罐内部分空气，使罐内气压低于外面大气压，借以将罐吸着于施术部位的皮肤上。火罐法其吸拔力的大小与罐具的大小和深度、罐内燃火的温度和方式、扣罐的时机与速度及空气在扣罐时再进入罐内的多少等因素有关。

1. 闪火法　用镊子或止血钳等挟住95%酒精棉球，点燃后在火罐内壁中段绕1~2圈，迅速退出并及时将罐扣在施术部位上。此法比较安全，不受体位限制，是常用的拔罐方法，须注意操作时不要烧罐口，以免灼伤皮肤。

2. 投火法　将纸条点燃后，投入罐内，然后迅速将罐扣在施术部位。此法多适用于侧面拔，需注意将纸投入罐内时，未燃的一端应向下。

（二）抽气法

先将备好的抽气罐紧扣在需拔罐的部位上，用抽气筒将罐内的空气抽出，使之产生所需负压，即能吸住，此法适用于任何部位拔罐。

（三）起罐

起罐亦称脱罐。用一手拿住火罐，另一手将火罐口边缘的皮肤轻轻按下，待空气缓缓进入罐内后，即可将罐取下。切不可硬拔，以免损伤皮肤。若起罐太快，易造成空气快速进入罐内，则负压骤减，易使患者产生疼痛。拔罐后局部红紫痕数日即消失。

Precautions

(1)Strict antisepsis is necessary to avoid infection.

(2)The patients always feel severe pain when needling the auricle,attention should be paid to prevent fainting.

(3)The ear acupuncture therapy is contraindicated in pregnant women with a history of habitual abortion.For the elderly,the overtired and patients with severe anaemia,the therapy should be cautiously used.

Section 8   Cupping Therapy

Indications

Cupping is a therapy causing local congestion and mildly subcutaneous bleeding to strengthen the activity of qi and blood and smooth the meridians.This method has the function of promoting the free flow of qi and relieving pain,dispersing swelling and dissipating binds,dispeling wind and cold,clearing heat and removing poison.Cupping therapy is widely used in diseases of internal medicine,surgery,gynedology,pediatrics,otorhinolaryngology and neurology.Cupping therapy has the characteristics of no-pain,non-invasive and safe to use,and is often used with the combination of needling.

Manipulations of Cupping

Fire cupping

Fire cupping is a therapy in which a jar is attached to the skin surface through expansion of part of the air and exclusion of part of the air to create the negative pressure by introducing heat in the form of an ignited material.The absorbing force of fire cupping method is decided by the size and depth of a cup,the temperature of the cup and the way ignite the fire,the timing and the speed of cup buckling,and air into the cup during cup buckling.

1. Flash-fire cupping method

Clamp a cotton ball soaked with 95% alcohol with the forceps or mippers,ignite it and put it into the cup,rotate it 1−2 circles inside the cup,and immediately take it out and palce the cup on the selected position.This method is relatively safe,without postural restriction,and it is a commonly used method of cupping.Pay attention that during the operation,do not burn the mouth of cup to avoid burning the patient's skin.

2. Fire-insertion cupping method

Throw a piece of ignited paper into the cup,and then rapidly place the mouth of the cup firmly against the skin on the desired location.This method is applied on the lateral side of the body.Pay attention that when throw the ignited paper into the cup,the unignited end should be towards the skin.

Suction cupping

Cup the prepared evacuating jar to the selected skin,and then remove the air to create the negative pressure by exhausting pump,making the cup absorb the skin.This method is used for any location.

Withdrawing cup

When withdrawing the cup,hold the cup with one hand,and press the skin around the rim of the cup with another hand to let air in,and then take the cup away.Do not remove the cup with strong force to avoid damaging the skin.If the cup is removed too fast,the air goes into the cup too fast and the negative pressure reduces too fast,this makes the patients feel pain.After cupping,the blood stasis at the local area will disappear in a few days.

三、拔罐注意事项

1. 拔罐时要选择适当体位和肌肉丰满的部位。若体位不当、移动、骨骼凸凹不平，毛发较多的部位均不适用。

2. 拔罐时要根据所拔部位的面积大小而选择大小适宜的罐。操作时必须迅速，才能使罐拔紧，吸附有力。

3. 用火罐时应注意勿灼伤或烫伤皮肤。

4. 皮肤有过敏、溃疡、水肿及大血管分布部位，不宜拔罐。高热抽搐者，以及孕妇的腹部、腰骶部位，亦不宜拔罐。

第九节 常见病证的针灸治疗

一、中风

中风是以突然昏仆、不省人事或伴口角㖞斜、半身不遂、语言不利等，或无昏仆仅以口歪、半身不遂为主要症状的疾病。因发病急骤，症见多端，病情变化迅速，与风的善行数变特点相似。古代文献有"卒中"、"厥证"、"偏枯"等名称。

本病包括现代医学的脑溢血、脑血栓形成、脑梗死等脑血管疾病。

（一）病因病机

中风是多种因素导致，风、火、痰浊、瘀血为主要病因。如正气不足，经络空虚，风邪入侵；烦劳过度，病后体虚，年老体衰，阴阳失调，内风旋动；饮食不节、劳倦内伤、脾失健运、聚湿生痰、痰瘀化热、阻滞经络、蒙蔽清窍；或肝阳素旺，木克脾土，脾失运化，内生痰浊；或内火炽盛，炼液为痰，以致肝风挟痰火窜扰经络，蒙蔽清窍而猝然昏倒，㖞僻不遂；五志过极，心火暴盛，风火相煽；或肝郁气滞，失于条达，气血瘀滞；或者暴怒伤肝，肝阳暴动，气血俱浮，上冲于脑，突发中风。

（二）辨证

中风多属于本虚标实之证，在本属肝肾不足，气血衰少；在标为风火相煽，痰浊雍盛，气血瘀阻。

辨病位浅深和病情轻重，分为中经络和中脏腑

1. 中经络　肌肤不仁，一侧手足麻木或偏身麻木，半身不遂、口眼㖞斜或语言不利。

2. 中脏腑　神志不清或昏迷，半身不遂，口眼㖞斜，或失语或头痛，项强，高

Precautions of Cupping

The areas where the muscles are abundant and elastic are selected. Otherwise, improper posture, inappropriate movement, the uneven site around the bone, and the areas with more hair are not selected for cupping.

Cups in different sizes are used according to the cupping location. The cupping manipulation should be rapid, so as to make the cup stick to the skin tightly.

When performing fire cupping, be careful not to burn the skin.

It is prohibited to apply cupping to the skin with allergy, ulcer, edema, or an area overlying large blood vessels. It is prohibited for hyperspasmia due to high fever, contraindicated in the abdominal and sacral regions of pregnant women.

Section 9   Acupuncture Therapy of the Common Diseases

Stroke

Stroke is an emergency case manifested by falling down in a fit with loss of consciousness, deviated mouth, hemiplegia, and slurred speech, or not a falling down but with deviated mouth and hemiplegia. It is characterized by abrupt onset with various pathological changes varying quickly like the wind, from which the term stroke comes. It is also termed as "apoplexy", "jue syndrome", and "hemiplegia" in the ancient literature.

Stroke includes cerebral hemorrhage, cerebral thrombosis, cerebral infarction, and other cerebrovascular diseases in modern medicine.

Etiology and Pathogenesis

Stroke is caused by various factors. Wind, fire, phlegm turbidity, and stasis are its main causes. It is caused by deficiency of healthy qi, empty of meridians, and wind evil attacks; or caused by vacuity wind stir internally due to being overtired, weakness after diseases, old age, and imbalance of yin and yang; or caused by irregular intake, internally injury, failure of the spleen's function of transportation and transformation, and phlegm and dampness accumulate to induce congestion of meridians to disturb clear orifice; or caused by excess of yang of the liver disturbing the function of the spleen, and phlegm turbidity is produced; or caused by excessively internal fire making humor into phlegm; or caused by the wind combined with phlegm and fire disturbs meridians and collaterals and clear orifice, causing sudden collapse; or caused by excess among the five minds; or caused by liver depression and qi stagnation and qi stagnation and blood stasis; or caused by the damage of the liver and hyperactivity of liver yang after a sudden violet anger, which causes qi and blood floating and upwards clash to the brain.

Differentiation

Stroke has the characteristic of root vacuity and tip repletion. The root is liver-kidney deficiency and dual deficiency of qi and blood, whereas the tip is wind combined with fire, excess of phlegm turbidity, and qi stagnation and blood stasis.

According to its conditions, stroke is divided into attack on the viscera and bowels and attack on the meridians and collaterals.

1. Attack on the meridians and collaterals

Insensitivity of the skin, hemiplegia, numbness of a side of the body, limbs and extremities, deviated mouth and eye, and slurring of speech.

2. Attack on the viscera and bowels

热，呼吸鼾鸣，喉中痰声漉漉，口角流涎等。根据病因、病机不同，又分为闭证和脱证。

（1）闭证：多因气火冲逆，血菀于上，肝风煽张，痰浊壅盛。症见神志昏昧，牙关禁闭，口噤不开，两手握固，面赤气粗，喉中痰鸣，二便闭结，脉弦滑有力。

（2）脱证：由于真阳衰微，元阳暴脱。症见目合口张，鼻鼾息微，手撒遗尿，四肢逆冷，脉细弱等，若见汗出如油，两颧淡红，脉微欲绝或浮大无根，为真阳外越之危候。

（三）治疗

1. 中经络　调和经脉，疏通气血。

（1）半身不遂：取手足阳明经穴为主，辅以太阳、少阳经穴。一般刺病侧穴。也可先针健侧，后针病侧，即"补患侧，泻健侧"的治法，适用于病程较久者。上肢：肩髃、曲池、手三里、外关、合谷；下肢：环跳、阳陵泉、足三里、解溪、昆仑。配穴：肩髎、阳池、后溪、风市、悬钟。毫针刺用补泻兼施法。

（2）口眼㖞斜：取手足阳明经穴为主，初起单刺病侧，病久左右均刺。

取穴：地仓、颊车、合谷、太冲、内庭。

2. 中脏腑　开闭泄热，醒脑开窍，回阳固脱。

（1）闭证：治法：取督脉和十二井穴为主，毫针刺用泻法或点刺出血。

处方：人中、十二井穴、太冲、丰隆、劳宫、内关。

（2）脱证：治法：取任脉经穴为主，用大艾炷灸。

处方：关元、神阙（隔盐灸）。

配合头皮针疗法，效果更佳。根据症状可选取运动区、感觉区、足运感区、语言一、二、三区等。

二、带状疱疹

带状疱疹是由水痘-带状疱疹病毒引起的急性炎症性皮肤病。主要侵犯皮肤及脊神经后根，引起该神经感受区内疼痛，并在相应的皮肤表面产生带状疱疹特有的节段性水疱丘疹。该病好发于春秋季节，成人多见。

Loss of consciousness, tightly and coma, hemiplegia, deviated mouth and eye, aphasia, headache, stiffness of the neck, high fever, coarse breathing, rattling in the throat, drooling from the corners of the mouth, retention of urine, constipation. According to the different etiology or pathogenesis, this type can be subdivided into block syndrome and collapse syndrome.

Block syndrome: the wind can be stirred up by the upsurge of liver yang, which, together with the accumulated phlegm fires, disturbs the mind, leading to sudden loss of consciousness with clenched jaws and tightly closed hands, flushed face, coarse breathing, rattling in the throat, retention of urine and constipation, string-like, and slippery and forceful pulse.

Collapse syndrome: severe weakness and exhaustion of primary yang, leading to mouth agape and eyes closed, snoring but feeble breathing, faccid paralysis of limbs, cold and spasm of extremities, small and weak pulse. If complicated with sweating like oil, flushed face, fading or big floating pulse, it is a critical case, indicating collapse of the isolated yang.

Treatment

Attack on the meridians and collaterals: harmonize the meridians and collaterals, reconcile qi and blood.

1. Hemiplegia

Mainly select the yangming meridian of hand and foot, combined with Taiyang and Shaoyang meridians. Usually needle the points opposite of the disorder side, or firstly needle the healthy side, and then needle the disorder side. Reinforce the disorder side and reduce the healthy side, and this method is for a long course of disease. Upper limbs: Jianyu(LI 15), Quchi(LI 11), Shousanli(LI 10), Waiguan(TE 5), Hegun(LI 4); and lower limbs: Huantiao(GB 30), Yanglingquan(GB 34), Zusanli(ST 36), Jiexi(ST 41), Kunlun(BL 60). Combined with Jianliao(TE 14), Yangchi(TE 4), Houxi(SI 3), Fengchi(GB 20), Xuanzhong(GB 39). Filiform needling therapy with the reinforcing and reducing manipulation.

2. Deviated mouth and eye

Mainly needle the Yangming meridians of foot and hand. Needle the disorder side at the stage of onset, needle both sides if it is chronic.

Acupuncture points: Dicang(ST 4), Jiache(ST 6), Hegu(LI 4), Taichong(LR 3), and Neiting(ST 44).

Attack on the viscera and bowels: open block and clear heat, wake the brain and open the orifice, and save yang to avoid collapse.

Block syndrome:

Treatment: Mainly puncture the Governor vessel and the twelve well points. Puncture with the reducing method or prick to induce bleeding.

Prescription: Renzhong(GV 20), the twelve well points, Taichong(LR 3), Fenglong(ST 40), Laogong(PC 8), and Neiguan(PC 6).

Collapse syndrome:

Treatment: mainly puncture the conception vessel. Moxibustion with big moxa cones.

Prescription: Guanyuan(CV 4) and Shenque(CV 8)(moxibustion with salt).

The therapeutic effects will be better if combination with scalp acupunture. In accordance with the symptoms, puncture the motor area, the sensory area, the foot motor sensory area, the and 1st, 2nd, 3rd speech areas.

Herpes zoster neuralgia

Herpes zoster neuralgia is an acute inflammatory skin disease caused by the varicella-zoster virus, mainly affecting the skin and spinal nerve root, causing pain in the nerve sensory area, and zoster-specific

（一）病因病机

本病多因情志不遂，肝经火盛，肝郁化火；饮食失调，过食辛辣厚味，以致脾失健运，湿浊内蓄，湿热搏结；或正气虚而外感湿毒而发。

（二）辨证施治

选取疱疹区穴位为主，选用针刺疗法、艾灸疗法、刺络拔罐、耳针和局部围刺法等。

主穴：合谷，依据疱疹所发部位的不同，选取发病侧相应节段的华佗夹脊穴。

1. 肝胆热盛型

【证候】局部皮损鲜红，疱壁紧张，灼热刺痛。自觉口苦咽干、口渴，烦闷易怒，食欲不佳。小便赤，大便干。舌质红，舌苔薄黄或黄厚，脉弦滑微数。

【治法】清利肝胆湿热。

【处方】主穴+阳陵泉、足临泣、行间、太冲、血海，毫针刺用泻法。

2. 脾虚湿蕴型

【证候】皮肤颜色较淡，疱壁松弛，疼痛略轻。口不渴或渴而不欲饮，不思饮食，食后腹胀，大便时溏，女性患者常见白带多。舌质淡红体胖，舌苔白厚或白腻，脉沉缓或滑。

【治法】健脾化湿。

【处方】主穴+阴陵泉、三阴交、足三里、曲池、血海，毫针刺用补泻兼施法。

3. 气滞血瘀型

【证候】皮疹消退后局部疼痛难忍，拒按。伴烦躁失眠，精神不振，胃纳不佳。舌暗红或有瘀点斑，苔薄白，脉弦细。

【治法】理气活血，通络止痛。

【处方】主穴+血海、膈俞，委中，毫针刺用泻法。

（三）其他疗法

1. 耳针　主穴：肺、神门；配穴：皮质下、内分泌、交感、肾上腺。

2. 艾灸法　在疱疹患处取"阿是穴"回旋灸，每穴施灸 5~7 分钟，每次灸 3~4 穴，每日或隔日 1 次。

3. 刺络拔罐法。

三、胃痛

胃痛是以上腹胃脘反复性发作性疼痛为主的病证。由于痛及心窝部，故文献中也称为"胃心痛"、"心下痛"等。

segmental vesicular papules in the related skin surface.This disease usually occurs in spring and autumn, and it is more common in adults.

Etiology and Pathogenesis

Herpes zoster neuralgia is caused by fire in the liver meridian due to affect-mind dissatisfaction, or liver depression transforming into fire, or caused by dysfunction of the spleen due to irregular intake of fatty and spicy food, causing dampness accumulation combined with heat; or caused by exogenous dampness and toxins in patients with the deficiency of healthy qi.

Differentiation and Treatment

Select the acupuncture points in the locations of herpes, with the reducing method, moxibustion, pricking and cupping, auricular acupuncture, and needling around the herpes.

Main Points: Hegu(LI 4) , in accordance with the location of blisters, select Hua Tuo's paravertebral points of the segment pertaining to the blisters.

1. Excessive heat of the liver and gallbladder

【Main manifestations】Red lesions in local skin with blisters wall tension, burning and tingling, bitterness in the mouth and dry throat, thirst, irritability, poor appetite, yellow urine, dry stools, red tongue with thin yellow or thick yellow tongue coating, string-like and wild rapid, or slippery and wild rapid pulse.

【Treatment】Clear heat and dispel dampness of the liver and gallbladder.

【Prescription】Main points together with Zulinqi(GB 41) , Xingjian(LR 2) , Taichong(LR 3) , and Xuehai(SP 10).Filiform needling with the reducing method.

2. Dampness accumulation due to spleen deficiency

【Main manifestations】Lighter skin color, blister wall relaxation, no severe pain, no thirst or thirst but do not want to drink, no appetite, abdominal distention after eating, runny stool, leukorrhagia for women patients, pale red and fat tongue with thick white or white greasy tongue, and sunken and slow pulse or slippery pulse.

【Treatment】Strengthen the spleen to dispel dampness.

【Prescription】Main points together with Yanglingquan (GB 34) , Sanyinjiao (SP 6) , Zusanli (ST 36) , Quchi(LI 11) , and Xuehai(SP 10).Filiform needling with the reinforcing and reducing method.

3. Qi stagnation and blood stasis

【Main manifestations】Local pain after the rash subsided, refused to press, with irritability, insomnia, lassitude, poor appetite, dark red tongue with ecchymosis and thin white tongue, and string-like and fine pulse.

【Treatment】Regulate qi and activate the blood, free the collaterals and relieve pain.

【Prescription】Main points together with Xuehai(SP 10) , Geshu(BL 17) , and Weizhong(BL 40). Filiform needling with the reducing method.

Other Therapies

(1) Main points: Pt. lung, Pt. shenmen, combined with Pt. subcortex, Pt. endocrine, Pt. sympathetic nerve and Pt.adrenal.

(2)Moxibustion: Circling moxibustion on the Ashi points around the herpes, 5−7minutes each point, 3−4 points each time, one time every day or every other day.

(3)Pricking and Cupping.

Stomach ache

Stomach ache is a common symptom, often characterized by repeated recurrence of epigastric pain. Since the pain is close to the cardia, it was also named"cardio-abdominal pain"or"cardiac pain"in TCM literature.

（一）病因病机

胃痛主要有三方面病因：外邪犯胃，包括寒热及饮食失节等；肝气犯胃，郁怒可致肝郁，致胃气滞；素体脾胃虚弱、劳倦过度及久病迁延等导致的脾胃虚弱。因脾胃相互表里，肝调节气机，胃痛还直接影响脾和肝。尽管胃痛原因多样，"不通则痛"仍是其常见病机。

（二）辨证施治

主穴：中脘、足三里、内关。

1. 寒邪客胃

【证候】胃痛暴作，痛势较剧，得温痛减，遇寒痛增，口和不渴，喜热饮；舌质淡红，苔薄白，脉弦紧。

【治法】散寒止痛。

【处方】主穴+阳陵泉、胃俞、公孙、梁丘；毫针刺用补泻兼施法，可灸。

2. 饮食停滞

【证候】胃痛，脘腹胀满，嗳腐吞酸，恶心呕吐，大便不爽；苔厚腻，脉滑或弦滑。

【治法】消导除积。

【处方】主穴+公孙、内庭、天枢；毫针刺用泻法。

3. 肝气犯胃

【证候】胃脘胀满，痛连胁或痛无定处，嗳气频繁，泛酸，每因恼怒、郁闷发作或加重；舌质暗红，苔薄白，脉沉弦或沉细。

【治法】疏肝理气和胃。

【处方】主穴+太冲、期门、章门；毫针刺用泻法。

4. 湿热中阻

【证候】胃脘灼热胀痛，得食则重，甚食入即吐，泛酸，口干口苦，口气重浊；舌质暗红，苔黄腻，脉滑数。

【治法】清热化湿。

【处方】主穴+内庭、厉兑、阴陵泉；毫针刺用泻法。

5. 脾胃虚寒

【证候】胃痛隐隐，喜温喜按，空腹痛甚，得食痛减，纳呆神疲，畏寒肢冷，大便溏薄；舌质淡红或舌体胖大，苔白而滑，脉细弱或迟缓。

【治法】健脾温中。

【处方】主穴+脾俞、胃俞、公孙；毫针刺用补法，可灸。

Etiology and Pathogenesis

There are three main causes:attack of stomach by pathogenic factors including cold,heat,improper diet,etc;invasion of the stomach by liver qi,stagnant liver qi due to mental depression or anger affects the stomach and blocks qi;spleen and gastric weakness due to constitutional weakness of the spleen and stomach,strain and stress,or long standing illness,etc.Since the spleen and stomach are interior-exteriorly related,and the liver regulates the flow of qi,epigastric pain directly influences the spleen and liver.Although there are many causes of stomach ache,"obstruction causes pain"is the common pathogenesis.

Differentiation and Treatment

Main points:Zhongwan(CV 12),Zusanli(ST 36),and Neiguan(PC 6).

1. Cold invading the stomach

【Main manifestations】A suddenly occurred severe stomach ache,which may be relieved by pressure and warmth,aggravated by coldness,no thirst,preference for hot water,pale red tongue with thin tongue fur,and string-like and tight pulse.

【Treatment】Dissipate cold to relieve pain.

【Prescription】Main points together with Yanglingquan(GB 34),Weishu(BL 21),Gongsun(SP 4),and Liangqiu(ST 34).Filiform needling with the reinforcing and reducing method.

2. Food accumulation

【Main manifestations】Epigastric pain,distention,belching with fetid odor,nausea and vomiting,uncomfortable stools,and thick and greasy tougue,and slippery pulse or string-like and splippery pulse.

【Treatment】Promote digestion and disperse stagnant food.

【Prescription】Main points together with Gongsun(SP 4),Neiting(ST 44),and Tianshu(ST 25).Filiform needling with the reducing method.

3. Liver qi invading the stomach

【Main manifestations】Fullness in the epigastrium,implicates the rib-side,radiating to the hypochondriac regions,frequent belching,acid regurgitation,occur or aggravated by anger or depression,dark red tongue with white thin tongue fur,and sunken and string-like pulse or sunken and fine pulse.

【Treatment】Soothe the liver and regulate qi to harmonize the stomach.

【Prescription】Main points together with Taichong(LR 3),Qimen(LR 14),and Zhangmen(LR 13).Filiform needling with the reducing method.

4. Dampness-heat in the middle energizer

【Main manifestations】Burning pain in the epigastrium,aggravated by intaking of food;in the severe cases,vomit right after food intake,acid regurgitation,dry mouth,bitter taste in the mouth,belching with fetid odor,dark red tongue with yellow greasy tongue coating,and rapid and slippery pulse.

【Treatment】Clear heat and resolve dampness.

【Prescription】Main points together with Neiting(ST 44),Lidui(ST 45),Yinlingquan(SP 9).Filiform needling with the reducing method.

5. Spleen-stomach deficiency cold

【Main manifestations】Dull pain in the epigastrium,which may be relieved by pressure and warmth,aggravated by hunger,alleviated by intake of food,torpid intake,fatigue,aversion to cold,cold of extremities,loose stools,pale red tongue or swollen tongue with white greasy tongue fur,fine and weak pulse or slow and moderate pulse.

【Treatment】Tonify the spleen and warm the middle.

【Prescription】Main points together with Pishu(BL 20),Weishu(BL 21),and Gongsun(SP 4).Filiform needling with the reinforcing method.Moxibustion is advisable.

（三）其他疗法

1. 耳穴贴压　胃、脾、肝、交感、神门。

2. 头针　胃区。

3. 火罐疗法　脾俞、胃俞、肝俞闪罐、留罐或走罐，以皮肤红润、充血或瘀血为度。

四、头痛

头痛是一种主观症状，常见于各种急慢性疾病，涉及范围很广。本病常见于西医学的高血压、偏头痛、神经血管性头痛、感染性发热性疾患、脑外伤以及眼、鼻、耳等病中。

（一）病因病机

头为"诸阳之会"，手足三阳经和足厥阴肝经均上头面，督脉直接与脑府相联系。本病的病因分外感、内伤两方面。"伤于风者，上先受之"，风邪袭络，上犯巅顶络脉，则气血不和，经络阻遏，久则络脉留瘀。暴怒伤肝，气机郁结，肝阳上亢，可致头痛。饮食不节，痰浊内生，清阳不升，浊阴不降；禀赋虚弱，气血不足，髓海精气不充；外伤血瘀阻络等，均可导致头痛。

（二）辨证施治

外感头痛　按头痛部位分经取穴。前头部：上星、头维、合谷、阿是穴；巅顶部：百会、通天、太冲、阿是穴；侧头部：率谷、太阳、外关、阿是穴；后头部：后顶、风池、昆仑、阿是穴。毫针刺用泻法。

内伤头痛　主穴：百会、风池、太阳。

1. 肝阳上亢

【证候】头痛目眩，心烦易怒，夜寐不宁，面赤口苦；舌红苔黄，脉弦数。

【治法】平肝潜阳。

【处方】主穴+太冲、阳陵泉；毫针刺用泻法。

2. 痰浊上扰

【证候】头痛昏蒙，胸脘满闷，呕吐痰涎；舌质暗红，舌苔白腻，脉滑。

【治法】祛痰化浊利窍。

【处方】主穴+头维、中脘、丰隆；毫针刺用泻法。

3. 肾精亏损

【证候】头痛且空，兼眩晕，腰痛酸软，神疲乏力，耳鸣，少寐；舌红少苔，脉细无力。

【治法】补肾填髓。

Other Therapies

(1)Paste and press ear points:Pt.stomach,Pt.spleen,Pt.liver,Pt.sympathetic,and Pt.shenmen.

(2)Scalp acupunture:the gastric area.

(3)Cupping therapy:flash-fire cupping,retained cupping or slide cupping in Pishu(BL 20),Weishu (BL 21),and Ganshu(BL 18),withdraw the cups when the skin around the points appears red,congestion,or stasis.

Headache

Headache is a subjective symptom,it can be induced by various acute and chronic diseases and covers a wide sphere.In conventional medicine,headache usually appears in diseases such as hypertension, migraine,neurovascular headache,infectious febrile disease,traumatic brain injury,as well as eyes,nose and ears diseases.

Etiology and Pathogenesis

The head is the place where all the Yang meridians of hand and foot meet,and the qi and blood all flow upward to the head.In addition,the Governor vessel connects with the brain.Attacks of endogenous or exogenous factors may cause headache.

Invasion of wind attacks the upper part of body.Invasion of pathogenic wind into the upper meridians and collaterals causes derangement and obstruction of qi and blood.Long lasting obstruction causes stasis in the collaterals.Headache may be caused by upsurge of the liver yang due to stagnation of qi or injury of the liver after anger.Irregular food intake causes excess internal phlegm,which prevents the clear yang from ascending and turbid yin from descending;the brain is lack of supplementation of essense and qi due to constitutional insufficiency and dual deficiency of qi and blood;blood stasis in the collaterals due to trauma,all the above mentioned cause headache.

Differentiation and Treatment

Headache due to invasion of pathogenic factors:select the points according to meridians of head.The anterior part of the head:Shangxin(GV 23),Touwei(ST 8),Hegu(LI 4),and Ashi points;the vertex part of the head:Baihui(GV 20),Tongtian(BL 7),Taichong(LR 3),and Ashi points;the lateral part of headache:Shuaigu(GB 8),Taiyang(EX-HN 5),Waiguan(TE 5),and Ashi point;and the posterior head: Houding(GV 19),Fengchi(GB 20),Kunlun(BL 60),and Ashi point.Filiform needling with reducing method.

Headache due to internal injuries:main points:Baihui(GV 20),Fengchi(GB 20),and Taiyang(EX-HN 5).

1. Ascendant hyperactivity of liver yang

【Main manifestations】Headache and blurred vision,irritability,hot temper,insomnia,flushed face, bitter taste in the mouth,red tongue with yellow tongue fur,string-like and rapid pulse.

【Treatment】Pacify the liver to subdue yang.

【Prescription】Main points together with Taichong(LR 3) and Yanglingquan(GB 34).Filiform needling with the reducing method.

2. Phlegm turbidity invading the head

【Main manifestations】Headache,daze,chest fullness,vomiting sputum,dark red tongue with white greasy tongue fur,and slippery pulse.

【Treatment】Resolve the phlegm and turbidity to open the orifices.

【Prescription】Main points together with Touwei(ST 8),Zhongwan(CV 12) and Fenglong(ST 40). Filiform needling with the reducing method.

3. Kidney essence deficiency

【处方】主穴+脑空、肾俞、悬钟、太溪；毫针刺用补法，可灸。

4. 气血亏虚

【证候】头痛绵绵，遇劳则甚；兼见心悸怔忡，神疲乏力，面色不华，食欲不振；舌淡苔白，脉细无力。

【治法】补益气血。

【处方】主穴+心俞、脾俞、足三里、三阴交；毫针刺用补法，可灸。

5. 瘀血阻络

【证候】头痛经久不愈，痛处固定不移，痛如锥刺；舌紫黯或有瘀斑，脉细涩或细弦。

【治法】活血化瘀，通络止痛。

【处方】主穴+阿是穴、合谷、血海、委中；毫针刺用泻法。

（三）其他疗法

1. 耳穴贴压　枕、额、脑、神门、肝。

2. 皮肤针　取穴：太阳、印堂、阿是穴。适用于肝阳上亢及瘀血阻络型。

五、坐骨神经痛

坐骨神经痛是指多种病因所致的沿坐骨神经分布区的疼痛，临床以臀部、大腿后侧，小腿后外侧、足外侧疼痛为主症。属于足太阳、足少阳经脉和经筋病证。

（一）病因病机

感受风寒湿邪，风寒水湿之邪浸渍经络，经络之气阻滞而发病。肾亏体虚，长期操劳过度，久坐久立，或因房劳过度，精气耗损，肾气虚惫也可导致。跌打外伤闪挫，经筋、络脉受损，瘀血阻滞致病。

（二）辨证施治

主穴：腰2~5华佗夹脊穴、阿是穴、环跳、委中、阳陵泉。

1. 风寒湿痹

【证候】腰腿冷痛，上下走窜，屈伸不便，遇阴雨寒冷气候加重，或伴下肢肿胀；舌质淡红，苔薄白或白腻，脉浮紧或沉。

【治法】祛风散寒，除湿止痛。

【处方】主穴+秩边、命门，毫针刺用泻法，可灸。

2. 瘀血阻滞

【证候】有腰部挫伤史，腰腿刺痛，痛处拒按，按之刺痛放散，夜间痛甚；舌紫暗或有瘀斑，脉涩。

【治法】活血通络。

【Main manifestations】Headache with empty sensation, vertigo, soreness and pain in the lower back, fatigue, tinnitus, insomnia, red tongue with scanty tongue fur, and fine and weak pulse.

【Treatment】Supplement the kidney and replenish the marrow.

【Prescription】Main points together with Naokong(GB 19), Shenshu(BL 23), Xuanzhong(GB 39), and Taixi(KI 3). Filiform needling with the reinforcing method. Moxibustion is advisable.

4. Dual deficiency of qi and blood

【Main manifestations】Chronic headache deteriorated after labour, concurrent with palpitation, fatigue, pale complexion, poor appetite, pale tongue with white fur, and fine and weak pulse.

【Treatment】Tonify qi and engender blood.

【Prescription】Main points together with Xinshu(BL 15), Pishu(BL 20), Zusanli(ST 36), and Sanyinjiao(SP 6). Filiform needling with the reinforcing method. Moxibustion is advisable.

5. Blood stasis obstructing the collaterals

【Main manifestations】Cone-thorn-like long lasting and fixed headache, dark purple tongue with ecchymosis, and fine and rough pulse or string-like and fine pulse.

【Treatment】Activate blood to dissipate stasis, free the collateral vessels to relieve pain.

【Prescription】Main points together with Hegu(LI 4), Xuehai(SP 10), and Weizhong(BL 40). Filiform needling with the reducing method.

Other Therapies

(1)Paste and press ear points: Pt.occiput, Pt.forehead, Pt.brain, Pt.shenmen, and Pt.liver.

(2)Dermal needle: Points: Taiyang(EX-HN 5), Yintang(GV 29), and Ashi points. Indicated for headache due to ascendant hyperactivity of liver yang and blood stasis obstructing the collaterals.

Sciatica

Sciatica refers to pain in the distribution region of the sciatic nerve due to various causes. Its main clinical manifestations include the radiating pain in the regions of the buttocks, the posterior side of the thigh, the posterior-lateral side of the leg and the lateral side of the dorsum of foot. It belongs to the diseases of the Foot-Taiyang meridian, Foot-Shaoyang meridian and the meridian sinews.

Etiology and Pathogenesis

The disease is caused by the invasion of pathogenic factors of wind, cold and dampness, which immerse in the meridians and collaterals and obstruct the meridian qi. It is also caused by kidney qi deficiency, which results from constitutional insufficiency of kidney, long-term overwork, sitting or standing for a long time, and consumption of essence and qi by excessive sexual activity. Sprain, contusion or injury also may cause damage of meridian sinews and collateral vessels, and blood stasis obstructing collateral vessels.

Differentiation and Treatment

Main points: the second to fifth lumbar Hua Tuo's paravertebral points, Ashi points, Huantiao(GB 30), Weizhong(BL 40), Yanglingquan(GB 34).

1. Wind-cold-dampness impediment

【Main manifestations】Pain and cold in the lower back and legs, radiating upwards and downwards, flexion inconvenience, aggravated in rainy cold days, or concurrent with swelling and edema in the lower limbs, pale red tongue with thin white coating or white greasy coating, floating and tight pulse or sunken pulse.

【Treatment】Dispel wind and dissipate cold, eliminate dampness to relieve pain.

【Prescription】Main points together with Zhibian(BL 54), and Mingmen(GV 4). Filiform needling with the reducing method. Moxibustion is advisable.

2. Blood stasis

【处方】主穴+膈俞、血海；毫针刺用泻法。

3. 气血不足

【证候】腰腿隐痛，反复发作，遇劳则甚，下肢萎软，恶风畏寒，喜揉喜按，神疲乏力，面色无华；舌淡苔少，脉沉细。

【治法】补益气血。

【处方】主穴+足三里、三阴交；毫针刺用补泻兼施法，可灸。

（三）其他疗法

1. 耳穴贴压　坐骨神经、臀、腰骶椎、肾。

2. 火罐疗法　阿是穴或相应穴位闪罐、留罐或走罐，以皮肤红润、充血或瘀血为度。

六、三叉神经痛

以眼、面颊部出现反复发作的、短暂的、阵发性、烧灼样抽掣疼痛，三叉神经分眼支、上颌支和下颌支，临床上以第二、第三支同时发病多见。

（一）病因病机

本病多由外感或内伤所致血脉壅闭、气血受阻而发生疼痛。外风侵袭面部的三阳经，导致头面部疼痛；内伤者或由肝胆风火上逆；或由胃火上炎；或由痰浊上扰，以致风火攻冲头面，上扰清窍而作痛。

（二）辨证施治

主穴：合谷、内庭、太冲。

【证候】触及面部某一点而突然发作，甚至不敢洗脸、漱口和进食。疼痛呈阵发样、闪电样剧痛，其痛如刀割、针刺、火灼，可伴有病侧部面部肌肉抽搐、流泪、流涎等现象。发作时间短暂，数秒钟或数分钟后可缓解。舌质暗红，苔白或薄黄，脉浮数或弦。

【处方】第一支痛：主穴+鱼腰、下关，可配阳白、上星等穴；第二、三支痛：主穴+四白、下关、地仓、承浆、颧髎等。

其中头面部穴位取患侧；合谷、内庭、太冲取双侧。毫针刺用补泻兼施法。针刺入穴位后，患侧面部出现触电样针感，这是取得疗效的关键。加强针感的传导刺激，则得气快，针感强，止痛效果显著。针刺鱼腰穴使针感放散至前额；四白穴针感放散至下睑、上唇及鼻翼处。

【Main manifestations】Have a history of lumbar sprain, stabbing pain in the lower back and legs, aversion to touch, and the pain radiates when pressed and becomes severe in the night, dark purplish tongue with ecchymosis, rough pulse.

【Treatment】Activate blood and free the collateral vessels.

【Prescription】Main points together with Geshu(BL 17), and Xuehai(SP 10).Filiform needling with the reducing method.

3. Dual deficiency of qi and blood

【Main manifestations】Recurrent dull pain in the lower back and legs, deterioration after labour, lower limb atrophy, aversion to wind and cold, preference to pressing and rubbing, fatigue, lusterless facial complexion, pale tongue with slim tongue coating, and sunken and fine pulse.

【Treatment】Supplement both qi and blood.

【Prescription】Main points together with Zusanli(ST 36), and Sanyinjiao(SP 6).Filiform needling with the reducing and reinforcing methods.Moxibustion is advisable.

Other Therapies

(1)Paste and press auricle points:Pt.sciatic nerve,Pt.buttock,Pt.lumbosacral vertebrae and Pt.kidney.

(2)Cupping therapy:flash-fire cupping,retained cupping or slide cupping in Ashi points and the related points,withdraw the cups when the skin around the points appears red,congestion and stasis.

Trigeminal neuralgia

Trigeminal neuralgia is a neuropathic disorder characterized by intensely recurrent, transient buring, and pulling-like pain in the eyes and cheek.Trigeminal nerve is composed by the ophthalmic, maxillary and mandibular branches.Clinically, the second and the third branches onset at the same time is more common.

Etiology and Pathogenesis

The disease is mainly caused by obstruction of blood vessels and blocked qi and blood due to the exogenous pathologic factors and internal injuries.The exogenous pathologic wind attacks the three yang meridians in the face,which induce the pain in the face and head.The internal injuries,such as,the ascending wind-heat of the liver and gallbladder,stomach fire bearing upward,or phlegm turbidity harassing the upper body,cause the fire and wind attacking the head and face,and harassing the upper orifices,therefore result in pain.

Differentiation and Treatment

Main Points:Hegu(LI 4),Neiting(ST 44),and Taichong(LR 3).

【Main manifestations】Sudden onset after a touch of the face,even can not wash face,gargle and eat. This kind of pain was paroxysmal,lightning-like pain,like cutting,needling and burning,may be associated with muscle twitching,tearing,salivation and other phenomena of the disease lateral face.The onset time is short,can be alleviated after a few seconds or minutes,red or dark purplish tongue with white coating or yellow thin coating,floating and rapid pulse or string-like pulse.

【Prescription】Pain in the first branch:Yuyao(EX-HN 4),Xiaguan(ST 7),Yangbai(GB 14), and Shangxing(GV 23).Pain in the second and third branches:Sibai(ST 2),Xiaguan(ST 7),Dicang(ST 4), Chengjiang(CV 24), and Quanliao(SI 13).When needling the acupuncture points,the patient has an electric shock-like feeling in the face of disease side,which is the key to obtain efficacy.Strengthening the conduction of acupuncture stimulation,will quicken the arrival of qi,strengthen the needle sensation and the therapeutic effect.Needling Yuyao(EX-HN 4) can diffuse the needle sensation to the forehead;while needling Sibai(ST 2) can diffuse the needle sensation to the lower eyelid,upper lip and nose.

（三）其他疗法

耳穴贴压：根据疼痛发作的不同部位选取穴位，常用的穴位有：牙、颌、面颊、颞、额、肝、胆、神门、皮质下等。

七、肩关节周围炎

肩关节周围炎是指肩关节周围的肌肉、肌腱、韧带、滑囊、关节囊等软组织发生无菌性炎症，有充血、渗出、水肿、粘连等改变，导致肩关节疼痛及功能障碍。可由急性损伤或慢性劳损所致的肱二头肌腱鞘炎、冈上肌炎、肩峰下滑囊炎等发展而来。中老年人上肢因外伤、手术或其他原因所致疼痛，肩关节较长时间不活动，也可诱发此病。

（一）病因病机

感受风寒湿邪，风寒水湿之邪浸渍肩部，经络之气阻滞而发病。或肾亏体虚，长期操劳过度，慢性劳损，跌扑外伤闪挫，经筋、络脉受损，瘀血阻滞所致。

（二）辨证施治

主穴：肩髃、肩贞、合谷。

1. 风寒湿痹

【证候】肩部疼痛，遇寒加重或日轻夜重，得温痛减，肩酸痛不举，动则痛剧；舌淡红，苔薄白，脉弦滑或弦紧。

【治法】祛风散寒，除湿止痛。

【处方】主穴+天宗、风门、曲池、外关，毫针刺用补泻兼施法。

2. 经脉失养

【证候】肩痛日久，肩臂肌肉挛缩，关节僵直，动作受限，酸痛乏力，局部得温痛减，受凉加剧；舌淡或有瘀点，脉沉细。

【治法】益气活血，疏通经脉。

【处方】主穴+气海、足三里、三阴交，毫针刺用补泻兼施法。肩内侧痛，加尺泽、阴陵泉；肩外侧痛，加臂臑、阳陵泉；肩后痛，加条口透承山。

（三）其他疗法

1. 耳穴贴压　肩、肩关节、肾上腺、压痛点。

2. 透针法　取穴：条口透承山、阳陵泉透阴陵泉。单肩病取健侧穴，双肩病则双侧取穴。本法适用于病程短者。

3. 火罐疗法　阿是穴或相应穴位闪罐、留罐或走罐，以皮肤红润、充血或瘀血为度。

八、周围性面神经麻痹

周围性面神经麻痹是以口、眼向一侧㖞斜为主症的病证。中医学称之为"口眼㖞

Other Therapies

Paste and press ear points: according to the location of pain, select corresponding points. Mainly used points: Pt. tooth, Pt. jaw, Pt. cheek, Pt. temple, Pt. forehead, Pt. liver, Pt. gallbladder, Pt. shenmen, Pt. subcortex.

Periarthritis of shoulder

Periarthritis of shoulder refers to aseptic inflammation of muscles around the shoulder, tendons, ligaments, bursa, joint capsule and other soft tissue, appearing congestion, exudation, edema, adhesions, resulting in shoulder pain and dysfunction. Periarthritis of shoulder can be caused by strain biceps tenosynovitis, supraspinatus and subacromial bursitis due to acute or chronic injuries. For the elderly, periarthritis of shoulder is caused by a long time of shoulder's inactivity caused by trauma, surgery, upper limb pain, or other reasons.

Etiology and Pathogenesis

Periarthritis of shoulder is caused by exogenous pathologic factors, the pathogenic factors of wind, cold and dampness immerse in the shoulder, then the meridian qi is blocked. It is also caused by kidney deficiency, or a long time overwork, chronic fatigue, trauma, sprain or injuries, which result in injured meridian sinews and collateral vessels, and blood stasis obstructing the collateral vessels.

Differentiation and Treatment

Main Points: Jianyu(LI 15), Jianzhen(SI 9), and Hegu(LI 4).

1. Wind-cold-dampness impediment

【Main manifestations】Shoulder pain, intensified in the day and alleviated in the night, or alleviated by warmth, hard to move due to soreness and pain, intensified by movement, pale red tongue with white thin tongue coating, string-like and slippery pulse or string-like and tight pulse.

【Treatment】Disperse wind and dissipate cold, remove dampness and relieve pain.

【Prescription】Main points together with Tianzong(SI 11), Fengchi(GB 20), and Waiguan(SJ 5). Filiform needling with the reducing and reinforcing methods.

2. Malnutrition of the meridians

【Main manifestations】Chronic pain in the shoulder, contraction of the shoulder muscles, stiffness of the joint, limited movement, soreness and pain, and fatigue, improved by warmth and intensified by coldness attacks; pale tongue, or with ecchymosis, sunken and fine pulse.

【Treatment】Supplement both qi and blood, soothe the meridians and collaterals.

【Prescription】Main points together with Qihai(CV 6), Zusanli(ST 36), and Sanyinjiao(SP 6). Filiform needling with the reducing and reinforcing methods. For pain in the interior side of the shoulder, plus Chize(LU 5) and Yanglingquan(GB 34); for pain in the exterior side of the shoulder, plus Binao(LI 13) and Yanglingquan(GB 34), for pain in the posterior part of the shoulder, plus Tiaokou(ST 38) and Chengshan(BL 57).

Other Therapies

(1) Paste and press ear points: Pt. shoulder, Pt. shoulder Joint, Pt. liver, Pt. adrenal and Ashi points.

(2) Penetration needling: Points: penetrate Tiaokou(ST 38) to Chengshan(BL 57), penetrate Yanglinquan(GB 34) to Yinlinquan(SP 9). Single shoulder select points in the healthy side, and for both shoulders select points in both sides. This method is applicable for cases with short course.

(3) Cupping therapy: flash-fire cupping, retained cupping or slide cupping in Ashi points and related points, withdraw when the skin around the points appears red, congestion and stasis.

Peripheral facial paralysis

Peripheral facial paralysis is the disease whose main symptom is that the mouth, eyes skew to the

斜"、"面瘫"，俗称"吊线风"。本病多因感受风寒、病毒导致面神经血管痉挛，局部缺血、水肿，使面神经受压，神经营养缺乏，甚至引起神经变性而发病。也有因疱疹病毒等引起的非化脓性炎症所致。

（一）病因病机

病邪侵犯面部经络，可导致本病的发生。本病多由脉络空虚，风寒之邪乘虚侵袭阳明、少阳脉络，以致经气阻滞、经筋失养、筋肌纵缓不收而发病。

（二）辨证施治

主穴：地仓、颊车、阳白、四白、内庭、合谷、太冲。

1. 风邪袭络

【证候】突然口眼㖞斜，面部感觉异常，耳后耳中隐痛，额纹浅或消失；鼓腮漏气，或有恶寒发热，鼻塞流涕；舌质淡红，苔薄白或薄黄，脉浮紧或浮数。

【治法】祛风通络。

【处方】主穴＋风池、翳风、外关，毫针刺用补泻兼施法。

2. 虚风内动

【证候】口眼㖞斜，面部麻紧感，面肌蠕动，每于说话或情绪激动时口眼抽动，或有头晕耳鸣，目涩无泪；舌淡或红，少苔，脉弦细。

【治法】滋补肝肾，熄风止痉。

【处方】主穴＋太溪、足三里、阳陵泉，毫针刺用补泻兼施法。

（三）其他疗法

1. 耳穴贴压　面颊区、肝、眼、口、下屏尖、额。

2. 火罐疗法　瘫痪侧面部相应穴位闪罐、留罐或走罐，以皮肤红润、充血或瘀血为度。

九、牙痛

牙痛是指牙齿因各种原因引起的疼痛，遇冷、热、酸、甜等刺激时牙痛发作或加重。常见于龋齿，急、慢性牙髓炎，牙周炎，根尖周围炎和牙本质过敏等；也见于三叉神经痛、周围性面神经炎等。

（一）病因病机

手、足阳明经脉分别入下齿、上齿，大肠、胃腑积热，或风邪外袭经络，郁于阳明而化火，火邪循经上炎而发为牙痛。肾主骨，齿为骨之余，肾阴不足，虚火上炎亦可引起牙痛。亦有多食甘酸之品，垢秽蚀齿而作痛。

（二）辨证施治

主穴：合谷、颊车、下关。

side.It is known as deviated eyes and mouth,facial paralysis,and hoisted-line wind in TCM.The disease mostly caused by invasion of wind-cold,or the virus that causes facial nerve vasospasm,ischemia,edema, compression of facial nerve,lack of nutrients leading to nerve degeneration.It is also caused by non-suppurative inflammation due to herpes viruses.

Etiology and Pathogenesis

When the exogenous pathologic factors attack meridians in the face,this disease may occurs.This disease is caused by the wind-cold attacking Yangming and Shaoyang meridians on the basis of empty of meridians and collaterals,which causing the congestion of meridian qi,malnutrition of the meridians.

Differentiation and Treatment

Main Points:Dicang(ST 4),Jiache(ST 6),Yangbai(GB 14),Sibai(ST 2),Neiting(ST 44),Hegu (LI 4) and Taichong(LR 3).

1. Pathologic wind attacks the collaterals

【Main manifestations】A sudden deviated eyes and mouth,facial paresthesia,dull pain in the ears, the veins of forehead shallow or disappear,or aversion to cold,fever,nasal congestion,running rose;pale red tongue with thin white or thin yellow tongue coating,and floating and tight or floating and rapid pulse.

【Treatment】Dispel wind and smooth collaterals.

【Prescription】Main points together with Fengchi(GB 20) and Waiguan(TE 5).Filiform needling with the reducing and reinforcing methods.

2. Vacuity wind stirring internally

【Main manifestations】Deviated eyes and mouth,numbness and tight sensation of facial muscle,facial muscle motility,eyes and mouth twitching when speak and be emotional,dizziness,tinnitus,dry eyes with no tears,pale tongue or red tongue,scanty tongue coating,and string-like and fine pulse.

【Treatment】Nourish both the liver and kidney,extinguish wind to arrest convulsions.

【Prescription】Main points together with Taixi(KI 3),Zusanli(ST 36),and Yanglingquan(GB 34). Filiform needling with the reducing and reinforcing methods.

Other Therapies

(1)Paste and press ear points:Pt.cheek,Pt.liver,Pt.eye,Pt.mouth,Pt.infratragic apex,and Pt.forehead.

(2)Cupping therapy:for face paralysis,flash-fire cupping,retained cupping or slide cupping in Ashi points and related points,withdraw when the skin around the points appears red,congestion,and stasis.

Toothache

Toothache refers to various reasons such as the stimulations of cold,heat,sour,and sweet.It commonly appears in acute and chronic pulpitis,periodontitis,periapical and dentine hypersensitivity,etc.It also appears in patients with trigeminal neuralgia,peripheral facial neuritis.

Etiology and Pathogenesis

The Hand and Foot-Yangming meridians go into the upper and lower gums,respectively.Toothache may be caused by flaring up along the meridians of the pathogenic fire transformed from pathogenic heat in the large intestine and stomach,or from exogenous pathogenic wind that attacks and accumulates in the Yangming meridians.The kidney controls bones,and the teeth are the odds and ends of the bones.Deficiency of the kidney yin with flaring up of the asthenic fire may also result in toothache.Sometimes toothache is due to dental caries caused by over-intake of sour and sweet food.

Differentiation and Treatment

Main points:Hegu(LI 4),Jiache(ST 6),and Xiaguan(ST 7).

1. Invasion of wind-fire

1．风热侵袭

【证候】牙痛突然发作，牙龈肿胀，寒战发热，口渴；舌红苔白或薄黄，脉浮数。

【治法】祛风清热。

【处方】主穴+风池、外关，毫针刺用泻法。

2．胃火上蒸

【证候】牙痛剧烈，牙龈红肿口臭，或出脓血，口渴，便秘，舌红苔黄燥；脉弦数或滑数。

【治法】清胃泻火。

【处方】主穴+二间、内庭，毫针刺用泻法。

3．虚火上炎

【证候】牙痛隐隐，时作时止，日轻夜重，牙龈暗红萎缩，牙根松动；腰膝酸软，五心烦热；舌嫩红少苔，脉细数。

【治法】滋阴清火。

【处方】主穴+太溪、照海、悬钟，毫针刺用补泻兼施法。

（三）其他疗法

1．耳针　牙痛点、神门、屏尖、上颌、下颌。

2．耳穴贴压　牙痛点、神门、屏尖、上颌、下颌。

十、痛经

痛经是妇女在行经期间或行经前后，出现周期性小腹或腰骶部疼痛或胀痛，甚则剧痛难忍，常可伴有面色苍白、头面冷汗淋漓、手足厥冷、泛恶呕吐等症。

（一）病因病机

本病多因行经期感受寒邪，饮食生冷，以致脉络凝滞，瘀血停滞胞中，经行受阻，不通则痛；或因情志郁结，气滞经行不畅而成。或因体质虚弱，或大病、久病之后，气血不足，渐至血海空虚，胞脉失养所致。

（二）辨证施治

主穴：三阴交、太冲、中极。

1．寒湿凝滞

【证候】经前或行经时小腹冷痛，重则连及腰背，得热痛减；伴经行量少，色暗有血块，畏寒便溏；舌苔白腻，脉沉紧。

【治法】祛寒除湿，活血止痛。

【处方】主穴+关元、地机、归来、血海，毫针刺用补泻兼施法，可灸。

【Main manifestations】Acute toothache with gingival swelling accompanied by chills and fever, thirst, red tongue with white or yellow thin coating, and floating and rapid pulse.

【Treatment】Dispel wind and clear heat.

【Prescription】Main points together with Fengchi(GB 20), Xiaguan(ST 7). Filiform needling with the reducing method.

2. Stomach fire bearing upward

【Main manifestations】Severe toothache accompanied by foul breath or bleeding, thirst, constipation, red tongue with yellow dry tongue coating, and string-like and rapid pulse or rapid and slippery pulse.

【Treatment】Clear stomach fire.

【Prescription】Main points together with Erjian(LI 2), Neiting(ST 44). Filiform needling with the reducing method.

3. Deficiency fire flaming upward

【Main manifestations】Dull pain off and on, severe in night, dark red gum atrophy, loose teeth, soreness and weakness in the lumbar and knees, heat sensation in chest, palms and soles, red tongue with scanty tongue coating, and fine and rapid pulse.

【Treatment】Nourish yin and clear fire.

【Prescription】Main points together with Taixi(KI 3), Zhaohai(KI 6), and Xuanzhong(GB 39). Filiform needling with the reinforcing and reducing method.

Other Therapies

(1) Ear acupuncture therapy: the toothache points, Pt.shenmen, Pt.tragic apex, Pt.upper jaw and Pt. lower jaw.

(2) Paste and press ear points: the toothache points, Pt.shenmen, Pt.tragic apex, Pt.upper jaw, and Pt.lower jaw.

Dysmenorrhea

Dysmenorrhea refers to the severe pain periodically appearing in the lower abdomen and lumbosacral region or distending pain during, before or after menstruation, accompanied by pale face, cold sweating in the head and face, reversal cold of extremities, vomiting and hiccup. The severe cases always suffer from unbearable pain.

Etiology and Pathogenesis

Dysmenorrhea is caused by affection of external cold or intake of cold drinks during menstrual periods, which hurts the lower energizer, and makes the cold retain in the uterus. It is due to stagnation of the liver qi, which fails to carry the free flow of the blood. In circumstances of qi and blood deficiency due to either weak body-build or chronic disease, menstruation drains up the seas of blood and deprives the uterus from nourishment, and then pain occurs.

Differentiation and Treatment

Main points: Sanyinjiao(SP 6), Taichong(LR 3), and Zhongji(CV 3).

1. Cold-dampness

【Main manifestations】Pain in the lower abdomen, usually starting before menstruation, implicate the lower back and back for severe cases, alleviated by warming, retarded and scanty and dark purple menses with clots, aversion of cold and diarrhea, white greasy tongue coating, and sunken and tight pulse.

【Treatment】Dissipate cold and remove dampness, activate blood to relieve pain.

【Prescription】Main points together with Guanyuan(CV 4), Diji(SP 8), Guilai(ST 29), and Xuehai (SP 10). Filiform needling with the reinforcing and reducing method. Moxibustion is advisable.

2. Liver qi stagnation

2. 肝郁气滞

【证候】经前或经期小腹胀痛，胀甚于痛，经中有瘀块，块下后疼痛减轻；月经量少，淋漓不畅，色黯，胸胁两乳作胀；舌质黯或有瘀斑，脉沉弦。

【治法】疏肝解郁，理气止痛。

【处方】主穴+曲泉、气海，毫针刺用泻法。

3. 肝肾亏损

【证候】月经后小腹隐痛，按之痛减；月经量少色淡，质稀，腰膝酸痛，头晕耳鸣；舌质淡苔薄白，脉沉细。

【治法】滋补肝肾。

【处方】主穴+关元、肝俞、肾俞、照海、足三里，毫针刺用补泻兼施法。

4. 肝郁湿热

【证候】经前或经期小腹疼痛，甚则痛及腰骶，或感腹内灼热；经行量多质稠，色鲜红或紫，有小血块，胁肋疼痛，小便短赤，带下黄稠；舌红，苔黄腻，脉弦数。

【治法】疏肝解郁，清热利湿。

【处方】主穴+期门、章门、次髎，毫针刺用泻法。

（三）其他疗法

1. 耳穴贴压　子宫、内分泌、交感、肾。

2. 头针　生殖区。

十一、肥胖症

肥胖症是人体内脂肪贮存过多，因体脂增加使体重超过标准体重20%称为肥胖症。如无明显病因可寻者称单纯性肥胖症；具有明确病因者称为继发性肥胖症。针灸减肥以治疗单纯性肥胖为主。

（一）病因病机

本病形成多由过食肥甘、膏粱厚味之品，加之久卧、久坐，膏脂内聚；七情所伤，肝气郁滞，脾失健运则浊脂内聚；脾肾气虚，肝胆失调，不仅造成膏脂、痰浊、水湿停蓄，也使气机失畅，而造成气滞或血瘀。因此，肥胖病的发病为本虚标实，本为气虚，标为湿、痰、脂（瘀）。

（二）辨证施治

主穴：中脘、足三里、天枢、水道、归来。

1. 痰湿阻滞

【证候】体型肥胖，嗜睡，疲倦，纳差，口淡无味，月经少或闭经，舌胖有齿痕，脉沉缓或滑。

【Main manifestations】Distending pain in the lower abdomen, usually starting before menstruation, implicate the lower back and back for severe cases, menses with clots, and the pain alleviated by clots out-flow, scant menstrual flow, dark color, distention of chest and rib-side, dark tongue with ecchymosis, sunken and string-like pulse.

【Treatment】Soothe the liver and resolve depression, regulate qi and relieve pain.

【Prescription】Main points together with Ququan(LR 8), and Qihai(CV 6). Filiform needling with the reducing method.

3. Liver-kidney deficiency

【Main manifestations】Dull pain in the lower abdomen after menstruation, alleviated by pressing; pale and thin quality menstruation, soreness and pain in the waist and knees, dizziness, tinnitus, pale tongue with white thin tongue coating, and sunken and fine pulse.

【Treatment】Nourish the liver and kidney.

【Prescription】Main points together with Guanyuan(CV 4), Ganshu(BL 18), Shenshu(BL 23), Zhaohai(RI 6), and Zusanli(ST 36). Filiform needling with the reinforcing and reducing method.

4. Liver stagnation with dampness-heat

【Main manifestations】Pain in the lower abdomen, usually starting before menstruation, or a feeling of heat in abdomen, dark and thick quality menstruation, clots, pain in rib-side, short voidings of reddish u-rine, yellow and thick vaginal discharge, red tongue with yellow greasy tongue coating, and string-like and rapid pulse.

【Treatment】Soothe the liver and resolve depression, clear heat, and resolve dampness.

【Prescription】Main points together with Qimen(LR 14), Zhangmen(LR 13), and Ciliao(BL 32). Filiform needling with the reinforcing and reducing method.

Other Therapies

(1) Paste and press ear points: Pt. uterus, Pt. sympathetic nerve, and Pt. kidney.

(2) Scalp acupunture: the reproduction area.

Obesity

Obesity is a medical condition in which excess body fat has accumulated to the extent that increased weight surpasses more than 20% of standard weight. The type that no obvious cause could be found is termed as simple obesity; while the one have a clear cause is called secondary obesity. Acupuncture treatment is mainly for the simple obesity.

Etiology and Pathogenesis

Obesity is caused by excessive intake of fatty, sweet foods, in addition with long lasting sitting and lying without movement, therefore, fat is accumulated internally; the stagnation of liver qi due to injuries from seven emotions, prevents the spleen's function of transmitting food, fat and turbidity is accumulated; spleen-kidney qi deficiency and disorder of liver and gallbladder cause accumulation of fat, phlegm-turbidity, water and dampness, and irregulation of qi flow, and result in qi stagnation or blood stasis. Thus, the onset of obesity has the characteristic of deficient root and excessive tip. The root is of qi deficiency, and the tip is of dampness, phlegm, and fat(stasis).

Differentiation and Treatment

Main points: Zhongwan(CV 12), Zusanli(ST 36), Tianshu(ST 25), Shuidao(ST 28), and Guilai(ST 29).

1. Phlegm-dampness obstruction

【Main manifestations】Obese, lethargy, fatigue, anorexia, pale and tasteless mouth, menstruation or a-menorrhea, swollen tongue with teeth marks, sunken and moderate pulse or slippery pulse.

【治法】祛痰化湿，健脾和胃。

【处方】主穴+脾俞、胃俞、阴陵泉、丰隆、中极、三阴交，毫针刺用补泻兼施法。

2. 胃火炽盛

【证候】体型肥胖，胃纳亢进，消谷善饥，舌质红，苔黄腻，脉滑数。

【治法】清胃泻火。

【处方】主穴+合谷、曲池、内庭，毫针刺用补泻兼施法。

（三）其他疗法

1. 耳穴贴压 胃、内分泌、三焦、缘中、大肠。方法：每次餐前30分钟按压耳穴3~5分钟，有灼热感为宜。

2. 火罐疗法 沿背部督脉、膀胱经走罐、留罐，以皮肤红润、充血或瘀血为度。

（孙 华 包 飞）

【Treatment】Resolve phlegm and dampness, strengthen the spleen and harmonize the stomach.

【Prescription】Main points together with Pishu(BL 20), Weishu(BL 21), Yinlinquan(SP 9), Fenglong(ST 40), Zhongji(CV 3), and Sanyinjiao(SP 6). Filiform needling with the reinforcing and reducing method.

2.Intense stomach fire

【Main manifestations】Obese, hyperorexia, hyperactivity of digestion with rapid hungering, red tongue with yellow greasy tongue coating, slippery and rapid pulse.

【Treatment】Clear the stomach fire.

【Prescription】Main points together with Hegu(LI 4), Quchi(LI 11), Neiting(ST 44). Filiform needling with the reinforcing and reducing method.

Other Therapies

(1) Paste and press ear points: Pt.stomach, Pt.endocrine, Pt.liver sanjiao, Pt.middle border and Pt. large inrestine. Method: press the related auricle points for 3−5 minutes, 30 minutes before each meal, until the related region has a burning sensation.

(2) Cupping therapy: slide cupping or retained cupping along the Governor vessel or the bladder meridian, withdraw when the skin around the points appears red, congestion and stasis.

(Piao Yuanlin   Zhang Wen   Sun Hua)

参考文献 References

［1］梁晓春，孙华. 中医学. 北京：中国协和医科大学出版社，2011.

［2］李家邦. 中医学. 第 7 版. 北京：人民卫生出版社，2008.

［3］陆付耳. 中医学. 北京：高等教育出版社，2006.

［4］郑守曾. 中医学. 北京：人民卫生出版社，1999.

［5］印会河. 中医基础理论. 上海：上海科学技术出版社，1984.

［6］邓铁涛. 中医诊断学. 上海：上海科学技术出版社，1984.

［7］高学敏. 中药学. 第 2 版. 北京：中国中药出版社，2007.

［8］国家药典委员会. 中华人民共和国药典（2000 年版一部）. 北京：化学工业出版社，2000.

［9］邱德文. 现代方剂学. 北京：中医古籍出版社，2006.

［10］王绵之. 方剂学讲稿. 北京：人民卫生出版社，2005.

［11］邱茂良. 针灸学. 上海：上海科学技术出版社，2004.

［12］杨甲三. 腧穴学. 上海：上海科学技术出版社，1984.

［13］石学敏. 针灸学. 北京：中国中医药出版社，2002.

［14］陈德兴. 方剂学. 第 2 版. 北京：人民卫生出版社，2007.

［15］Giovanni Maciocia. The practice of Chinese medicine：the treatment of diseases with acupuncture and Chinese herbs. 2nd edition. Churchill Livingstone：Elsevier，2008.

［16］Chen Keji. Advanced textbook on traditional Chinese medicine and pharmacology. Beijing：New World Press，1996.

［17］欧明. 汉英中医辞典. 广州：广东科技出版社，1986.

［18］谢竹藩. 汉英中医药分类辞典. 北京：新世界出版社，1994.

［19］WHO. WHO international standard terminologies on traditional medicine in the western pacific region. 2007.